# Fruits and Their Roles in Nutraceuticals and Functional Foods

Adequate intake of fruits has been linked with the reduction in the risk of chronic diseases and maintenance of body weight. *Fruits and Their Roles in Nutraceuticals and Functional Foods* covers recent research related to the bioactive compounds present in a variety of fruits. Novel techniques and methodologies used in the extraction, isolation, and identification of bioactive compounds of functional fruits are discussed in detail.

Written by various experts in the field, the book examines a variety of fruits including apple, pear, mango, pomegranate, papaya, watermelon, pineapple, banana, and orange, among others.

**Key Features**

- Covers all aspects related to the role of fruits in nutraceutical and functional foods

- Examines the health elements of bioactive compounds as a treatment for various chronic disorders

- Provides an insight on the global regulatory aspects for the utilization of fruits in nutraceuticals and functional foods

# Fruits and Their Roles in Nutraceuticals and Functional Foods

Edited by
Sajad Ahmad Wani
Jasmeet Kour
Raees ul Haq
Mohamed S. Elshikh

CRC Press
Taylor & Francis Group
Boca Raton  New York  London

CRC Press is an imprint of the
Taylor & Francis Group, an **informa** business

First edition published 2023
by CRC Press
6000 Broken Sound Parkway NW, Suite 300, Boca Raton, FL 33487-2742

and by CRC Press
4 Park Square, Milton Park, Abingdon, Oxon, OX14 4RN

*CRC Press is an imprint of Taylor & Francis Group, LLC*

---

**Library of Congress Cataloging-in-Publication Data**

---

Names: Wani, Sajad Ahmad, editor. | Kour, Jasmeet, editor. | Haq, Raees ul,
editor.
Title: Fruits and their roles in nutraceuticals and functional foods /
edited by Sajad Ahmad Wani, Jasmeet Kour, Raees ul Haq.
Description: First edition. | Boca Raton : Taylor & Francis, 2023. |
Includes bibliographical references and index.
Identifiers: LCCN 2022040982 (print) | LCCN 2022040983 (ebook) | ISBN
9781032194462 (hardback) | ISBN 9781032194912 (paperback) | ISBN
9781003259213 (ebook)
Subjects: MESH: Fruit | Functional Food | Dietary Supplements
Classification: LCC RA784 (print) | LCC RA784 (ebook) | NLM WB 430 | DDC
613.2--dc23/eng/20230119
LC record available at https://lccn.loc.gov/2022040982
LC ebook record available at https://lccn.loc.gov/2022040983

---

ISBN: 9781032194462 (hbk)
ISBN: 9781032194912 (pbk)
ISBN: 9781003259213 (ebk)

DOI: 10.1201/9781003259213

Typeset in Palatino
by KnowledgeWorks Global Ltd.

# Contents

# Preface

Fruits are the mature ovary and other allied parts. They possess lots of health-promoting agents. Adequate intake of fruits has been linked with a reduction in the risk of chronic diseases and maintenance of body weight. These agents are generally referred to as bioactive compounds. The presence of bioactive compounds with health-promising and disease-preventing benefits makes fruits functional foods. This book covers the most recent research-related role of fruits in nutraceuticals and functional foods and provides information related to bioactive compounds present in functional fruits. The book also covers the health elements of fruits. The novel techniques and methodologies used in the extraction, isolation, identification, and characterization of bioactive compounds in fruits are discussed. Accumulating such information related to functional fruits in a book to attract an audience towards their role in nutraceuticals, functional foods, and bioactive compounds thus paves the way for researchers, readers, and scientists, which is the main aim of this book.

# Editors

**Sajad Ahmad Wani** is currently working as a post-doctoral fellow in the Department of Food Technology, Islamic University of Science and Technology, Awantipora, J&K, India. He completed his master's degree in food technology from IUST, Awantipora, J&K, India and PhD from Sant Longowal Institute of Engineering and Technology, Punjab, India. The Qualified National Eligibility Test (2015) (NET) was conducted by the Indian Council of Agricultural Research (ICAR) in December 2015. He has published more than 35 research/review articles, 10 book chapters, and 2 books. He has also written articles for the popular magazines *Food & Beverage News* (India's First Magazine for the Food & Beverage Industry). He has attended 50 national and 20 international conferences, seminars, and workshops throughout the world. Dr. Wani has participated in various faculty development programmes. Dr. Wani serves as Honorary Associate Editor of the esteemed *International Journal of Food Science and Technology*, Wiley. He is a potential peer reviewer of reputed international journals related to food science and technology that belong to popular publishing houses, including Elsevier, Taylor & Francis, Wiley, and Springer. He also works as a member of various associations like IFT, IFERP, the International Association for Agricultural Sustainability, AFSTI, the Asia Society of Researchers, and Asian Council of Science Editors. Dr. Wani is the recipient of prestigious fellowships, including the "D. S. Kothari Postdoctoral Fellowship: 2021" and the Maulana Azad National Fellowship (MANF-2013-14), from the University Grant Commission, India.

**Jasmeet Kour** completed her master's degree in food science and technology from the Government College for Women, Gandhi Nagar, Jammu University, Jammu and Kashmir, India. She was awarded a doctoral degree from Sant Longowal Institute of Engineering and Technology, Longowal, Sangrur, Punjab, India, from the Department of Food Engineering and Technology. She has been serving as an Assistant Professor at the Department of Food Science and Technology, Government College for Women, Gandhi Nagar, Jammu and Kashmir since 2009. She has conducted her vast research in various prominent nutraceuticals derived from plant origin and her work has been published in reputed journals with high-impact factors in eminent publishing houses in the field of food science. She has done research and review paper presentations in various national and international conferences. She has authored as well as co-authored numerous book chapters and scientific articles published in international books with prestigious publishing names such as Elsevier and Springer. She is also a part of various international projects. As her research work left a great imprint, she was cordially invited to share her newest research findings at Tokyo University of Agriculture, Japan at the 6th International Conference on Agricultural and Biological Sciences (ABS 2020). She is currently working as an editorial board member and peer reviewer of various journals of international repute. Lastly, she has already submitted a book entitled *Nutraceuticals and Health Care* in none other than the Elsevier publishing house. Apart from this, she has another pivotal mega-book project entitled *Handbook of Plant and Animal Toxins in Food: Occurrence, Toxicity, and Prevention* in press in CRC Press/Taylor & Francis.

**Raees ul Haq** was awarded a PhD degree from the Department of Food Engineering and Technology of Sant Longowal Institute of Engineering and Technology, Longowal, Sangrur, Punjab, India. He has completed his master's degree in food technology from Islamic University of Science and Technology, Awantipora, J&K, India. He has authored as well as co-authored different chapters for edited books published by prominent international publishers. Dr. Raees has presented his research work at various national and international conferences, seminars, and workshops. He is actively engaged with the scientific community by publishing his work as well as working as an editorial member and peer reviewer of reputed international journals. He has been the recipient of a Maulana Azad National Fellowship awarded by the University Grants Commission (UGC) and has published a number of research as well as review articles in reputed journals.

**Mohamed S. Elshikh** is a PhD researcher at King Saud University, College of Science, Botany and Microbiology Department. He completed his master's degree in 2016 and is currently pursuing his PhD in plant taxonomy and bioinformatics from King Saud University, Riyadh, Saudi Arabia. He has attended 15 national and 10 international conferences, seminars, and workshops throughout the world. He has published more than 120 papers in ISI journals. He is a potential peer reviewer of various reputed international journals related to botany and biotechnology that belong to popular publishing houses, including Elsevier, Taylor & Francis, Wiley, and Springer.

# Contributors

**Muhammad Afzaal**
Department of Food Sciences
Government College University
Faisalabad, Pakistan

**Anees Ahmed Khali**
University Institute of Diet and
    Nutritional Sciences
The University of Lahore
Lahore Pakistan

**Ammar Ahmed Khan**
University Institute of Diet and
    Nutritional Sciences
The University of Lahore
Lahore Pakistan

**Huma Bader Ul Ain**
University Institute of Diet and
    Nutritional Sciences
University of Lahore
Lahore, Pakistan

**Mohammed Shafiq Alam**
Department of Processing and
    Food Engineering
Punjab Agricultural University
Ludhiana, India

**Ahmad Ali**
Department of Life Sciences
University of Mumbai, Vidyanagari
Mumbai, India

**Poonam Baniwal**
Food Corporation of India
New Delhi, India

**Mehvish Bashir**
Sher-e-Kashmir University of
    Agricultural Sciences and
    Technology of Kashmir
Division of Fruit Science, Shalimar
Srinagar, India

**Shahid Bashir**
University Institute of Diet and
    Nutritional Sciences
University of Lahore
Lahore, Pakistan

**A. Tabish Jehan Been**
Sher-e-Kashmir University of
    Agricultural Sciences and
    Technology of Kashmir
Division of Fruit Science, Shalimar
Srinagar, India

**Abida Bhat**
Department of Immunology and
    Molecular Medicine
Sher-e-Kashmir Institute of
    Medical Sciences
Srinagar, India

**Rifat Bhat**
Sher-e-Kashmir University of
    Agricultural Sciences and
    Technology of Kashmir
Division of Fruit Science,
    Shalimar
Srinagar, India

**Hitesh Chopra**
Chitkara College of Pharmacy
Chitkara University
Rajpura, India

**Monika Choudhary**
Department of Food and Nutrition
Punjab Agricultural University
Ludhiana, India

**Subhamoy Dhua**
Department of Food Engineering
    and Technology
Tezpur University
Assam, India

**Mohamed S. Elshikh**
Department of Botany and
    Microbiology College of Science
King Saud University
Riyadh, Saudi Arabia

**Arun Kumar Gupta**
Department of Food Engineering
    and Technology
Tezpur University
Assam, India

**Maha Hameed**
Afro-Asian Institute Lahore
Lahore, Pakistan

**Sharbat Hussian**
Sher-e-Kashmir University of
    Agricultural Sciences and
    Technology of Kashmir
Division of Fruit Science,
    Shalimar
Srinagar, India

**Amarjeet Kaur**
Department of Food and Nutrition
Punjab Agricultural University
Ludhiana, India

**Gurjeet Kaur**
Department of Processing and
    Food Engineering
Punjab Agricultural University
Ludhiana, India

**Mahaldeep Kaur**
Department of Microbial
    Biotechnology
Punjab University
Chandigarh, India

**Parneet Kaur**
School of Biotechnology
Faculty of Applied Sciences and
    Biotechnology
Shoolini University
Solan, India

**Sandaldeep Kaur**
Post Graduate Government
    College for Girls
Chandigarh, India

**Rekha Kaushik**
Department of Food Science and
    Technology (Hotel Management)
Maharishi Markandeshwar (Deemed
    to Be University)
Ambala, India

**Jasmeet Kour**
Govt. PG College for Women
    Gandhi Nagar
Jammu, India

**Saurabh Kulshreshtha**
School of Biotechnology
Faculty of Applied Sciences and
    Biotechnology
Shoolini University
Solan, India

**Amarjeet Kumar**
Department of Home Science
Rohtas Mahila College Sasaram
Veer Kunwar Singh University
Arrah, Bihar, India

**Shiv Kumar**
Department of Food Science and
    Technology (Hotel Management)
Maharishi Markandeshwar
    (Deemed to Be University)
Ambala, India

**Varun Kumar**
Department of Home Science
RJMC, Bhupendra Narayan Mandal
    University
Madhepura, Bihar

**Lembe Samukelo Magwaza**
Discipline of Crop Science
School of Agricultural, Earth and
    Environmental Sciences
University of KwaZulu-Natal
Scottsville Pietermaritzburg,
    South Africa

**Rahul Mehra**
Department of Food Science and
    Technology (Hotel Management)
Maharishi Markandeshwar (Deemed
    to Be University)
Ambala, India

**Mohammad Amin Mir**
Sher-e-Kashmir University of
    Agricultural Sciences and
    Technology
Kashmir Division of Fruit Science,
    Shalimar
Srinagar, India

**Poonam Mishra**
Department of Food Engineering
    and Technology
Tezpur University
Assam, India

**Bharti Mittu**
National Institute of Pharmaceutical
    Education and Research (NIPER)
S.A.S. Nagar, Mohali, India

**Bindu Naik**
Department of Life Sciences (Food
    Technology)
Graphic Era Deemed to Be University
Dehradun, India

**Khyali Ncama**
Crop Science Department
Food Security and Safety Niche Area
Faculty of Natural and Agricultural
    Sciences
North-West University
Mmabatho, South Africa

**Santwana Palai**
Department of Veterinary
    Pharmacology & Toxicology
College of Veterinary Science and
    Animal Husbandry
Odisha University of Agriculture and
    Technology
Bhubaneswar, India

**Jessica Pandohee**
Centre for Crop and Disease
    Management School of Molecular
    and Life Sciences
Curtin University
Bentley, Australia

**Deependra Rajoriya**
Department of Food Technology
Rajiv Gandhi University
Arunachal Pradesh, India

**Breetha Ramaiyan**
Athletebit Healthcare Pvt. Ltd.
R&D Office
Mysore, India

**Farhan Saeed**
Department of Food Sciences
Government College University
Faisalabad, Pakistan

**Sangeeta**
Food Processing Department
Guru Nanak College
Budhlada, Mansa, India

**Rabia Shabbir**
Afro-Asian Institute Lahore
Lahore, Pakistan

**Anuj Sharma**
School of Biotechnology
Faculty of Applied Sciences and
    Biotechnology
Shoolini University
Solan, India

**Kanchan Sharma**
Department of Home Science
University of Jammu
Jammu, India

**Renu Sharma**
Department of Chemistry
Akal Degree College
Mastuana Sahib Sangrur, India

**Sugandha Sharma**
Department of Food Science
    and Technology (Hotel
    Management)
Maharishi Markandeshwar
    (Deemed to Be University)
Ambala, India

**Nkanyiso J. Sithole**
Department of Crop Science
Food Security and Safety
    Niche Area
Faculty of Natural and Agricultural
    Sciences
North-West University
Mmabatho, South Africa

**Rahul Thakur**
Department of Food Process
    Engineering
National Institute of Technology
Rourkela, India

**Sheetal Thakur**
Department of Food Science
    and Technology (Hotel
    Management)
Maharishi Markandeshwar
    (Deemed to Be University)
Ambala, India

**Tabussam Tufail**
University Institute of Diet and
    Nutritional Sciences
University of Lahore
Lahore, Pakistan

**Shahla Yasmin**
Department of Zoology
Patna Women's College
Patna University
Patna, India

**Ruchika Zalpouri**
Department of Processing and Food
    Engineering
Punjab Agricultural University
Ludhiana, India

# 1 Introduction to the Role of Fruits in Nutraceutical and Functional Foods

*Hitesh Chopra, Sangeeta, and Mohamed S. Elshikh*

## CONTENTS

## 1.1 INTRODUCTION

Dr. Stephen De Felice (founder and head of the Foundation for Innovation in Medicine [FIM] in Cranford, New Jersey) was the first to introduce the word "nutraceutical" in 1989. (Brower 1998). The definition of a nutraceutical by De Felice is as follows: "A food (or component of a meal) that delivers medical or health advantages, such as disease prevention and/or treatment." (Brower 1998). Simply put, nutraceuticals may help prevent and treat a wide range of diseases and disorders, including anemia. In contrast to dietary supplements, nutraceuticals are ingested as part of a typical meal or as the only component of a diet. (Kalra 2003). Nutraceuticals are products that are supplemented with nutrients, such as milk or orange juice (Kalra 2003).

A diet abundant in fruits and vegetables has been linked to a decreased incidence of chronic illnesses because of its high vitamin and mineral content and the presence of health-protective components, such as antioxidants and anti-inflammatory molecules (Donno et al. 2013). Plants produce these substances as secondary metabolites. Metabolites that are helpful to both humans and animals are found in abundance. These include UV radiation, parasites, oxidants, appealing odors, and colors, and inter-species rivalry (Kaur and Das 2011).

Inflammation is the result of an organism's response to potentially harmful stimuli. When treating a wide variety of inflammatory diseases, traditional medicine makes considerable use of anti-inflammatory medications. Fruits and vegetables, particularly their essential oils and monoterpenes, are becoming more recognized as a rich source of natural bioactive anti-inflammatory compounds (Cássia Da Silveira E Sá, Andrade, and De Sousa 2013). Polyphenols account for 10 times the amount of vitamin C found in the diet, making them the most abundant bioactive chemicals in the body (Scalbert, Hercberg, and Galan 2005; Shahidi and Ambigaipalan 2015). Extrinsic and intrinsic variables such as plant genetics, soil composition, growing circumstances, maturity stage, and postharvest conditions may all impact polyphenol content and quality in plant foods (Jeffery et al. 2003). Regarding phenolic consumption, eating habits, and tastes are important factors to consider (Shahidi and Ambigaipalan 2015).

DOI: 10.1201/9781003259213-1

Simple phenolics may be found in wide variety of foods and drinks (hydroxycinnamic acid conjugates and flavonoids) (Rice-Evans, Miller, and Paganga 1997). In vitro investigations have shown that these compounds possess a broad spectrum of antioxidant properties, suggesting that they may be beneficial in the prevention of cancer and heart disease. This list contains substances ranging from the most basic (such as vitamin C and phenolic acids) to the most heavily polymerized (like lutein). Flavonoids and phenolic acids are the phenolic chemicals found in the greatest abundance in plants (Tabart et al. 2011, 2012). Because of the differences in their structure and chemistry, organic acids have a variety of action mechanisms (Eyduran et al. 2015; Komes et al. 2011). However, due to their rich antioxidant content, they are very beneficial to overall well-being (Figure 1.1).

The main aim of the chapter is to highlight the recent findings on fruits for human use. Fruits have been an indispensable part of the human diet for ages, but not as a primary food. Secondary metabolites are found in plants' biochemistry (i.e., chemical compounds produced within the plants that are not directly involved in the normal growth, development, or reproduction of the organism). These metabolites have positive impacts on both people and animals. In addition to their high vitamin and mineral content, fruits contain molecules that have health-protective properties, such as antioxidant and anti-inflammatory substances. This has been linked to a decreased risk of chronic illnesses. Many degenerative illnesses may be prevented or even reversed with a plant-based diet high in fiber and other phytonutrients. These include but are not limited to: Type 2 diabetes and obesity, cardiovascular disease, and cancer. Many other benefits of fruits and their nutraceutical use are described in the following chapters.

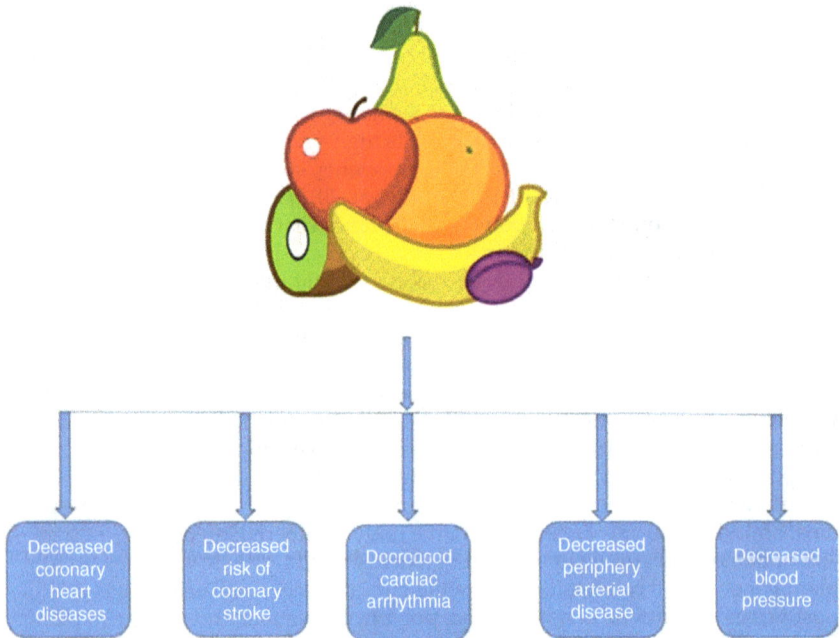

**Figure 1.1**  Benefits of fruits as nutraceuticals.

## 1.2 NUTRACEUTICAL PROPERTIES OF FRUITS

Plants, particularly fruits, are one of the most significant sources of human nourishment and have been used for thousands of years as a natural source of therapeutic chemicals. Natural goods and health-promoting foods have attracted much attention lately, thanks to recent developments in medical and nutrition sciences. Phytonutrients, phytomedicines, and phytotherapy are gaining importance in our daily lives (Bagchi 2006; Berger and Shenkin 2006; Bland 1996) and are playing a positive role in enhancing medical benefits and further improving immune function to prevent specific diseases with the promise of fewer side effects. Some of the fruits with nutraceutical properties are discussed below.

The Appalachian Mountains are home to the pawpaw (*Asimina triloba* L. Dunal), a tree fruit unique to the region. In the United States and Canada, pawpaws have been eaten for centuries by Native Americans, European explorers and settlers, and now by rural residents. Pawpaws have a high concentration of phytochemicals and other health-promoting components. When it comes to dietary fiber, iron, copper, and manganese, apples, and oranges are very similar to one another. They may have antioxidant activity on par with other fruits, if not more. Among the nutrients included in these meals are potassium (3,000–3,800 mg/kg), essential amino acids (40 mg/kg protein), riboflavin (0.06–0.15 mg/kg), niacin (10–12 mg/kg), calcium (500–800 mg/kg), phosphorus (400–500 mg/kg), zinc (10–12 mg/kg), and riboflavin. Fruits such as mangoes include polyphenols that are either equivalent to or greater in quantity than those found in other fruits. Caffeic acid, vitamin C, ellagic acid, ferulic acid, and quercetin are among those found in mangoes (*Mangifera indica* L.). The antioxidant content of ananas and guavas is comparable (Kobayashi, Wang, and Pomper 2008). These products, which include Paw Paw Cell Reg and Graviola Max, as well as Royal Graviola and Graviola liquid extract, have been the subject of clinical trials and animal investigations (Coothankandaswamy et al. 2010).

Goji (*Lycium barbarum*) is a brilliant orange-red ellipsoid berry shrub native to China, Tibet, and other areas in Asia. The fruits are harvested from late summer to early fall. Vitamins (C, B, and E), flavonoids, phenolic acids, minerals, trace elements, 18 amino acids (including eight essential amino acids), alkaloids, and fats are among the nutrients and phytochemicals found in *Lycium* fruits. Glaucoma, immunomodulation, cytoprotection, and antioxidant activities of the goji fruit have been studied. Traditional Chinese medicine uses *L. barbarum* and *L. chinense* fruits, which are also marketed as nutritional supplements or nutraceuticals for long-term use. Some researchers claim that the health-promoting compounds in goji berry reduce oxidative stress and fight free radicals.

*Amelanchier canadensis* is a sweet serviceberry whose products have grown dramatically over the past two decades (Michigan). For centuries, fruits have been used to make wine, beer, and tea. Much research has been done into the health advantages of serviceberries, particularly as a source of minerals (such as manganese) and carotenoids (such as β-carotenes). Nutraceuticals, such as phenolics, are also present in the fruit (e.g., anthocyanins, chlorogenic acid, catechins, and rutin). Sterols and unsaturated fatty acids may also be found in the oil produced from the seeds of *Amelanchier* spp. (Juríková et al. 2013). Serviceberry juice, for example, was historically used in Canada to treat stomach and intestine problems. Ripe serviceberries were also used to make eye and ear drops, as well as other products. Additionally, if pregnant mothers experienced an injury, they could drink the boiled tree bark to prevent miscarriage.

Traditional Native American cultures utilize twigs to make tea for new mothers, and the bark of the tree is used as a placenta aid. Numerous *Amelanchier* spp. cultivars have been shown to contain antioxidant and free radical scavenging characteristics in addition to their antiviral activity against enteric coronavirus. Finally, serviceberry fruits are antidiabetic and modulate lipid metabolism and energy expenditure (Bakowska-Barczak, Marianchuk, and Kolodziejczyk 2007; Bakowska-Barczak and Kolodziejczyk 2008).

Rutaceae is a family of plants that includes citrus fruits such as oranges, mandarins, limes, lemons, grapefruits, and citrons. Lemons and oranges have their origins in the Mediterranean. For fruits to be considered organoleptic or commercially viable (i.e., tasty), they need to have a variety of distinct characteristics (García-Salas et al. 2013). Fresh, juiced, or preserved segments of citrus fruits are the most common methods of citrus fruit consumption. There is a range of uses for citrus fruits as chemoprophylactic drugs and chemoprophylactic additives and spices (He et al. 2011; Kelebek and Selli 2011). Vitamin C and fiber content in citrus fruits are particularly noteworthy. In addition to sugars, fruits are rich sources of dietary fiber and a wide range of minerals and vitamins, including folate, thiamine, niacin, and vitamin B6 as well as phosphorus, magnesium, copper, riboflavin, and pantothenic acid (Economos and Clay 1999). Secondary metabolites, on the other hand, are a popular topic right now as pharmacologically active but non-essential phytochemicals may be found in plants. Citrus fruits contain an array of phytonutrients and compounds, such as flavonoids and alkaloids, as well as carotenoids and other pigments. Some of these active secondary metabolites have antioxidant properties that are beneficial to human health and other bioactivities such as cardiovascular and neuroprotective properties.

The pomegranate is native to the Mediterranean region. Because of its high drought resilience, pomegranate is an excellent fruit crop for arid climates. Arils (40%), seeds (10%), and the fruit's skin (the remaining 50%) are all edible parts of the fruit. More than 85% of arils' makeup consists of sugars and pectin, organic acids, and flavonoids, the bulk of which are anthocyanins, as well as water. This group includes linolenic and linoleic acids, punicic, olive, stearic, and palmitic acids (Viuda-Martos, Fernández-Lóaez, and Pérez-álvarez 2010). This meal is high in vitamin E. Ellagitannins and gallotannins are the two forms of hydrolyzable tannins. Ellagitannins are found in the pericarp, seeds, flowers, and bark, while gallotannins are found in the leaf and other parts of the plant. Pomegranate and its derivatives, which impact the stomach's flora, may be used to make an antibacterial agent. Bacteria metabolize ellagic acid in the intestines, which results in the formation of urolithin A and B (Finegold et al. 2014). It is the prebiotic qualities of the pomegranate that are responsible for this. Pomegranate juice and extracts may have a prebiotic effect on the bacteria in the human stomach. Using lactic acid bacteria to simulate gastrointestinal digestion of various juices, the prebiotic impact of ellagitannin, epicatechin, and catechin metabolism was studied, resulting in the increased bio-accessibility of phenolic compounds as well as improved survival of lactic acid bacteria (Valero-Cases, Nuncio-Jáuregui, and María José Frutos 2017). Anti-carcinogenic properties of pomegranate extracts have been investigated in recent years (Rettig et al. 2008). The use of pomegranate extracts as dietary supplements may be effective in treating persons with small, localized kidney tumors who otherwise would not be candidates for nephrolithotomy surgery. Punicalagin, a polyphenol derived from the pomegranate fruit, has been shown to have antiproliferative activity in prostate cancer cells by inducing apoptosis (Adaramoye et al. 2017; Deng et al. 2017).

Fruits like bananas are enjoyed by billions of people worldwide every year. They have a low protein content, a high carbohydrate content (hemicellulose, starch, and pectin), and a healthy dosage of vitamins A and C, in addition to minerals and vitamins such as potassium, calcium, sodium, and magnesium. Traditional and indigenous medicine practitioners in Africa, Asia, and the Pacific have been using a range of banana parts for hundreds of years to treat a number of ailments (Pereira and Maraschin 2015). Snake bite, inflammation, colitis, dysentery, and diarrhea are all conditions that have been successfully treated with these medicinal plant constituents in the past. While bananas are now being investigated for their potential involvement in reducing carbohydrate-digesting enzymes (glucosidase and amylase) and glucose absorption, they also possesses antioxidant characteristics worth noting (Famakin et al. 2016; Jaber et al. 2013). They are a nutritional powerhouse when it comes to fiber content. Known for its high concentration of amino acids and antioxidants such as carotenoids and polyphenols, banana peel, and pulp make for a delicious culinary and dessert component. Sugars, carbs, fiber, and cellulose components may be found in banana pulp. The peels of bananas are particularly rich in fiber. Phytochemicals are known to have anticancer and chemopreventive agents (Ketron and Osheroff 2014). In addition to bioactive chemicals such as phenolics and carotenoids, berries also include glycosides, phlobatannins, and other types of tannin (Singh et al. 2016). Additionally, berries may include several additional substances, such as steroids and saponins (Mathew and Negi 2017). The pulp and peel of bananas contain provitamin A as well as antioxidants. Banana peel has a greater concentration of antioxidants when compared to banana pulp (Kondo, Kittikorn, and Kanlayanarat 2005; Vu, Scarlett, and Vuong 2018). Banana contains biogenic amines, phenolics, phytosterols, and carotenoids (Gonzalez-Aguilar et al. 2008). These chemicals are very beneficial to consumers owing to their many health benefits due to their antioxidative characteristics, which effectively reduce oxidative stress. Banana pulp contains antitumor and antioxidant properties (Borges et al. 2014). Bananas are beneficial to muscles owing to their high K content. Banana is generally recommended for anemia sufferers due to their high Fe content. Its low Na content helps regulate blood pressure (Singh et al. 2016). Bananas contain syringic acid (Muthukumaran et al. 2013). This antidiabetic drug may be utilized to treat glycoprotein abnormalities(Muthukumaran et al. 2013). Increased plasma antioxidant activity and fat oxidation are all benefits of eating catechin-rich bananas (Williamson and Manach 2005). Banana gallic acid has been shown to be hepatoprotective (Rasool et al. 2010). It contains dopamine and ascorbic acid, which reduce plasma oxidative stress and increase resistance to oxidative modification of low-density lipoproteins (LDLs) (Bennett et al. 2010; Hosein Farzaei et al. 2015). As an ingredient in many energy beverages and dried banana bars, the banana is an excellent energy source for sportsmen. The fruit's vitamin K and Mg content have been utilized to reduce muscle contractions in athletes.

Grapes are grown in temperate climates. They are rich sources of flavonoids. Flavonoids are potent antioxidants, anti-inflammatory, anticancer, and antibacterial nutraceuticals found in foods and phytopharmaceuticals (Groot and Rauen 1998; Hertog et al. 1995; Knekt et al. 1996; Marchand 2002). Thus, understanding grape flavonoids' biological activity, bioavailability, and metabolism is critical for human health. The tradition of frequent red wine drinking has been linked to a reduced risk of cardiovascular disease (Renaud et al. 1992). Red wine flavonoids are the most likely compounds to blame (Formica and Regelson 1995).

Grape is a rich source of important phytonutrients with outstanding beneficial effects on human health (Nassiri-Asl and Hosseinzadeh 2009; Vislocky and Fernandez 2013; Xia et al. 2010). Phytochemicals in grapes include simple phenolics, flavonoids, anthocyanins, stilbenes, proanthocyanins, and vitamin E (Ali et al. 2010). Pigments include hydroxycinnamic acid (p-coumaric, caffeic, and ferulic acids) and hydroxybenzoic acid (gallic, gentisic). Same has been shown to contain 7–10 times the gallic acid concentration of European grapes (*Vitis vinifera* L., "*Chardonnay*" and "*Merlot*" var.) (Yilmaz and Toledo 2004). Gallic acid possesses antioxidant, anticancer, anti-inflammatory, antifungal, and antiviral effects (Nguyen et al. 2013; Sameermahmood et al. 2010; Shabir et al. 2013). Grapes contain a large number of physiologically active chemicals, including flavonoids, stilbenes, and proanthocyanins. The grape is one of the fruits highest in polyphenols. There are several flavonoids in grapes that have been shown to have cardioprotective, neurological, antibacterial, and antiaging effects. Most flavonoids are found in the grape skin, whereas 60–70% of total polyphenols are found in grape seeds (Capanoglu et al. 2013). In grape juice preparation, only 2% of anthocyanins are removed with the cell sap (Capanoglu et al. 2013). The polymeric compounds produced by fermentation/maceration include proanthocyanins, pyranoanthocyanins (vitamin A and vitamin B), and oligostilbenes (Proantocianidinas and Vinho 2005). However, over 70% of grape polyphenols remain in the pomace (a by-product of wine/grape juice production), making it a rich source of health-promoting nutraceuticals (Ratnasooriya and Vasantha Rupasinghe 2012). Grape seeds may also be extracted from the pomace and utilized to produce grape seed oil or as dietary supplements in the form of powder or extracts (Chamorro et al. 2012). Grape peels also provide flavonoid-rich compounds (Greenspan et al. 2005; Jeong et al. 2012).

Mulberries are important as far as their nutraceutical properties are concerned. *Morus alba, Morus nigra,* and *Morus rubra* are the three most promising mulberry species since they contain the highest medicinal characteristics of any other mulberry species. As a result of mulberry's extraordinary medicinal capabilities, the numerous vegetative components of the plant are of enormous interest to researchers today. Currently, mulberries are a big issue because of their remarkable nutraceutical importance. Mulberries are recognized for their therapeutic benefits, including their ability to alleviate fatigue, tiredness, and anemia, as well as support the liver and kidneys. Sore throat, sadness, and fever are some of the conditions it is used to treat in the elderly and those who are anemic. More research shows that mulberry fruit juice may improve health by soothing the nervous system, increasing alcohol metabolism, and improving the immune system. Carbohydrates can be found in large quantities in mulberries and may be ingested in various ways, from juice to wine to tea to jams and jellies (Jan et al. 2021; Singhal et al. 2010). Vitamins and minerals in the mulberry fruit have the potential to cure a wide range of chronic illnesses. Nutraceuticals such as amino acids, carbs, lipids, vitamins, and minerals abound in mulberry fruit, making it a valuable addition to a healthy diet. Mulberries are also known to include anthocyanins, phloridzin, quercetin, chlorogenic acid, resveratrol, and rutin, among other beneficial phytochemicals (Gundogdu et al. 2011; Shrikanta, Kumar, and Govindaswamy 2015; Tomas et al. 2015). Anticancer, antioxidant, neuroprotective, hepatoprotective, antibacterial, anti-obesity, and hypolipidemic properties may be attributed to the mulberry's high concentration of phytochemicals and nutraceuticals (Jiang et al. 2013). Plant-based sources of nutrition and phytochemicals are important. Getting those chemicals to where they are meant to be used in the body is more important. The bioavailability of nutrients and phytochemicals is more important than understanding where they come from, and a few studies have shown that mulberry fruits are excellent sources of bioavailability. The bioavailability of mulberries, which has been overlooked in most assessments of mulberries, is also addressed in this chapter. Because of their therapeutic capabilities, mulberries have the potential to become a new functional food and a current focus of attention for many nutritionists. Tonics for blood, kidney, and liver disorders may be nourished by drinking mulberry fruit juice, one of the exceptional by-products of mulberries. Juice from mulberry fruits contains carbs, protein, oil (omega-6-polyunsaturated fatty acids such as linoleic acid), free acids, fiber, and minerals that may improve human health. When stored in the refrigerator, the mulberry juice retains its characteristics for up to 3 months.

Inhibiting apoptosis and matrix metalloproteinase, the active components in mulberries, helps to halt the growth of cancer (Huang, Ou, and Wang 2013). Antioxidants in mulberries, such as anthocyanins, enhance vision by encouraging the death of cancerous cells (Fallis 2013).

## 1.3 BENEFITS OF FRUITS IN VARIOUS DISEASE STATES

Fruits are rich in dietary fiber and are a good source of important vitamins and minerals. Fruits also include a variety of health-promoting antioxidants, such as flavonoids. A fruit-rich diet can lower one's chance of acquiring a variety of ailments, including heart disease, cancer, inflammation, diabetes, and others. Fruits are considered "powerhouses" due to their dense nutritional value and low calorie content. Some of the health benefits of fruits are discussed in Table 1.1.

### 1.3.1 In Cognition and Brain

Medicinal uses for grapes and their derivatives date back millennia, making them one of the most popular and well-researched berry fruits (Singh, Liu, and Ahmad 2015). A preliminary study involving 35 young smokers (mean age 26 years) found no acute effect of Concord grape juice (10 mL/kg) on cognition in a double-blind, placebo-controlled crossover (Hendrickson and Mattes 2008). Then again, subsequent studies in older adults have proven effective. Twelve older people (mean age 78.2 years) with mild memory decline drank Concord grape juice (6–9 mL/kg/d) or a placebo in a randomized, double-blind, placebo-controlled study (Krikorian et al. 2010). Participants who drank grape juice showed an increase in verbal learning and a trend toward an increase in verbal recall after 12 weeks of supplementation. Twenty-one older men and women (mean age 76.9 years) with mild cognitive impairment who were being treated for hypertension participated in a randomized, double-blind, placebo-controlled study (Krikorian et al. 2010) to compare cognition before and after 16 weeks of supplementation with Concord grape juice (6.3–7.8 mL/kg/d). When it came time to perform a word list learning task, participants who had consumed grape juice performed significantly better than placebo controls in terms of making fewer intrusion errors, a sign of improved executive function. Functional magnetic resonance imaging (fMRI) showed that participants who drank grape juice had greater activation in two brain areas linked to working memory (right superior parietal and right middle frontal cortices) than those who drank a placebo. After 12 weeks of daily Concord grape juice (335 mL) or placebo consumption in a randomized, double-blind, crossover trial, 25 working mothers (40–50-years-old) completed a battery of cognitive tests and were evaluated in a driving simulator. Grape juice treatment improved spatial learning and driving simulator accuracy, compared to placebo treatment, according to the results of a spatial learning test. Many prospective studies have shown that adherence to a Mediterranean Diet (MedDiet) is associated with reduced cognitive decline, improved cognitive

## Table 1.1: Biological Activities of Various Fruits

| Fruit Extracts/ Bioactive Compound | Experimental Models/ Subjects | Results | References |
|---|---|---|---|
| Red orange | Human keratinocytes (HaCaT) cell line | • Efficiently counteracted UVB-induced response.<br>• Prevent inflammation by inhibiting NF-κB and AP-1 translocation and procaspase-3 cleavage. | (Cimino et al. 2007) |
| Orange peel extract | Human esophageal cancer cell (YM1) | • Reduces the systemic toxicity of chemotherapeutic agents like doxorubicin. | (Tajaldini et al. 2020) |
| Orange peel extract | 10 *ApcMin/+* mice (4 weeks old) per group | • Inhibits intestinal tumor growth. | (Fan et al. 2007) |
| Orange extract | N2 wild-type *Caenorhabditis elegans* | • Increased the mean lifespan (dose-dependently).<br>• Improves motility. | (Wang et al. 2020) |
| Orange peel | Xenografts 5 male mice (6–8 weeks old) | • Reduces the size of tumors. | (Tajaldini et al. 2020) |
| Red orange extract | 20 Caucasian subjects with skin erythema induced by UV irradiation (aged 26–47 years) | • Significant reduction in the skin erythema degree. | (Puglia et al. 2014) |
| Red orange extract | 25 volunteers with tanning skin homogeneity (aged 45–70 years) | • Improvement in pigmentation and skin appearance. | |
| Red orange | 32 patients with Type 2 diabetes and 28 healthy volunteers | • Decreases serum free radical levels in patients with high blood oxidative stress status. | (Bonina et al. 2002) |
| Freeze-dried strawberry | Breast (MCF-7 and T47-D) and cervical (CaSki and SiHa) cancer cell lines | • Significantly suppresses the cervical cancer cells but has less effect on breast cancer cells. | (Wedge et al. 2001) |
| Strawberry-rich extracts | Human oral (KB, CAL-27), prostate (LNCaP), colon (HT-29, HCT-116), and breast (MCF-7) tumor cell lines | • Inhibits cancer cell proliferation. | (Seeram et al. 2006) |
| Crude extracts and purified compounds | Human oral (CAL-27, KB), prostate (LNCaP, DU145), and colon (HT-29 and HCT-116) cancer cells | • Inhibits cell proliferation. | (Zhang et al. 2008) |
| Kaempferol | HT-29 colon cancer cells | • Induces cell cycle arrest.<br>• Inhibits cancer cells growth and proliferation. | (Cho and Park 2013) |
| Freeze-dried strawberry | AOM/DSS induced male Crj: CD-1 mice | • Decreases pro-inflammatory mediators and oncogenic signaling pathways. | (Shi et al. 2015) |
| Quercetin | HT1080 human fibrosarcoma cells | • Suppresses phenazine methosulfate (PMS)-induced intracellular ROS formation.<br>• Decreases matrix metalloproteinase activity. | (Lee et al. 2013) |

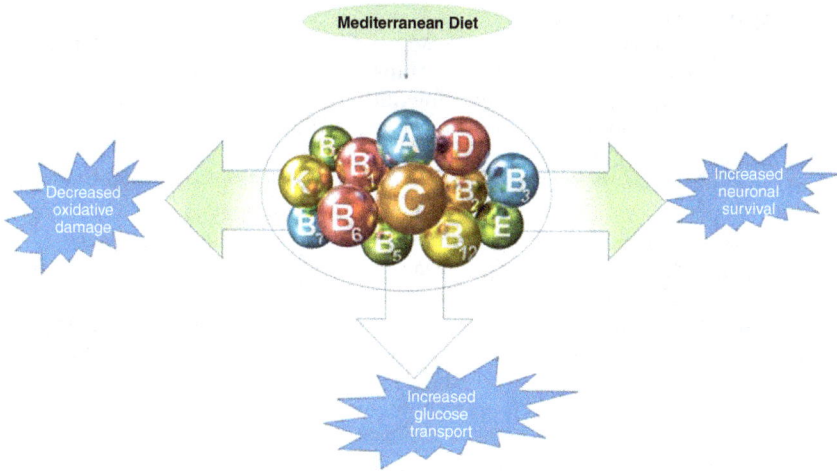

**Figure 1.2** Benefits of the Mediterranean Diet in reducing health risks.

outcomes (independent of cardiovascular disease risk factors), and preservation of cognitive function in populations at risk for Alzheimer's disease (Figure 1.2) (Hardman et al. 2016; Knight, Bryan, and Murphy 2016; Trichopoulou et al. 2015). A recent qualitative evaluation and systematic review of longitudinal and prospective trials has been conducted to examine the effect of long-term MedDiet on cognitive function by Hardman and co-workers. Various aspects of memory, executive function, and visual constructs were found to be enhanced by MedDiet (e.g., delayed recognition, long-term memory, and working memory) (Hardman et al. 2016).

According to research, cellular signaling can be altered and protection provided by berry fruits and their chemical constituents. Human monoamine oxidases (MAOs) A and B, expressed in *baculovirus*-infected insect cells, were studied by Dreiseitel and colleagues in relation to anthocyanins and related compounds (anthocyanidins, proanthocyanidins, etc.) (Dreiseitel et al. 2009). Because MAOs are tissue-specific, they can only be found in the brain, where they are found in the neurons and glia of the catecholaminergic (MAO A34) and serotonergic (MAO B35) systems, respectively (Levitt, Pintar, and Breakefield 1982; Shih, Chen, and Ridd 1999). AD is associated with elevated levels of MAO activity (Kennedy et al. 2003; Thomas 2000). In vitro, it was discovered that anthocyanins inhibited both subtypes. By blocking the enzymes that break down the amines in the brain, anthocyanins, and other phenolic compounds, which are known to inhibit MAOs, may help treat neurological disorders caused by low levels of amines in the brain (Hou et al. 2005; Lee et al. 2001; Yáñez et al. 2006). The neurotransmitter acetylcholine is involved in memory and learning. Neuronal mAChRs become less sensitive with age, and patients with Alzheimer's disease have the most significant decrease in this sensitivity (Terry 2001). Using fluorescence imaging, our lab has found that mAChR (M1 subtype) transfected COS-7 cells show impaired calcium buffering when exposed to either amyloid-42 (A), the protein that accumulates in the brain during AD, or dopamine, a neurotransmitter that induces oxidative stress in high doses, prior to depolarization. Cell viability and A42- and dopamine-induced calcium dysregulation were prevented by pretreatment of cells with a variety of berry extracts (Joseph et al. 2004). The mAChR i3 domain appears to play a role in berry protection in the M1 and M3 subtypes. In the presence of blueberry extract, dopamine-treated, transfected cells showed altered activation of signaling critical to learning and memory, resulting in decreased activation of PKC-gamma and phosphorylated CREB, and increased activation of extracellular signal-regulated kinase 1/2 (ERK1/2).

Intake of polyphenols, found in fruits and vegetables, has been linked to improvements in cognitive function (Sofi et al. 2010; Tangney et al. 2011). More polyphenol consumption was linked to better language and episodic memory in healthy middle-aged adults (45–60 years old) and to better baseline cognitive performance and less decline in non-demented adults aged 70 and over (Kesse-Guyot et al. 2012). Non-demented adults aged 70 and over who ate more anthocyanins from blueberries and strawberries had a lower rate of cognitive decline (Devore et al. 2012). Several studies have found that blueberries have a significant effect on short- and long-term memory; animal studies have shown that improvements in spatial memory can be seen within 3 weeks, which is the equivalent of about three years in humans. There is evidence that the catechins in green tea (0.025%–0.010% of the weight of the tea leaf) and pure epicatechin (0.025%–0.010% of the weight of the tea leaf) help mice (8–10 weeks old) retain their spatial memory (Li et al. 2009). The dentate gyrus (DG) appears to play a role in the mechanisms (Burke and Barnes 2006; Casadesus et al. 2004). Polyphenol-rich foods may be able to improve memory through a link between hippocampal neurogenesis, cognitive performance, and aging (Stangl and Thuret 2009). Despite this, epidemiological and pre-clinical investigations have shown that polyphenols may have neurocognitive benefits, although results from human intervention trials are less certain (Scholey et al. 2010). More research is needed to corroborate these early findings (Vauzour et al. 2017).

### 1.3.2 As Antiaging

A process known as oxidative stress is responsible for the majority of aging-related malfunctions and illnesses, and many colorful fruits and vegetables have been thoroughly researched for their ability to neutralize free radicals that may harm DNA and cell membranes via this method (Figure 1.3) (Gupta et al. 2019). However, although some fruits like blueberries, grapes, and cranberries do not contain a cure-all, they do include a range of health-promoting components such as vitamins, fiber, and antioxidants (Paredes-López et al. 2010; Nile and Park 2014). Vitamin C and other antioxidants in fruits seem to have the most important function in slowing the progression of aging-related illnesses. Raspberries have been linked to health advantages by nutritionists in labs across the globe (Beekwilder, Hall, and De Vos 2005). A study in 2018 looked at the effects of blueberry supplementation on *Caenorhabditis elegans* longevity and stress tolerance. A dose-dependent increase in lifetime was seen when the extract was applied to the worms for 4 days at 50, 100, and 200 mg/mL of blueberry extract, respectively. Compared to untreated *Caenorhabditis* worms, blueberry-treated *Caenorhabditis elegans* had higher resilience to heat, paraquat, and ultraviolet-B radiation (Wang et al. 2018).

### 1.3.3 As Antihypertensive Agents

It has been shown that whole freeze-dried blueberries may reduce the risk of obesity and hypertension in rats given a high-fat diet for 3 months by 5% or 10% (w/w). Blueberries have been shown to reduce inflammation in the body and prevent hypertension. Adding 3% blueberry to the diet for 2 weeks lowered plasma ACE (angiotensin-converting enzyme) activity in spontaneously

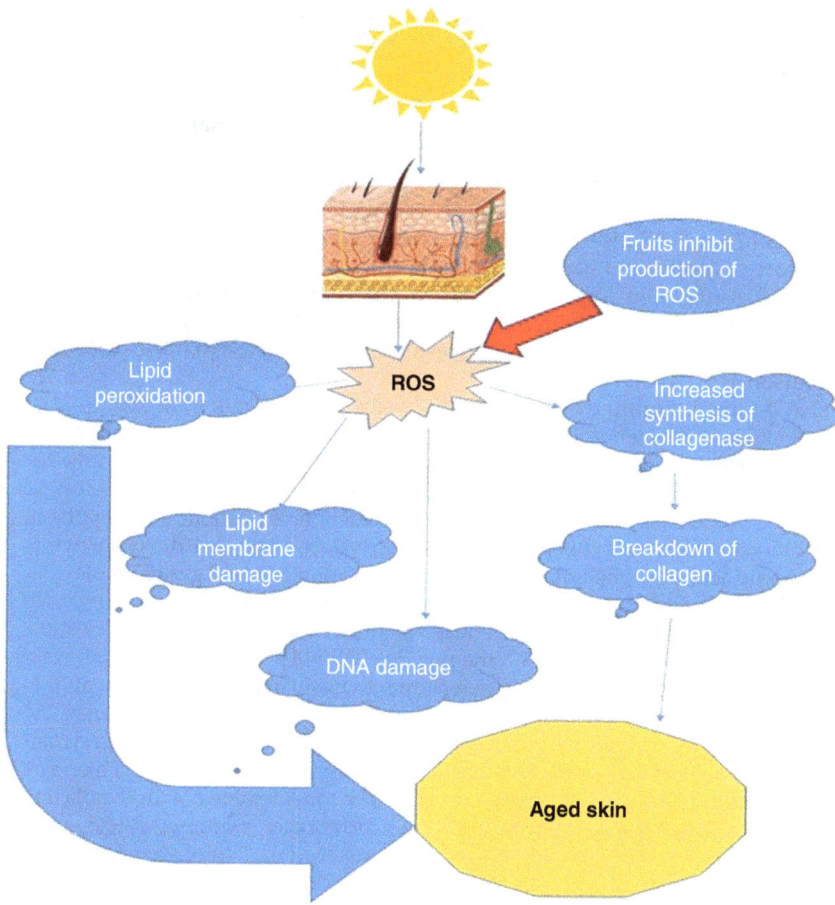

**Figure 1.3**  Benefits of fruits in reducing the aging of the skin.

hypertensive stroke-prone rats (SHRSP), which is in line with the findings of this research (Wiseman et al. 2011). Blueberry intake (250 gm daily) for 3 weeks showed no impact on ACE activity, blood pressure, or plasma antioxidant levels in chronic smokers; this was ascribed to smokers' low polyphenol intake, which is thought to be the cause of the lack of effect (McAnulty et al. 2014). Wild blueberry drink intake had no significant impact on vascular function indicators, total nitric oxide levels, or blood pressure, according to previous research by Riso et al. (2013). Because anthocyanins had a short bioavailability period of between 1 and 3 hours, it was pointed out that their lack of effect was related to this.

It has been shown that blueberries lower blood pressure in both animal and human trials. The effects of polyphenols on nicotinamide adenine dinucleotide phosphate (NADPH) oxidase inhibition and increased nitric oxide bioavailability in rats fed a high fat and cholesterol diet led to a drop in blood pressure and an improvement in endothelial dysfunction, according to research published in 2013 (Rodriguez-Mateos et al. 2013). SHRSP and normal rats were fed a diet enhanced with 3% blueberry extract for 8 weeks. Consumption of blueberries reduced systolic blood pressure in SHRSP by 19% at week 4, and by 30% at week 6. The reactive oxygen species (ROS) scavenging capacity of blueberry reduced urine protein and nitrite levels in the kidney, as well (Stull et al. 2015).

Blueberry freeze-dried extract was given to postmenopausal women with pre- and stage 1 hypertension in randomized, double-blind, placebo-controlled research for 8 weeks, and blood pressure, arterial stiffness, C-reactive protein, nitric oxide, and superoxide dismutase were examined. As measured by the brachial-ankle pulse wave velocity (baPWV), which is a composite measure of central and peripheral arterial stiffness, the systolic and diastolic blood pressures were lowered, but the carotid-femoral pulse wave velocity (cfPWV), the arterial pressure, and the heart rate did not change significantly. Furthermore, the activation of eNOS resulted in an increase in nitric oxide levels (Johnson et al. 2015).

N(G)-nitro-L-arginine methyl ester (L-NAME)-treated rats were given blueberries fermented with *Lactobacillus plantarum*, DSM 15313, to examine their antihypertensive properties. By regulating the NO-dependent pathway, the ingestion of fermented blueberries reduced blood pressure significantly. An antihypertensive effect was found in the production of phenolic acids by the probiotic bacteria in fermented goods (hydroxyllactic acid, 3, 4-dioxyphenyl-propionic acid, and phenyllactic acid). Consumption of 1 or 2 gm of whole wild blueberry powder or 200 mg extract (which provides 2.7, 5.4, or 14 mg of anthocyanins daily) for 6 weeks reduced systolic blood pressure significantly, but no impact was detected with the powder (Whyte et al. 2018). Ellagitannins isolated from strawberries have been shown to have an anti-ACE action at 50 mg/mL (da Silva Pinto et al. 2010). Individuals at risk for cardiovascular disease were shown to have lower blood pressure, increased HDL (high-density lipoprotein) cholesterol, and decreased platelet function after taking a blend of berry supplements. Some studies have shown a considerable rise in the plasma levels of polyphenols such as quercetin and caffeic acid, p-coumaric acid, and vanillic acid. For hyperglycemia and hypertension, a variety of strawberry cultivars were tested, which showed different ACE inhibitory actions but were effective in managing hypertension (Cheplick et al. 2010). In rats, Hellström et al. (2010) found that a combination of black chokeberry polyphenols somewhat inhibited ACE activity (Hellström et al. 2010). They hypothesized that these chemicals may have an effect on NO production through an ACE-independent mechanism and by stimulating the endothelial nitric oxide enzyme (eNO) in the blood vessels. This reaffirmed the findings of a research that found black chokeberry extract to be beneficial in the production of NO. Chokeberry extracts activated eNOS in bovine coronary artery endothelial cells by phosphorylating the activation site, serine 1,177, according to the research findings. After 10 minutes of stimulation with the extract, the maximal level of enzyme activity was achieved, and long-term exposure to the extract (48 hours) had no significant influence on NOS levels. This is only one of several probable mechanisms of action besides ACE inhibitory activity. Endothelin-1 alterations have been shown to boost NO generation and vasorelaxation activity as well as to have greater antioxidative potential. For example, the results of tests on animal models indicate that antioxidative activity has an influence on blood pressure and that eating products containing chokeberries have an effect on total antioxidant capacity and endogenous glutathione levels.

Atherosclerosis is caused by high blood pressure, which affects the internal organs. Experiments have shown that chokeberry extract has an anti-inflammatory effect on the heart and renal tissue. Endothelial progenitor cells

(EPC), which play a critical role in postnatal vasculogenesis and cardiovascular system function, have been shown to be negatively affected by angiotensin II (Ciocoiu et al. 2013). According to a study published in 2015, black chokeberry extracts increased EPC functions by increasing EPC proliferation; decreasing the progression of cell senescence; and changing EPC migratory and adhesion qualities. Antihypertensive effects of red raspberry red ethyl acetate extract were studied by Jia and colleagues (2011), and they found that the extract decreased blood pressure after 1 week and that the effects remained until the fifth week (Jia et al. 2011). People with pre-hypertension were shown to have lower systolic blood pressure when they took 2.5 gm of black raspberry powder every day for 8 weeks, compared to those who took the same amount of powder every day. Results of anthocyanin intake by 15 athletes who took anthocyanin-rich black currant extract for 12 days demonstrated that only the two highest anthocyanin concentrations were effective at lowering arterial blood pressure (ABP) (Cook et al. 2017). Black currant juice with 40 mg of anthocyanin a day for 6 weeks had no impact on blood pressure in the research of 66 overweight persons (Khan et al. 2014).

### 1.3.4 In Cancer

Nearly 10 million people die each year from cancer, making it a serious public health concern. Numerous studies have shown a high correlation between fruit consumption and decreased rates of several types of cancer (Van't Veer et al. 2000). Polyphenolic extracts (triterpenoids, proanthocyanidin oligomers, and flavonols) from cranberries and their derivatives have been demonstrated in several in vitro and in vivo investigations to inhibit tumor development and multiplication in the lungs, prostate, colon, and breast (Neto 2007). Numerous studies have shown that a diet high in phytochemicals, such as that found in fresh fruits and vegetables, lowers the risk of developing a variety of malignancies in humans (Karasawa and Mohan 2018). There is evidence that berries may protect cancer cells and animal models from the harmful effects of oxidative stress and carcinogens. A study found that raspberry phytochemicals may inhibit cancer cell growth and proliferation in vitro by influencing the PTEN/AKT pathway (Zhang et al. 2018a). Strawberry, blueberry, and cranberry have been demonstrated to inhibit cancer formation by modulating many pathways, including Wnt/-catenin, ERK/MAPK, JAK/STAT, NF-B, and PI3K/ AKT/mTOR (Afrin et al. 2016; Bishayee et al. 2016; Chu et al. 2014), which alters cellular processes linked in growth, multiplication, and metastasis. Carcinogen metabolism is influenced by berries, resulting in lower rates of DNA damage caused by carcinogens. Pre-malignant cell development is slowed, apoptosis is boosted, and angiogenesis is inhibited due to these measures (Stoner et al. 2007). There are a lot of methods fruits polyphenols can fight cancer, including activating metabolizing enzymes, gene expression regulation, influencing cell proliferation, cell signal transduction pathways, and the death of cells.

### 1.3.5 In Diabetes

The antidiabetic properties of various berries are primarily due to their high anthocyanin content, which has been linked to a variety of distinct anti-hyperglycemic pathways. As a first step, anthocyanins are natural antioxidants that have been shown to reduce the ROS level in pancreatic β-cells, protecting them from oxidative stress. Due to their limited antioxidant capacity, islets are vulnerable to oxidative damage. Chinese bayberry C3G significantly improved mouse islets' antioxidant capacity and NPI (Li et al. 2017). Dietary anthocyanin extracts exhibited significant antioxidant activity against STZ-induced oxidative stress, which was substantially ascribed to their antidiabetic benefits in vivo (Sun et al. 2012; Zhang et al. 2013). It has been shown that the significant antioxidant ability of anthocyanins may up-regulate the expression of the insulin transcription factor and the levels of insulin, and reduce insulin resistance and metabolic syndrome (Noratto, Chew, and Atienza 2017). Because of this, anthocyanins may be used as an additional antioxidant therapy for people with diabetes.

Secondly, anthocyanins have been shown to block digestive enzymes such as α-amylase, β-glucosidase, or maltase, which may result in lower postprandial blood glucose levels (Zhang et al. 2018b). In vitro, significant β-glucosidase inhibitory activity was found in mulberry anthocyanin extract (Wang et al. 2013), blueberry fruit and fermented beverages (Johnson et al. 2011; 2016), cranberry powders rich in anthocyanins (Pinto et al. 2010), and blackberry (Spínola et al. 2019).

## 1.4 CONCLUSION

As the incidence of oxidative stress-mediated aging and other chronic diseases rises, there is a need to boost the body's defensive system with the fewest adverse effects possible. In order to meet this demand, powerful antioxidants have been used (naturally occurring compounds). Furthermore, polyphenolic substances in fruits have antioxidant properties. A free radical scavenger is a natural antioxidant that protects the body from oxidative damage caused by free radicals. Antioxidants, including anthocyanins, phenolics, vitamins, minerals, and other antiaging phytochemicals like resveratrol and quercetin found in fruits like apples, oranges, berries, grapes, and cherries may help delay the aging process and improve health. The scientific community and the general public have a tremendous interest in these fruits. There is still a lot of work to be done to understand how phytochemicals identified recently may help in the fight against aging in humans.

## REFERENCES

Adaramoye, Oluwatosin, Bettina Erguen, Bianca Nitzsche, Michael Höpfner, Klaus Jung, and Anja Rabien. 2017. "Punicalagin, a Polyphenol from Pomegranate Fruit, Induces Growth Inhibition and Apoptosis in Human PC-3 and LNCaP Cells." *Chemico-Biological Interactions* 274. https://doi.org/10.1016/j.cbi.2017.07.009.

Afrin, Sadia, Massimiliano Gasparrini, Tamara Y. Forbes-Hernandez, Patricia Reboredo-Rodriguez, Bruno Mezzetti, Alfonso Varela-López, Francesca Giampieri, and Maurizio Battino. 2016. "Promising Health Benefits of the Strawberry: A Focus on Clinical Studies." *Journal of Agricultural and Food Chemistry*. https://doi.org/10.1021/acs.jafc.6b00857.

Ali, Kashif, Federica Maltese, Young Hae Choi, and Robert Verpoorte. 2010. "Metabolic Constituents of Grapevine and Grape-Derived Products." *Phytochemistry Reviews*. https://doi.org/10.1007/s11101-009-9158-0.

Bagchi, Debasis. 2006. "Nutraceuticals and Functional Foods Regulations in the United States and around the World". *Toxicol* 221: 1–3.

Bakowska-Barczak, Anna M., and Paul Kolodziejczyk. 2008. "Evaluation of Saskatoon Berry (*Amelanchier alnifolia* Nutt.) Cultivars for their Polyphenol

Content, Antioxidant Properties, and Storage Stability." *Journal of Agricultural and Food Chemistry* 56 (21). https://doi.org/10.1021/jf801887w.

Bakowska-Barczak, Anna M., Myles Marianchuk, and Paul Kolodziejczyk. 2007. "Survey of Bioactive Components in Western Canadian Berries." *Canadian Journal of Physiology and Pharmacology* 85 (11). https://doi.org/10.1139/Y07-102.

Proantocianidinas, E. E. D. U. E. and D. Vinho. 2005. "Quantitative Extraction and Analysis of Grape and Wine Proanthocyanidins and Stilbenes." *Cílncia e Tècnica Vitivinìcola* 20 (2): 59–89.

Beekwilder, Jules, Robert D. Hall, and C. H. Ric De Vos. 2005. "Identification and Dietary Relevance of Antioxidants from Raspberry." *BioFactors* 23. https://doi.org/10.1002/biof.5520230404.

Bennett, Richard N., Tánia M. Shiga, Neuza M. A. Hassimotto, Eduardo A. S. Rosa, Franco M. Lajolo, and Beatriz R. Cordenunsi. 2010. "Phenolics and Antioxidant Properties of Fruit Pulp and Cell Wall Fractions of Postharvest Banana (*Musa acuminata* Juss.) Cultivars." *Journal of Agricultural and Food Chemistry* 58 (13). https://doi.org/10.1021/jf1008692.

Berger, Mette M., and Alan Shenkin. 2006. "Vitamins and Trace Elements: Practical Aspects of Supplementation." *Nutrition* 22: 952–955.

Bhattacharya, Tanima, Giselle Amanda Borges e Soares, Hitesh Chopra, Md. Mominur Rahman, Ziaul Hasan, Shasank S. Swain, and Simona Cavalu. 2022. "Applications of Phyto-Nanotechnology for the Treatment of Neurodegenerative Disorders." *Materials* 15 (3): 804. https://doi.org/10.3390/MA15030804.

Bishayee, Anupam, Yennie Haskell, Chau Do, Kodappully Sivaraman Siveen, Nima Mohandas, Gautam Sethi, and Gary D. Stoner. 2016. "Potential Benefits of Edible Berries in the Management of Aerodigestive and Gastrointestinal Tract Cancers: Preclinical and Clinical Evidence." *Critical Reviews in Food Science and Nutrition* 56 (10). https://doi.org/10.1080/10408398.2014.982243.

Bland, J. S. 1996. "Phytonutrition, Phytotherapy and Phytopharmacology." *Alternative Therapies in Health and Medicine* 2: 73–76.

Bonina, F. P., C. Leotta, G. Scalia, C. Puglia, D. Trombetta, G. Tringali, A. M. Roccazzello, P. Rapisarda, and A. Saija. 2002. "Evaluation of Oxidative Stress in Diabetic Patients after Supplementation with a Standardised Red Orange Extract." *Diabetes, Nutrition and Metabolism – Clinical and Experimental* 15 (1): 14–19.

Borges, Cristine Vanz, Vanusia Batista De Oliveira Amorim, Fernanda Ramlov, Carlos Alberto Da Silva Ledo, Marcela Donato, Marcelo Maraschin, and Edson Perito Amorim. 2014. "Characterisation of Metabolic Profile of Banana Genotypes, Aiming at Biofortified *Musa* spp. Cultivars." *Food Chemistry* 145. https://doi.org/10.1016/j.foodchem.2013.08.041.

Brower, V. 1998. "Nutraceuticals: Poised for a Healthy Slice of the Healthcare Market?" *Nature Biotechnology*. https://doi.org/10.1038/nbt0898-728.

Burke, Sara N., and Carol A. Barnes. 2006. "Neural Plasticity in the Ageing Brain." *Nature Reviews Neuroscience.* https://doi.org/10.1038/nrn1809.

Capanoglu, Esra, Ric C. H. De Vos, Robert D. Hall, Dilek Boyacioglu, and Jules Beekwilder. 2013. "Changes in Polyphenol Content during Production of Grape Juice Concentrate." *Food Chemistry* 139 (1–4). https://doi.org/10.1016/j.foodchem.2013.01.023.

Casadesus, Gemma, Barbara Shukitt-Hale, Heather M. Stellwagen, Xiongwei Zhu, Hyoung Gon Lee, Mark A. Smith, and James A. Joseph. 2004. "Modulation of Hippocampal Plasticity and Cognitive Behavior by Short-Term Blueberry Supplementation in Aged Rats." *Nutritional Neuroscience* 7 (5–6). https://doi.org/10.1080/10284150400020482.

Cássia Da Silveira E Sá, Rita De, Luciana Nalone Andrade, and Damião Pergentino De Sousa. 2013. "A Review on Anti-Inflammatory Activity of Monoterpenes." *Molecules.* https://doi.org/10.3390/molecules18011227.

Chamorro, Susana, Isabel Goñi, Deysy Hervert-Hernández, Agustín Viveros, and Agustín Brenes. 2012. "Changes in Polyphenolic Content and Antioxidant Activity after Thermal Treatments of Grape Seed Extract and Grape Pomace." *European Food Research and Technology* 234 (1). https://doi.org/10.1007/s00217-011-1621-7.

Cheplick, Susan, Young-In Kwon, Prasanta Bhowmik, and Kalidas Shetty. 2010. "Phenolic-Linked Variation in Strawberry Cultivars for Potential Dietary Management of Hyperglycemia and Related Complications of Hypertension." *Bioresource Technology* 101 (1). https://doi.org/10.1016/j.biortech.2009.07.068.

Cho, Han Jin, and Jung Han Yoon Park. 2013. "Kaempferol Induces Cell Cycle Arrest in HT-29 Human Colon Cancer Cells." *Journal of Cancer Prevention* 18 (3). https://doi.org/10.15430/jcp.2013.18.3.257.

Chopra, Hitesh, Protity Shuvra Dey, Debashrita Das, Tanima Bhattacharya, Muddaser Shah, Sidra Mubin, Samka Peregrine Maishu, et al. 2021. "Curcumin Nanoparticles as Promising Therapeutic Agents for Drug Targets." *Molecules.* https://doi.org/10.3390/molecules26164998.

Chu, Shu Chen, Yih Shou Hsieh, Li Sung Hsu, Kuo Shuen Chen, Chien Cheng Chiang, and Pei Ni Chen. 2014. "*Rubus idaeus* L Inhibits Invasion Potential of Human A549 Lung Cancer Cells by Suppression Epithelial-to-Mesenchymal Transition and Akt Pathway In Vitro and Reduces Tumor Growth In Vivo." *Integrative Cancer Therapies* 13 (3). https://doi.org/10.1177/1534735413510559.

Cimino, Francesco, Mariateresa Cristani, Antonina Saija, Franco Paolo Bonina, and Fabio Virgili. 2007. "Protective Effects of a Red Orange Extract on UVB-Induced Damage in Human Keratinocytes." *BioFactors* 30 (2). https://doi.org/10.1002/biof.5520300206.

Ciocoiu, Manuela, Laurentiu Badescu, Anca Miron, and Magda Badescu. 2013. "The Involvement of a Polyphenol-Rich Extract of Black Chokeberry in Oxidative

Stress on Experimental Arterial Hypertension." *Evidence-Based Complementary and Alternative Medicine* 2013. https://doi.org/10.1155/2013/912769.

Cook, Matthew David, Stephen David Myers, Mandy Lucinda Gault, Victoria Charlotte Edwards, and Mark Elisabeth Theodorus Willems. 2017. "Cardiovascular Function during Supine Rest in Endurance-Trained Males with New Zealand Blackcurrant: A Dose-Response Study." *European Journal of Applied Physiology* 117 (2): 247–254. https://doi.org/10.1007/S00421-016-3512-X.

Coothankandaswamy, Veena, Yang Liu, Shui Chun Mao, J. Brian Morgan, Fakhri Mahdi, Mika B. Jekabsons, Dale G. Nagle, and Yu Dong Zhou. 2010. "The Alternative Medicine Pawpaw and Its Acetogenin Constituents Suppress Tumor Angiogenesis via the HIF-1/VEGF Pathway." *Journal of Natural Products* 73 (5). https://doi.org/10.1021/np100228d.

Deng, Yuanle, Yali Li, Fangfang Yang, Anqi Zeng, Shuping Yang, Yi Luo, Yiwen Zhang, et al. 2017. "The Extract from *Punica granatum* (Pomegranate) Peel Induces Apoptosis and Impairs Metastasis in Prostate Cancer Cells." *Biomedicine and Pharmacotherapy* 93. https://doi.org/10.1016/j.biopha.2017.07.008.

Devore, Elizabeth E., Jae Hee Kang, Monique M. B. Breteler, and Francine Grodstein. 2012. "Dietary Intakes of Berries and Flavonoids in Relation to Cognitive Decline." *Annals of Neurology* 72 (1). https://doi.org/10.1002/ana.23594.

Donno, Donno, Manuela Cavanna, Gabriele Loris Beccaro, Gabriella M. Mellano, Daniela Torello Marinoni, Alessandro Kim Cerutti, and Giancarlo Bounous. 2013. "Currants and Strawberries as Bioactive Compound Sources: Determination of Antioxidant Profiles with HPLC-DAD/MS." *Journal of Applied Botany and Food Quality* 86 (1). https://doi.org/10.5073/JABFQ.2013.086.001.

Dreiseitel, Andrea, Gabriele Korte, Peter Schreier, Anett Oehme, Sanja Locher, Martina Domani, Goeran Hajak, and Philipp G. Sand. 2009. "Berry Anthocyanins and Their Aglycons Inhibit Monoamine Oxidases A and B." *Pharmacological Research* 59 (5). https://doi.org/10.1016/j.phrs.2009.01.014.

Economos, Christine., and William D. Clay. 1999. "Nutritional and Health Benefits of Citrus Fruits." *Food, Nutrition and Agriculture – FAO* 24.

Eyduran, S. P., S. Ercisli, M. Akin, O. Beyhan, M. K. Gecer, E. Eyduran, and Y. E. Erturk. 2015. "Organic Acids, Sugars, Vitamin C, Antioxidant Capacity, and Phenolic Compounds in Fruits of White (*Morus alba* L.) and Black (*Morus nigra* L.) Mulberry Genotypes." *Journal of Applied Botany and Food Quality* 88. https://doi.org/10.5073/JABFQ.2015.088.019.

Fallis, A. G. 2013. "Wild Crop Relatives, Genomic and Breeding Resources Vegetables." *Journal of Chemical Information and Modeling* 53.

Famakin, Opeyemi, Akindele Fatoyinbo, Oluwole Steve Ijarotimi, Adebanjo Ayobamidele Badejo, and Tayo Nathaniel Fagbemi. 2016. "Assessment of Nutritional Quality, Glycaemic Index, Antidiabetic and Sensory Properties of Plantain (*Musa paradisiaca*)-Based Functional Dough Meals." *Journal of Food Science and Technology* 53 (11). https://doi.org/10.1007/s13197-016-2357-y.

Fan, Kunhua, Naoto Kurihara, Sadanori Abe, Chi Tang Ho, Geetha Ghai, and Kan Yang. 2007. "Chemopreventive Effects of Orange Peel Extract (OPE) I. OPE Inhibits Intestinal Tumor Growth in ApcMin/+ Mice." *Journal of Medicinal Food* 10 (1). https://doi.org/10.1089/jmf.2006.0214.

Finegold, Sydney M., Paula H. Summanen, Karen Corbett, Julia Downes, Susanne M. Henning, and Zhaoping Li. 2014. "Pomegranate Extract Exhibits In Vitro Activity against *Clostridium difficile*." *Nutrition* 30 (10). https://doi.org/10.1016/j.nut.2014.02.029.

Formica, J. V., and W. Regelson. 1995. "Review of the Biology of Quercetin and Related Bioflavonoids." *Food and Chemical Toxicology*. https://doi.org/10.1016/0278-6915(95)00077-1.

García-Salas, Patricia, Ana María Gómez-Caravaca, David Arráez-Román, Antonio Segura-Carretero, Eduardo Guerra-Hernández, Belén García-Villanova, and Alberto Fernández-Gutiérrez. 2013. "Influence of Technological Processes on Phenolic Compounds, Organic Acids, Furanic Derivatives, and Antioxidant Activity of Whole-Lemon Powder." *Food Chemistry* 141 (2). https://doi.org/10.1016/j.foodchem.2013.02.124.

Gonzalez-Aguilar, G., R. M. Robles-Sánchez, M. A. Martínez-Téllez, G. I. Olivas, E. Alvarez-Parrilla, and L. A. De La Rosa. 2008. "Bioactive Compounds in Fruits: Health Benefits and Effect of Storage Conditions." *Stewart Postharvest Review*. https://doi.org/10.2212/spr.2008.3.8.

Greenspan, Phillip, John D. Bauer, Stanley H. Pollock, J. David Gangemi, Eugene P. Mayer, Abdul Ghaffar, James L. Hargrove, and Diane K. Hartle. 2005. "Antiinflammatory Properties of the Muscadine Grape (*Vitis rotundifolia*)." *Journal of Agricultural and Food Chemistry* 53 (22). https://doi.org/10.1021/jf058015+.

Groot, H. De, and U. Rauen. 1998. "Tissue Injury by Reactive Oxygen Species and the Protective Effects of Flavonoids." *Fundamental and Clinical Pharmacology*. https://doi.org/10.1111/j.1472-8206.1998.tb00951.x.

Gundogdu, M., F. Muradoglu, R. I. Gazioglu Sensoy, and H. Yilmaz. 2011. "Determination of Fruit Chemical Properties of *Morus nigra* L., *Morus Alba* L. and *Morus rubra* L. by HPLC." *Scientia Horticulturae* 132 (1). https://doi.org/10.1016/j.scienta.2011.09.035.

Gupta, Bhanushree, Bhupesh Kumar, Anshuman Sharma, Deeksha Sori, Rahul Sharma, and Saumya Mehta. 2019. "Nutraceuticals for Antiaging." *Nutraceuticals in Veterinary Medicine*. https://doi.org/10.1007/978-3-030-04624-8_25.

Hardman, Roy J., Greg Kennedy, Helen Macpherson, Andrew B. Scholey, and Andrew Pipingas. 2016. "Adherence to a Mediterranean-Style Diet and Effects on Cognition in Adults: A Qualitative Evaluation and Systematic Review of Longitudinal and Prospective Trials." *Frontiers in Nutrition*. https://doi.org/10.3389/fnut.2016.00022.

He, Dongxiu, Yang Shan, Yuehui Wu, Guozhu Liu, Bo Chen, and Shouzhuo Yao. 2011. "Simultaneous Determination of Flavanones, Hydroxycinnamic Acids and Alkaloids in Citrus Fruits by HPLC-DAD-ESI/MS." *Food Chemistry* 127 (2). https://doi.org/10.1016/j.foodchem.2010.12.109.

Hellström, Jarkko K., Alexander N. Shikov, Marina N. Makarova, Anne M. Pihlanto, Olga N. Pozharitskaya, Eeva Liisa Ryhänen, Pirjo Kivijärvi, Valery G. Makarov, and Pirjo H. Mattila. 2010. "Blood Pressure-Lowering Properties of Chokeberry (*Aronia mitchurinii*, var. Viking)." *Journal of Functional Foods* 2 (2). https://doi.org/10.1016/j.jff.2010.04.004.

Hendrickson, Sara J., and Richard D. Mattes. 2008. "No Acute Effects of Grape Juice on Appetite, Implicit Memory and Mood." *Food and Nutrition Research* 52. https://doi.org/10.3402/fnr.v52i0.1891.

Hertog, Michaël G. L., Daan Kromhout, Christ Aravanis, Henry Blackburn, Ratko Buzina, Flaminio Fidanza, Simona Giampaoli, et al. 1995. "Flavonoid Intake and Long-Term Risk of Coronary Heart Disease and Cancer in the Seven Countries Study." *Archives of Internal Medicine* 155 (4). https://doi.org/10.1001/archinte.1995.00430040053006.

Hosein Farzaei, Mohammad, Roja Rahimi, Fatemeh Farzaei, and Mohammad Abdollahi. 2015. "Traditional Medicinal Herbs for the Management of Diabetes and Its Complications: An Evidence-Based Review." *International Journal of Pharmacology*. https://doi.org/10.3923/ijp.2015.874.887.

Hou, Wen Chi, Rong Dih Lin, Cheng Tang Chen, and Mei Hsien Lee. 2005. "Monoamine Oxidase B (MAO-B) Inhibition by Active Principles from *Uncaria rhynchophylla*." *Journal of Ethnopharmacology* 100 (1–2). https://doi.org/10.1016/j.jep.2005.03.017.

Huang, Hui Pei, Ting Tsz Ou, and Chau Jong Wang. 2013. "Mulberry (Sang Shèn Zǐ) and Its Bioactive Compounds, the Chemoprevention Effects and Molecular Mechanisms in Vitro and in Vivo." *Journal of Traditional and Complementary Medicine* 3 (1). https://doi.org/10.4103/2225-4110.106535.

Jaber, Hwaida, Elias Baydoun, Ola EL-Zein, and Sawsan Ibrahim Kreydiyyeh. 2013. "Anti-Hyperglycemic Effect of the Aqueous Extract of Banana Infructescence Stalks in Streptozotocin-Induced Diabetic Rats." *Plant Foods for Human Nutrition* 68 (1). https://doi.org/10.1007/s11130-013-0341-5.

Jan, Bisma, Rabea Parveen, Sultan Zahiruddin, Mohammad Umar Khan, Sradhanjali Mohapatra, and Sayeed Ahmad. 2021. "Nutritional Constituents of Mulberry and Their Potential Applications in Food and Pharmaceuticals: A Review." *Saudi Journal of Biological Sciences*. https://doi.org/10.1016/j.sjbs.2021.03.056.

Jeffery, E. H., A. F. Brown, A. C. Kurilich, A. S. Keck, N. Matusheski, B. P. Klein, and J. A. Juvik. 2003. "Variation in Content of Bioactive Components in Broccoli." *Journal of Food Composition and Analysis*. https://doi.org/10.1016/S0889-1575(03)00045-0.

Jeong, Yoo Seok, Joo Heon Hong, Kyung Hyun Cho, and Hee Kyoung Jung. 2012. "Grape Skin Extract Reduces Adipogenesis- and Lipogenesis-Related

Gene Expression in 3T3-L1 Adipocytes through the Peroxisome Proliferator-Activated Receptor-γ Signaling Pathway." *Nutrition Research* 32 (7). https://doi.org/10.1016/j.nutres.2012.06.001.

Jia, Han, Ji Wen Liu, Halmurat Ufur, Geng Sheng He, Hai Liqian, and Peipei Chen. 2011. "The Antihypertensive Effect of Ethyl Acetate Extract from Red Raspberry Fruit in Hypertensive Rats." *Pharmacognosy Magazine* 7 (25). https://doi.org/10.4103/0973-1296.75885.

Jiang, Dong Qing, Ying Guo, Dian Hong Xu, Ya Si Huang, Ke Yuan, and Zhi Qiang Lv. 2013. "Antioxidant and Anti-Fatigue Effects of Anthocyanins of Mulberry Juice Purification (MJP) and Mulberry Marc Purification (MMP) from Different Varieties Mulberry Fruit in China." *Food and Chemical Toxicology* 59. https://doi.org/10.1016/j.fct.2013.05.023.

Johnson, Michelle H., Anita Lucius, Tessa Meyer, and Elvira Gonzalez De Mejia. 2011. "Cultivar Evaluation and Effect of Fermentation on Antioxidant Capacity and In Vitro Inhibition of α-Amylase and α-Glucosidase by Highbush Blueberry (*Vaccinium corombosum*)." *Journal of Agricultural and Food Chemistry* 59 (16). https://doi.org/10.1021/jf201720z.

Johnson, Michelle H., Matthew Wallig, Diego A. Luna Vital, and Elvira G. de Mejia. 2016. "Alcohol-Free Fermented Blueberry-Blackberry Beverage Phenolic Extract Attenuates Diet-Induced Obesity and Blood Glucose in C57BL/6J Mice." *Journal of Nutritional Biochemistry* 31. https://doi.org/10.1016/j.jnutbio.2015.12.013.

Johnson, Sarah A., Arturo Figueroa, Negin Navaei, Alexei Wong, Roy Kalfon, Lauren T. Ormsbee, Rafaela G. Feresin, et al. 2015. "Daily Blueberry Consumption Improves Blood Pressure and Arterial Stiffness in Postmenopausal Women with Pre- and Stage 1-Hypertension: A Randomized, Double-Blind, Placebo-Controlled Clinical Trial." *Journal of the Academy of Nutrition and Dietetics* 115 (3). https://doi.org/10.1016/j.jand.2014.11.001.

Joseph, James A., Derek R. Fisher, Amanda Carey, and Aleksandra Szprengiel. 2004. "The M3 Muscarinic Receptor I3 Domain Confers Oxidative Stress Protection on Calcium Regulation in Transfected COS-7 Cells." *Aging Cell* 3 (5). https://doi.org/10.1111/j.1474-9728.2004.00123.x.

Juríková, Tunde, Stefan Balla, Jiri Sochor, Miroslav Pohanka, Jiri Mlcek, and Mojmir Baron. 2013. "Flavonoid Profile of Saskatoon Berries (*Amelanchier alnifolia* Nutt.) and Their Health Promoting Effects." *Molecules*. https://doi.org/10.3390/molecules181012571.

Kalra, Ekta K. 2003. "Nutraceutical – Definition and Introduction." *AAPS PharmSci* 5 (3). https://doi.org/10.1208/ps050325.

Karasawa, Marines Marli Gniech, and Chakravarthi Mohan. 2018. "Fruits as Prospective Reserves of Bioactive Compounds: A Review." *Natural Products and Bioprospecting*. https://doi.org/10.1007/s13659-018-0186-6.

Kaur, Sumeet, and Madhusweta Das. 2011. "Functional Foods: An Overview." *Food Science and Biotechnology*. https://doi.org/10.1007/s10068-011-0121-7.

Kelebek, Hasim, and Serkan Selli. 2011. "Determination of Volatile, Phenolic, Organic Acid and Sugar Components in a Turkish cv. Dortyol (*Citrus sinensis* L. Osbeck) Orange Juice." *Journal of the Science of Food and Agriculture* 91 (10). https://doi.org/10.1002/jsfa.4396.

Kennedy, B. P., M. G. Ziegler, M. Alford, L. A. Hansen, L. J. Thal, and E. Masliah. 2003. "Early and Persistent Alterations in Prefrontal Cortex MAO A and B in Aizheimer's Disease." *Journal of Neural Transmission* 110 (7). https://doi.org/10.1007/s00702-003-0828-6.

Kesse-Guyot, Emmanuelle, Léopold Fezeu, Valentina A. Andreeva, Mathilde Touvier, Augustin Scalbert, Serge Hercberg, and Pilar Galan. 2012. "Total and Specific Polyphenol Intakes in Midlife are Associated with Cognitive Function Measured 13 Years Later." *Journal of Nutrition* 142 (1). https://doi.org/10.3945/jn.111.144428.

Ketron, Adam C., and Neil Osheroff. 2014. "Phytochemicals as Anticancer and Chemopreventive Topoisomerase II Poisons." *Phytochemistry Reviews*. https://doi.org/10.1007/s11101-013-9291-7.

Khan, Faisel, Sumantra Ray, Angela M. Craigie, Gwen Kennedy, Alexander Hill, Karen L. Barton, Jane Broughton, and Jill J. F. Belch. 2014. "Lowering of Oxidative Stress Improves Endothelial Function in Healthy Subjects with Habitually Low Intake of Fruit and Vegetables: A Randomized Controlled Trial of Antioxidant- and Polyphenol-Rich Blackcurrant Juice." *Free Radical Biology and Medicine* 72. https://doi.org/10.1016/j.freeradbiomed.2014.04.006.

Knekt, Paul, Ritva Järvinen, Antti Reunanen, and Jouni Maatela. 1996. "Flavonoid Intake and Coronary Mortality in Finland: A Cohort Study." *British Medical Journal* 312 (7029). https://doi.org/10.1136/bmj.312.7029.478.

Knight, Alissa, Janet Bryan, and Karen Murphy. 2016. "Is the Mediterranean Diet a Feasible Approach to Preserving Cognitive Function and Reducing Risk of Dementia for Older Adults in Western Countries? New Insights and Future Directions." *Ageing Research Reviews*. https://doi.org/10.1016/j.arr.2015.10.005.

Kobayashi, Hideka, Changzheng Wang, and Kirk W. Pomper. 2008. "Phenolic Content and Antioxidant Capacity of Pawpaw Fruit (*Asimina triloba* L.) at Different Ripening Stages." *HortScience* 43 (1). https://doi.org/10.21273/hortsci.43.1.268.

Komes, Draženka, Ana Belščak-Cvitanović, Dunja Horžić, Gordana Rusak, Saša Likić, and Marija Berendika. 2011. "Phenolic Composition and Antioxidant Properties of Some Traditionally Used Medicinal Plants Affected by the Extraction Time and Hydrolysis." *Phytochemical Analysis* 22 (2). https://doi.org/10.1002/pca.1264.

Kondo, Satoru, Monrudee Kittikorn, and Sirichai Kanlayanarat. 2005. "Preharvest Antioxidant Activities of Tropical Fruit and the Effect of Low Temperature Storage on Antioxidants and Jasmonates." *Postharvest Biology and Technology* 36 (3). https://doi.org/10.1016/j.postharvbio.2005.02.003.

Krikorian, Robert, Tiffany A. Nash, Marcelle D. Shidler, Barbara Shukitt-Hale, and James A. Joseph. 2010. "Concord Grape Juice Supplementation Improves

Memory Function in Older Adults with Mild Cognitive Impairment." *British Journal of Nutrition* 103 (5). https://doi.org/10.1017/S0007114509992364.

Lee, Dong Eun, Min Yu Chung, Tae Gyu Lim, Won Bum Huh, Hyong Joo Lee, and Ki Won Lee. 2013. "Quercetin Suppresses Intracellular Ros Formation, MMP Activation, and Cell Motility in Human Fibrosarcoma Cells." *Journal of Food Science* 78 (9). https://doi.org/10.1111/1750-3841.12223.

Lee, M. H., R. D. Lin, L. Y. Shen, L. L. Yang, K. Y. Yen, and W. C. Hou. 2001. "Monoamine Oxidase B and Free Radical Scavenging Activities of Natural Flavonoids in *Melastoma candidum* D. Don." *Journal of Agricultural and Food Chemistry* 49 (11). https://doi.org/10.1021/jf010622j.

Levitt, P., J. E. Pintar, and X. O. Breakefield. 1982. "Immunocytochemical Demonstration of Monoamine Oxidase B in Brain Astrocytes and Serotonergic Neurons." *Proceedings of the National Academy of Sciences of the United States of America* 79 (20 I). https://doi.org/10.1073/pnas.79.20.6385.

Li, Chao, Bin Yang, Zhihao Xu, Eric Boivin, Mazzen Black, Wenlong Huang, Baoyou Xu, et al. 2017. "Protective Effect of Cyanidin-3-O-Glucoside on Neonatal Porcine Islets." *Journal of Endocrinology* 235 (3). https://doi.org/10.1530/JOE-17-0141.

Li, Q., H. F. Zhao, Z. F. Zhang, Z. G. Liu, X. R. Pei, J. B. Wang, M. Y. Cai, and Y. Li. 2009. "Long-Term Administration of Green Tea Catechins Prevents Age-Related Spatial Learning and Memory Decline in C57BL/6 J Mice by Regulating Hippocampal Cyclic Amp-Response Element Binding Protein Signaling Cascade." *Neuroscience* 159 (4). https://doi.org/10.1016/j.neuroscience.2009.02.008.

Marchand, Loïc Le. 2002. "Cancer Preventive Effects of Flavonoids – A Review." *Biomedicine and Pharmacotherapy* 56 (6). https://doi.org/10.1016/S0753-3322(02)00186-5.

Mathew, Nimisha Sarah, and Pradeep Singh Negi. 2017. "Traditional Uses, Phytochemistry and Pharmacology of Wild Banana (*Musa acuminata* Colla): A Review." *Journal of Ethnopharmacology*. https://doi.org/10.1016/j.jep.2016.12.009.

McAnulty, Lisa S., Scott R. Collier, Michael J. Landram, D. Stanton Whittaker, Sydeena E. Isaacs, Jason M. Klemka, Sarah L. Cheek, Jennifer C. Arms, and Steven R. McAnulty. 2014. "Six Weeks Daily Ingestion of Whole Blueberry Powder Increases Natural Killer Cell Counts and Reduces Arterial Stiffness in Sedentary Males and Females." *Nutrition Research* 34 (7). https://doi.org/10.1016/j.nutres.2014.07.002.

Muthukumaran, Jayachandran, Subramani Srinivasan, Rantham Subramaniyam Venkatesan, Vinayagam Ramachandran, and Udaiyar Muruganathan. 2013. "Syringic Acid, a Novel Natural Phenolic Acid, Normalizes Hyperglycemia with Special Reference to Glycoprotein Components in Experimental Diabetic Rats." *Journal of Acute Disease* 2 (4). https://doi.org/10.1016/s2221-6189(13)60149-3.

Nassiri-Asl, Marjan, and Hossein Hosseinzadeh. 2009. "Review of the Pharmacological Effects of *Vitis vinifera* (Grape) and Its Bioactive Compounds." *Phytotherapy Research*. https://doi.org/10.1002/ptr.2761.

Neto, Catherine C. 2007. "Cranberry and Its Phytochemicals: A Review of In Vitro Anticancer Studies." *Journal of Nutrition* 137. https://doi.org/10.1093/jn/137.1.186s.

Nguyen, Dang Minh Chanh, Dong Jun Seo, Hyang Burm Lee, In Seon Kim, Kil Yong Kim, Ro Dong Park, and Woo Jin Jung. 2013. "Antifungal Activity of Gallic Acid Purified from *Terminalia nigrovenulosa* Bark against *Fusarium solani.*" *Microbial Pathogenesis* 56. https://doi.org/10.1016/j.micpath.2013.01.001.

Nile, Shivraj Hariram, and Se Won Park. 2014. "Edible Berries: Bioactive Components and Their Effect on Human Health." *Nutrition.* https://doi.org/10.1016/j.nut.2013.04.007.

Noratto, Giuliana D., Boon P. Chew, and Liezl M. Atienza. 2017. "Red Raspberry (*Rubus idaeus* L.) Intake Decreases Oxidative Stress in Obese Diabetic (Db/Db) Mice." *Food Chemistry* 227. https://doi.org/10.1016/j.foodchem.2017.01.097.

Paredes-López, Octavio, Martha L. Cervantes-Ceja, Mónica Vigna-Pérez, and Talía Hernández-Pérez. 2010. "Berries: Improving Human Health and Healthy Aging, and Promoting Quality Life–A Review." *Plant Foods for Human Nutrition.* https://doi.org/10.1007/s11130-010-0177-1.

Pereira, Aline, and Marcelo Maraschin. 2015. "Banana (*Musa* spp.) from Peel to Pulp: Ethnopharmacology, Source of Bioactive Compounds and Its Relevance for Human Health." *Journal of Ethnopharmacology.* https://doi.org/10.1016/j.jep.2014.11.008.

Pinto, Marcia Da Silva, Reza Ghaedian, Rahul Shinde, and Kalidas Shetty. 2010. "Potential of Cranberry Powder for Management of Hyperglycemia Using In Vitro Models." *Journal of Medicinal Food* 13 (5). https://doi.org/10.1089/jmf.2009.0225.

Puglia, Carmelo, Alessia Offerta, Antonella Saija, Domenico Trombetta, and Cardile Venera. 2014. "Protective Effect of Red Orange Extract Supplementation against UV-Induced Skin Damages: Photoaging and Solar Lentigines." *Journal of Cosmetic Dermatology* 13 (2). https://doi.org/10.1111/jocd.12083.

Rasool, Mahaboob Khan, Evan Prince Sabina, Segu R. Ramya, Pranatharthiharan Preety, Smita Patel, Niharika Mandal, Punya P. Mishra, and Jaisy Samuel. 2010. "Hepatoprotective and Antioxidant Effects of Gallic Acid in Paracetamol-Induced Liver Damage in Mice." *Journal of Pharmacy and Pharmacology* 62 (5). https://doi.org/10.1211/jpp.62.05.0012.

Ratnasooriya, Charmila C., and H. P. Vasantha Rupasinghe. 2012. "Extraction of Phenolic Compounds from Grapes and Their Pomace Using β-Cyclodextrin." *Food Chemistry* 134 (2). https://doi.org/10.1016/j.foodchem.2012.02.014.

Renaud, S. C., A. D. Beswick, A. M. Fehily, D. S. Sharp, and P. C. Elwood. 1992. "Alcohol and Platelet Aggregation: The Caerphilly Prospective Heart Disease Study." *American Journal of Clinical Nutrition* 55 (5). https://doi.org/10.1093/ajcn/55.5.1012.

Rettig, Matthew B., David Heber, Jiabin An, Navindra P. Seeram, Jian Y. Rao, Huiren Liu, Tobias Klatte, et al. 2008. "Pomegranate Extract Inhibits

Androgen-Independent Prostate Cancer Growth through a Nuclear Factor-KB-Dependent Mechanism." *Molecular Cancer Therapeutics* 7 (9). https://doi.org/10.1158/1535-7163.MCT-08-0136.

Rice-Evans, Catherine A., Nicholas J. Miller, and George Paganga. 1997. "Antioxidant Properties of Phenolic Compounds." *Trends in Plant Science*. https://doi.org/10.1016/S1360-1385(97)01018-2.

Riso, Patrizia, Dorothy Klimis-Zacas, Cristian Del Bo', Daniela Martini, Jonica Campolo, Stefano Vendrame, Peter Møller, Steffen Loft, Renata De Maria, and Marisa Porrini. 2013. "Effect of a Wild Blueberry (*Vaccinium angustifolium*) Drink Intervention on Markers of Oxidative Stress, Inflammation and Endothelial Function in Humans with Cardiovascular Risk Factors." *European Journal of Nutrition* 52 (3). https://doi.org/10.1007/s00394-012-0402-9.

Rodriguez-Mateos, Ana, Catarina Rendeiro, Triana Bergillos-Meca, Setareh Tabatabaee, Trevor W. George, Christian Heiss, and Jeremy P. E. Spencer. 2013. "Intake and Time Dependence of Blueberry Flavonoid-Induced Improvements in Vascular Function: A Randomized, Controlled, Double-Blind, Crossover Intervention Study with Mechanistic Insights into Biological Activity." *American Journal of Clinical Nutrition* 98 (5). https://doi.org/10.3945/ajcn.113.066639.

Sameermahmood, Zaheer, Lenin Raji, Thangavel Saravanan, Ashok Vaidya, Viswanathan Mohan, and Muthuswamy Balasubramanyam. 2010. "Gallic Acid Protects RINm5F β-Cells from Glucolipotoxicity by Its Antiapoptotic and Insulin-Secretagogue Actions." *Phytotherapy Research* 24 (SUPPL. 1). https://doi.org/10.1002/ptr.2926.

Scalbert, Augustin, Ian T. Johnson, and Mike Saltmarsh. 2005. "Polyphenols: Antioxidants and Beyond." *American Journal of Clinical Nutrition*. https://doi.org/10.1093/ajcn/81.1.215s.

Scholey, Andrew B., Stephen J. French, Penelope J. Morris, David O. Kennedy, Anthea L. Milne, and Crystal F. Haskell. 2010. "Consumption of Cocoa Flavanols Results in Acute Improvements in Mood and Cognitive Performance during Sustained Mental Effort." *Journal of Psychopharmacology* 24 (10). https://doi.org/10.1177/0269881109106923.

Seeram, Navindra P., Lynn S. Adams, Yanjun Zhang, Rupo Lee, Daniel Sand, Henry S. Scheuller, and David Heber. 2006. "Blackberry, Black Raspberry, Blueberry, Cranberry, Red Raspberry, and Strawberry Extracts Inhibit Growth and Stimulate Apoptosis of Human Cancer Cells In Vitro." *Journal of Agricultural and Food Chemistry* 54 (25). https://doi.org/10.1021/jf061750g.

Shabir, Ahmad, A. Sarumathi, S. Anbu, and N. Saravanan. 2013. "Gallic Acid Protects Against Immobilization Stress-Induced Changes in Wistar Rats." *Journal of Stress Physiology & Biochemistry* 9 (1).

Shahidi, Fereidoon, and Priyatharini Ambigaipalan. 2015. "Phenolics and Polyphenolics in Foods, Beverages and Spices: Antioxidant Activity and Health Effects – A Review." *Journal of Functional Foods*. https://doi.org/10.1016/j.jff.2015.06.018.

Shi, Ni, Steven K. Clinton, Zhihua Liu, Yongquan Wang, Kenneth M. Riedl, Steven J. Schwartz, Xiaoli Zhang, Zui Pan, and Tong Chen. 2015. "Strawberry Phytochemicals Inhibit Azoxymethane/Dextran Sodium Sulfate-Induced Colorectal Carcinogenesis in Crj: CD-1 Mice." *Nutrients* 7 (3). https://doi.org/10.3390/nu7031696.

Shih, J. C., K. Chen, and M. J. Ridd. 1999. "Monoamine Oxidase: From Genes to Behavior." *Annual Review of Neuroscience.* https://doi.org/10.1146/annurev.neuro.22.1.197.

Shrikanta, Akshatha, Anbarasu Kumar, and Vijayalakshmi Govindaswamy. 2015. "Resveratrol Content and Antioxidant Properties of Underutilized Fruits." *Journal of Food Science and Technology* 52 (1). https://doi.org/10.1007/s13197-013-0993-z.

da Silva Pinto, Marcia, Joao Ernesto de Carvalho, Franco Maria Lajolo, Maria Inés Genovese, and Kalidas Shetty. 2010. "Evaluation of Antiproliferative, Anti-Type 2 Diabetes, and Antihypertension Potentials of Ellagitannins from Strawberries (*Fragaria × ananassa* Duch.) Using In Vitro Models." *Journal of Medicinal Food* 13 (5). https://doi.org/10.1089/jmf.2009.0257.

Singh, Balwinder, Jatinder Pal Singh, Amritpal Kaur, and Narpinder Singh. 2016. "Bioactive Compounds in Banana and Their Associated Health Benefits – A Review." *Food Chemistry.* https://doi.org/10.1016/j.foodchem.2016.03.033.

Singh, Chandra K., Xiaoqi Liu, and Nihal Ahmad. 2015. "Resveratrol, in Its Natural Combination in Whole Grape, for Health Promotion and Disease Management." *Annals of the New York Academy of Sciences* 1348 (1). https://doi.org/10.1111/nyas.12798.

Singhal, Brij Kishore, Mohammad Ashraf Khan, Anil Dhar, Farooq Mohammad Baqual, and Bharat Bushan Bindroo. 2010. "Approaches to Industrial Exploitation of Mulberry (*Mulberry* Sp.) Fruits." *Journal of Fruit Ornamental Plant Research* 18 (1).

Sofi, Francesco, Rosanna Abbate, Gian Franco Gensini, and Alessandro Casini. 2010. "Accruing Evidence on Benefits of Adherence to the Mediterranean Diet on Health: An Updated Systematic Review and Meta-Analysis." *American Journal of Clinical Nutrition.* https://doi.org/10.3945/ajcn.2010.29673.

Spínola, Vítor, Joana Pinto, Eulogio J. Llorent-Martínez, Helena Tomás, and Paula C. Castilho. 2019. "Evaluation of *Rubus grandifolius* L. (Wild Blackberries) Activities Targeting Management of Type-2 Diabetes and Obesity Using In Vitro Models." *Food and Chemical Toxicology* 123. https://doi.org/10.1016/j.fct.2018.11.006.

Stangl, Doris, and Sandrine Thuret. 2009. "Impact of Diet on Adult Hippocampal Neurogenesis." *Genes and Nutrition.* https://doi.org/10.1007/s12263-009-0134-5.

Stoner, Gary D., Li Shu Wang, Nancy Zikri, Tong Chen, Stephen S. Hecht, Chuanshu Huang, Christine Sardo, and John F. Lechner. 2007. "Cancer Prevention with Freeze-Dried Berries and Berry Components." *Seminars in Cancer Biology.* https://doi.org/10.1016/j.semcancer.2007.05.001.

Stull, April J., Katherine C. Cash, Catherine M. Champagne, Alok K. Gupta, Raymond Boston, Robbie A. Beyl, William D. Johnson, and William T. Cefalu. 2015. "Blueberries Improve Endothelial Function, but Not Blood Pressure, in Adults with Metabolic Syndrome: A Randomized, Double-Blind, Placebo-Controlled Clinical Trial." *Nutrients* 7 (6). https://doi.org/10.3390/nu7064107.

Sun, Chong De, Bo Zhang, Jiu Kai Zhang, Chang Jie Xu, Yu Lian Wu, Xian Li, and Kun Song Chen. 2012. "Cyanidin-3-Glucoside-Rich Extract from Chinese Bayberry Fruit Protects Pancreatic β Cells and Ameliorates Hyperglycemia in Streptozotocin-Induced Diabetic Mice." *Journal of Medicinal Food* 15 (3). https://doi.org/10.1089/jmf.2011.1806.

Tabart, Jessica, Claire Kevers, Danièle Evers, and Jacques Dommes. 2011. "Ascorbic Acid, Phenolic Acid, Flavonoid, and Carotenoid Profiles of Selected Extracts from *Ribes nigrum*." *Journal of Agricultural and Food Chemistry* 59 (9). https://doi.org/10.1021/jf104445c.

Tabart, Jessica, Thierry Franck, Claire Kevers, Joël Pincemail, Didier Serteyn, Jean Olivier Defraigne, and Jacques Dommes. 2012. "Antioxidant and Anti-Inflammatory Activities of *Ribes nigrum* Extracts." *Food Chemistry* 131 (4). https://doi.org/10.1016/j.foodchem.2011.09.076.

Tajaldini, Mahboubeh, Firooz Samadi, Ayyoob Khosravi, Azim Ghasemnejad, and Jahanbakhsh Asadi. 2020. "Protective and Anticancer Effects of Orange Peel Extract and Naringin in Doxorubicin Treated Esophageal Cancer Stem Cell Xenograft Tumor Mouse Model." *Biomedicine and Pharmacotherapy* 121. https://doi.org/10.1016/j.biopha.2019.109594.

Tangney, Christine C., Mary J. Kwasny, Hong Li, Robert S. Wilson, Denis A. Evans, and Martha Clare Morris. 2011. "Adherence to a Mediterranean-Type Dietary Pattern and Cognitive Decline in a Community Population." *American Journal of Clinical Nutrition* 93 (3). https://doi.org/10.3945/ajcn.110.007369.

Terry, Robert D. 2001. "Copernicus Revisited: Amyloid Beta in Alzheimer Disease." *Neurobiology of Aging*. https://doi.org/10.1016/S0197-4580(00)00210-4.

Thomas, Tom. 2000. "Monoamine Oxidase-B Inhibitors in the Treatment of Alzheimers Disease." In *Neurobiology of Aging* 21. https://doi.org/10.1016/S0197-4580(00)00100-7.

Tomas, Merve, Gamze Toydemir, Dilek Boyacioglu, Robert Hall, Jules Beekwilder, and Esra Capanoglu. 2015. "The Effects of Juice Processing on Black Mulberry Antioxidants." *Food Chemistry* 186. https://doi.org/10.1016/j.foodchem.2014.11.151.

Trichopoulou, Antonia, Andreas Kyrozis, Marta Rossi, Michalis Katsoulis, Dimitrios Trichopoulos, Carlo La Vecchia, and Pagona Lagiou. 2015. "Mediterranean Diet and Cognitive Decline over Time in an Elderly Mediterranean Population." *European Journal of Nutrition* 54 (8). https://doi.org/10.1007/s00394-014-0811-z.

Valero-Cases, Estefanía, Nallely Nuncio-Jáuregui, and María José Frutos. 2017. "Influence of Fermentation with Different Lactic Acid Bacteria and In Vitro Digestion on the Biotransformation of Phenolic Compounds in Fermented

Pomegranate Juices." *Journal of Agricultural and Food Chemistry* 65 (31). https://doi.org/10.1021/acs.jafc.6b04854.

Van't Veer, Pieter, Margje Cjf Jansen, Mariska Klerk, and Frans J. Kok. 2000. "Fruits and Vegetables in the Prevention of Cancer and Cardiovascular Disease." *Public Health Nutrition* 3 (1). https://doi.org/10.1017/s1368980000000136.

Vauzour, David, Maria Camprubi-Robles, Sophie Miquel-Kergoat, Cristina Andres-Lacueva, Diána Bánáti, Pascale Barberger-Gateau, Gene L. Bowman, et al. 2017. "Nutrition for the Ageing Brain: Towards Evidence for an Optimal Diet." *Ageing Research Reviews.* https://doi.org/10.1016/j.arr.2016.09.010.

Vislocky, Lisa M., and Maria Luz Fernandez. 2013. "Grapes and Grape Products: Their Role in Health." *Nutrition Today.* https://doi.org/10.1097/NT.0b013e31823db374.

Viuda-Martos, M., J. Fernández-Lóaez, and J. A. Pérez-álvarez. 2010. "Pomegranate and Its Many Functional Components as Related to Human Health: A Review." *Comprehensive Reviews in Food Science and Food Safety* 9 (6). https://doi.org/10.1111/j.1541-4337.2010.00131.x.

Vu, Hang T., Christopher J. Scarlett, and Quan V. Vuong. 2018. "Phenolic Compounds within Banana Peel and Their Potential Uses: A Review." *Journal of Functional Foods.* https://doi.org/10.1016/j.jff.2017.11.006.

Wang, Huailing, Jie Liu, Tong Li, and Rui Hai Liu. 2018. "Blueberry Extract Promotes Longevity and Stress Tolerance via DAF-16 in *Caenorhabditis elegans.*" *Food and Function* 9 (10). https://doi.org/10.1039/c8fo01680a.

Wang, Jing, Na Deng, Hong Wang, Tong Li, Ling Chen, Bisheng Zheng, and Rui Hai Liu. 2020. "Effects of Orange Extracts on Longevity, Healthspan, and Stress Resistance in *Caenorhabditis elegans.*" *Molecules* 25 (2). https://doi.org/10.3390/molecules25020351.

Wang, Yihai, Limin Xiang, Chunhua Wang, Chao Tang, and Xiangjiu He. 2013. "Antidiabetic and Antioxidant Effects and Phytochemicals of Mulberry Fruit (*Morus Alba* L.) Polyphenol Enhanced Extract." *PLoS ONE* 8 (7). https://doi.org/10.1371/journal.pone.0071144.

Wedge, D. E., K. M. Meepagala, J. B. Magee, S. H. Smith, G. Huang, and L. L. Larcom. 2001. "Short Communication: Anticarcinogenic Activity of Strawberry, Blueberry, and Raspberry Extracts to Breast and Cervical Cancer Cells." *Journal of Medicinal Food* 4 (1). https://doi.org/10.1089/10966200152053703.

Whyte, Adrian R., Nancy Cheng, Emilie Fromentin, and Claire M. Williams. 2018. "A Randomized, Double-Blinded, Placebo-Controlled Study to Compare the Safety and Efficacy of Low Dose Enhanced Wild Blueberry Powder and Wild Blueberry Extract (Thinkblue™) in Maintenance of Episodic and Working Memory in Older Adults." *Nutrients* 10 (6). https://doi.org/10.3390/nu10060660.

Williamson, Gary, and Claudine Manach. 2005. "Bioavailability and Bioefficacy of Polyphenols in Humans. II. Review of 93 Intervention Studies." *American Journal of Clinical Nutrition.* https://doi.org/10.1093/ajcn/81.1.243s.

Wiseman, Waylon, Jennifer M. Egan, Jennifer E. Slemmer, Kevin S. Shaughnessy, Katherine Ballem, Katherine T. Gottschall-Pass, and Marva I. Sweeney. 2011. "Feeding Blueberry Diets Inhibits Angiotensin II-Converting Enzyme (ACE) Activity in Spontaneously Hypertensive Stroke-Prone Rats." *Canadian Journal of Physiology and Pharmacology* 89 (1). https://doi.org/10.1139/Y10-101.

Xia, En Qin, Gui Fang Deng, Ya Jun Guo, and Hua Bin Li. 2010. "Biological Activities of Polyphenols from Grapes." *International Journal of Molecular Sciences.* https://doi.org/10.3390/ijms11020622.

Yáñez, Matilde, Nuria Fraiz, Ernesto Cano, and Francisco Orallo. 2006. "Inhibitory Effects of Cis- and Trans-Resveratrol on Noradrenaline and 5-Hydroxytryptamine Uptake and on Monoamine Oxidase Activity." *Biochemical and Biophysical Research Communications* 344 (2). https://doi.org/10.1016/j.bbrc.2006.03.190.

Yilmaz, Yusuf, and Romeo T. Toledo. 2004. "Major Flavonoids in Grape Seeds and Skins: Antioxidant Capacity of Catechin, Epicatechin, and Gallic Acid." *Journal of Agricultural and Food Chemistry* 52 (2). https://doi.org/10.1021/jf030117h.

Zhang, Bo, Miranbieke Buya, Wenjie Qin, Chongde Sun, Haolei Cai, Qiuping Xie, Bing Xu, and Yulian Wu. 2013. "Anthocyanins from Chinese Bayberry Extract Activate Transcription Factor Nrf2 in β Cells and Negatively Regulate Oxidative Stress-Induced Autophagy." *Journal of Agricultural and Food Chemistry* 61 (37). https://doi.org/10.1021/jf4012399.

Zhang, Haopeng, Jiaren Liu, Guodong Li, Jiufeng Wei, Hongsheng Chen, Chunpeng Zhang, Jinlu Zhao, et al. 2018a. "Fresh Red Raspberry Phytochemicals Suppress the Growth of Hepatocellular Carcinoma Cells by PTEN/AKT Pathway." *International Journal of Biochemistry and Cell Biology* 104. https://doi.org/10.1016/j.biocel.2018.09.003.

Zhang, Jizhen, Xianqing Li, Xueqing Zhang, Min Zhang, Gangshi Cong, Guangwu Zhang, and Feiyu Wang. 2018b. "Geochemical and Geological Characterization of Marine–Continental Transitional Shales from Longtan Formation in Yangtze Area, South China." *Marine and Petroleum Geology* 96. https://doi.org/10.1016/j.marpetgeo.2018.05.020.

Zhang, Yanjun, Navindra P. Seeram, Rupo Lee, Lydia Feng, and David Heber. 2008. "Isolation and Identification of Strawberry Phenolics with Antioxidant and Human Cancer Cell Antiproliferative Properties." *Journal of Agricultural and Food Chemistry* 56. https://doi.org/10.1021/jf071989c.

# 2 Current Trends and Techniques in the Nutraceutical Industry

*Mohammed Shafiq Alam, Gurjeet Kaur, and Ruchika Zalpouri*

## CONTENTS

## 2.1 INTRODUCTION

The modern world is struggling with poor air quality, non-drinkable water, contaminated foods, and a polluted environment owing to the tremendous population growth and industrialization. According to the World Health Organization, lifestyle, and diet patterns are major contributors to develop diabetes, coronary heart disease, cancer, obesity, and osteoporosis (WHO 2003). Consumers and food processors have realized the beneficial effects of foods based upon the principle of Hippocrates (the father of modern medicine) "Let food be thy medicine, thy medicine shall be thy food" (El Sohaimy 2012). Therefore, to uplift their health status, people consume various dietary supplements or nutraceuticals and functional foods. Although the phrases "functional food" and "nutraceutical food" are used interchangeably in the food sector, these terms are significantly different.

Functional foods are considered part of the normal diet with beneficial nutrients whose effects go beyond the well-known conventional nutritional effects (Roberfroid 2002). The European Food Information Council defined functional foods as foods containing bioactive components that have the potential to optimize physical and mental well-being and which may also reduce the risk of disease (Daliri and Lee 2015). For example: Raw fruits and

DOI: 10.1201/9781003259213-2

vegetables containing bioactive compounds such as polyphenols, antioxidants, dietary fibers, vitamins, and minerals. Nutraceutical is a combination of two words such as "nutrition" and "pharmaceutical". Thus, along with providing the required nutrients, nutraceutical foods protect the human body from serious illnesses. According to (DeFelice 1995), nutraceutical foods or a part of food exhibit several health benefits by preventing or treating a disease. These foods are derived from natural foods and consumed in the form of tablets, powders, capsules, and solutions. These foods carry a concentrated form of a bioactive component derived from food with the function of improving health in excess of what could be achieved from common foods (Zeisel 1999).

## 2.2 CLASSIFICATION SYSTEMS

There are numerous systems to categorize nutraceuticals. Some commonly used classification systems are discussed next.

### 2.2.1 Nutrients, Dietary Supplements, and Herbal Foods

*Nutrients:* These constituents are present in foods at an intensity that exhibits the potential to support life and growth. The chief nutrients are carbohydrates, fats, minerals, and protein. Water soluble and insoluble vitamins and various antioxidants play a pivotal role in human health and well-being. These compounds are naturally present in foods such as fruits, vegetables, dairy, various types of meats, and cereals. Consumption of these foods protects the human body from many diseases, including cardiovascular diseases, obesity, diabetes, various types of cancer, osteoporosis, and osteoarthritis (Kumar and Kumar 2015).

*Dietary supplements:* These essential ingredients are generally vitamins, minerals, herbs, and amino acids are used in the form of concentrates, extracts, or metabolites of these ingredients. These supplements, when incorporated into foods, provide several therapeutic effects. Out of available dietary supplements (approximately 50,000), the most familiar are multivitamins. The presence of probiotic bacteria such as *Lactobacillus acidophilus* and *bifidobacteria* are leading the sector of yogurts as these microorganisms aid in digestion by improving gut health (Dolkar et al. 2017). Some dietary supplements are meant for sports persons to meet excessive energy demands, whereas some of these help in weight control. Ketogenic diets, which are low in carbohydrates and high in proteins and fats, help control epilepsy, a disease related to nerve cells (Gupta et al. 2010), and weight loss.

*Herbal foods:* Ancient history holds a plethora of information about to the health benefits of herbal products (Singh et al. 2017). An Indian tradition, "Ayurveda" contains natural remedies for acute and chronic diseases to ensure health care. With this concept, herbal concentrates or extracts are being used as nutraceuticals to cure or prevent disorders. Aloe vera gel acts as an anti-inflammatory agent and helps heal wounds (Singh et al. 2017).

*Potential or established nutraceuticals:* Potential nutraceuticals are intended to be used as nutraceuticals by promising a health benefit. These nutraceuticals become established once they are clinically tested to analyze that benefit. Most nutraceuticals fall under the potential nutraceutical category while waiting to be categorized as established nutraceuticals (DeFelice 1995).

### 2.2.2 Bioactive Components

This is the widely used classification system for nutraceuticals. The presence of biologically active compounds in different food groups plays a significant role in maintaining the health of humans, as shown in Table 2.1.

## Table 2.1: Bioactive Compounds and Their Health Benefits

| Source | Bioactive Compound | Health Benefits |
|---|---|---|
| | **Polyphenolic Compounds** | |
| Blueberries, apple, onion, tea, broccoli | Flavonols (Quercetin, Myricetin, Isorhamnetin, Kaempfero) | • Antioxidant<br>• Anti-inflammatory<br>• Antimicrobial<br>• Anticancer<br>• Antidiabetic |
| Citrus peels, thyme, celery, parsley | Flavones (Luteolin, Apigenin) | • Anti-inflammatory<br>• Neuroprotective<br>• Anti-metastatic |
| Citrus fruits | Flavanones (Hesperetin, Naringenin) | • Antioxidant<br>• Anticancer |
| Soy foods | Isoflavones (Diadzein, Glycitein, Genistein) | • Decrease low-density lipoproteins (LDLs) and menopause symptoms<br>• Prevent breast cancer and endometrial cancer |
| Mango, banana, berries, grapes, peaches, wine, beer, chocolate, tea, spices, onions, plums, peas, cabbage, nuts, barley | Anthocyanidins and proanthocyanidins (Delphinidin, Malvidin, Pelargonidin, Cyanidin, etc.) | • Anti-carcinogenic<br>• Neutralization of free radicals |
| Turmeric | Curcumin | • Anti-inflammatory<br>• Antioxidant<br>• Anti-clotting agent |
| Strawberries, rose, coffee, wine, basil, rosemary, rice | Phenolic acid | • Anti-inflammatory<br>• Anticancer<br>• Antioxidant<br>• Help in weight loss<br>• Reduce low-density lipoproteins |
| Berries, peanuts, and grapevine | Stilbenes (Resveratrol) | • Protect against cardiovascular disease, cancer, and neurodegenerative diseases |
| Tea, mustard, rapeseed | Catechins | • Antioxidant<br>• Anti-carcinogenic |
| Oilseeds, nuts, and cereals | Phytosterols and Phytotanols | • Consumed as non-pharmacologic serum and low-density lipoprotein |
| Bananas, potatoes, legumes | Non-digestible carbohydrates | • Act as prebiotics by adding bulk to stool, reducing LDL cholesterol, coronary heart diseases |
| Soybeans, chickpeas, quinoa | Saponins | • Antibiotic<br>• Anticancer<br>• Control cholesterol<br>• Antioxidant |
| Plant sterols | | |
| Soy, wheat, corn | Stanol ester | • Prevent cholesterol absorption |
| Phytoestrogen | | |
| Maize, soybean, seeds (flax, lentil) | Isoflavones (Daidzein, genistein) | • Control menopause symptoms<br>• Strengthen bone and brain functioning |
| Vegetables, flax seeds, rye | Lignans | • Anticancer<br>• Lower risk of heart-related disorders |

*(Continued)*

**31**

## Table 2.1: Bioactive Compounds and Their Health Benefits (*Continued*)

| Source | Bioactive Compound | Health Benefits |
|---|---|---|
| **Carotenoids** | | |
| Mango, carrots, papaya | β-carotene | • Neutralization of free radicals |
| Eggs, vegetables, and citrus fruits | Lutein | • Enhance vision |
| Tomato | Lycopene | • Prevent prostate cancer |
| Palm oil, different grains | Tocotrienol | • Improve cardiovascular health<br>• Protect against breast cancer |
| **Dietary fiber** | | |
| Bran (wheat, rice) and fruits | Insoluble dietary fiber | • Lower risk of breast cancer<br>• Improve digestion |
| Cereals, oats | Whole grain, β-glucan | • Protection from cardiovascular diseases |
| **Fatty acids** | | |
| Dairy and meat products | Conjugated linoleic acid | • Anticancer |
| Fish, flax seeds | Omega-3 fatty acids | • Anti-inflammatory<br>• Control brain functioning and dispositioning of cholesterol |
| Tree nuts | Monosaturated fatty acids | • Prevent coronary heart diseases |
| Fruits | Polyols (xylitol, sorbitol) | • Prevent tooth cavity |
| **Prebiotics/Probiotics** | | |
| Dairy and non-dairy products | *Lactobacillus*, biofidobacteria | • Improve the functioning of the gastrointestinal system |
| Onions, artichokes, shallots | Fructooligosaccharides | • Improve the functioning of the gastrointestinal system |

## 2.3 CURRENT TRENDS AND TECHNIQUES IN NUTRACEUTICAL INDUSTRY

The demand for nutraceutical foods is exerting pressure on food processing industries and posing a great challenge to meet the expectations of consumers for food items that are relishing along with healthy ingredients (Shah 2007). Before developing a functional product, food industries consider various parameters such as sensory acceptability, shelf stability, cost, nutritional composition and properties (Granato et al. 2010). Betoret et al. (2003) classified the techniques used in development of these foods as follows:

■ Blending and characterization

■ Biological modifications

■ Microencapsulation

■ Edible coatings and films

■ Vacuum impregnation

### 2.3.1 Blending and Characterization

While developing nutraceutical foods, the first operation involves the extraction of the biologically active ingredients from various natural foods. These extracts are used in the concentrated form after dehydration processes with or without a carrier. The formulation of nutraceutical foods includes the blending of various components and trace elements. According to the daily requirements, all the ingredients of nutraceutical foods must be precisely blended. An additive effect is obtained by combining nutraceuticals if the total combined effect is equivalent to the individual effect of components. When the combination of nutraceuticals provides a greater effect as compared to the sum of the individual parts, it is termed as a synergistic effect. On the other hand, if this combined effect is less than the sum, it is called an antagonistic effect. Another term, potentiation, is related to an effect when an inactive component improves the impact of another active compound (Efferth and Koch 2011).

The key factors which need to be considered while blending and formulation nutraceutical foods are:

- Particle size of active ingredients
- Flowability and compressibility
- Properties of single as well as combined ingredients
- Dosage requirement
- Manufacturing process

### 2.3.2 Biological Modifications

Biotechnology involves using living organisms (or their parts) to produce or transform plants, animals, or microorganisms for improved yields, nutritional quality, and disease tolerance. It involves selective breeding in which two plants' genetic materials are exchanged to produce a new offspring. This offspring possesses the desired traits to fulfill specific purposes. However, for this process, the parent plants used must be related to each other. This process is lengthy and not very precise, and results in the absence of required interesting characteristics. This problem is overcome by modern biotechnology with precise and fast results along with potential sources to obtain desirable traits (Persley and Siedow 1999). This technique developed new plant varieties with improved nutrition during the 20th century(Zimmermann and Hurrell 2002) with a major focus on environmental stress management, protection against insects/pests (Borlaug 2000), and improvement of sensory characteristics as in tomato (Lewinsohn et al. 2001). Recently, studies have been documented on enhancing the nutritional content by introducing minerals and vitamins.

### 2.3.3 Microencapsulation

Micronutrients such as iron, calcium, zinc, vitamins, and minerals are required in our body in significantly less amounts, but their deficiency can result in severe health issues such as anemia, short-sightedness, osteoporosis, weak bone density, etc. Similarly, bioactive compounds such as flavonoids, polyphenols, omega-3 fatty acids, prebiotics, and probiotics are vital to the well-being of humans. Thus, these compounds must reach their target and effectively deliver, release, and function. Therefore, efficient delivery systems such as microencapsulation are currently being used to make their availability at the appropriate locations in the human body.

Microencapsulation is a technique in which micronutrients or nutraceuticals are entrapped inside a food-grade coating, called a shell, to protect them from heat, oxygen, light, and other reactive compounds. Table 2.2 demonstrates the recent studies on microencapsulation of nutraceuticals documented by various researchers. The health-promoting material which is being encapsulated is

## Table 2.2: Microencapsulation Applications in Fruits

| Fruit | Shell Material | Technique Used | Nutraceutical | Reference |
|---|---|---|---|---|
| Cornelian cherry | Soy protein and maltodextrin | Freeze and spray drying | Anthocyanin | Dumitraşcu et al. (2021) |
| Guava pulp | Inulin and maltodextrin | Spray-drying | Carotenoid, antioxidant activity | Rivas, Cabral and da Rocha-Leão (2021) |
| Jabuticaba peel | Chitosan | Spray-drying | Phenolic extract | Cabral et al. (2018) |
| Purple cactus pear | Maltodextrins, canola oil, and polyglycerol | Spray-drying | Phenolic compounds, antioxidant capacity | Toledo-Madrid, Gallardo-Velázquez, and Osorio-Revilla (2018) |
| Passion fruit juice | Maltodextrin and/or inulin | Spray-drying | Probiotic | Dias et al. (2018) |
| Dragon fruit peel | Maltodextrin | Freeze-drying | Betacyanin | Handayani et al. (2018) |
| Grape skin extract | Maltodextrin, gum arabic, and skim milk powder | Spray-drying | Anthocyanin and phenol | Kalušević et al. (2017) |
| Jussara | Maltodextrin inulinoligofructose | Spray-drying | Probiotic | Paim et al. (2016) |
| Jussara pulp | Gum arabic, modified starch | Spray-drying | Anthocyanins | Santana et al. (2016) |
| Strawberry | β-cyclodextrin | Coacervation, vacuum-drying | *Rosmarinus officinalis* and *Thymus vulgaris* | Alikhani and DaraeiGarmakhany (2012) |
| Blueberry | Maltodextrin | Ultrasonic nozzle and freeze-drying | Total phenolic content and antioxidant activity | Turan, Cengiz, and Kahyaoglu (2015) |
| Juçara | Gelatin, gum arabic, and maltodextrin | Spray-drying | Anthocyanin | Bicudo et al. (2015) |
| Banana passion fruit | Maltodextrin, modified starch | Spray-drying | Phenolic compounds | Gil et al. (2014) |
| Andes berry | Maltodextrin, arabic gum, cornstarch, and hi-cap™ | Spray-drying | Anthocyanin | Villacrez, Carriazo, and Osorio (2014) |
| Garcinia cowa (rind) | Whey protein isolate | Spray-drying | Hydroxycitric acid | Parthasarathi et al. (2013) |
| Pequi | Arabic gum | Spray-drying | Vitamin c and carotenoids | Santana et al. (2013) |
| Jaboticaba peel | Arabic gum maltodextrin and capsul™ | Spray-drying | Anthocyanins | Silva et al. (2013) |
| Black currant | Maltodextrin and corn syrup solids | Spray-drying | Polyphenols | Bakowska-Barczak and Kolodziejczyk (2011) |

known as an active or core ingredient (Ghosh 2006). This process generally follows the following stages (Oxley 2014).

*Core and shell ingredient formation:* Core or active ingredients are generally formed before encapsulation using grinding, granulation, or milling techniques. When core ingredients are in liquid form, emulsification is carried out to generate droplets. Moreover, surfactants or viscosity modifiers are used to easily process the core material in microcapsules. Shell or matrix material is used in liquid form to cover the core ingredients. These materials are selected based on suitability to microencapsulation technique, efficiency, and availability of encapsulated material. Derivatives of starch, sugars, gums, proteins, cellulose, and lipids are commonly used for this purpose.

*Encapsulation techniques:* To form a microcapsule by combining core and matrix material, several encapsulation techniques are used in the food industry. The most common methods are:

*Atomization:* This is a process of aerosol formation in which air is the gaseous phase and droplets are a mixture of core and shell material. Atomization of this mixture takes place once it passes through the nozzle. The resulting mixture contains core ingredients dispersed in the shell.

*Spray coating:* This process is also known as granulation, fluid-bed coating, or pan coating, in which the atomized mixture deposits over a solid material. The aerosol particles containing core material come in contact with solid particles suspended in air or rotating in a drum. The resulting droplets are dried to form a shell around the solid core material.

*Emulsions:* The above-discussed techniques are based upon atomization to form droplets. In emulsion formation, the core material in a liquid state is dispersed into another liquid containing dissolved shell or matrix material.

*Coacervation:* This technique is referred to as "phase separation", as it separates the liquid phases into polymer-rich concentrated and polymer-depleted dilute phases (Dziezak 1988). This technique can be classified as simple or complex.

*Extrusion:* This technique is most suitable for volatiles and flavors. These sensitive materials are encapsulated in a glassy carbohydrate shell, which enhances the shelf stability of volatile and flavoring compounds. This technique, also known as annular jet atomization, uses a concentric nozzle system to form a microcapsule by the axis symmetric breakdown of an annular jet. The encapsulating system consists of a cylinder with a concentric feed tube. Core material enters through the central tube, whereas coating or shell materials pass through the outer tube. As the attached rotating shaft head moves, core, and coating materials get co-extruded in the form of a rod as they pass out through the nozzles. This rod breaks down into small particles (*Diameter*: 150–2,000 mm) with the action of centrifugal force (Desai and Park 2005).

*Centrifugal suspension:* This recent microencapsulation technique involves adding a mixture of core and shell materials to a rotating disk. The core materials get coated with the residual liquid as they leave the rotating disk and are then dried.

*Co-crystallization:* In this technique, sucrose is used to form a matrix to incorporate core materials. Sucrose syrup is processed until it reaches supersaturated condition and is maintained at a high temperature to avoid crystal formation. After the addition of core material in this syrup, the resultant material is mechanically agitated to initiate nucleation and then crystallization. This process continues until the agglomerated material discharges from the container. The resulting microencapsulated products are dried to the required moisture content.

*Molecular inclusion complexation:* This process occurs at the molecular level with α-cyclodextrin as encapsulating medium. α-cyclodextrin is obtained enzymatically from partially hydrolyzed starch. The outer part of the cyclodextrin is hydrophilic, and the inner part is hydrophobic. Non-polar molecules such as essential oils and flavors can be entrapped through hydropic interaction within the inner cavity.

### 2.3.4 Edible Coatings or Films

A material that is coated or wrapped around food and suitable to be eaten along with food is considered edible coating or film (Pavlath and Orts 2009). These materials serve the purpose of limiting gas or vapor migration, surface browning, texture alterations, microbial contamination, and physiological disorders (Baldwin et al. 1996). Apart from including certain food additives, flavors, colors, anti-browning, and antimicrobial agents (Pranoto, Salokhe, and Rakshit 2005), these films and coatings have great potential to include nutraceuticals or functional ingredients to enhance the nutritional uptake by humans. Khalifa et al. (2017) reported that film obtained using olive leaf and pomace extracts incorporated into Chitosan was used for apple coating. The addition of olive leaf extracts in the film prevented the deterioration of flavonoids, antioxidants, and phenolic compounds and pomace extract recorded minimum influence on anthocyanins. Frassinetti et al. (2020) evaluated the effectiveness of coatings prepared from gelatin wastes and blueberry juice against flavonoids, carotenoids, polyphenols, antioxidant, and antimicrobial activity of tomatoes. The results indicated that the coating maintained nutritional quality and reduced mesophilic and coliform bacteria growth after 7 days of storage. Tampucci et al. (2021) aimed at the diffusion of the polyphenolic compound tyrosol infused in chitosan coating and transferred to tomato peel. An active transfer was recorded on the basis of reduced tyrosol content in the tomato peel and increased concentration in the flesh resulting in the development of a functional fruit.

### 2.3.5 Vacuum Impregnation

Vacuum impregnation techniques imply the exchange of gaseous or liquid present in the pores of a material with an external liquid by a hydrodynamic mechanism enhanced by pressure variation (Fito and Pastor 1994). The system contains a chamber, pressure control valves and sensors, a vacuum pump, a data acquisition system, and a circulation system for external solutions (Lima et al. 2016).

This process is comprising of two stages based on pressure (Kubzdela, Marecik, and Kidoń 2014):

- *Vacuum stage:* Once the material is immersed in a tank containing liquid, 50–100 mbar vacuum pressure ($p_1$) is applied for time $t_1$ on this closed tank to elevate expansion and discharge of internal gases. As gases are released, pores are filled with native liquid.

- *Atmospheric stage:* As pressure restores to atmospheric ($p_2$) for time $t_2$, compression reduces the volume of remaining gas in pores of material (see Figure 2.1). This further leads to an influx of external fluid. The scope of this technique in the food processing sector is prominent based on enhancement of quality and saving energy.

Fruits and vegetables are sensitive to handling techniques and processing temperatures. This technique is a gentle treatment without causing any damage to

**Fresh fruit**

↓

| Vacuum impregnation |
| --- |
| Stage 1 ($p_1$,$t_1$) |
| Stage 2 ($p_2$,$t_2$) |

**External liquid** ⟶ □ ⟶ **Residual liquid**

↓

Storage of vacuum-impregnated food

↓

**Heated air** ⟶ Drying of vacuum-impregnated food ⟶ **Humid air**

↓

Storage

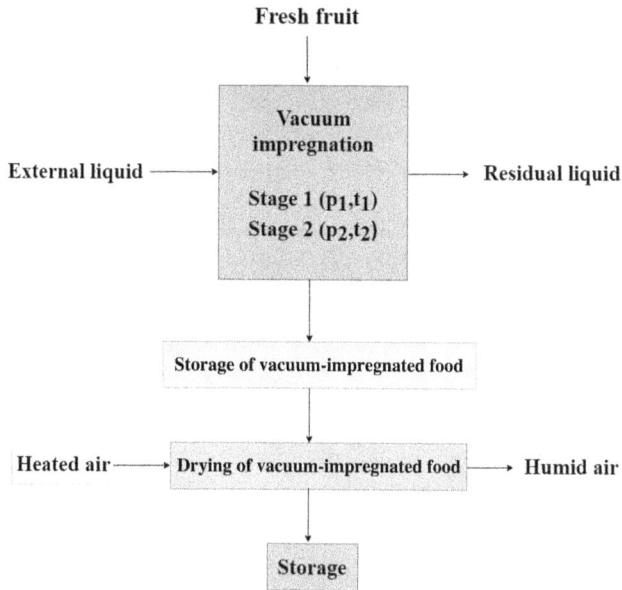

**Figure 2.1**  Flowchart showing vacuum impregnation of probiotics in fruit products.

tissues, color, flavor, aroma, and nutrients. Energy savings are achieved through the removal of water without heat treatment and subsequently less energy required for the removal of remaining water in foods (Zhao and Xie 2004). The vacuum impregnation technique has been adopted to include ingredients in porous food materials for modifications of composition to enhance stability and quality. The various applications of this technology include salting, drying pretreatment, calorie densification, fortification, and thermal properties modification (Ashitha and Prince 2018). As fruit structure is porous, this technology holds exclusive scope for improving the nutritional composition by the addition of nutraceuticals. Gooseberry (*Physalis peruviana* L.) samples were subjected to an emulsion technique containing calcium, vitamin D$_3$, vitamin E, vitamin B$_9$, and soybean protein while undergoing vacuum impregnation, and were subsequently freeze-dried. This combination provided a product with an excellent amount of vitamin D and good amounts of calcium and vitamins B$_9$, C, and E based on daily reference values (Cortés, Herrera, and Rodríguez 2015). Bioactive ingredients, such as β-carotene and lutein, were added to fruit salads using the vacuum impregnation technique by Moreira et al. (2018). From the optimized conditions, it was clear that 7 minutes of vacuum impregnation treatment was adequate to provide recommended daily intake of carotenoids from 25 g of fruit salad.

## 2.4  EXTRACTION OF NUTRACEUTICAL COMPOUNDS FROM FRUITS

Extraction is a fundamental procedure to separate and recover bioactive components from plant sources. Bioactive compounds present in fruits can be extracted using numerous ways. These techniques differ depending on the process factors such as frequency, temperature, electromagnetic waves, and pH. The method also relies on the type of fruit, sensitivity, chemical, and functional properties, and final use (Pattnaik et al. 2021). Traditional methods performed for extraction viz. digestion, percolation, maceration, decoction, was time-consuming, inefficient, and required high amounts of solvents (as in solvent extraction). Thus, to overcome these issues and meet the consumer demand for high-quality nutrient dense foods, advanced techniques adopted by the food industry are discussed below.

### 2.4.1 Solvent Extraction

Solvent extraction (SE) is a technique used to extract specific compounds from various materials, including sediments, soil, polymers, bacteria, fungi, algae, and microalgae, and, more commonly, plants (Hattab et al. 2007; Plaza, Cifuentes, and Ibáñez 2008). In general, pretreated raw material is exposed to various solvents, which absorb compounds of interest and other agents (flavor and colorings). Typically, samples are centrifuged and filtered to remove solid residue, and the extract may be used as an additive, food supplement, or in the preparation of functional foods (Starmans and Nijhuis 1996). Hexane, ether, chloroform, acetonitrile, benzene, and ethanol are some of the most commonly used solvents in extraction procedures, and they are commonly used in various ratios with water (Li and Zhang 2013). These organic solvents can be used to extract both polar and nonpolar organic compounds such as alkaloids, organochlorine pesticides, phenols, aromatic hydrocarbons, fatty acids, and oils (Hattab et al. 2007; Plaza et al. 2008; Starmans and Nijhuis 1996; Villa-Rodríguez et al. 2011). SE is superior to other methods due to its low processing cost and ease of use. However, this method employs toxic solvents, necessitates an evaporation/concentration step for recovery, and typically necessitates large amounts of solvent and a lengthy time frame (Miron et al. 2011). Furthermore, due to the high temperatures of the solvents during the long extraction times, the possibility of thermal degradation of natural bioactive compounds cannot be ignored.

In general, the art of separation is improving, with new methods and procedures being developed at a rapid pace. Other methods, such as Soxhlet, ultrasound, microwave extraction, and SFE, among others, have been used to improve SE yields (Szentmihályi et al. 2002).

### 2.4.2 Microwave-Assisted Extraction

Microwaves have electromagnetic fields from 300 MHz to 300 GHz. When microwaves come in contact with polar molecules in food, it gets heated up due to the absorption of microwave energy (Figure 2.2(a)). This heating process is carried out by ionic conduction and dipole movements (dielectric heating). Microwave-assisted extraction (MAE) is a technique that can be performed using two conditions. In the first condition, extraction occurs in a closed vessel with controlled temperature and pressure. In contrast, in the second condition, an open vessel is used at atmospheric pressure and maximum boiling temperature of the solvent. A solvent having high dielectric properties is utilized to extract biologically active ingredients. During this process, the polar molecules, such as water, absorb microwaves and give rise to localized heating. These further leads to the expansion and rupture of the food cell wall by disturbing the forces of attraction between solutes and plant matrix. The ruptured walls allow the movement of solvent into the food matrix and functional components into the solvent. This technique is highly efficient, time-saving, and requires less solvent than traditional methods of extraction.

Ferreres et al. (2017) optimized the condition for microwave-assisted extraction (MAE) of high-value components from pitaya fruit peel. The obtained product contained phenolic compounds such as 18 cinnamoyl, 17 flavonoid derivatives, and 4 betacyanins, showing the potential of using bioproducts as a

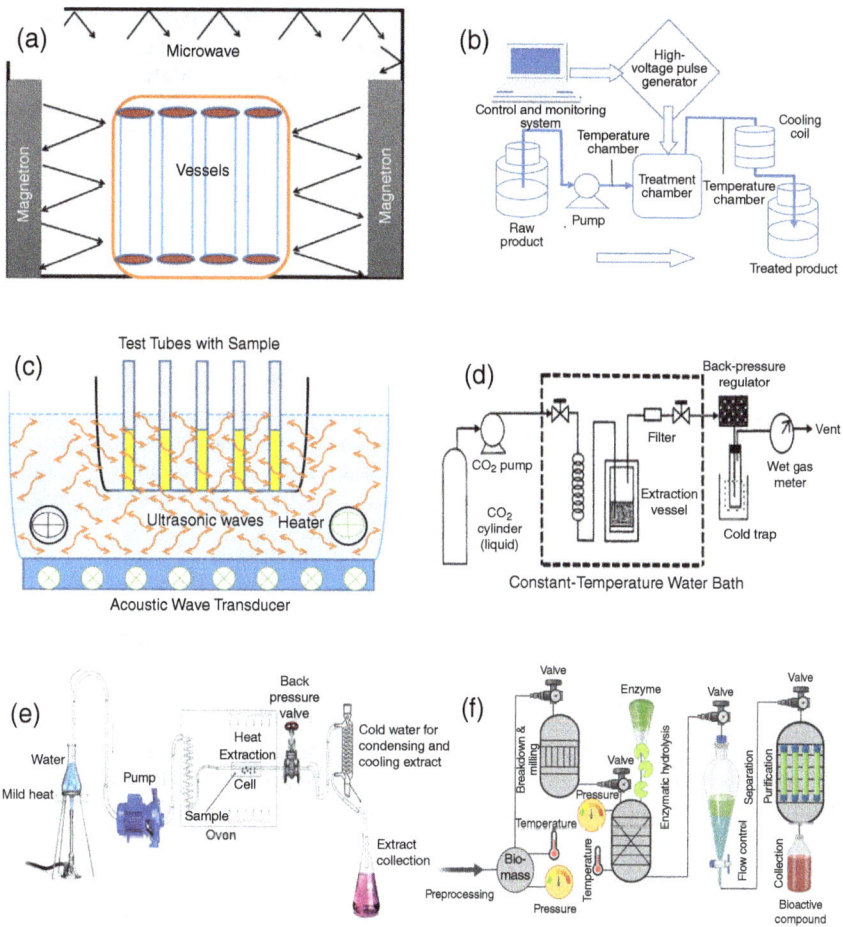

**Figure 2.2** Latest techniques used for extraction: (a) Microwave-assisted extraction (Belwal et al. 2018); (b) pulsed electric field extraction; (c) ultrasound-assisted extraction (Belwal et al. 2018); (d) supercritical fluid extraction (Markom, Singh, and Hasan 2001); (e) subcritical water extraction (Gbashi et al. 2017); (f) enzyme-assisted extraction.

source of nutritionally beneficial compounds. *Morus nigra* L., i.e., black mulberry fruits rich in phenolic compounds, were subjected to microwave-assisted extraction by Koyu et al. (2018). The outcomes of this study demonstrated that better extraction yield was found for anthocyanin and tyrosinase inhibitory activity in contrast to the traditional method. Thirugnanasambandham and Sivakumar (2017) estimated the extracted betalain content using the microwave technique from dragon fruit. From the optimized conditions viz. temperature (35°C), sample (20 g), and treatment time (8 min), the betalain content of 9 mg/L was extracted. The microwave-assisted technique has primarily been used to recover phenolic compounds (Li et al. 2011) and carotenoids (Zhao et al. 2006), and bioactive compounds, such as terpenoids, alkaloids, and saponins (Zhang, Yang, and Wang 2011). The majority of these studies concluded that using MAE reduced solvent consumption and extraction times while providing better

39

antioxidant capacity and equivalent or higher extraction yields than other methods. Compared to rotary extraction, peel extracts of citrus mandarin (Hayat et al. 2009) and tomatoes (Li et al. 2012) produced higher yields and higher antioxidant activity. MAE of natural bioactive compounds can be influenced by a wide range of factors, including microwave power, frequency, and time, moisture content, and particle size of the sample matrix, solvent type, and concentration, solid-liquid ratio, extraction temperature, extraction pressure, and the number of extraction cycles (Li and Zhang 2013).

### 2.4.3 Pulsed Electric Field Extraction

This non-thermal technique is quite popular for extracting heat-sensitive compounds. As the name suggests, short pulses generated by two electrodes with electric field strength (0.1–50 kV/cm) are passed through a food sample placed in a treatment chamber as shown in Figure 2.2(b). Food cell membranes accumulate charges on both sides and develop trans-membrane potential. As trans-membrane potential crosses a critical value, membrane electroporation starts at weaker areas. It enhances the permeability of the membrane resulting migration of intracellular components through the membrane. This technology improves yield at less energy consumption and has little effect on the environment. El Kantar et al. (2018) used this technique to extract polyphenolic compounds from oranges, lemons, and pomelos. Along with the enhancement of juice yield from these citrus fruits using the pulsed electric field technique, polyphenols extraction also elevated up to 22 mg gallic acid equivalent/g of dry mass. Another research on date palm fruits by Siddeeg et al. (2019) evaluated the impact of this technology on the extraction of biologically active compounds and physicochemical. It resulted in improved amounts of flavonoids, carotenoids, anthocyanins, volatile components, and antioxidant activity compared to untreated samples. Redondo et al. (2018) studied the potential of thinned peach fruits to provide nutritional entities. A pulsed electric field extraction along with methanol and water as solvents was analyzed. Observations recorded for the extraction efficiency of these combinations suggested pulsed electric field-assisted extraction with water provided a better number of bioactive compounds. Blueberry was analyzed for juice yield and anthocyanins (from press cake) after treatment with the pulsed electric field process. Extracts were obtained from the press cake of PEF-treated blueberries at 10kJ/kg field strength. Anthocyanin content and antioxidant capacities were 75% and 71% (by FRAP), and 109% (by DPPH), which was significantly higher than non-treated extracts of berries.

### 2.4.4 Ultrasound-Assisted Extraction

Ultrasound regions have sound frequencies greater than 20 kHz, which is far beyond human detection. For effective extraction of biologically active components from foods, 20–100 kHz is considered best as it results in strong physical forces (Cravotto et al. 2008). This technique facilitates mass transfer and influx of solvents into the food matrix based on vibrations, mixing, and acoustic cavitations. When ultrasound energy passes through any liquid medium, it induces the growth of bubbles from cavitation (Figure 2.2(c)). These bubbles collapse and generate shockwaves and turbulence. These effects lead to the breakdown of the food cell wall, the formation of holes on the surface, and oozing of intracellular plant material in the surrounding solvent such as water, methanol, hexane, etc. (Wen et al. 2018a). Moreover, these waves give rise to regions of high and low pressure termed acoustic pressure. The cavitation bubbles expand in the negative pressure cycle and diffuse vapors to inner parts.

The positive pressure cycle causes contraction and hence diffusion of vapors to the outer side of the bubbles (Alzorqi and Manickam 2016). This diffusion phenomenon leads to deposit mass on the bubble surface with time and hence their growth. As soon as bubbles attain a critical size known as resonance, they collapse. A low-frequency range, i.e., 16–100 kHz, is considered a power ultrasound zone as bubbles of resonance size collapse with high intensity and produce intense physical effects (Leong, Martin, and Ashokkumar 2017). This ultrasound-assisted extraction (UAE) facilitates low-temperature extraction, less solvent volume, and pure and efficient extraction. It has been used to extract proteins, sugars, polysaccharides-protein complexes, and oil (Adam et al. 2012; Karki et al. 2010; Qu et al. 2012).

### 2.4.5 Supercritical Fluid Extraction

Currently, supercritical fluid extraction (SCFE) and subcritical fluid extraction are being seen as green approaches for the extraction of functional compounds owing to their negligible impact on the environment. In contrast to traditional methods, these are quicker, highly selective, and high-quality pure outputs using cheap, eco-friendly, and safe solvents (García-Pérez et al. 2020; Zacconi et al. 2017).

The supercritical fluid extraction technique (SCFE) has been widely adopted for heat-sensitive and high-value food products. SCFE is based on fluid properties such as density, diffusivity, dielectric constant, and viscosity, and usually modifies pressure and temperature to achieve a supercritical fluid (SF) (Herrero et al. 2010). As SF has similar density and viscosity to that of a liquid and gas, respectively, it is classified as a fluid under these conditions. As a result, the supercritical state of a fluid is the state in which the liquid and gas are identical to one another (Wang and Weller 2006). During this extraction, the raw material is kept in a chamber containing fluid, as shown in Figure 2.2(d). This fluid is pressurized by a pump which regulates the temperature. Supercritical fluids (SFs) possess the property not to attain a gaseous or liquid state once they cross critical temperature and critical pressure. Such property is fruitful to the influx of these fluids in the food matrix like a gas and dissolves compounds of interest like a liquid. Despite the fact that many compounds (ethylene, methane, nitrogen, xenon, or fluorocarbons) can be used as SFs, most separation systems use carbon dioxide ($CO_2$) due to its safety and low cost (Daintree, Kordikowski, and York 2008). $CO_2$ serves as an ideal supercritical fluid due to its non-toxic and non-explosive nature, along with its effectiveness in extracting non-polar, partially polar, oxygenated medium molecular weight compounds (Cvjetko Bubalo et al. 2018). Moreover, the critical temperature of $CO_2$ is 31°C, which is close to room temperature. The critical pressure of $CO_2$ is 74 bars, which enable it to be used at a moderate pressure range, i.e., 100–450 bar (García-Pérez et al. 2020). Various solvent compounds require small quantities of additives to improve the process's solubility and selectivity, this phenomenon is known as the "cosolvent effect" (Daintree, Kordikowski, and York 2008). Because of lower toxicity and miscibility in $CO_2$, ethanol is recommended as a cosolvent in SCFE (Wang and Weller 2006). The dissolved components in the fluid are transferred to separating units where fluids are recycled, leaving the components at the bottom (Shimojo et al. 2006). This process is unique in terms of capacity, diffusivity, and less viscosity of supercritical fluids over the other, which makes this process to complete in short time with high yields (Soquetta, Terra, and Bastos 2018). SCFE is now widely used in various industrial applications, such as coffee decaffeination, fatty acid refining, and the extraction of essential oils and flavors from natural sources, with potential applications in nutraceuticals and functional foods (Daintree, Kordikowski, and York 2008).

### 2.4.6 Supercritical Antisolvent Fractionation

This is another technique that employs supercritical fluids as antisolvent. This process aims to recover high molecular weight compounds that are not soluble in $CO_2$ and collect them in separators. Contact between supercritical fluid and polar compounds in a pressurized chamber leads to the precipitation of polar components. A $CO_2$-containing non-polar entity is depressurized in a downstream process to recover these compounds. This system can be operated at low temperatures, oxygen-deficient conditions, and in the presence of light. Using this technique, Maran, Priya, and Manikandan (2014) investigated anthocyanins and phenolic components in jamun fruits. The optimal process conditions were 162 bar pressure, 50°C temperature, and 2.0 g/min flow rate of solvent. Experimental values complied with predicted values using these conditions. Akay, Alpak, and Yesil-Celiktas (2011) worked on *Arbutus unedo* fruits to optimize total phenolic yield using supercritical fluid extraction. Using the optimum conditions of pressure- 60 bar, temperature- 48°C, total phenols were quantified as 25.72 mg gallic acid equivalent (GAE)/g extract and 99.9% radical scavenging, which were high corresponding to the observations recorded from water (24.89 mg/g; 83.8%) and ethanol (15.12 mg/g; 95.8%) extractions.

### 2.4.7 Subcritical Water Extraction

Another environment-friendly and less toxic technique popular these days is subcritical water extraction (SWE), also known as pressurized liquid extraction [Figure 2.2(e)]. The basic principle of this technique is to reduce the dielectric constant of water, which behaves like commonly used solvents such as methanol and ethanol, having 33 and 24 dielectric constants, respectively. For this purpose, water is heated to attain a temperature between 100–320°C and maintaining pressure (approximately 20–150 bar). SWE has several advantages over traditionally used extraction techniques as it is faster, produces higher yields, and uses less solvent amount (Plaza et al. 2010b). When the liquid state is maintained, solvent parameters such as dielectric constant, solubility, and temperature are affected. As a result, while the dielectric constant of water is nearly 80 at room temperature, it can be reduced to around 30 at 250°C. Under these conditions, a value similar to that of some organic solvents, such as ethanol or methanol, is obtained. The solubility parameter also decreases, approaching the value obtained for less polar compounds (Adil et al. 2007). As a result, this technique can be used to replace organic solvents in the extraction of nonpolar natural bioactive compounds. However, the variability of dielectric constants for different types of compounds must be considered. SWE has been used successfully to extract various natural bioactive compounds from a variety of fruits. This technique was applied by Lachos-Perez et al. (2018) to extract flavones from orange peel. The yields demonstrated that this method is highly efficient in recovering bioactive compounds. Kheirkhah, Baroutian, and Young Quek (2019) aimed to recover the phenolic entities from kiwifruit pomace by subcritical water extraction. Maximum recovery (60.53 mgCaE/g DW) was obtained at 150°C and process time 90 min having (+)-catechin, protocatechuic chlorogenic acid, p-coumaric acid, and caffeic acid. Citrus pomaces were another vegetable matrix used by SWE to extract bioactive compounds (Kim et al. 2009). In general, using SWE has several advantages, including shorter extraction times, higher product quality, lower cost of extracting agent, and is an environment-friendly technique. This method can be applied to nutraceuticals that provide health benefits.

### 2.4.8 Enzyme-Assisted Extraction

The basic approach of this technique is to pretreat a sample to easily extract the bonded compounds [Figure 2.2(f)]. When the common solvent cannot access the compounds bonded with strong forces, enzymes assist in delinking these compounds. The presence of polysaccharides, such as pectins, cellulose, and hemicelluloses, hinder the release of intracellular functional entities. This can be overcome by hydrolyzing these polysaccharides by breaking cell walls using pectinase, cellulose, xylanase, and β-glucosidase enzymes (Moore et al. 2006). The remarkable features of this process include easy product recovery, less energy requirement, high product yield, easy isolation, and recovery, safer, easier to do, and recyclable (Alam et al. 2017; Fleurence et al. 1995; Shen et al. 2008). Enzyme-assisted solvent extraction was applied to extract phenolic compounds from watermelon rind Mushtaq et al. (2015) using optimized conditions viz. enzyme concentration: 0.5–6.5%, pH: 6–9, temperature: 25–75°C, and time: 30–90 min. The outcomes indicated that this process enhanced the release of phenolic compounds three times in contrast to conventional solvent extraction, with total phenolics on a fresh weight basis (173.70 mg gallic acid equivalent/g), Trolox equivalent antioxidant capacity of 279.96 mg TE/g and 2,2-diphenyl-1-picrylhydrazyl (DPPH) radical scavenging activity (IC50) 112.27 mg/mL, used different solvents to extract lycopene and analyzed the impact of enzyme treatments. Industrial waste, peels, pulp, and whole tomato fruit were first subjected to enzyme treatment, then solvent extraction. Maximum lycopene content was found in tomato peel (417.97 g/g), industrial waste (195.74 g/g), and whole fruit (83.85 g/g); and the minimum was found in the pulp (47.6 g/g).

### 2.4.9 Instant Controlled Pressure Drop-Assisted Extraction

Pressurized liquid extraction (PLE) is gaining popularity and is widely used to extract natural bioactive compounds from natural sources (Miron et al. 2011). A thermo-chemical mechanism enhances the mass transfer and hence the extraction of nutritional compounds. This process starts with exposing the raw material to saturated steam for a short time period. A sudden fall in pressure close to the vacuum results in the vaporization of volatile components and the cooling effect, which prevents the thermal deterioration of compounds. This technology is widely accepted for the extraction of antioxidants (Allaf et al. 2013) and volatile compounds (Berka-Zougali et al. 2010). This also facilitates the enhanced recovery of the components by expanding the cell walls of the material (Allaf et al. 2013). Due to these facts, it is appropriate to recover essential oils. The high pressure speeds up the filling of the extraction cells and forces liquid into the solid matrix. Compared to traditional SE, these new techniques allow for faster extraction with fewer solvents and higher yields. Furthermore, using PLE enables the production of food-grade extracts, which are only obtained when water or other GRAS (generally recognized as safe) solvents, such as ethanol, are used (Plaza et al. 2010a). Despite its advantages over traditional methods, this method is not suitable for thermolabile compounds because high temperatures can have negative effects on their structure and functional activity (Ajila et al. 2011).

Various factors must be considered before selecting an adequate method of extraction. These factors include the type of plant, sample collection time,

## Table 2.3: Extraction Techniques for Bioactive Compounds from Different Parts of Plants

| Bioactive Compound | Plant Part Used | Extraction Technique |
|---|---|---|
| Anthocyanins | Leaves | Supercritical fluid extraction |
| | Fruits | Microwave-assisted extraction |
| Alkaloids | Leaves | Supercritical fluid extraction |
| | Roots | Microwave-assisted extraction |
| Carotenoids | Leaves | Supercritical fluid extraction |
| | Fruits | Subcritical water extraction |
| Flavonoids | Leaves | Supercritical fluid extraction |
| | Fruits | Microwave-assisted extraction |
| Oils | Leaves | Supercritical fluid extraction |
| | Fruits | Instant controlled pressure drop-assisted extraction |
| Polyphenols | Fruits | Supercritical fluid extraction |
| | Leaves | Microwave-assisted extraction |
| Polysaccharides | Roots | Microwave-assisted extraction |
| | Fruits | Ultrasound-assisted extraction |
| Saponins | Leaves | Supercritical fluid extraction |
| | Fruits | Microwave-assisted extraction |

*Source:* Modified from Belwal et al. (2018).

pre-processing methods, solvents for the desired compound, extraction runs, temperature, pressure, extractor design, etc. The various methods in trend for different functional/bioactive compounds and part of the plant used are summarized in Table 2.3.

### 2.5 TECHNIQUES OF ISOLATION AND IDENTIFICATION OF NUTRACEUTICALS OF FRUITS

The extracted compounds from plants are generally associated with different types of phytochemicals or functional ingredients. Due to such complexity, the isolation and identification of these compounds are a challenge for nutraceutical industries. Isolation and characterization of these compounds can be done by different chromatographic techniques such as thin-layer chromatography, high-performance liquid chromatography, gas-liquid chromatography, column chromatography, and spectroscopic techniques viz. UV-visible, nuclear magnetic resonance, infrared, mass spectroscopy, and Fourier-transform infrared spectroscopy, as shown in Table 2.4.

### 2.5.1 Chromatographic Techniques

Chromatography is ideal for separating compounds from a mixture based on their differential partitioning depending upon their affinity towards phases. Two phases are common in all types of chromatographic techniques: Stationary phase, which is either solid or liquid applied on a solid base, and a mobile phase, which comprises a liquid or a gas. The mixture to be separated and dissolved in the mobile phase moves through the stationary phase. The various components of the extract mixture travel different distances at different speeds. This leads to the separation of compounds by calculating the retention factor, i.e., $R_f$.

## Table 2.4: Isolation and Identification Techniques for Nutraceuticals from Functional Fruits

| Fruit | Technique Used | Purpose | Reference |
|---|---|---|---|
| Mahlab cherry | High-pressure liquid chromatography-diode array detector (HPLC-DAD) and gas chromatography-mass spectrometry (GC-MS) | Characterization of anthocyanins | Ozturk et al. (2014) |
| Jujube | Reversed-phase chromatography | Separation of organic acids | Cosmulescu et al. (2018) |
| Saskatoon berry | High-pressure liquid chromatography and ultra-high performance liquid chromatography (UHPLC) | Quantification of organic acids, sugars, and bioactive compounds | Lachowicz et al. (2019) |
| Brazilian exotic fruit residues Achachairu, Araça-boi, and Bacaba | UHPLC-qqq-MS/MS | Identification and quantification of the phenolic compounds | Barros et al. (2017) |
| Hungarian sour cherry | High-performance liquid chromatography (HPLC) | Monitoring of anthocyanins | Gitta et al. (2005) |
| Chinese firethorn | Hplc-qtof-ms/ms | Identification of phytochemicals | Wang et al. (2019) |
| Noni | High-pressure liquid chromatography (HPLC) | Detection of quercetin, scopoletin, rutin | Deng, West, and Jensen (2010) |
| American cranberry | HPLC and LC-MS/MS | Identification and quantification of anthocyanins, flavonol, glycosides, proanthocyanidins, and organic acids | Wang et al. (2017) |
| Pomegranate | High-performance liquid chromatography coupled with photodiode array and mass spectrometry detection (HPLC-PDA-ESI/MS) | Analysis of phenolic compounds | Russo et al. (2018) |
| Blood orange | High-performance liquid chromatography (HPLC) | Analysis of limonoids and flavonoids | Russo et al. (2021) |
| Pomegranate | High-performance liquid chromatography coupled with diode-array detection (HPLC-DAD) | Investigation of phenolic compounds | Ali et al. (2014) |
| Gooseberry | Column chromatography and Thin-layer chromatography, MS, NMR | Isolation and identification of more bioactive compounds to determine the molecular weight of each compound | Luo et al. (2009) |
| Giant Sacha Inch or Giant Inca Peanut | Gas chromatography (GC)/ mass spectrometry (MS) | Identification of phytocompound | Seukep et al. (2020) |
| Black chokeberries, elderberries, red raspberries, and black raspberries | UV-Visible spectroscopy (UV/Vis) | Determination of total anthocyanins | Viskelis et al. (2010) |

*(Continued)*

**45**

## Table 2.4: Isolation and Identification Techniques for Nutraceuticals from Functional Fruits (*Continued*)

| Fruit | Technique Used | Purpose | Reference |
|---|---|---|---|
| Manga-beira | High-performance liquid chromatography coupled with diode array detector (HPLC-DAD) and Liquid chromatography coupled with Mass spectrometry (LC-MS) | Identification of bioactive compounds | Torres-Rêgo et al. (2016) |
| White and red guava | Gas chromatography (GC)/ Mass spectrometry (MS) | Determination of volatile compounds | Thuaytong and Anprung (2011) |
| Kiwi | Mass spectrometry (MS) | Determination of bioactive compounds | Park et al. (2014) |
| | Fourier transform infrared (FT-IR) | Analysis of interaction between polyphenols and human serum albumin (HSA) | Leontowicz et al. (2016) |
| | Nuclear magnetic resonance ($^1$H NMR) | Determination of various groups present in metabolites | Abdul Hamid et al. (2017) |
| Mulberry | Nuclear magnetic resonance (NMR) and Liquid chromatography-Mass spectrometry (LC/MS) | Identification and quantification of bioactive metabolites | Lee et al. (2018) |
| Bur | High-pressure liquid chromatography-quadrupole time-of-flight Mass spectrometry (HPLC-QTOFMS) and HPLC | Identification of polyphenolic compounds | Kim et al. (2019) |
| Mango | Visible spectrometry and HPLC-tandem mass spectrometry | Quantification of β-carotene and mangiferin | Hewavitharana et al. (2013) |
| Chokeberry | High-performance liquid chromatography (HPLC) coupled with a Tandem mass spectrometer and a Photodiode-array detector (LC-PDA-ESI-MS/MS), and UPLC-MS/MS (using a Q/TOF detector and a PDA detector) | Identification and quantification of polyphenols | Oszmiański and Lachowicz (2016) |
| Sweet cherry | Ultra-high-pressure liquid chromatograph Mass spectrometry analysis a Q-Exactive Orbitrap LC-MS/MS | Qualitative and quantitative profile of polyphenolic compounds | di Matteo et al. (2017) |
| Goji berry | High-performance liquid chromatography–diode array detector-Tandem mass spectrometry (HPLC-DAD-MS/MS) | Characterization of phenolic compounds | Tripodo et al. (2018) |
| Juçara | The ripening of juçara fruit by HPLC-ESI-MS/MS | Identification of phenolic compounds | Schulz et al. (2015) |

(*Continued*)

## Table 2.4: Isolation and Identification Techniques for Nutraceuticals from Functional Fruits (*Continued*)

| Fruit | Technique Used | Purpose | Reference |
|---|---|---|---|
| Durian | Fourier transform infrared (FTIR) | Determination of bioactive compounds | Paśko et al. (2019) |
| Victoria plums | Fourier transform infrared spectroscopy (FTIR) Gas chromatography/Mass spectrometry (GC/MS) | Detection of structural changes in bioactive compounds and analysis of volatile compounds | Rahaman et al. (2019) |
| Apricot | Gas chromatography/Mass spectrometry (GC/MS) Fourier-transform infrared spectroscopy (FTIR) | Detection of structural changes in bioactive compounds and analysis of volatile compounds | Rahaman et al. (2020) |
| Crabapples | Liquid chromatography mass spectrometry (LC-MS), ultra high-pressure liquid chromatography with diode array detector (UPLC) and Nuclear magnetic resonance (NMR) | Isolation and identification bioactive compounds | Wen et al. (2018b) |
| Date | Nuclear magnetic resonance ($^1$H NMR) | Determination of bioactive metabolites | Kadum et al. (2019) |

It is calculated as the ratio of the distance traveled by the compound from the starting point, i.e., solvent front, to the distance traveled by the solvent from the starting point.

*Thin-layer and column chromatography* are widely used techniques at the lab scale due to convenience, economic viability, and options for the stationary phase. The separation is based on the interaction of materials with a thin adsorbent layer affixed to a plate (Dhandhukia and Thakker 2011). This method works best for molecules with a low weight. This approach has the benefit over paper chromatography in that it is more adaptable, sensitive, and rapid in informing the researcher of the amount of chemicals present in a sample (Sasidharan et al. 2011). Thin-layer chromatography has numerous applications in phytochemistry and biochemistry and in formulating health-promoting products (Kumar, Jyotirmayee, and Sarangi 2013). Screening of separated components is done by spraying reagents, which give a unique color in accordance with the bioactive compound present in the plant extract (Sasidharan et al. 2011).

*High-performance liquid chromatography (HPLC)* is also a highly efficient, accurate, and fast method. It is used for the isolation, identification, and quantification of compounds, as mentioned in Table 2.4. It is different from column chromatography in terms of the pressurized flow of the mobile phase. HPLC instruments consist of a pump, injector, column, detector, recorder, and column heater. The small porous granular material is used as a stationary phase in a separation column. The plant extract, along with the mobile phase, is injected into a stainless steel capillary. Subsequently, the individual components of the plant extract migrate through the column at different rates because of their different degree of retention due to interaction with the stationary phase. A detector detects the separated components as they leave the column and receives them as a signal at the data acquisition unit. The most popular detectors are UV as they provide high sensitivity (Li, Jiang, and Chen 2004). This feature is a bonus if the component to be identified is present in a small quantity. There are other methods that provide the detection of phytochemicals, such as a diode array detector (DAD) attached to a mass spectrometer (MS) (Tsao and Deng 2004). For complex mixtures of plant extracts, liquid chromatography coupled with mass spectrometry (LC/MS) is a highly effective technique (He 2000; Cai et al. 2002)

*High-performance thin-layer chromatography* is more advanced than TLC, with higher efficiency and resolution, automatic spot visualization, and the capacity to perform quantitative analysis (Reich and Schibli 2005). The separation plates are contained in chambers rather than columns in this technique. HPTLC is made with plate adsorbents that are between 5–7 microns in size and a coating layer that is between 150–200 microns thick, which is thicker than TLC. Using constant pressure, the mobile phase is pushed over the plates. HPTLC is sometimes utilized in conjunction with spectroscopic techniques to optimize the analytical potential of these techniques (Attimarad et al. 2011).

*Optimum performance lamina chromatography* technique combines TLC and HPLC principles to create a preparative and analytical tool that may be used in both research and quality control laboratories. A liquid mobile phase is pushed through a column encased in a solid silica stationary phase or bonded phase media (amino, diol, cyano, ion exchange, C8, and C18). The mobile phase can be pushed through the planar columns at a constant velocity with a pressure of up to 50 bars (Ingle et al. 2017). Purification may employ one or more of the processes listed above, depending on convenience, ease of separation owing to the nature of the compounds involved, and availability of materials and tools.

### 2.5.1.1 *Other Liquid Chromatographic Techniques*

Phase states and mechanisms, phase polarities, separation zone geometries, the gradient of experimental parameters, and duration and column dimensions are all used to characterize chromatographic procedures. These are as follows:

*Adsorption chromatography* is also known as liquid/solid or displacement chromatography since it is based on solute interactions with active sites on the solid stationary phase. The stationary phase uses non-polar contacts, non-covalent bonds, hydrophobic interactions, and Van-Der-Waals forces to engage with specific functional groups in the mobile phase (Reich and Schibli 2005). The mobile phase compounds are sorted based on how similar they are to the stationary phase compounds, with loosely bound molecules eluting first.

*Partition chromatography* is also known as liquid/liquid chromatography. This is based on the interaction of the molecules to be separated with two immiscible liquid phases based on their solubility, with the stationary liquid phase adsorbed on a solid. The components that are soluble in one are held strongly by it; if mobile phase, they are the first to be eluted; nevertheless, if the stationary phase holds them more strongly, they will be delayed within the system (Akter et al. 2018).

*Affinity chromatography and ion chromatography* involve the stationary phase, where the extracts are injected into the columns and interact with the ligands. If they have a strong affinity for the ligands, they will be drawn to the stationary phase. They can be quickly washed away if they have a low or no affinity by using buffers with a different pH or a higher ionic strength, resulting in early elution. The ligands are frequently linked to the desired components (Ingle et al. 2017). On the other hand, ion chromatography uses electrical characteristics to separate ionic components from polar molecules in extracts. In the stationary phase, ion resins are utilized (Weiss 2016; Mtewa et al. 2018).

*Size exclusion chromatography* is also known as gel permeation, molecular sieve, or gel filtration chromatography, and it is based on the widths of the permeation spaces on the stationary phases. It may be used to determine molecular weights and their distribution in substances, particularly polymeric compounds (Uliyanchenko 2014). Interstices are created by the liquid stationary phase on a polymeric solid. To achieve phase equilibrium, sieving or partitioning might be utilized (Pirok et al. 2017). There is no chemical contact with this procedure.

*Bonded phases* method has the stationary phase, which involves organic species bonded to a solid surface. If the mobile phase is a liquid, the method is known as liquid-bonded phase equilibrium, and it is based on the partition of the liquid and the bonded surface (Bocian, Nowaczyk, and Buszewski 2012). If the mobile phase is a gas, the method is known as a gas-bonded phase, and the equilibrium is based on the partition between the gas and the bonded surface (Bocian, Nowaczyk, and Buszewski 2015).

*Gas chromatographic techniques* are used to separate volatile and stable compounds in situations where the species are distributed between the gas (mobile) and liquid (stationary) phases. Samples are vaporized and injected into a chromatographic column, where they are carried by an inert gas. The stationary phase is embedded in a solid material that is inert. The distribution of species in the test sample provides a measure of separation, as some get well mingled into the stationary phase and either delay or do not elute with the gas phase at all, whereas those that distribute well into the gas phase elute as the gas does (König and Hochmuth 2004). Gas chromatography is divided into three major categories based on phase states and mechanisms. The gas-bonded phase has already been discussed in the section on bonded phases. The second is gas-liquid, in which a liquid adsorbed onto a solid act as the stationary phase, and equilibrium is achieved through partitioning between gas and liquid. The final technique is the gas-solid technique, in which a solid serves as the stationary phase, and equilibrium is achieved through adsorption (Mtewa et al. 2018).

### 2.5.2 Non-Chromatographic Techniques

Spectroscopic techniques are used to provide the structural arrangement of certain molecules, and this work is purely based on the propagation of electromagnetic energy through the organic molecules. As some of the radiation is absorbed by the sample, a spectrum is produced according to the number of absorbed radiations. The structure of molecules can be identified on the basis of spectra, as these are particular to bonds in a molecule. The structures are identified through spectral interpretation or by searching and comparing with previously discovered, identified, and known data from spectral libraries. ChemSpider (Williams 2008) and PubChem (Wang et al. 2009), as well as drug and metabolism databases such as HMDB (Wishart et al. 2009), DrugBank (Wishart 2008), KEGG (Kanehisa et al. 2008), MZedDB (Draper et al. 2009), and ChEBI (Degtyarenko et al. 2008), offer a web-based search of formulae and masses of molecular compounds already known with any of their available biological test results (Brown et al. 2009).

*Nuclear Magnetic Resonance Spectroscopy (NMR)* works as a nucleus having magnetic moment ($^1H$ or $^{13}C$) experiences an intensive magnetic field; it will start the process just like a spinning top due to the excitation of nuclei to higher energy levels. At this moment, the application of radio waves of the same frequency, which matches the precession frequency, leads to develop the NMR spectrum. This technique provides extensive knowledge about the structure of molecules and connections in atoms. Time Domain NMR, which provides information on molecular dynamics in solutions, is another type of NMR. If the sample is solid, Solid-State NMR can be used to directly determine the structure of the solid sample. Because of their versatility, NMR techniques are increasingly replacing X-ray crystallography techniques in industrial applications (Ingle et al. 2017).

*Mass Spectrometry (MS)* is used to identify unknown compounds by determining molecular weight and find out the structure and chemical properties of individual molecules. This is accomplished by the conversion of molecules to ions which can be well-processed under electric and magnetic fields. The important phenomenon occurring in a mass spectrometer is:

*Ionization* of sample generally to cations. Sample molecules are bombarded by electrons released from a heat source. Sorting and separation of ions on the basis of mass and charge. These cations are moved away by charged plate and passed as a beam through slits. Measurement of ions and display on chart. As the beam passes, a perpendicular magnetic field deflects it giving an arc whose radius is related to the mass of ions.

*UV-Visible Spectroscopy (UV-Vis)* works based on the Beer-Lambert law, which states that the absorbance of a solution is directly proportional to the path length and concentration of the absorbing molecules within the solution. The UV-Vis region falls within the 200–350 nm and 350–700 nm range of the electromagnetic spectrum, respectively. Adsorption of light by molecules within the UV-Vis region results in electronic transitions in which electrons excite from bonding and/or nonbonding orbital to ant bonding orbital. Consequently, it facilitates information related to double or triple bonds and conjugated $\pi$ arrangements. It is primarily performed for qualitative analysis and the identification of various types of compounds on the basis of the fixed path.

*Infrared Spectroscopy (IR)* works on the principle that when a component is exposed to IR radiations, its molecules tend to absorb some part of it. The intensity of radiation absorption is specific to the polarity of bonds in an organic compound. This absorption develops vibrational motion in molecules. The vibrational frequencies vary according to the bonding type, hence identifying different functional groups which can be detected from frequency bands (4,000–1,300 $cm^{-1}$) in the spectrum obtained (Urbano et al. 2006). The most popular, rapid, and high-resolution technique based on IR spectroscopy is *Fourier Transform Infrared Spectroscopy (FTIR)* which identifies chemical components and clarifies the structure. FTIR can analyze all frequencies simultaneously instead of individually in a sequence for each component as in a simple IR spectrophotometer.

*Immunoassay* is used for monoclonal antibodies against low molecular mass bioactive natural compounds and drugs (Eberhardt et al. 2007). They are extremely sensitive to receptor binding analyses, qualitative, and quantitative analyses, and enzyme assays. In most cases, enzyme-linked immunosorbent assays (ELISA) are more sensitive than chromatography (Sasidharan et al. 2011). This method is efficient, but it is time-consuming to obtain reagents, ethical clearance for in vivo assays, and expensive for in vitro assays on cell lines.

## 2.6 FUTURE PROSPECTS OF NUTRACEUTICALS AND FUNCTIONAL FOODS WITH FRUITS

There has been ever-growing interest in nutraceuticals as witnessed by various studies described in the above sections. An average growth rate of 8.3% of CAGR over the period 2020–2027 is expected to bring the global nutraceuticals market size to USD 722.49 billion. Improving medical conditions such as cardiovascular diseases and malnutrition is the major driving force to uplift the dietary supplements market. The functional foods industry is anticipated to grow owing to increased medical care costs and the rise in the geriatric population across the globe. Moreover, the outbreak of the global pandemic COVID-19 is another fact for the consistent growth of the nutraceuticals industry to help people boost their immune systems. Expanding the body of scientific research that validates the effectiveness and safety of these new products will stimulate further investment in the technology and application. Apart from this, the innovations in storage, increased consumer awareness, improved health concerns, harmful effects of prolonged medications, and high costs of medicine are anticipated to stimulate the demand for nutraceuticals and functional foods in the coming years. The creativity of food technology might also contribute to further advances in developing food products that can support optimum health. People are more concerned about calorie intake and weight management, particularly in the United States, China, and India. This trend will probably improve the consumption of nutraceuticals, which, in turn, will significantly impact the growth of the industry. The United States holds the first rank in the largest and rapidly growing nutraceuticals market. It has been suggested that around 50% of the food market is related to the utilization of nutraceuticals and functional foods. The important points related to nutraceuticals and functional food markets are:

- Prebiotics and probiotics segment is expected to grow with a CAGR of 10.1% in the future as they have the potential to avoid illness from harmful microorganisms.

- The largest segment of dietary supplements, i.e., vitamins and minerals held a 40.71% share in 2019, as consumers are well aware of the relationship between diet and health

- Asia Pacific region is contributing to industry growth, as is retail chain expansion in countries viz. India, Japan, and China led to an increase in the consumption of dietary supplements and functional foods.

- The key market participants in nutraceuticals and functional foods manufacturing and development include Cargill, Incorporated, DuPont Nestle S.A., Archer Daniels Midland Company, WR Grace, Danone, General Mills, Innophos, and Amway Corporation.

In the case of fruits, the total market share of processed fruits in the fruits and vegetables sector is 65%. These include frozen, canned, dried fruit and vegetables, and others. Thus, one-third of natural foods gets wasted due to a lack of processing and storage facilities, and the perishable nature of foods. Research suggests that the wastage from these perishable plant products, particularly fruits, is a vital source of biologically active compounds. This shows that fruits and their by-products can play a vital role in the development of nutraceuticals along with waste management. Rudra et al. (2015) have reviewed various by-products of the fruit processing industry, such as seeds, stones, and peels, as prominent sources of dietary fibers, antioxidants, phytochemicals, antibiotics, vitamins, etc. According to Donno and Turrini (2020), local growers have an opportunity to improve their income by growing alternative and under utilized fruits with high nutritional value and capable of protecting humans from degenerative diseases. The formulation of new products by incorporating special ingredients of these fruits to improve the stability of foods could provide further applications of fruits in the nutraceuticals industry. Thus, the future of nutraceuticals and functional foods relies on the following factors:

- Adoption of innovative techniques to extract phytochemicals to the maximum extent without negative effects on the quality of fruit.

- Advancement in technologies for identifying and quantifying extracted compounds to make their effective use in nutraceuticals intended to prevent life-threatening diseases.

- Investment in secondary industries by food manufacturers to effectively utilize fruit-based by-products.

- Development of new techniques and measures to adopt waste reclamation to encourage the use of fruit wastage.

- Validation of effectiveness and safety of products by the expansion of scientific research

## 2.7 CONCLUSION

The struggle of the current world to achieve good air quality, drinkable water, fresh foods, and a clean environment is tremendously growing along with population growth and industrialization. Therefore, to achieve healthy living, people are leaning towards the consumption of dietary supplements or nutraceuticals and functional foods. Nutraceuticals are the best option as, along with providing the required nutrients, nutraceutical foods protect the human body from serious illness. Various nutrients such as vitamins, minerals, fats, proteins, etc., dietary supplements, viz. multivitamins, prebiotics, and herbal products, are vital sources of nutraceutical compounds.

The common techniques used in the food industries to produce nutraceuticals include blending and characterization, biological modifications, microencapsulation, edible coatings, and vacuum impregnation. Apart from these, the extraction of bioactive or functional compounds from fruits involves several processes with the most traditional techniques varying from solvent extraction to advanced such as microwave-assisted extraction, pulsed electric field extraction, ultrasound-assisted extraction, supercritical fluid extraction, supercritical antisolvent fractionation, subcritical water extraction, enzyme assisted extraction, instant controlled pressure drop-assisted extraction. After the extraction of these compounds, various chromatographic, and non-chromatographic techniques are being adopted industrially to isolate and identify these bioactive compounds. The future use of these compounds in human diets depends upon the adoption of innovative techniques of extraction, advanced technologies for identification and quantification, innovations in storage facilities, increased consumer awareness, improved health concerns, harmful effects for prolonged medications, and high costs of medicine.

## REFERENCES

Abdul Hamid, N. A., A. Mediani, M. Maulidiani, F. Abas, Y. S. Park, H. Leontowicz, M. Leontowicz, J. Namiesnik, and S. Gorinstein. 2017. "Characterization of Metabolites in Different Kiwifruit Varieties by NMR and Fluorescence Spectroscopy." *Journal of Pharmaceutical and Biomedical Analysis* 138 (May). Elsevier: 80–91. doi:10.1016/J.JPBA.2017.01.046.

Adam, F., M. Abert-Vian, G. Peltier, and F. Chemat. 2012. "'Solvent-Free' Ultrasound-Assisted Extraction of Lipids from Fresh Microalgae Cells: A Green, Clean and Scalable Process." *Bioresource Technology* 114 (June): 457–465. doi:10.1016/j.biortech.2012.02.096.

Adil, I. H., H. I. Çetin, M. E. Yener, and A. Bayindirli. 2007. "Subcritical (Carbon Dioxide + Ethanol) Extraction of Polyphenols from Apple and Peach Pomaces, and Determination of the Antioxidant Activities of the Extracts." *Journal of Supercritical Fluids* 43 (1). Elsevier: 55–63. doi:10.1016/J.SUPFLU. 2007.04.012.

Ajila, C. M., S. K. Brar, M. Verma, R. D. Tyagi, S. Godbout, and J. R. Valéro. 2011. "Extraction and Analysis of Polyphenols: Recent Trends." *Critical Reviews in Biotechnology* 31 (3). Taylor & Francis: 227–249. doi:10.3109/07388551. 2010.513677.

Akay, S., I. Alpak, and O. Yesil-Celiktas. 2011. "Effects of Process Parameters on Supercritical $CO_2$ Extraction of Total Phenols from Strawberry (*Arbutus unedo* L.) Fruits: An Optimization Study." *Journal of Separation Science* 34 (15). John Wiley & Sons, Ltd: 1925–1931. doi: https://doi.org/10.1002/jssc.201100361.

Akter, F., S. Saito, Y. Tasaki-Handa, and M. Shibukawa. 2018. "Partition/Ion-Exclusion Chromatographic Ion Stacking for the Analysis of Trace Anions in Water and Salt Samples by Ion Chromatograph." *Analytical Sciences* 34: 369–373.

Ali, S. I., F. K. El-Baz, G. A. E. El-Emary, E. A. Khan, and A. A. Mohamed. 2014. "HPLC-Analysis of Polyphenolic Compounds and Free Radical Scavenging Activity of Pomegranate Fruit (*Punica granatum* L.)." *International Journal of Pharmaceutical and Clinical Research* 6: 348–355. https://www.researchgate.net/publication/287291310.

Alikhani, M., and A. DaraeiGarmakhany. 2012. "Effect of Microencapsulated Essential Oils on Storage Life and Quality of Strawberry (*Fragaria ananassa* cv. Camarosa)." *Quality Assurance and Safety of Crops and Foods* 4 (2): 106–112. doi:10.1111/j.1757-837X.2012.00128.x.

Allaf, T., V. Tomao, K. Ruiz, and F. Chemat. 2013. "Instant Controlled Pressure Drop Technology and Ultrasound Assisted Extraction for Sequential Extraction of Essential Oil and Antioxidants." *Ultrasonics Sonochemistry* 20 (1). Elsevier: 239–246. doi:10.1016/J.ULTSONCH.2012.05.013.

Alam M. A., M. Z. I. Sarker, K. Ghafoor et al. 2017. "Bioactive Compounds and Extraction Techniques." In Nguyen V. T. (ed.), *Recovering Bioactive Compounds from Agricultural Wastes*, 33–53. Chichester: Wiley.

Alzorqi, I., and S. Manickam. 2016. "Ultrasonic Process Intensification for the Efficient Extraction of Nutritionally Active Ingredients of Polysaccharides from Bioresources." In *Handbook of Ultrasonics and Sonochemistry*, 1271–1286. Singapore: Springer Singapore. doi:10.1007/978-981-287-278-4_65.

Ashitha, G. N., and M. V. Prince. 2018. "Vacuum Impregnation: Applications in Food Industry." *International Journal of Food and Fermentation Technology* 8 (December). New Delhi Publishers: 141–151. doi:10.30954/2277-9396.02.2018.3.

Attimarad, M., K. K. M. Ahmed, B. E. Aldhubaib, and S. Harsha. 2011. "High-Performance Thin Layer Chromatography: A Powerful Analytical Technique in Pharmaceutical Drug Discovery." *Pharmaceutical Methods* 2 (2). EManuscript Services: 71–75. doi:10.4103/2229-4708.84436.

Bakowska-Barczak, A. M., and P. P. Kolodziejczyk. 2011. "Black Currant Poly-phenols: Their Storage Stability and Microencapsulation." *Industrial Crops and Products* 34 (2). Elsevier: 1301–1309. doi:10.1016/J.INDCROP.2010.10.002.

Baldwin, E. A., M. O. Nisperos, X. Chen, and R. D. Hagenmaier. 1996. "Improving Storage Life of Cut Apple and Potato with Edible Coating." *Postharvest Biology and Technology* 9 (2). Elsevier: 151–163. doi:10.1016/S0925-5214(96)00044-0.

Barros, R. G. C., J. K. S. Andrade, M. Denadai, M. L. Nunes, and N. Narain. 2017. "Evaluation of Bioactive Compounds Potential and Antioxidant Activity in Some Brazilian Exotic Fruit Residues." *Food Research International* 102 (December). Elsevier: 84–92. doi:10.1016/J.FOODRES.2017.09.082.

Belwal, T., S. M. Ezzat, L. Rastrelli, I. D. Bhatt, M. Daglia, A. Baldi, et al. 2018. "A Critical Analysis of Extraction Techniques Used for Botanicals: Trends, Priorities, Industrial Uses and Optimization Strategies." *TrAC Trends in Analytical Chemistry* 100: 82–102.

Berka-Zougali, B., A. Hassani, C. Besombes, and K. Allaf. 2010. "Extraction of Essential Oils from Algerian Myrtle Leaves Using Instant Controlled Pressure Drop Technology." *Journal of Chromatography A* 1217 (40). Elsevier: 6134–6142. doi:10.1016/J.CHROMA.2010.07.080.

Betoret, N., L. Puente, M. J. Díaz, M. J. Pagán, M. J. García, M. L. Gras, J. Martínez-Monzó, and P. Fito. 2003. "Development of Probiotic-Enriched Dried Fruits by Vacuum Impregnation." *Journal of Food Engineering* 56 (2–3). Elsevier: 273–277. doi:10.1016/S0260-8774(02)00268-6.

Bicudo, M. O. P., J. Jó, G. A. Oliveira, F. P. Chaimsohn, M. R. Sierakowski, R. A. Freitas, and R. H. Ribani. 2015. "Microencapsulation of Juçara (*Euterpe edulis* M.) Pulp by Spray Drying Using Different Carriers and Drying Temperatures." *Drying Technology* 33 (2). Taylor & Francis: 153–161. doi:10.1080/07373937.2014. 937872.

Bocian, S., A. Nowaczyk, and B. Buszewski. 2012. "New Alkyl-Phosphate Bonded Stationary Phases for Liquid Chromatographic Separation of Biologically Active Compounds." *Analytical and Bioanalytical Chemistry* 404 (August): 731–740. doi:10.1007/s00216-012-6134-0.

Bocian, S., A. Nowaczyk, and B. Buszewski. 2015. "Synthesis and Characterization of Ester-Bonded Stationary Phases for Liquid Chromatography." *Talanta* 131. Elsevier B.V.: 684–692. doi:10.1016/j.talanta.2014.07.069.

Borlaug, N. E. 2000. "Ending World Hunger. The Promise of Biotechnology and the Threat of Antiscience Zealotry." *Plant Physiology* 124: 487–490. https://academic. oup.com/plphys/article/124/2/487/6098810.

Brown, M., W. B. Dunn, P. Dobson, Y. Patel, C. L. Winder, S. Francis-Mcintyre, P. Begley, et al. 2009. "Mass Spectrometry Tools and Metabolite-Specific Databases for Molecular Identification in Metabolomics." *Analyst* 134. Royal Society of Chemistry: 1322–1332. doi:10.1039/b901179j.

Cabral, B. R. P., P. M. de Oliveira, G. M. Gelfuso, T. S. C. Quintão, J. A. Chaker, M. G. O. Karnikowski, and E. F. Gris. 2018. "Improving Stability of Antioxidant Compounds from *Plinia cauliflora* (Jabuticaba) Fruit Peel Extract by Encapsulation in Chitosan Microparticles." *Journal of Food Engineering* 238 (December). Elsevier: 195–201. doi:10.1016/J.JFOODENG.2018.06.004.

Cai, Z., F. S. C. Lee, X. R. Wang, and W. J. Yu. 2002. "A Capsule Review of Recent Studies on the Application of Mass Spectrometry in the Analysis of Chinese Medicinal Herbs." *Journal of Mass Spectrometry* 37 (10). John Wiley & Sons, Ltd: 1013–1024. doi: https://doi.org/10.1002/jms.370.

Cortés, M., E. Herrera, and E. Rodríguez. 2015. "Experimental Optimization of the Freeze Dry Process of Cape Gooseberry Added with Active Compounds by Vacuum Impregnation." *Vitae* 22(1): 47–56.

Cosmulescu, S., I. Trandafir, V. Nour, G. Achim, M. Botu, and O. Iordanescu. 2018. "Variation of Bioactive Compounds and Antioxidant Activity of Jujube (*Ziziphus jujuba*) Fruits at Different Stages of Ripening." *Notulae Botanicae Horti Agrobotanici Cluj-Napoca* 46 (1). Academic Press: 134–137. doi:10.15835/ nbha46110752.

Cravotto, G., L. Boffa, S. Mantegna, P. Perego, M. Avogadro, and P. Cintas. 2008. "Improved Extraction of Vegetable Oils under High-Intensity Ultrasound and/or Microwaves." *Ultrasonics Sonochemistry* 15 (5). Elsevier: 898–902. doi:10.1016/ J.ULTSONCH.2007.10.009.

Cvjetko Bubalo, M., S. Vidović, I. Radojčić Redovniković, and S. Jokić. 2018. "New Perspective in Extraction of Plant Biologically Active Compounds by Green Solvents." *Food and Bioproducts Processing* 109 (May). Elsevier: 52–73. doi:10.1016/J.FBP.2018.03.001.

Daintree, L. S., A. Kordikowski, and P. York. 2008. "Separation Processes for Organic Molecules Using SCF Technologies." *Advanced Drug Delivery Reviews*. doi:10.1016/j.addr.2007.03.024.

Daliri, E. B., and B. H. Lee. 2015. "Current Trends and Future Perspectives on Functional Foods and Nutraceuticals." In *Beneficial Microorganisms in Food and Nutraceuticals, Microbiology*, 221–244. Springer International Publishing Switzerland. doi:10.1007/978-3-319-23177-8_10.

DeFelice, S. L. 1995. "The Nutraceutical Revolution: Its Impact on Food Industry R&D." *Trends in Food Science & Technology* 6 (2). Elsevier: 59–61. doi:10.1016/S0924-2244(00)88944-X.

Degtyarenko, K., P. de matos, M. Ennis, J. Hastings, M. Zbinden, A. Mcnaught, R. Alcántara, M. Darsow, M. Guedj, and M. Ashburner. 2008. "ChEBI: A Database and Ontology for Chemical Entities of Biological Interest." *Nucleic Acids Research* 36 (January): D344–D350. doi:10.1093/nar/gkm791.

Deng, S., B. J. West, and C. J. Jensen. 2010. "A Quantitative Comparison of Phytochemical Components in Global Noni Fruits and Their Commercial Products." *Food Chemistry* 122 (1). Elsevier: 267–270. doi:10.1016/J.FOODCHEM.2010.01.031.

Desai, K. G. H., and H. J. Park. 2005. "Recent Developments in Microencapsulation of Food Ingredients." *Drying Technology* 23 (7). Taylor & Francis: 1361–1394. doi:10.1081/DRT-200063478.

Dhandhukia, P. C., and J. N. Thakker. 2011. "Quantitative Analysis and Validation of Method Using HPTLC." In *High-Performance Thin-Layer Chromatography (HPTLC)*, 203–221. Springer Berlin Heidelberg. doi:10.1007/978-3-642-14025-9_12.

di Matteo, Antonio, Rosa Russo, Giulia Graziani, Alberto Ritieni, and Claudio di Vaio. 2017. "Characterization of Autochthonous Sweet Cherry Cultivars (*Prunus avium* L.) of Southern Italy for Fruit Quality, Bioactive Compounds and Antioxidant Activity." *Journal of the Science of Food and Agriculture* 97 (9). John Wiley & Sons, Ltd: 2782–2794. doi: https://doi.org/10.1002/jsfa.8106.

Dias, C. O., J. S. O. de Almeida, S. S. Pinto, F. C. O. Santana, S. Verruck, C. M. O. Müller, E. S. Prudêncio, and R. D. M. C. Amboni. 2018. "Development and Physico-Chemical Characterization of Microencapsulated Bifidobacteria in Passion Fruit Juice: A Functional Non-Dairy Product for Probiotic Delivery." *Food Bioscience* 24 (August). Elsevier: 26–36. doi:10.1016/J.FBIO.2018.05.006.

Dolkar, D., P. Bakshi, V. K. Wali, V. Sharma, and R. A. Shah. 2017. "Fruits as Nutraceuticals." *Ecology, Environment and Conservation* 23: S113–S118.

Donno, D., and F. Turrini. 2020. "Plant Foods and Underutilized Fruits as Source of Functional Food Ingredients: Chemical Composition, Quality Traits, and Biological Properties." *Foods* MDPI AG. doi:10.3390/foods9101474.

Draper, J., D. P. Enot, D. Parker, M. Beckmann, S. Snowdon, W. Lin, and H. Zubair. 2009. "Metabolite Signal Identification in Accurate Mass Metabolomics Data with MZedDB, an Interactive m/z Annotation Tool Utilising Predicted Ionisation Behaviour 'Rules.'" *BMC Bioinformatics* 10 (July). doi:10.1186/1471-2105-10-227.

Dumitraşcu, L., N. Stănciuc, D. Borda, C. Neagu, E. Enachi, V. Barbu, and I. Aprodu. 2021. "Microencapsulation of Bioactive Compounds from Cornelian Cherry Fruits Using Different Biopolymers with Soy Proteins." *Food Bioscience* 41 (June). Elsevier: 101032. doi:10.1016/J.FBIO.2021.101032.

Dziezak, J. D. 1988. "Microencapsulation and Encapsulated Ingredients." *Food Technology* 42 (January): 136–151.

Eberhardt, T. L., X. Li, T. F. Shupe, and C. Y. Hse. 2007. "Chinese Tallow Tree (*Sapium sebiferum*) Utilization: Characterization of Extractives and Cell-Wall Chemistry." *Wood and Fiber Science* 39 (2): 319–324. https://www.researchgate.net/publication/251870157.

Efferth, T., and E. Koch. 2011. "Complex Interactions between Phytochemicals. The Multi-Target Therapeutic Concept of Phytotherapy." *Current Drug Targets* 12: 122–132.

El Kantar, S., N. Boussetta, N. Lebovka, F. Foucart, H. N. Rajha, R. G. Maroun, N. Louka, and E. Vorobiev. 2018. "Pulsed Electric Field Treatment of Citrus Fruits: Improvement of Juice and Polyphenols Extraction." *Innovative Food Science & Emerging Technologies* 46 (April). Elsevier: 153–161. doi:10.1016/J.IFSET.2017.09.024.

El Sohaimy, S. A. 2012. "Functional Foods and Nutraceuticals-Modern Approach to Food Science." *World Applied Sciences Journal* 20 (5): 691–708. doi:10.5829/idosi.wasj.2012.20.05.66119.

Ferreres, F., C. Grosso, A. Gil-Izquierdo, P. Valentão, A. T. Mota, and P. B. Andrade. 2017. "Optimization of the Recovery of High-Value Compounds from Pitaya Fruit By-Products Using Microwave-Assisted Extraction." *Food Chemistry* 230 (September). Elsevier Ltd: 463–474. doi:10.1016/j.foodchem.2017.03.061.

Fleurence, J., L. Massiani, O. Guyader, and S. Mabeau. 1995. "Use of Enzymatic Cell Wall Degradation for Improvement of Protein Extraction from *Chondrus crispus*, *Gracilaria verrucosa* and *Palmaria palmata*." *Journal of Applied Phycology* 7:393–397.

Fito, P., and R. Pastor. 1994. "Non-Diffusional Mechanisms Occurring during Vacuum Osmotic Dehydration." *Journal of Food Engineering* 21 (4). Elsevier: 513–519. doi:10.1016/0260-8774(94)90070-1.

Frassinetti, S., A. Castagna, M. Santin, L. Pozzo, I. Baratto, V. Longo, and A. Ranieri. 2020. "Gelatin-Based Coating Enriched with Blueberry Juice Preserves the Nutraceutical Quality and Reduces the Microbial Contamination of Tomato Fruit." *Natural Product Research*, September. Taylor & Francis: 1–5. doi:10.1080/14786419.2020.1824224.

García-Pérez, J. S., S. P. Cuéllar-Bermúdez, A. Arévalo-Gallegos, C. Salinas-Salazar, J. Rodríguez-Rodríguez, R. de la Cruz-Quiroz, H. M. N. Iqbal, and R. Parra-Saldívar. 2020. "Influence of Supercritical $CO_2$ Extraction on Fatty Acids Profile, Volatile Compounds and Bioactivities from *Rosmarinus officinalis*." *Waste and Biomass Valorization* 11 (4): 1527–1537. doi:10.1007/s12649-018-0408-5.

Gbashi, S., Adebo, O. A., Piater, L., Madala, N. E., & Njobeh, P. B. 2017. Subcritical water extraction of biological materials. *Separation & Purification Reviews* 46(1): 21–34.

Ghosh, S. K. 2006. "Functional Coatings and Microencapsulation: A General Perspective." In *Functional Coatings*. Weinheim, FRG: Wiley-VCH Verlag GmbH & Co. KGaA. doi:10.1002/3527608478.ch1.

Gil, M., A. Restrepo, L. Millán, L. Alzate, and B. Rojano. 2014. "Microencapsulation of Banana Passion Fruit (*Passiflora tripartita* var. *mollissima*): A New Alternative as a Natural Additive as Antioxidant." *Food and Nutrition Sciences* 5. Scientific Research Publishing, Inc: 671–682. doi:10.4236/fns.2014.58078.

Gitta, F., G. Végvári, G. Sándor, M. Stéger-Máté, E. Kállay, S. Szügyi, and M. Tóth. 2005. "HPLC Evolution of Anthocyanin Components in the Fruits of Hungarian Sour Cherry Cultivars during Ripening." *Journal of Food, Agriculture & Environment* 9 (1): 132–137. https://www.researchgate.net/publication/262232669.

Granato, D., G. F. Branco, F. Nazzaro, A. G. Cruz, and J. A. F. Faria. 2010. "Functional Foods and Nondairy Probiotic Food Development: Trends, Concepts, and Products." *Comprehensive Reviews in Food Science and Food Safety* 9: 292–302.

Gupta, S., D. Chauhan, K. Mehla, P. Sood, and A. Nair. 2010. "An Overview of Nutraceuticals: Current Scenario." *Journal of Basic and Clinical Pharmacy* 1 (2): 55–62. www.jbclinpharm.com.

Handayani, M. N., I. Khoerunnisa, D. Cakrawati, and A. Sulastri. 2018. "Microencapsulation of Dragon Fruit (*Hylocereus polyrhizus*) Peel Extract Using Maltodextrin." In *IOP Conference Series: Materials Science and Engineering*. 288. Institute of Physics Publishing. doi:10.1088/1757-899X/288/1/012099.

Hattab, M. E., G. Culioli, L. Piovetti, S. E. Chitour, and R. Valls. 2007. "Comparison of Various Extraction Methods for Identification and Determination of Volatile Metabolites from the Brown Alga *Dictyopteris* membranacea." *Journal of Chromatography A* 1143 (March): 1–7. doi:10.1016/j.chroma.2006.12.057.

Hayat, K., S. Hussain, S. Abbas, U. Farooq, B. Ding, S. Xia, C. Jia, X. Zhang, and W. Xia. 2009. "Optimized Microwave-Assisted Extraction of Phenolic Acids from Citrus Mandarin Peels and Evaluation of Antioxidant Activity In Vitro." *Separation and Purification Technology* 70 (November): 63–70. doi:10.1016/j.seppur.2009.08.012.

He, X. G. 2000. "On-Line Identification of Phytochemical Constituents in Botanical Extracts by Combined High-Performance Liquid Chromatographic–Diode Array Detection–Mass Spectrometric Techniques." *Journal of Chromatography A* 880 (1–2). Elsevier: 203–232. doi:10.1016/S0021-9673(00)00059-5.

Herrero, M., J. A. Mendiola, A. Cifuentes, and E. Ibáñez. 2010. "Supercritical Fluid Extraction: Recent Advances and Applications." *Journal of Chromatography A*. doi:10.1016/j.chroma.2009.12.019.

Hewavitharana, A. K., Z. W. Tan, R. Shimada, P. N. Shaw, and B. M. Flanagan. 2013. "Between Fruit Variability of the Bioactive Compounds, β-Carotene and Mangiferin, in Mango (*Mangifera indica*)." *Nutrition & Dietetics* 70 (2). John Wiley & Sons, Ltd: 158–163. doi: https://doi.org/10.1111/1747-0080.12009.

Ingle, K. P., A. G. Deshmukh, D. A. Padole, M. S. Dudhare, M. P. Moharil, and V. C. Khelurkar. 2017. "Phytochemicals: Extraction Methods, Identification and Detection of Bioactive Compounds from Plant Extracts." *Journal of Pharmacognosy and Phytochemistry* 6 (1): 32–36.

Kadum, H., A. A. Hamid, F. Abas, N. S. Ramli, A. K. S. Mohammed, B. J. Muhialdin, and A. H. Jaafar. 2019. "Bioactive Compounds Responsible for Antioxidant Activity of Different Varieties of Date (*Phoenix dactylifera* L.) Elucidated by 1H-NMR Based Metabolomics." *International Journal of Food Properties* 22 (1). Taylor & Francis: 462–476. doi:10.1080/10942912.2019.1590396.

Kalušević, A. M., S. M. Lević, B. R. Čalija, J. R. Milić, V. B. Pavlović, B. M. Bugarski, and V. A. Nedović. 2017. "Effects of Different Carrier Materials on Physicochemical Properties of Microencapsulated Grape Skin Extract." *Journal of Food Science and Technology* 54 (11). Springer India: 3411–3420. doi:10.1007/s13197-017-2790-6.

Kanehisa, M., M. Araki, S. Goto, M. Hattori, M. Hirakawa, M. Itoh, T. Katayama, et al. 2008. "KEGG for Linking Genomes to Life and the Environment." *Nucleic Acids Research* 36 (January): D480–D484. doi:10.1093/nar/gkm882.

Karki, B., B. P. Lamsal, S. Jung, J. van Leeuwen, A. L. Pometto, D. Grewell, and S. K. Khanal. 2010. "Enhancing Protein and Sugar Release from Defatted Soy Flakes Using Ultrasound Technology." *Journal of Food Engineering* 96 (2): 270–278. doi:10.1016/j.jfoodeng.2009.07.023.

Khalifa, I., H. Barakat, H. A. El-Mansy, and S. A. Soliman. 2017. Preserving Apple (*Malus domestica* var. *Anna*) Fruit Bioactive Substances Using Olive Wastes Extract-Chitosan Film Coating." *Information Processing in Agriculture* 4 (1). Elsevier: 90–99. doi:10.1016/J.INPA.2016.11.001.

Kheirkhah, H., S. Baroutian, and S. Y. Quek. 2019. "Evaluation of Bioactive Compounds Extracted from Hayward Kiwifruit Pomace by Subcritical Water Extraction." *Food and Bioproducts Processing* 115: 143–153.

Kim, D. W., W. J. Lee, Y. A. Gebru, H. S. Choi, S. H. Yeo, Y. J. Jeong, S. Kim, Y. H. Kim, and M. K. Kim. 2019. "Comparison of Bioactive Compounds and Antioxidant Activities of *Maclura tricuspidata* Fruit Extracts at Different Maturity Stages." *Molecules* 24 (3). MDPI AG. doi:10.3390/molecules24030567.

Kim, J., T. Nagaoka, Y. Ishida, T. Hasegawa, K. Kitagawa, and S. Lee. 2009. "Subcritical Water Extraction of Nutraceutical Compounds from Citrus Pomaces." *Separation Science and Technology* 44 (11). Taylor & Francis: 2598–2608. doi:10.1080/01496390903014375.

König, W. A., and D. H. Hochmuth. 2004. "Enantioselective Gas Chromatography in Flavor and Fragrance Analysis: Strategies for the Identification of Known and Unknown Plant Volatiles." *Journal of Chromatographic Science* 42: 423–439.

Koyu, H., A. Kazan, S. Demir, M. Z. Haznedaroglu, and O. Yesil-Celiktas. 2018. "Optimization of Microwave Assisted Extraction of *Morus nigra* L. Fruits Maximizing Tyrosinase Inhibitory Activity with Isolation of Bioactive

Constituents." *Food Chemistry* 248 (May). Elsevier: 183–191. doi:10.1016/J.FOODCHEM.2017.12.049.

Kubzdela, E. R., R. B. Marecik, and M. Kidoń. 2014. "Applicability of Vacuum Impregnation to Modify Physico-Chemical, Sensory and Nutritive Characteristics of Plant Origin Products—A Review." *International Journal of Molecular Sciences*. MDPI AG. doi:10.3390/ijms150916577.

Kumar, K., and S. Kumar. 2015. "Role of Nutraceuticals in Health and Disease Prevention: A Review." *South Asian Journal of Food Technology and Environment* 1 (2). Society for World Environment, Food and Technology: 116–121. doi:10.46370/sajfte.2015.v01i02.02.

Kumar, S., K. Jyotirmayee, and M. Sarangi. 2013. "Thin Layer Chromatography: A Tool of Biotechnology for Isolation of Bioactive Compounds from Medicinal Plants." *International Journal of Pharmaceutical Sciences Review and Research* 18 (1): 126–132.

Lachos-Perez, D., A. M. Baseggio, P. C. Mayanga-Torres, M. R. M. Junior, M. A. Rostagno, J. Martínez, and T. Forster-Carneiro. 2018. "Subcritical Water Extraction of Flavanones from Defatted Orange Peel." *Journal of Supercritical Fluids* 138: 7–16.

Lachowicz, S., J. Oszmiański, R. Wiśniewski, Ł. Seliga, and S. Pluta. 2019. "Chemical Parameters Profile Analysis by Liquid Chromatography and Antioxidative Activity of the Saskatoon Berry Fruits and Their Components." *European Food Research and Technology* 245 (9). Springer Verlag: 2007–2015. doi:10.1007/s00217-019-03311-2.

Lee, D., J. S. Yu, S. R. Lee, G. S. Hwang, K. S. Kang, J. G. Park, H. Y. Kim, K. H. Kim, and N. Yamabe. 2018. "Beneficial Effects of Bioactive Compounds in Mulberry Fruits against Cisplatin-Induced Nephrotoxicity." *International Journal of Molecular Sciences* 19 (4). MDPI AG. doi:10.3390/ijms19041117.

Leong, T. S. H., G. J. O. Martin, and M. Ashokkumar. 2017. "Ultrasonic Encapsulation – A Review." *Ultrasonics Sonochemistry* 35 (March). Elsevier: 605–614. doi:10.1016/J.ULTSONCH.2016.03.017.

Leontowicz, H., M. Leontowicz, P. Latocha, I. Jesion, Y. S. Park, E. Katrich, D. Barasch, A. Nemirovski, and S. Gorinstein. 2016. "Bioactivity and Nutritional Properties of Hardy Kiwi Fruit *Actinidia arguta* in Comparison with *Actinidia deliciosa* 'Hayward' and *Actinidia eriantha* 'Bidan.'" *Food Chemistry* 196 (April). Elsevier: 281–291. doi:10.1016/J.FOODCHEM.2015.08.127.

Lewinsohn, E., F. Schalechet, J. Wilkinson, K. Matsui, Y. Tadmor, K. H. Nam, O. Amar, et al. 2001. "Enhanced Levels of the Aroma and Flavor Compound S-Linalool by Metabolic Engineering of the Terpenoid Pathway in Tomato Fruits." *Plant Physiology* 127. American Society of Plant Biologists: 1256–1265. doi:10.1104/pp.010293.

Li, H. B., Y. Jiang, and F. Chen. 2004. "Separation Methods Used for *Scutellaria baicalensis* Active Components." *Journal of Chromatography B* 812 (1–2). Elsevier: 277–290. doi:10.1016/J.JCHROMB.2004.06.045.

Li, H., Z. Deng, T. Wu, R. Liu, S. Loewen, and R. Tsao. 2012. "Microwave-Assisted Extraction of Phenolics with Maximal Antioxidant Activities in Tomatoes." *Food Chemistry* 130 (February): 928–936. doi:10.1016/j.foodchem. 2011.08.019.

Li, S., and Q. H. Zhang. 2013. "Technologies for Extraction and Production of Bioactive Compounds to be Used as Nutraceuticals and Food Ingredients: An Overview." *Comprehensive Reviews in Food Science and Food Safety* 12 (1): 5–23. doi:10.1111/1541-4337.12005.

Li, Y., G. K. Skouroumounis, G. M. Elsey, and D. K. Taylor. 2011. "Microwave-Assistance Provides Very Rapid and Efficient Extraction of Grape Seed Polyphenols." *Food Chemistry* 129 (November): 570–576. doi:10.1016/j.foodchem. 2011.04.068.

Lima, M. M., G. Tribuzi, J. A. R. Souza, I. G. Souza, J. B. Laurindo and B. A. M. Carciofi. 2016. "Vacuum Impregnation and Drying of Calcium-Fortified Pineapple Snacks." *Lebensmittel-Wissenschaft & Technologie - Food Science and Technology* 72: 501–509.

Luo, W., M. Zhao, B. Yang, G. Shen, and G. Rao. 2009. "Identification of Bioactive Compounds in *Phyllenthus emblica* L. Fruit and Their Free Radical Scavenging Activities." *Food Chemistry* 114 (2). Elsevier: 499–504. doi:10.1016/J.FOODCHEM.2008.09.077.

Maran, J. P., B. Priya, and S. Manikandan. 2014. "Modeling and Optimization of Supercritical Fluid Extraction of Anthocyanin and Phenolic Compounds from *Syzygium cumini* Fruit Pulp." *Journal of Food Science and Technology* 51 (9): 1938–1946. doi:10.1007/s13197-013-1237-y.

Markom, M., H. Singh, and M. Hasan. 2001. "Supercritical $CO_2$ Fractionation of Crude Palm Oil." *Journal of Supercritical Fluids* 20 (1): 45–53.

Miron, T. L., M. Plaza, G. Bahrim, E. Ibáñez, and M. Herrero. 2011. "Chemical Composition of Bioactive Pressurized Extracts of Romanian Aromatic Plants." *Journal of Chromatography A* 1218 (July): 4918–4927. doi:10.1016/j.chroma.2010.11.055.

Moore, J., Z. Cheng, L. Su, and L. Yu. 2006. "Effects of Solid-State Enzymatic Treatments on the Antioxidant Properties of Wheat Bran." *Journal of Agricultural and Food Chemistry* 54 (24). American Chemical Society: 9032–9045. doi:10.1021/jf0616715.

Moreira, M. S., D. A Paula, E. M. F. Martins, É. N. R. Vieira, A. M. Ramos, and P. C. Stringheta. 2018. "Vacuum Impregnation of β-Carotene and Lutein in Minimally Processed Fruit Salad." *Journal of Food Processing and Preservation* 42 (March). Blackwell Publishing Ltd: e13545. doi:10.1111/jfpp.13545.

Mtewa, A. G., S. Deyno, F. M. Kasali, A. Annu, and D. C. Sesaazi. 2018. "General Extraction, Isolation and Characterization Techniques in Drug Discovery: A Review." *International Journal of Sciences: Basic and Applied Research* 38 (1): 10–24. http://gssrr.org/index.php?journal=JournalOfBasicAndApplied.

Mushtaq, M., B. Sultana, H. N. Bhatti, and M. Asghar. "RSM Based Optimized Enzyme-Assisted Extraction of Antioxidant Phenolics from Underutilized Watermelon (*Citrullus lanatus* Thunb.) Rind." *Journal of Food Science and Technology* 2015. 52(8): 5048–5056. doi: 10.1007/s13197-014-1562-9.

Oszmiański, J., and S. Lachowicz. 2016. "Effect of the Production of Dried Fruits and Juice from Chokeberry (*Aronia melanocarpa* L.) on the Content and Antioxidative Activity of Bioactive Compounds." *Molecules* 21 (8). MDPI AG. doi:10.3390/molecules21081098.

Oxley, J. 2014. "Overview of Microencapsulation Process Technologies." In *Microencapsulation in the Food Industry*, 35–46. Academic Press doi:10.1016/B978-0-12-404568-2.00004-2.

Ozturk, I., S. Karaman, M. Baslar, M. Cam, O. Caliskan, O. Sagdic, and H. Yalcin. 2014. "Aroma, Sugar and Anthocyanin Profile of Fruit and Seed of Mahlab (*Prunus mahaleb* L.): Optimization of Bioactive Compounds Extraction by Simplex Lattice Mixture Design." *Food Analytical Methods* 7 (4): 761–773. doi:10.1007/s12161-013-9679-4.

Paim, D. R. S. F., S. D. O. Costa, E. H. M. Walter, and R. V. Tonon. 2016. "Microencapsulation of Probiotic Jussara (*Euterpe edulis* M.) Juice by Spray Drying." *LWT* 74 (December). Academic Press: 21–25. doi:10.1016/J.LWT.2016.07.022.

Park, Y. S., J. Namiesnik, K. Vearasilp, H. Leontowicz, M. Leontowicz, D. Barasch, A. Nemirovski, S. Trakhtenberg, and S. Gorinstein. 2014. "Bioactive Compounds and the Antioxidant Capacity in New Kiwi Fruit Cultivars." *Food Chemistry* 165 (December). Elsevier: 354–361. doi:10.1016/J.FOODCHEM.2014.05.114.

Parthasarathi, S., P. N. Ezhilarasi, B. S. Jena, and C. Anandharamakrishnan. 2013. "A Comparative Study on Conventional and Microwave-Assisted Extraction for Microencapsulation of Garcinia Fruit Extract." *Food and Bioproducts Processing* 91 (2). Elsevier: 103–110. doi:10.1016/J.FBP.2012.10.004.

Paśko, P., M. Tyszka-Czochara, S. Trojan, S. Bobis-Wozowicz, P. Zagrodzki, J. Namieśnik, R. Haruenkit, S. Poovarodom, P. Pinsirodom, and S. Gorinstein. 2019. "Glycolytic Genes Expression, Proapoptotic Potential in Relation to the Total Content of Bioactive Compounds in Durian Fruits." *Food Research International* 125 (November). Elsevier: 108563. doi:10.1016/J.FOODRES.2019.108563.

Pattnaik, M., P. Pandey, G. J. O. Martin, H. N. Mishra, and M. Ashokkumar. 2021. "Innovative Technologies for Extraction and Microencapsulation of Bioactives from Plant-Based Food Waste and Their Applications in Functional Food Development." *Foods*. MDPI AG. doi:10.3390/foods10020279.

Pavlath, A. E., and W. Orts. 2009. "Edible Films and Coatings: Why, What, and How?" In *Edible Films and Coatings for Food Applications*. New York, NY: Springer New York. doi:10.1007/978-0-387-92824-1_1.

Persley, G. J., and J. N. Siedow. 1999. "Applications of Biotechnology to Crops: Benefits and Risks." *CAST* 12.

Pirok, B. W. J., P. Breuer, S. J. M. Hoppe, M. Chitty, E. Welch, T. Farkas, S. van der Wal, R. Peters, and P. J. Schoenmakers. 2017. "Size-Exclusion Chromatography Using Core-Shell Particles." *Journal of Chromatography A* 1486 (February). Elsevier B.V.: 96–102. doi:10.1016/j.chroma.2016.12.015.

Plaza, M., M. Amigo-Benavent, M. D. del Castillo, E. Ibáñez, and M. Herrero. 2010a. "Neoformation of Antioxidants in Glycation Model Systems Treated under Subcritical Water Extraction Conditions." *Food Research International* 43 (4). Elsevier: 1123–1129. doi:10.1016/J.FOODRES.2010.02.005.

Plaza, M., M. Amigo-Benavent, M. D. del Castillo, E. Ibáñez, and M. Herrero. 2010b. "Facts about the Formation of New Antioxidants in Natural Samples after Subcritical Water Extraction." *Food Research International* 43 (10). Elsevier: 2341–2348. doi:10.1016/J.FOODRES.2010.07.036.

Plaza, M., A. Cifuentes, and E. Ibáñez. 2008. "In the Search of New Functional Food Ingredients from Algae." *Trends in Food Science and Technology* 19 (January): 31–39. doi:10.1016/j.tifs.2007.07.012.

Pranoto, Y., V. M. Salokhe, and S. K. Rakshit. 2005. "Physical and Antibacte Rial Properties of Alginate-Based Edible Film Incorporated with Garlic Oil." *Food Research International* 38 (3). Elsevier: 267–272. doi:10.1016/J.FOODRES.2004.04.009.

Qu, W., H. Ma, J. Jia, R. He, L. Luo, and Z. Pan. 2012. "Enzymolysis Kinetics and Activities of ACE Inhibitory Peptides from Wheat Germ Protein Prepared with SFP Ultrasound-Assisted Processing." *Ultrasonics Sonochemistry* 19 (5). Elsevier B.V.: 1021–1026. doi:10.1016/j.ultsonch.2012.02.006.

Rahaman, A., X. A. Zeng, A. Kumari, M. Rafiq, A. Siddeeg, M. F. Manzoor, Z. Baloch, and Z. Ahmed. 2019. "Influence of Ultrasound-Assisted Osmotic Dehydration on Texture, Bioactive Compounds and Metabolites Analysis of Plum." *Ultrasonics Sonochemistry* 58 (November). Elsevier: 104643. doi:10.1016/J.ULTSONCH.2019.104643.

Rahaman, A., X. Zeng, M. A. Farooq, A. Kumari, M. A. Murtaza, N. Ahmad, M. F. Manzoor, et al. 2020. "Effect of Pulsed Electric Fields Processing on Physiochemical Properties and Bioactive Compounds of Apricot Juice." *Journal of Food Process Engineering* 43 (8). John Wiley & Sons, Ltd: e13449. doi:https://doi.org/10.1111/jfpe.13449.

Redondo, D., M. E. Venturini, E. Luengo, J. Raso, and E. Arias. 2018. "Pulsed Electric Fields as a Green Technology for the Extraction of Bioactive Compounds from Thinned Peach By-Products." *Innovative Food Science & Emerging Technologies* 45 (February). Elsevier: 335–343. doi:10.1016/J.IFSET.2017.12.004.

Reich, E., and A. Schibli. 2005. "Stationary Phases for Planar Separations – Plates for Modern TLC." *LC-GC North America* 23 (May): 458–469.

Rivas, J. C., L. M. C. Cabral, and M. H. M. da Rocha-Leão. 2021. "Microencapsulation of Guava Pulp Using Prebiotic Wall Material." *Brazilian Journal of Food Technology* 24. Instituto de Tecnologia de Alimentos - ITAL: e2020213. doi:10.1590/1981-6723.21320.

Roberfroid, M. B. 2002. "Global View on Functional Foods: European Perspectives." *British Journal of Nutrition* 88 (S2). Cambridge University Press: S133–S138. doi:10.1079/BJN2002677.

Rudra, S. G., J. Nishad, N. Jakhar, and C. Kaur. 2015. "Food Industry Waste: Mine of Nutraceuticals." *International Journal of Science, Environment and Technology* 4: 205–229. www.ijset.net.

Russo, M., I. L. Bonaccorsi, A. Arigò, F. Cacciola, L. de Gara, P. Dugo, and L. Mondello. 2021. "Blood Orange (*Citrus sinensis*) as a Rich Source of Nutraceuticals: Investigation of Bioactive Compounds in Different Parts of the Fruit by HPLC-PDA/MS." *Natural Product Research* 35 (22). Taylor & Francis: 4606–4610. doi:10.1080/14786419.2019.1696329.

Russo, M., C. Fanali, G. Tripodo, P. Dugo, R. Muleo, L. Dugo, L. de Gara, and L. Mondello. 2018. "Analysis of Phenolic Compounds in Different Parts of Pomegranate (*Punica granatum*) Fruit by HPLC-PDA-ESI/MS and Evaluation of Their Antioxidant Activity: Application to Different Italian Varieties." *Analytical and Bioanalytical Chemistry* 410 (15): 3507–3520. doi:10.1007/s00216-018-0854-8.

Santana, A. A., D. M. Cano-Higuita, R. A. de Oliveira, and V. R. N. Telis. 2016. "Influence of Different Combinations of Wall Materials on the Microencapsulation of Jussara Pulp (*Euterpe edulis*) by Spray Drying." *Food Chemistry* 212 (December). Elsevier: 1–9. doi:10.1016/J.FOODCHEM.2016.05.148.

Santana, A. A., L. E. Kurozawa, R. A. de Oliveira, and K. J. Park. 2013. "Influence of Process Conditions on the Physicochemical Properties of Pequi Powder Produced by Spray Drying." *Drying Technology* 31 (7). Taylor & Francis: 825–836. doi:10.1080/07373937.2013.766619.

Sasidharan, S., Y. Chen, D. Saravanan, K. M. Sundram, and L. Y. Latha. 2011. "Extraction, Isolation and Characterization of Bioactive Compounds from Plants' Extracts." *African Journal of Traditional, Complementary, and Alternative Medicines* 8 (1): 1–10.

Schulz, M., G. S. C. Borges, L. V. Gonzaga, S. K. T. Seraglio, I. S. Olivo, M. S. Azevedo, P. Nehring, et al. 2015. "Chemical Composition, Bioactive Compounds and Antioxidant Capacity of Juçara Fruit (*Euterpe edulis* Martius) during Ripening." *Food Research International* 77 (November). Elsevier: 125–131. doi:10.1016/J.FOODRES.2015.08.006.

Seukep, A. J., M. Fan, S. D. Sarker, V. Kuete, and M. Q. Guo. 2020. "*Plukenetia huayllabambana* Fruits: Analysis of Bioactive Compounds, Antibacterial Activity and Relative Action Mechanisms." *Plants* 9 (9). MDPI AG: 1–14. doi:10.3390/plants9091111.

Shah, N. P. 2007. "Functional Cultures and Health Benefits." *International Dairy Journal* 17 (11). Elsevier: 1262–1277. doi:10.1016/J.IDAIRYJ.2007.01.014.

Shen, L., X. Wang, Z. Wang et al. 2008. "Studies on Tea Protein Extraction Using Alkaline and Enzyme Methods." *Food Chemistry* 107:929–938.

Shimojo, K., K. Nakashima, N. Kamiya, and M. Goto. 2006. "Crown Ether-Mediated Extraction and Functional Conversion of Cytochrome c in Ionic Liquids." *Biomacromolecules* 7 (1). American Chemical Society: 2–5. doi:10.1021/bm050847t.

Siddeeg, A., M. F. Manzoor, M. H. Ahmad, N. Ahmad, Z. Ahmed, M. K. I. Khan, A. A. Maan, U. N. Mahr, X. A. Zeng, and A. F. Ammar. 2019. "Pulsed Electric Field-Assisted Ethanolic Extraction of Date Palm Fruits: Bioactive Compounds, Antioxidant Activity and Physicochemical Properties." *Processes* 7 (9). MDPI AG. doi:10.3390/pr7090585.

Silva, P. I., P. C. Stringheta, R. F. Teófilo, and I. R. N. de Oliveira. 2013. "Parameter Optimization for Spray-Drying Microencapsulation of Jaboticaba (*Myrciaria jaboticaba*) Peel Extracts Using Simultaneous Analysis of Responses." *Journal of Food Engineering* 117 (4). Elsevier: 538–544. doi:10.1016/J.JFOODENG.2012.08.039.

Singh, J., A. K. Rahul, N. Nama, and S. P. Singh. 2017. "A Review on Food Supplement-Nutraceuticals." *Asian Journal of Pharmaceutical Research and Development* 5 (3): 1–7. www.ajprd.com.

Soquetta, M. B., L. M. Terra, and C. P. Bastos. 2018. "Green Technologies for the Extraction of Bioactive Compounds in Fruits and Vegetables." *CYTA – Journal of Food*. Taylor and Francis Ltd. doi:10.1080/19476337.2017.1411978.

Starmans, D. A. J., and H. H. Nijhuis. 1996. "Extraction of Secondary Metabolites from Plant Material: A Review." *Trends in Food Science & Technology* 7: 191–197.

Szentmihályi, K., P. Vinklera, B. Lakatos, V. Illés, and M. Then. 2002. "Rose Hip (*Rosa canina* L.) Oil Obtained from Waste Hip Seeds by Different Extraction Methods." *Bioresource Technology* 82: 195–201.

Tampucci, S., A. Castagna, D. Monti, C. Manera, G. Saccomanni, P. Chetoni, E. Zucchetti, et al. 2021. "Tyrosol-Enriched Tomatoes by Diffusion across the Fruit Peel from a Chitosan Coating: A Proposal of Functional Food." *Foods* 10 (2). MDPI AG. doi:10.3390/foods10020335.

Thirugnanasambandham, K., and V. Sivakumar. 2017. "Microwave Assisted Extraction Process of Betalain from Dragon Fruit and Its Antioxidant Activities." *Journal of the Saudi Society of Agricultural Sciences* 16 (1). Elsevier: 41–48. doi:10.1016/J.JSSAS.2015.02.001.

Thuaytong, W, and P Anprung. 2011. "Bioactive Compounds and Prebiotic Activity in Thailand-Grown Red and White Guava Fruit (*Psidium guajava* L.)." *Food Science and Technology International* 17 (3). SAGE Publications Ltd STM: 205–212. doi:10.1177/1082013210382066.

Toledo-Madrid, K., T. Gallardo-Velázquez, and G. Osorio-Revilla. 2018. "Microencapsulation of Purple Cactus Pear Fruit (*Opuntia ficus indica*) Extract by the Combined Method W/O/W Double Emulsion-Spray Drying and Conventional Spray Drying: A Comparative Study." *Processes* 6 (10). MDPI AG: 189. doi:10.3390/pr6100189.

Torres-Rêgo, M., A. A. Furtado, M. A. O. Bitencourt, M. C. J. S. Lima, R. C. L. C. de Andrade, Eduardo Pereira de Azevedo, T. C. Soares, et al. 2016. "Anti-Inflammatory Activity of Aqueous Extract and Bioactive Compounds Identified from the Fruits of *Hancornia speciosa* Gomes (Apocynaceae)." *BMC Complementary and Alternative Medicine* 16 (1). BioMed Central Ltd. doi:10.1186/s12906-016-1259-x.

Tripodo, G., E. Ibáñez, A. Cifuentes, B. Gilbert-López, and C. Fanali. 2018. "Optimization of Pressurized Liquid Extraction by Response Surface Methodology of Goji Berry (*Lycium barbarum* L.) Phenolic Bioactive Compounds." *ELECTROPHORESIS* 39 (13). John Wiley & Sons, Ltd: 1673–1682. doi: https://doi.org/10.1002/elps.201700448.

Tsao, R., and Z. Deng. 2004. "Separation Procedures for Naturally Occurring Antioxidant Phytochemicals." *Journal of Chromatography B* 812 (1–2). Elsevier: 85–99. doi:10.1016/J.JCHROMB.2004.09.028.

Turan, F. T., A. Cengiz, and T. Kahyaoglu. 2015. "Evaluation of Ultrasonic Nozzle with Spray-Drying as a Novel Method for the Microencapsulation of Blueberry's Bioactive Compounds." *Innovative Food Science & Emerging Technologies* 32 (December). Elsevier: 136–145. doi:10.1016/J.IFSET.2015.09.011.

Uliyanchenko, E. 2014. "Size-Exclusion Chromatography—from High-Performance to Ultra-Performance." *Analytical and Bioanalytical Chemistry* 406 (25): 6087–6094. doi:10.1007/s00216-014-8041-z.

Urbano, M., M. D. Luque De Castro, P. M. Pérez, J. García-Olmo, and M. A. Gómez-Nieto. 2006. "Ultraviolet–Visible Spectroscopy and Pattern Recognition Methods for Differentiation and Classification of Wines." *Food Chemistry* 97 (1). Elsevier: 166–175. doi:10.1016/J.FOODCHEM.2005.05.001.

Villacrez, J. L., J. G. Carriazo, and C. Osorio. 2014. "Microencapsulation of Andes Berry (*Rubus glaucus* Benth.) Aqueous Extract by Spray Drying." *Food and Bioprocess Technology* 7 (5): 1445–1456. doi:10.1007/s11947-013-1172-y.

Villa-Rodríguez, J. A., F. J. Molina-Corral, J. F. Ayala-Zavala, G. I. Olivas, and G. A. González-Aguilar. 2011. "Effect of Maturity Stage on the Content of Fatty Acids and Antioxidant Activity of 'Hass' Avocado." *Food Research International* 44 (June): 1231–1237. doi:10.1016/j.foodres.2010.11.012.

Viskelis, P., M. Rubinskienė, R. Bobinaitė, and E. Dambrauskienė. 2010. "Bioactive Compounds and Antioxidant Activity of Small Fruits in Lithuania." *Journal of Food, Agriculture and Environment* 8: 259–263. https://www.researchgate.net/publication/282766756.

Wang, H., Y. Ye, H. Wang, J. Liu, Y. Liu, and B. Jiang. 2019. "HPLC-QTOF-MS/MS Profiling, Antioxidant, and α-Glucosidase Inhibitory Activities of *Pyracantha fortuneana* Fruit Extracts." *Journal of Food Biochemistry* 43 (5). John Wiley & Sons, Ltd: e12821. doi: https://doi.org/10.1111/jfbc.12821.

Wang, L., and C. L. Weller. 2006. "Recent Advances in Extraction of Nutraceuticals from Plants." *Trends in Food Science and Technology* 17 (6): 300–312. doi:10.1016/j.tifs.2005.12.004.

Wang, Y., J. Johnson-Cicalese, A. P. Singh, and N. Vorsa. 2017. "Characterization and Quantification of Flavonoids and Organic Acids over Fruit Development in American Cranberry (*Vaccinium macrocarpon*) Cultivars Using HPLC and APCI-MS/MS." *Plant Science* 262 (September). Elsevier: 91–102. doi:10.1016/J.PLANTSCI.2017.06.004.

Wang, Y., J. Xiao, T. O. Suzek, J. Zhang, J. Wang, and S. H. Bryant. 2009. "Pub-Chem: A Public Information System for Analyzing Bioactivities of Small Molecules." *Nucleic Acids Research* 37: W623–W633. doi:10.1093/nar/gkp456.

Weiss, J. 2016. *Handbook of Ion Chromatography, 3 Volume Set.* 1. John Wiley & Sons.

Wen, C., D. Wang, X. Li, T. Huang, C. Huang, and K. Hu. 2018b. "Targeted Isolation and Identification of Bioactive Compounds Lowering Cholesterol in the Crude Extracts of Crabapples Using UPLC-DAD-MS-SPE/NMR Based on Pharmacology-Guided PLS-DA." *Journal of Pharmaceutical and Biomedical Analysis* 150 (February). Elsevier: 144–151. doi:10.1016/J.JPBA.2017.11.061.

Wen, C., J. Zhang, H. Zhang, C. Se. Dzah, M. Zandile, Y. Duan, H. Ma, and X. Luo. 2018a. "Advances in Ultrasound Assisted Extraction of Bioactive Compounds from Cash Crops – A Review." *Ultrasonics Sonochemistry* 48 (November). Elsevier: 538–549. doi:10.1016/J.ULTSONCH.2018.07.018.

WHO, 2003. https://www.who.int/news/item/04-04-2022-billions-of-people-still-breathe-unhealthy-air-new-who-data

Williams, A. J. 2008. "A Perspective of Publicly Accessible/Open-Access Chemistry Databases." *Drug Discovery Today* 13 (11–12): 495–501. doi:10.1016/j.drudis.2008.03.017.

Wishart, D. S. 2008. "DrugBank and Its Relevance to Pharmacogenomics." *Pharmacogenomics*. Future Medicine Ltd. doi:10.2217/14622416.9.8.1155.

Wishart, D. S., C. Knox, A. C. Guo, R. Eisner, N. Young, B. Gautam, D. D. Hau, et al. 2009. "HMDB: A Knowledgebase for the Human Metabolome." *Nucleic Acids Research* 37: D603–D610. doi:10.1093/nar/gkn810.

Zacconi, F. C., A. L. Cabrera, F. Ordoñez-Retamales, J. M. del Valle, and J. C. de la Fuente. 2017. "Isothermal Solubility in Supercritical Carbon Dioxide of Solid Derivatives of 2,3-Dichloronaphthalene-1,4-Dione (Dichlone): 2-(Benzylamino)-3-Chloronaphthalene-1,4-Dione and 2-Chloro-3-(Phenethylamino)Naphthalene-1,4-Dione." *Journal of Supercritical Fluids* 129 (November). Elsevier: 75–82. doi:10.1016/J.SUPFLU.2016.09.014.

Zeisel, S. H. 1999. "Regulation of 'Nutraceuticals.'" *Science* 285: 1853–1855. doi:10.1126/science.285.5435.1853.

Zhang, H. F., X. H. Yang, and Y. Wang. 2011. "Microwave Assisted Extraction of Secondary Metabolites from Plants: Current Status and Future Directions." *Trends in Food Science and Technology*. doi:10.1016/j.tifs.2011.07.003.

Zhao, L., G. Zhao, F. Chen, Z. Wang, J. Wu, and X. Hu. 2006. "Different Effects of Microwave and Ultrasound on the Stability of (All-E)-Astaxanthin." *Journal of Agricultural and Food Chemistry* 54 (21). American Chemical Society: 8346–8351. doi:10.1021/jf061876d.

Zhao, Y., and J. Xie. 2004. "Practical Applications of Vacuum Impregnation in Fruit and Vegetable Processing." *Trends in Food Science & Technology* 15 (9). Elsevier: 434–451. doi:10.1016/J.TIFS.2004.01.008.

Zimmermann, M. B., and R. F. Hurrell. 2002. "Improving Iron, Zinc and Vitamin A Nutrition through Plant Biotechnology." *Current Opinion in Biotechnology* 13 (2). Elsevier Current Trends: 142–145. doi:10.1016/S0958-1669(02)00304-X.

# 3 Apple

*Jessica Pandohee, Parneet Kaur, Anuj Sharma, Ahmad Ali, Shahla Yasmin,
and Saurabh Kulshreshtha*

## CONTENTS

## 3.1 INTRODUCTION

The apple fruit (also known as *Malus domestica*) is an edible fruit, which is
cultivated across the world. While the first species (*Malus sieversii*) of apples
is thought to originate in Central Asia, the common apple (*M. domestica*) is the
result of several decades of hybridisation. To date, there are over 7,000 varieties
of apples, some of which are best consumed raw, cooked or as a substrate for the
manufacture of cider, jelly, and jam. The consumption of apples is believed to be
associated with multiple health benefits. While centuries ago, the proverb "an
apple a day keeps the doctor away" was recited to young children to encourage
the consumption of fruits, nowadays, increasing research has shown that
apple contains bioactive compounds with antioxidant and anti-inflammatory
properties (Biedrzycka and Amarowicz, 2008; Choi, 2019).

    Apples contain more than 4,000 flavonoids and other phytochemicals. The
biological properties of apple are due to the amount of polyphenols (including
flavonoids and phenolic acids). The concentration of these is often affected by
many factors, such as cultivar, harvest, storage, and processing of the apples.
For example, apples collected from higher altitude regions contain the highest
polyphenols and antioxidants (Bahukhandi et al., 2018). The concentration
of phytochemicals also varies greatly between the apple peels and the apple
flesh (Hyson, 2011). The peel of apple has been shown to contain the most
significant amount of total phenolic and flavonoid compounds, whereas the
flesh only comprises a subset of the phenolic compounds present in the peel
(Wolfe et al., 2003).

    Epidemiological studies have shown that phytochemicals are qualitatively
better antioxidants as compared to nutrient antioxidants such as Vitamin C and
E (Jan et al., 2010). According to Eberhardt et al. (2000), the amount of bioactive

DOI: 10.1201/9781003259213-3

compounds extracted from 0.1 mg of fresh apple has proven antioxidant and anticancer characteristics against colon and liver cancer cells. This chapter outlines the role of apples as a nutraceutical and functional food.

## 3.2 CHEMICAL COMPOSITION OF APPLE

Apples contain many biochemicals which are essential for the human health including phenolic compounds, organic acids, amino acids, vitamins, and phytochemicals (Zhang et al., 2010). The major phytochemicals present in apples are quercetin, catechin, phloridzin, and chlorogenic acid. These are all also strong antioxidants (Boyer and Liu, 2004).

### 3.2.1 Major Nutritional Components
#### 3.2.1.1 Carbohydrates

Carbohydrates are essential for growth as they are the structural component and also provide energy (Cheng et al., 2004). About 90% of the dry weight of apple consists of carbohydrates. Carbohydrates are classified into two types: Dietary fibre and digestible carbohydrates. Both are present in apples (Suni et al., 2000). In addition, apples have been shown to contain simple carbohydrates such as glucose, fructose, sucrose, xylose, galactose, starch, maltose, and ribose and its derivatives (sorbitol and myo-inositol) (Zhang et al., 2010). In apple varieties, the fructose content is much higher than the glucose content, and the fructose levels in apple are mainly affected by exogenous factors (Hermann and Bordewick-Dell, 2018). The fructose in apples causes an increase in plasma urate (Lotito and Frei, 2004), whereas free fructose has a more functional role in the gut as the latter contains bacteria that would feed on fructose resulting in fermentation (Skinner et al., 2018). Moreover, it has been shown that the apple seed contains about 24% of carbohydrates and about 4.9% of its dry weight and also some sugars and glycosides are present in the apple seed (Yu et al., 2007).

#### 3.2.1.2 Dietary Fibres

Dietary fibres are made up of soluble and insoluble fibres. The insoluble fibres constitute about 33.8%–60% and soluble fibres are about 13.5%–14.6% of total dietary fibres. Diets high in dietary fibre also improve the gut health and threat of serious diseases such as cancer (Bradbury et al., 2014; Park et al., 2013). Moreover, it was found that apple pomace contains more carbohydrates than the apple (Shalini et al., 2009); only one hundred grams provides about half of a person's necessary daily fibre consumption as it has high fibre content present in it (Skinner et al., 2018). The pectin present in the apple also reduces the cholesterol absorption as well as triglycerides in the blood and liver (Kumar and Chauhan, 2010).

#### 3.2.1.3 Proteins

The proteins in apples have been shown to be bioactive and have a functional role in the diet of humans. The apples are also a rich source of proteins, and it has been found that about 34% of the protein content is present in the apple seed (Yu et al., 2007). Furthermore, it was found that in apple, 53 of the proteins were identified and they play an important role in stress response and defence (49%), energy and metabolism (34%), synthesis of protein (3.8%), and cell structure and signal transduction (3.8%) (Shi et al., 2014). It is found that the interactions between polyphenols, especially flavonoids and plasma proteins, play an important role. The apples also contain various other nutritional constituents such as vitamins and antioxidants, which are also essential for human health and protect them from various diseases.

### 3.2.1.4 Vitamins

Apples are rich in vitamins C and E. It has been found that non-enzymatic antioxidants, vitamins C and E, are effective scavengers of reactive oxygen species (García-Closas et al., 2004). Apples also possess an antiproliferative effect on cancer cells due to their strong antioxidant bioactivity (Sun et al., 2002). Apple seed contains high values of vitamin E, which plays an important role in antioxidant activity and prevents chronic diseases (García-Closas et al., 2004). It has also been found that apple pomace contains vitamin C, which has the second highest free radical scavenging activity (Skinner et al., 2018).

### 3.2.1.5 Lipids

Fruit cells contain lipids and fatty acids, which are key structural and metabolic components. They are crucial components of biomembranes and play an important role in the majority of physical and chemical events that occur in a fruit cell (Duroňová et al., 2012). In a recent study, it was found that *Annurca* apple plays a vital role in the regulation of plasma cholesterol levels and *Annurca* flesh procyanidins which generally aggregate in the intestinal lumen, where they can potentially hinder cellular cholesterol uptake (Tenore et al., 2013).

### 3.2.2 Bioactive Compounds in Apple

### 3.2.2.1 Phenolic Compounds

Apples are a reliable source of various phenolic compounds (Sun et al., 2002). Polyphenols are phytochemicals that are well-known for their antioxidant qualities, which are beneficial for health. Procyanidins are the most prevalent class of phenolic compounds in apples (40%–89%) (Khanizadeh et al., 2008). Other phytochemicals detected in apples include hydroxycinnamic acids, dihydrochalcones, flavanols, anthocyanins, and flavan-3-ols. Polyphenols were found to be antimutagenic and anti-carcinogenic in nature (Miller and Evans, 1997). In a recent study, it was found that apple peels are the only source of anthocyanins, which also contribute to the red colour of the apple fruit (Sun et al., 2002).

### 3.2.2.2 Isoflavanoids

The peel of an apple includes a variety of flavonoid components, including procyanidins, catechins, epicatechins, chlorogenic acid, phloridzin, and quercetin conjugates (Schieber et al., 2001). The apple peel has a higher concentration of flavonoids than apple flesh. The flavonoids possess antioxidant benefits which aid the cardiovascular system. In a different study, it was found that quercetin improves the endothelial dysfunction and blood pressure, making more nitric oxide available in the system (Gunathilake and Considine, 2018). The antioxidant activity of apple pomace was due to the presence of high quantities of phloridzin, procyanidin B2, rutin + isoquercitrin, protocatechuic acid, and hyperin, according to the recent study (García et al., 2009).

### 3.2.2.3 Phytosterols

Apple also contains a number of substances with significant pharmacological potential. Triterpenic acids and phytosterols are two of the most important low-polarity bioactive chemicals found in apples. The triterpenic acid is present in the cuticle, which covers the aerial parts of plants (Woźniak et al., 2015). The phytosterols are best acknowledged for their ability to decrease cholesterol levels. In a recent study, it was found that the consumption of 1–3 g of phytosterols and their derivatives, like phytostanols, on a daily basis lowers the cholesterol levels. This has tremendous benefits to people who are prone to heart illness (Moreau et al., 2002). Apple pomace also contains many bioactive hydrophobic compounds including urosolic acid, oleanolic acid, and β-sitosterol, which are also essential for the metabolic health of human beings (Woźniak et al., 2018).

### 3.2.2.4 Carotenoids

Carotenoids are lipophilic chemicals that give fruits and vegetables their red, orange, and yellow colours, and they are also employed as food additives and give dishes their yellow-reddish colour (Moo-Huchin et al., 2017). Apple contains esterified carotenoids (violaxanthin, neoxanthin), β-carotene, lutein, zeaxanthin, antheraxanthin, etc. (Vondráková et al., 2020). Carotenoids are considered a potent antioxidant and singlet oxygen quencher which is involved in photoprotection (Merzlyak et al., 2003). They are also an essential component of the plant photosynthetic apparatus and play a role in light harvesting, stabilisation of thylakoid membranes, energy distribution, and dissipation in pigment protein complexes and photoprotection (Merzlyak and Solovchenko, 2002).

### 3.2.3 Volatile Organic Compounds

Apples are climacteric fruits that show an increase in the respiration and ethylene production after harvest, resulting in yellowing, decreased firmness, lower acidity, and the generation of volatile chemicals (Mattheis et al., 1991; Song and Bangerth, 1996). The apple sweetness depends on several volatile chemicals, including esters and farnesene. Sucrose, fructose, glucose, xylose, and sorbitol are the most common sugars and sugar alcohols found in apples. The apple sweetness can be enhanced more by the amount of sorbitol and organic acids than by the ratio of total sugar to organic acid concentration (Aprea et al., 2017). The main organic acids in apple are malic acid, which is approximately 90% of the acid content (Ackermann et al., 1992). Aprea et al. (2017) showed that in apples, more than half of the volatile compounds are esters (40 compounds) and alcohols (19 compounds) (Aprea et al., 2017).

### 3.3 BIOLOGICAL ACTIVITIES

#### 3.3.1 Antioxidant Properties

Oxidative stress is a phenomenon caused by an imbalance between production and accumulation of reactive oxygen species (ROS) in the cells and tissues. ROS is considered to cause oxidative damage, leading to occurrence of aging and related diseases. Polyphenols act as scavengers of reactive oxygen species. Inclusion of different nutraceuticals rich in polyphenols into the daily diet can potentially slow down the aging process (Piper and Bartke, 2008). Apple is considered an excellent source of polyphenol antioxidants (Lamperi et al., 2008). Apple polyphenol supplementation in fruit flies at 10 mg/mL prolonged the mean life span by 10% compared with the control (Peng et al., 2011). Similarly, Sunagawa et al. (2011) found apple procyanidins extended the mean life span of *Caenorhabditis elegans* by 8%–12%. In humans, it has been found that plasma ROS generation was suppressed in blood plasma within 30 minutes after apple juice consumption, and this radical scavenging effect was maintained for around two hours post-consumption (Ko et al., 2005). Vieira et al. (2012) described an increase of the antioxidant activity in human serum after apple consumption (300 mL apple juice—comparable to five apples—single dose).

Flavonoids such as quercetin, epicatechin, and procyanidin B2 contribute significantly to the total antioxidant activity of apples (Duda-Chodak et al.,

2011; Lee et al., 2003). Unripe apples, apple seeds, and peels have been found to have free radical scavenging properties (tested with ABTS and DPPH assays). The antioxidant activity of polyphenols is mainly due to their redox properties, which allow them to act as reducing agents, hydrogen donators, singlet oxygen quenchers, and metal chelators (Rice-Evans et al., 1996). Wang et al. (2019) showed that one of the apple polyphenols, phlorizin, had antioxidant and antiaging effects in fruit flies (*Drosophila melanogaster*). Another apple polyphenol phloretin has been widely investigated for its antioxidant, anti-inflammatory, and anticancer activities (Choi, 2019). Even flour prepared from apple residues obtained from pulp industries showed antioxidant activity (Lima et al., 2018).

Apple juice preparations may reduce important markers, including DNA damage markers (Barth et al., 2005). The whole fruit juice may have more effective antioxidant activity as compared to the individual components of juice. Extracts of whole apples cause significant dose-dependent reduction in the number and onset of mammary tumours in rats (Liu et al., 2005).

### 3.3.2 Anti-Inflammatory Properties

Inflammation is caused in response to infection, injury, or irritation. Most of the chronic diseases like cancer, diabetes, and cardiovascular and neurological disorders are related to both oxidative stress and inflammation. Inflammation results due to the breakdown of hyaluronic acid by hyaluronidase. Butkeviciute et al. (2021) have shown that apple extracts can inhibit hyaluronidase leading to reduction in the breakdown of hyaluronic acid and decrease of inflammation. Similarly, Espley et al. (2014) found that dietary flavonoids isolated from apples reduced the inflammation-related markers like interleukin-11 and interleukin-2 in intestinal tissue of mice. One of the apple polyphenols, quercetin, has also been attributed with anti-inflammatory activities (Jan et al., 2010). Apple cider vinegar (ACV), made from fermented apple juice, has low acidity (5% acetic acid) and contains organic acids, flavonoids, polyphenols, vitamins, and minerals. ACV inhibits pro-inflammatory cytokine secretion from human monocytes infected with *Escherichia coli*, *Candida albicans*, and *Staphylococcus aureus* and upregulates monocyte phagocytic capacity. This plays a key role in the functioning of innate immunity (Yagnik et al., 2018).

### 3.3.3 Antimicrobial and Antifungal Properties

Flavonoids are known to be synthesised by plants in response to microbial infection; therefore, they have been found in vitro to be effective antimicrobial substances against a wide array of microorganisms (Alberto et al., 2006). One of the apple polyphenols, quercetin, has also been attributed with antibacterial and antiviral activities (Jan et al., 2010). Similarly, the antibacterial activity of apple extracts was evaluated and confirmed against *Escherichia coli*, *Listeria monocytogenes*, *Salmonella Typhimurium*, and *Staphylococcus aureus* (Raphaelli et al., 2019). According to Sun et al. (2010), apple polyphenols are applicable as a natural antimicrobial agent and can be used as a safe food bacteriostat.

Apple cider vinegar has been found to have multiple antimicrobial potential with clinical therapeutic implications. Antimicrobial capacity of ACV against *Escherichia coli*, *Candida albicans*, and *Staphylococcus aureus* has been established (Yagnik et al., 2018). Various enzymes involved in growth, gene regulation, and metabolism of these microbes were impaired. In fact, apple cider vinegar in combination with honey was used in the past to combat infection and protect open skin wounds.

## 3.4 HEALTH BENEFITS OF APPLE CONSUMPTION

Apples are a rich source of phytochemicals which include quercetin, catechin, and phloridzin. The fruits are high in antioxidants, prevent chronic diseases and oxidative stress and lower ageing (Boyer and Liu, 2004). It is found that apples are among the most popular and frequently consumed fruit globally (Skinner et al., 2018). The consumption of apple decreases the risk of obesity, cancer, cardiovascular diseases, asthma, inflammation, high blood pressure, hyperglycaemia and diabetes. In a recent study, it was also found that the seed oil obtained from apple pomace contains a high amount of unsaturated fatty acids and is also effective against the proliferation of cancer cells of human lung carcinoma (A549) and human cervical cancer cells (SiHa) (Walia et al., 2014). The polyphenols present in apple provide antioxidant protection, preventing lipid, and DNA oxidation and cancer (Eberhardt et al., 2000). Figure 3.1 shows a schematic illustration of various health benefits of apple.

### 3.4.1 Modulation of the Immune System

The immune functions defend the body against the attack of pathogens and thus play an important role in the maintenance of health. The consumption of food with immune-modulating activity prevents the decline of the immune system and reduces the risk of diseases and cancer (Kaminogawa and Nanno, 2004). The consumption of polyphenols derived from plants reduces coronary heart diseases, age-related degradation, and cancers (Stevenson and Hurst, 2007). A well-functioning immune system is the backbone of the system. Apples are rich in polyphenols which provide antioxidant properties, mediation of cellular processes such as inflammation and modulation of gut microbiota. Apples and apple products are the major source of polyphenolics (Chun et al., 2007). The apples are also being evaluated for the reduction of atopic dermatitis and respiratory allergies. It was found that apple extracts reduce the effect of food allergens (Zuercher et al., 2010). In a recent study, it was also found that the seed extracts of apple have immunomodulatory activities on macrophages (Byun, 2013). The methanolic extract of *Aegle marmelos* (golden apple) fruit produces immunomodulatory activity by neutrophil adhesion

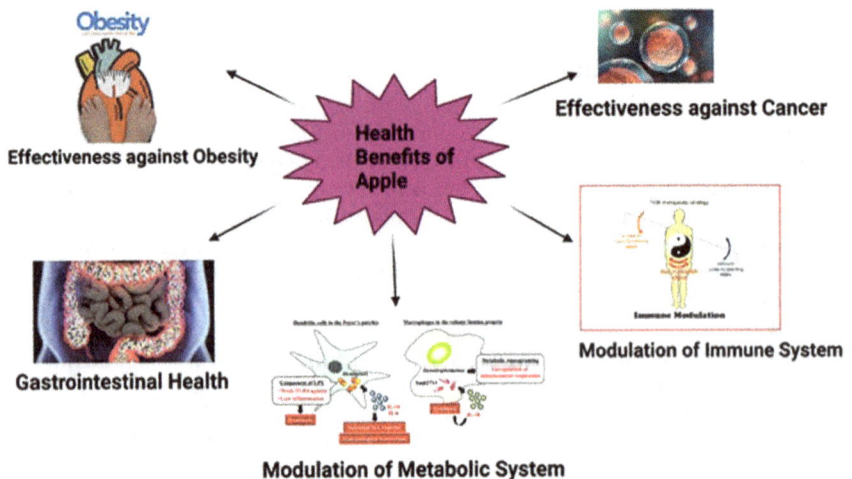

**Figure 3.1**   Various health benefits of apple.

test and carbon clearance assay (Bhar et al., 2019). The various studies were performed to analyse the immunomodulatory activity of the apple. Kim and Shin (2019) isolated a crude polysaccharide (KAV-0) from Korean apple vinegar which is novel in its origin. It was found that KAV-0 promoted the proliferation of peritoneal macrophages and RAW264.7 cells and also produced various cytokinin such as IL-6, IL012, and TNF, and the polysaccharide isolated has anti-metastatic activity and immunomodulatory activity which is beneficial to human health (Kim and Shin, 2019).

### 3.4.2 Modulation of the Metabolic System

Nowadays, obesity and metabolic disorders have emerged as a major health concern (Hoyt et al., 2014; Sassi et al., 2009). The main causes of metabolic disorders are unhealthy diet, lifestyle, and genetics. The fruits and extracts which are rich in polyphenols reduces the risk of inflammation, diabetes, and hepatic disorders. The metabolic syndrome is a serious result of diabetes which is characterised by serious cardiovascular risks. Therefore, in a diet enriched in nutritional quality, antioxidants are beneficial. In a study by Jiang et al., the potential effect of apple-derived pectin for weight gain, gut microbiota, and metabolic endotoxemia were evaluated in rats (Jiang et al., 2016). The results showed that the apple-derived pectin can modulate the gut microbiota, attenuate metabolic endotoxemia, and inflammation and also suppress weight gain and obesity (Jiang et al., 2016). To increase the nutritional food consumption by the body, biomarkers of food intake have been designed, and the identification of polyphenol microbial metabolite suggests that apple consumption mediates the gut microbial metabolic activity (Ulaszewska et al., 2020). Thus, several polyphenol metabolites can be used as a biomarker of food intake. It has also been reported that the cloudy apple juice induces metabolic alterations by reducing the levels of ALT and SDH and plays an important role in the protection against liver damage (Krajka-Kuźniak et al., 2015). The studies have shown that fruits such as apples and cherries, and their phytochemical extracts, are effective for decreasing the risks related to metabolic disorders such as abdominal fat accumulation, type 2 diabetes, heart disease, and inflammation (Hyson, 2011; McCune et al., 2010).

In a recent experiment, apple cedar vinegar was evaluated, and the results showed that the apple cedar vinegar is beneficial for the suppression of obesity-induced oxidative stress in HFD rats through the modulating antioxidant defence systems (Halima et al., 2018). Apple polyphenols were evaluated, and they were able to induce gene expression of enzymes related to tumour suppression, cell cycle arrest, regulation of cell cycle, apoptosis signalling, stress, and signal transduction and, in particular, detoxification enzymes systems (GST and UGT) in LT97 adenoma cells. It was also reported that lower concentrations were more effective and can act as chemo protectants (Veeriah et al., 2008). The regular consumption of apple juice decreases the total cholesterol and low-density lipoprotein (LDL) cholesterol levels (only for men), and also significantly increases high-density lipoprotein (HDL), cholesterol, and total antioxidant (Habanova et al., 2019). Hence, apple juice can play an important role in reducing the risk of cardiovascular diseases by positive modulation of the lipid profile and other health attributes in adults.

### 3.4.3 Gastrointestinal Health

The intestinal microbial community (microbiota) plays an essential role in the health and immunity of humans. The alterations or any changes in the microbiota cause a number of gastrointestinal disorders and metabolic diseases.

Fruits are the important constituents of our diet as they contain various nutrients such as vitamin C, carotenoids, and amino acids (Choi et al., 2016). The polyphenols present in apple extract has antioxidant activity. In a study, it was found that the apple peel polyphenol extract provides protection against macro and microscopic damage against the gastrointestinal tract and also has anti-inflammatory effects by preventing neutrophil infiltration in mucosa (Carrasco-Pozo et al., 2011). A study by Espley et al. (2014) evaluated that the apple was used to find out the dietary flavonoids on inflammation and gut microbiota and the results obtained showed that high flavonoid apples were associated with a decrease in the inflammation markers and changes in gut microbiota when supplemented to healthy mice. The pectin isolated from apples has a role on gastric emptying (GE), passage rate, and short chain fatty acid production along the porcine gastrointestinal tract, and short chain fatty acid content was increased significantly in the isolated pectin (Low et al., 2021).

To study the antioxidant ability during gastrointestinal digestion, the commonly consumed daily fruits such as apple, kiwi, grape, orange, and pomelo were selected and analysed. The results showed that the total phenolic content of the five fruit juices was generally stable or increased after gastric digestion, but the total phenolic content of apple juice significantly decreased during intestinal digestion due to the transition from lower pH conditions to a mildly alkaline intestinal environment (Quan et al., 2018).

### 3.4.4 Effectiveness against Obesity

Obesity is the most common nutritional disorder and is linked with certain diseases such as type 2 diabetes and atherosclerosis, which is the major risk factor for cardiovascular disease worldwide (Samout et al., 2016). Apples provide protection against the risk of obesity, arteriosclerosis, and diabetes due to the presence of soluble fibres and polyphenols present in them (Markowski et al., 2009). The consumption of apple and its products such as whole apples, apple sauces, and apple juice possess higher diet qualities and lower prevalence of obesity (O'Neil et al., 2015). Obesity is directly linked to diabetes. Apples also play an important role in protection against diabetes. The apple juice and apple peel extracts exhibit the antihyperglycemic effect by reducing inflammatory response and mitigating oxidative stress, which shows that they can be used as therapeutic agent for the treatment of the complication due to diabetes mellitus (Fathy and Drees, 2016).

Apple peel contains a high amount of quercetin which decreases the risk of type 2 diabetes (Boyer and Liu, 2004). In a recent study, it was examined that the unripe apple contains a high number of polyphenols which have anti-obesity effects, and the results showed that the unripe apple suppresses the increase in white adipose tissue mass, plasma, and liver triglyceride levels and also plays a role in the anti-obesity effect through the modulation of fatty acid metabolism in the liver and inhibition of absorption of fatty acids and carbohydrates (Azuma et al., 2013). Thus, high levels of polyphenols in unripe apple can act as a prophylactic for obesity. A recent study was performed to evaluate the potential of plant extracts such as almond, apple, cinnamon, orange, lime blossom, and grape vine and it was found that only apple extracts and cinnamon have anti-obesogenic potential because of their body fat lowering effects, and apple polyphenols also reduce the obesity-related metabolic complications (Boqué et al., 2013). Thus, it can be concluded that the apple and the extracts derived from apple are effective against obesity due to the high number of polyphenols present in them. Samout et al. (2016) evaluated the effect of apple pectin molecule on obesity. It was estimated that pectin molecule from apple decreased the total cholesterol level, triglycerides, uric acid, ASAT, LHD, ALP, and UREA, and increased the creatinine levels, superoxide dismutase, glutathione peroxidase, and catalase activities by 39%, 14% and 16% in liver; 5%, 7% and 31% in kidney; and 9%, 32%, and 22% in blood serum (Samout et al., 2016). It was determined that the interaction of the pectin molecule with both polysaccharide and the enzyme led to the anti-obesity effect of the pectin in several organ systems.

### 3.4.5 Effectiveness against Cancers

The consumption of fruits and vegetables decreases the risk of developing cancer and diabetes. The fruits contain the phytochemicals such as polyphenols which have anticancerous activity. The pectic oligosaccharides present in the apple induces cell cycle arrest and caspase dependent apoptosis in MDA-MB-231 cells of human breast cancer (Delphi and Sepehri, 2016). Colorectal cancer is the second most diagnosed cancer in women and is highly influenced by the lifestyle. In a recent study, it was found that the *Pelingo* apple is rich in components that can inhibit in vitro tumorigenesis and growth of human breast cancer cells and has potential chemo preventive activity (Schiavano et al., 2015). The phenolics present in fruits are the promising anti-carcinogenic agents. In a study by de Oliveira Raphaelli et al. it was found that phenolic extracts from apple *M. domestica* are used in the formulation of cosmetics, medicines for the protection of cellular DNA against UV radiations, and for the treatment of melanoma (de Oliveira Raphaelli et al., 2021).

Apple polyphenols possess anticancer, antioxidation, and anti-inflammation activity. Kao et al. (2015) found that apple phenols reduce cell viability, cause cell cycle arrest in G2/M phase, and cause apoptosis and mitotic catastrophe in human bladder cancer cells. Apples are the common source of dietary flavonoids. Apple peel flavonoid fraction 4 (AF4) is an ethanolic extract that contains numerous polyphenolic compounds, flavanols, and phenolic. In a recent study, it was found that a novel triterpenoid, named 3β-trans-cinnamoyloxy-2α-hydroxy-urs-12-en-28-oic acid (CHUA), from apple peels has a potential in vitro antitumour activity against human breast cancer cell lines and also induced apoptosis in (MDA- MB-231) cells via mitochondrial pathways and caspase-independent pathways (Qiao et al., 2015).

## 3.5 CONCLUSION AND FUTURE PERSPECTIVES

Several epidemiological studies have proven that the high antioxidant activity of phytochemicals in apple decreases the risk of cardiovascular diseases, asthma, and cancer. The antioxidation potential of apple plays a very important role in combatting these diseases. However, it is an indirect mechanism reported based on phytochemical fingerprints and radical scavenging activity of apple extracts. There may be other novel mechanisms involved which are required to be investigated. In addition, many studies have also suggested beneficial outcomes of apple consumption on Alzheimer's disease, diabetes, and factors accompanying the normal aging process. If this is indeed plausible, it indicates that the phytochemicals in apple act on a cellular as well as a metabolic level to prevent diseases. It also encourages reasoning that those phytochemicals in apple exhibit more complex mechanisms in suppression or modulation of mediator factors of above diseases and during the process of aging.

Although much research has been documented on the efficacy of phytochemicals in apple, there is rare documentation on the interaction of individual phytochemicals with each other, their bioavailability and mechanisms of action. Above other factors, more in-depth research in these areas may be helpful in giving insights to the potential mechanisms and role of diet in promoting overall health. In turn, it may prove to be helpful in minimising our dependence on nutrient supplements to boost our immunity.

## REFERENCES

Ackermann J, Fischer M, Amado R. Changes in sugars, acids, and amino acids during ripening and storage of apples (cv. Glockenapfel). *Journal of Agricultural and Food Chemistry.* 1992 Jul; 40(7):1131–4.

Alberto MR, Canavosio MAR, Manca De Nadra MC. Antimicrobial effect of polyphenols from apple skins on human bacterial pathogens. *Electronic Journal of Biotechnology.* 2006; 9(3).

Aprea E, Charles M, Endrizzi I, Corollaro ML, Betta E, Biasioli F, Gasperi F. Sweet taste in apple: The role of sorbitol, individual sugars, organic acids and volatile compounds. *Scientific Reports.* 2017 Mar 21; 7(1):1–0.

Azuma T, Osada K, Aikura E, Imasaka H, Handa M. Anti-obesity effect of dietary polyphenols from unripe apple in rats. *Nippon Shokuhin Kagaku Kogaku Kaishi.* 2013; 60(4):184–92.

Bahukhandi A, Dhyani P, Bhatt ID, Rawal RS. Variation in polyphenolics and antioxidant activity of traditional apple cultivars from West Himalaya, Uttarakhand. *Horticultural Plant Journal.* 2018; 4(4) :151–157.

Barth SW, Fähndrich C, Bub A, Dietrich H, Watzl B, Will F, Briviba K, Rechkemmer G. Cloudy apple juice decreases DNA damage, hyperproliferation and aberrant crypt foci development in the distal colon of DMH-initiated rats. *Carcinogenesis.* 2005; 26(8) :1414–21.

Bhar K, Mondal S, Suresh P. An eye-catching review of *Aegle marmelos* L. (golden apple). *Pharmacognosy Journal.* 2019; 11(2) :207–224.

Biedrzycka E, Amarowicz R. Diet and health: Apple polyphenols as antioxidants. *Food Reviews International.* 2008; 24(2). https://doi.org/10.1080/87559120801926302.

Boqué N, Campión J, de la Iglesia R, de la Garza AL, Milagro FI, San Román B, Bañuelos Ó, Martínez JA. Screening of polyphenolic plant extracts for anti-obesity properties in Wistar rats. *Journal of the Science of Food and Agriculture.* 2013 Mar 30; 93(5):1226–32.

Boyer J, Liu RH. Apple phytochemicals and their health benefits. *Nutrition Journal.* 2004 Dec; 3(1):1–5.

Bradbury KE, Appleby PN, Key TJ. Fruit, vegetable, and fiber intake in relation to cancer risk: Findings from the European prospective investigation into cancer and nutrition (EPIC). *American Journal of Clinical Nutrition.* 2014 Jul 1; 100(suppl_1):394S–8S.

Butkeviciute A, Petrikaite V, Jurgaityte V, Liaudanskas M, Janulis V. Antioxidant, anti-inflammatory, and cytotoxic activity of extracts from some commercial apple cultivars in two colorectal and glioblastoma human cell lines. *Antioxidants.* 2021; 10(7):1098.

Byun MW. Immunomodulatory activities of apple seed extracts on macrophage. *Journal of the Korean Society of Food Science and Nutrition.* 2013; 42(9):1513–7.

Carrasco-Pozo C, Speisky H, Brunser O, Pastene E, Gotteland M. Apple peel polyphenols protect against gastrointestinal mucosa alterations induced by indomethacin in rats. *Journal of Agricultural and Food Chemistry.* 2011 Jun 22; 59(12):6459–66.

Cheng L, Ma F, Ranwala D. Nitrogen storage and its interaction with carbohydrates of young apple trees in response to nitrogen supply. *Tree Physiology.* 2004 Jan 1; 24(1):91–8.

Choi BY. Biochemical basis of anticancer-effects of phloretin—A natural dihydrochalcone. *Molecules.* 2019.

Choi SH, Kozukue N, Kim HJ, Friedman M. Analysis of protein amino acids, non-protein amino acids and metabolites, dietary protein, glucose, fructose, sucrose, phenolic, and flavonoid content and antioxidative properties of potato tubers, peels, and cortexes (pulps). *Journal of Food Composition and Analysis.* 2016; 50:77–87.

Chun OK, Chung SJ, Song WO. Estimated dietary flavonoid intake and major food sources of US adults. *Journal of Nutrition.* 2007 May 1; 137(5):1244–52.

de Oliveira Raphaelli C, Azevedo JG, dos Santos Pereira E, Vinholes JR, Camargo TM, Hoffmann JF, Ribeiro JA, Vizzotto M, Rombaldi CV, Wink MR, Braganhol E. Phenolic-rich apple extracts have photoprotective and anticancer effect in dermal cells. *Phytomedicine Plus.* 2021 Nov 1; 1(4):100112.

Delphi L, Sepehri H. Apple pectin: A natural source for cancer suppression in 4T1 breast cancer cells in vitro and express p53 in mouse bearing 4T1 cancer tumors, in vivo. *Biomedicine & Pharmacotherapy.* 2016 Dec 1; 84:637–44.

Duda-Chodak A, Tarko T, Tuszyński T. Antioxidant activity of apples – An impact of maturity stage and fruit part. *Acta Scientiarum Polonorum, Technologia Alimentaria.* 2011; 10(4).

Duroňová K, Márová I, Čertík M, Obruča S. Changes in lipid composition of apple surface layer during long-term storage in controlled atmosphere. *Chemical Papers.* 2012 Oct 1; 66(10):940–8.

Eberhardt M, Lee C, Liu RH. Antioxidant activity of fresh apples. *Nature.* 2000 Jun 22;405:903–4.

Espley RV, Butts CA, Laing WA, Martell S, Smith H, McGhie TK, Zhang J, Paturi G, Hedderley D, Bovy A, Schouten HJ. Dietary flavonoids from modified apple reduce inflammation markers and modulate gut microbiota in mice. *Journal of Nutrition.* 2014 Feb 1; 144(2):146–54.

Fathy SM, Drees EA. Protective effects of Egyptian cloudy apple juice and apple peel extract on lipid peroxidation, antioxidant enzymes and inflammatory status in diabetic rat pancreas. *BMC Complement Al-Tern Med.* 2016; 16:8.

García YD, Valles BS, Lobo AP. Phenolic and antioxidant composition of by-products from the cider industry: Apple pomace. *Food Chemistry.* 2009 Dec 15; 117(4):731–8.

García-Closas R, Berenguer A, Tormo MJ, Sánchez MJ, Quiros JR, Navarro C, Arnaud R, Dorronsoro M, Chirlaque MD, Barricarte A, Ardanaz E. Dietary sources of vitamin C, vitamin E and specific carotenoids in Spain. *British Journal of Nutrition.* 2004 Jun; 91(6):1005–11.

Gunathilake DM, Considine M. Flavonoids rich apple for healthy life. *MOJ Food Processing & Technology.* 2018; 6(3):00149.

Habanova M, Saraiva JA, Holovicova M, Moreira SA, Fidalgo LG, Haban M, Gazo J, Schwarzova M, Chlebo P, Bronkowska M. Effect of berries/apple mixed juice consumption on the positive modulation of human lipid profile. *Journal of Functional Foods.* 2019 Sep 1; 60:103417.

Halima BH, Sonia G, Sarra K, Houda BJ, Fethi BS, Abdallah A. Apple cider vinegar attenuates oxidative stress and reduces the risk of obesity in high-fat-fed male Wistar rats. *Journal of Medicinal Food.* 2018 Jan 1; 21(1):70–80.

Hermann K, Bordewick-Dell U. Fructose in different apple varieties. Implications for apple consumption in persons affected by fructose intolerance. *Ernährungs Umschau.* 2018; 65:48–52.

Hoyt CL, Burnette JL, Auster-Gussman L. Obesity is a disease: Examining the self-regulatory impact of this public-health message. *Psychological Science.* 2014; 25:997–1002.

Hyson DA. A comprehensive review of apples and apple components and their relationship to human health. *Advances in Nutrition.* 2011; 2(5):408–20.

Jan AT, Kamli MR, Murtaza I, Singh JB, Arif A, Haq QMR. Dietary flavonoid quercetin and associated health benefits—An overview. *Food Reviews International.* 2010; 26(3):302–17.

Jiang T, Gao X, Wu C, Tian F, Lei Q, Bi J, Xie B, Wang HY, Chen S, Wang X. Apple-derived pectin modulates gut microbiota, improves gut barrier function, and attenuates metabolic endotoxemia in rats with diet-induced obesity. *Nutrients.* 2016 Mar; 8(3):126.

Kaminogawa S, Nanno M. Modulation of immune functions by foods. *Evidence-Based Complementary and Alternative Medicine.* 2004 Aug; 1(3):241–50.

Kao YL, Kuo YM, Lee YR, Yang SF, Chen WR, Lee HJ. Apple polyphenol induces cell apoptosis, cell cycle arrest at G2/M phase, and mitotic catastrophe in human bladder transitional carcinoma cells. *Journal of Functional Foods.* 2015 Apr 1; 14:384–94.

Khanizadeh S, Tsao R, Rekika D, Yang R, Charles MT, Rupasinghe HV. Polyphenol composition and total antioxidant capacity of selected apple genotypes for processing. *Journal of Food Composition and Analysis*. 2008 Aug 1; 21(5):396–401.

Kim HW, Shin KS. Immunomodulatory and anti-metastatic activities of a crude polysaccharide isolated from Korean apple vinegar. *Korean Journal of Food Science and Technology*. 2019; 51(2):152–9.

Ko SH, Seong Won C, Ye SK, Cho BL, Hyun Sook K, Chung MH. Comparison of the antioxidant activities of nine different fruits in human plasma. *Journal of Medicinal Food*. 2005; 8(1): 41–6.

Krajka-Kuźniak V, Szaefer H, Ignatowicz E, Ad-amska T, Markowski J, Baer-Dubowska W. Influence of cloudy apple juice on N-nitrosodiethylamine-induced liver injury and phases I and II biotransformation enzymes in rat liver. *Acta Poloniae Pharmaceutica*. 2015; 72:267–76.

Kumar A, Chauhan GS. Extraction and characterization of pectin from apple pomace and its evaluation as lipase (steapsin) inhibitor. *Carbohydrate Polymers*. 2010 Sep 5; 82(2):454–9.

Lamperi L, Chiuminatto U, Cincinelli A, Galvan P, Giordani E, Lepri L, del Bubba M. Polyphenol levels and free radical scavenging activities of four apple cultivars from integrated and organic farming in different Italian areas. *Journal of Agricultural and Food Chemistry*. 2008; 56(15):6536–46.

Lee KW, Kim YJ, Kim DO, Lee HJ, Lee CY. Major phenolics in apple and their contribution to the total antioxidant capacity. *Journal of Agricultural and Food Chemistry*. 2003; 51(22):1–4.

Lima DS, Almeida Duarte NB, Costa Barreto DL, de Oliveira GP, Takahashi JA, Fabrini SP, Sande D. Passion fruit and apple: From residues to antioxidant, antimicrobial and anti-Alzheimer's potential. *Ciencia Rural*. 2018; 48(9).

Liu RH, Liu J, Chen B. Apples prevent mammary tumors in rats. *Journal of Agricultural and Food Chemistry*. 2005; 53(6). https://doi.org/10.1021/jf058010c.

Lotito SB, Frei B. The increase in human plasma antioxidant capacity after apple consumption is due to the metabolic effect of fructose on urate, not apple-derived antioxidant flavonoids. *Free Radical Biology and Medicine*. 2004 Jul 15; 37(2):251–8.

Low DY, Pluschke AM, Flanagan B, Sonni F, Grant LJ, Williams BA, Gidley MJ. Isolated pectin (apple) and fruit pulp (mango) impact gastric emptying, passage rate and short chain fatty acid (SCFA) production differently along the pig gastrointestinal tract. *Food Hydrocolloids*. 2021 Sep 1; 118:106723.

Markowski J, Baron A, Mieszczakowska M, Płocharski W. Chemical composition of French and Polish cloudy apple juices. *Journal of Horticultural Science and Biotechnology*. 2009; (ISAFRUIT Special Issue 84):6874.

Mattheis JP, Fellman JK, Chen PM, Patterson ME. Changes in headspace volatiles during physiological development of Bisbee Delicious apple fruits. *Journal of Agricultural and Food Chemistry.* 1991 Nov; 39(11):1902–6.

McCune LM, Kubota C, Stendell-Hollis NR, Thomson CA. Cherries and health: A review. *Critical Reviews in Food Science and Nutrition.* 2010 Dec 30; 51(1):1–2.

Merzlyak MN, Solovchenko AE. Photostability of pigments in ripening apple fruit: A possible photoprotective role of carotenoids during plant senescence. *Plant Science.* 2002 Oct 1; 163(4):881–8.

Merzlyak MN, Solovchenko AE, Gitelson AA. Reflectance spectral features and non-destructive estimation of chlorophyll, carotenoid and anthocyanin content in apple fruit. *Postharvest Biology and Technology.* 2003 Feb 1; 27(2):197–211.

Miller NJ, Rice-Evans CA. The relative contributions of ascorbic acid and phenolic antioxidants to the total antioxidant activity of orange and apple fruit juices and blackcurrant drink. *Food Chemistry.* 1997 Nov 1; 60(3):331–7.

Moo-Huchin VM, Gonzlez-Aguilar GA, Moo-Huchin M, Ortiz-V E. Carotenoid composition and antioxidant activity of extracts from tropical fruits. Science Faculty of Chiang Mai University. 2017.

Moreau RA, Whitaker BD, Hicks KB. Phytosterols, phytostanols, and their conjugates in foods: Structural diversity, quantitative analysis, and health-promoting uses. *Progress in Lipid Research.* 2002 Nov 1; 41(6):457–500.

O'Neil CE, Nicklas TA, Fulgoni III VL. Consumption of apples is associated with a better diet quality and reduced risk of obesity in children: National Health and Nutrition Examination Survey (NHANES), 2003–2010. *Nutrition Journal.* 2015; 14:48.

Park KH, Lee KY, Lee HG. Chemical composition and physicochemical properties of barley dietary fiber by chemical modification. *International Journal of Biological Macromolecules.* 2013 Sep 1; 60:360–5.

Peng C, Edwin Chan HY, Huang Y, Yu H, Chen ZY. Apple polyphenols extend the mean lifespan of *Drosophila melanogaster. Journal of Agricultural and Food Chemistry.* 2011; 59(5):2097–2106.

Piper MDW, Bartke A.. Diet and aging. *Cell Metabolism.* 2008; 8(2):99–104. https://doi.org/10.1016/j.cmet.2008.06.012.

Qiao A, Wang Y, Xiang L, Wang C, He X. A novel triterpenoid isolated from apple functions as an anti-mammary tumor agent via a mitochondrial and caspase-independent apoptosis pathway. *Journal of Agricultural and Food Chemistry.* 2015 Jan 14; 63(1):185–91.

Quan W, Tao Y, Lu M, Yuan B, Chen J, Zeng M, Qin F, Guo F, He Z. Stability of the phenolic compounds and antioxidant capacity of five fruit (apple, orange, grape, pomelo and kiwi) juices during in vitro-simulated gastrointestinal digestion. *International Journal of Food Science & Technology.* 2018 May; 53(5):1131–9.

Raphaelli CO, Dannenberg G, Dalmazo GO, Pereira ES, Radünz M, Vizzotto M, Fiorentini AM, Gandra EA, Nora L. Antibacterial and antioxidant properties of phenolic-rich extracts from apple (*Malus domestica* cv. Gala). *International Food Research Journal.* 2019; 26(4):1133–42.

Rice-Evans CA, Miller NJ, Paganga G. Structure-antioxidant activity relationships of flavonoids and phenolic acids. *Free Radical Biology and Medicine.* 1996; 20(7):933–56.

Samout N, Bouzenna H, Dhibi S, Ncib S, ElFeki A, Hfaiedh N. Therapeutic effect of apple pectin in obese rats. *Biomedicine & Pharmacotherapy.* 2016 Oct 1; 83:1233–8.

Sassi F; Devaux M; Cecchini M; Rusticelli E. *The Obesity Epidemic: Analysis of Past and Projected Future Trends in Selected OECD Countries*; OECD Health Working Papers; Organisation for Economic Cooperation and Development (OECD): Paris, France. 2009.

Schiavano GF, De Santi M, Brandi G, Fanelli M, Bucchini A, Giamperi L, Giomaro G. Inhibition of breast cancer cell proliferation and in vitro tumorigenesis by a new red apple cultivar. *PLoS One.* 2015 Aug 18; 10(8):e0135840.

Schieber A, Keller P, Carle R. Determination of phenolic acids and flavonoids of apple and pear by high-performance liquid chromatography. *Journal of Chromatography A.* 2001 Mar 2; 910(2):265–73.

Shalini R, Gupta DK, Singh A. Drying kinetics of apple pomace cake. *Journal of Food Science and Technology.* 2009 Sep 1; 46(5):477.

Shi Y, Jiang L, Zhang L, Kang R, Yu Z. Dynamic changes in proteins during apple (*Malus x domestica*) fruit ripening and storage. *Horticulture Research.* 2014 Jan 22; 1(1):1–21.

Skinner RC, Gigliotti JC, Ku KM, Tou JC. A comprehensive analysis of the composition, health benefits, and safety of apple pomace. *Nutrition Reviews.* 2018 Dec 1; 76(12):893–909.

Song J, Bangerth F. The effect of harvest date on aroma compound production from 'Golden Delicious' apple fruit and relationship to respiration and ethylene production. *Postharvest Biology and Technology.* 1996 Sep 1; 8(4):259–69.

Stevenson DE, Hurst RD. Polyphenolic phytochemicals–just antioxidants or much more? *Cellular and Molecular Life Sciences.* 2007 Nov; 64(22):2900–16.

Sun J, Chu YF, Wu X, Liu RH. Antioxidant and antiproliferative activities of common fruits. *Journal of Agricultural and Food Chemistry.* 2002 Dec 4; 50(25):7449–54.

Sun HN, Sun AD, Su YJ, Gao XJ, Hu XD, Chen J. Antimicrobial effect of apple polyphenols. *Beijing Linye Daxue Xuebao/Journal of Beijing Forestry University.* 2010; 32(4).

Sunagawa T, Shimizu T, Kanda T, Tagashira M, Sami M, Shirasawa T. Procyanidins from apples (*Malus pumila* Mill.) extend the lifespan of *Caenorhabditis elegans*. *Planta Medica*. 2011; 77(2).

Suni M, Nyman M, Eriksson NA, Björk L, Björck I. Carbohydrate composition and content of organic acids in fresh and stored apples. *Journal of the Science of Food and Agriculture*. 2000 Aug; 80(10):1538–44.

Tenore GC, Campiglia P, Stiuso P, Ritieni A, Novellino E. Nutraceutical potential of polyphenolic fractions from Annurca apple (*M. pumila* Miller cv Annurca). *Food Chemistry*. 2013 Oct 15; 140(4):614–22.

Ulaszewska MM, Koutsos A, Trošt K, Stanstrup J, Garcia-Aloy M, Scholz M, Fava F, Natella F, Scaccini C, Vrhovsek U, Tuohy K. Two apples a day modulate human: Microbiome co-metabolic processing of polyphenols, tyrosine and tryptophan. *European Journal of Nutrition*. 2020 Dec; 59(8):3691–714.

Veeriah S, Miene C, Habermann N, Hofmann T, Klenow S, Sauer J, Böhmer F, Wölfl S, Pool-Zobel BL. Apple polyphenols modulate expression of selected genes related to toxicological defence and stress response in human colon adenoma cells. *International Journal of Cancer*. 2008 Jun 15; 122(12):2647–55.

Vieira, FGK, di Pietro PF, da Silva EL, Borges GSC, Nunes EC, Fett R. Improvement of serum antioxidant status in humans after the acute intake of apple juices. *Nutrition Research*. 2012; 32(3):229–32.

Vondráková Z, Trávníčková A, Malbeck J, Haisel D, Černý R, Cvikrová M. The effect of storage conditions on the carotenoid and phenolic acid contents of selected apple cultivars. *European Food Research and Technology*. 2020 Sep; 246(9):1783–94.

Walia M, Rawat K, Bhushan S, Padwad YS, Singh B. Fatty acid composition, physicochemical properties, antioxidant and cytotoxic activity of apple seed oil obtained from apple pomace. *Journal of the Science of Food and Agriculture*. 2014; 94:929–34.

Wang H, Sun Z, Liu D, Li X, Rehman RUR, Wang H, Wu Z. Apple phlorizin attenuates oxidative stress in *Drosophila melanogaster*. *Journal of Food Biochemistry*. 2019; 43(3). https://doi.org/10.1111/jfbc.12744.

Wolfe K, Wu X, Liu RH. Antioxidant activity of apple peels. *Journal of Agricultural and Food Chemistry*. 2003; 51(3):609–14.

Woźniak Ł, Skąpska S, Marszałek K. Ursolic acid—A pentacyclic triterpenoid with a wide spectrum of pharmacological activities. *Molecules*. 2015 Nov; 20(11):20614–41.

Woźniak Ł, Szakiel A, Pączkowski C, Marszałek K, Skąpska S, Kowalska H, Jędrzejczak R. Extraction of triterpenic acids and phytosterols from apple pomace with supercritical carbon dioxide: Impact of process parameters, modelling of kinetics, and scaling-up study. *Molecules*. 2018 Nov; 23(11):279.

Xiao J, Kai G. A review of dietary polyphenol-plasma protein interactions: Characterization, influence on the bioactivity, and structure-affinity relationship. *Critical Reviews in Food Science and Nutrition.* 2012 Jan 1; 52(1):85–101.

Yagnik D, Serafin V, Shah AJ. Antimicrobial activity of apple cider vinegar against *Escherichia coli, Staphylococcus aureus* and *Candida albicans*; downregulating cytokine and microbial protein expression. *Scientific Reports.* 2018; 8(1). https://doi.org/10.1038/s41598-017-18618-x.

Yu X, Van De Voort FR, Li Z, Yue T. Proximate composition of the apple seed and characterization of its oil. *International Journal of Food Engineering.* 2007 Oct 25; 3(5).

Zhang Y, Li P, Cheng L. Developmental changes of carbohydrates, organic acids, amino acids, and phenolic compounds in 'Honeycrisp' apple flesh. *Food Chemistry.* 2010 Dec 15; 123(4):1013–8.

Zuercher AW, Holvoet S, Weiss M, Mercenier A. Polyphenol-enriched apple extract attenuates food allergy in mice. *Clinical & Experimental Allergy.* 2010 Jun; 40(6):942–50.

# 4 Bioactives in Pear

*Kanchan Sharma*

## CONTENTS

## 4.1 INTRODUCTION

Pear plants have been cultivated by men since ancient times. Fresh pear and its processed products are consumed worldwide. It has also been used as an ancient remedy against certain ill health conditions in many countries. Pear is basically native to Asia and Europe, and in the seventeenth century people of North America started cultivating it (Reiland and Slavin 2015). Pear is a nutritious fruit and resembles much with apple in its nutritional properties due to its botanical relationship with it. The genus *Pyrus*, from the Rosaceae family, is commonly used for both pears and apples, though the genus *Malus* is most frequently used for apples, while *Pyrus* is used for pears. They are one of the highest fibre containing fruits at 4.1 g fibre per medium size pear (Hong et al. 2021). There are many cultivars of pear existing across the globe but among these only a hundred varieties are grown for commercial purpose. Most common pear cultivars are European or French pear, Asian pear which is commonly known as apple pear due to the resemblance of its texture with that of apple, Chinese white pear, etc. It is also known as pome fruit which means a fruit having a characteristic compartment core (Reiland and Slavin 2015). Figure 4.1 shows the Asian and European pear.

DOI: 10.1201/9781003259213-4

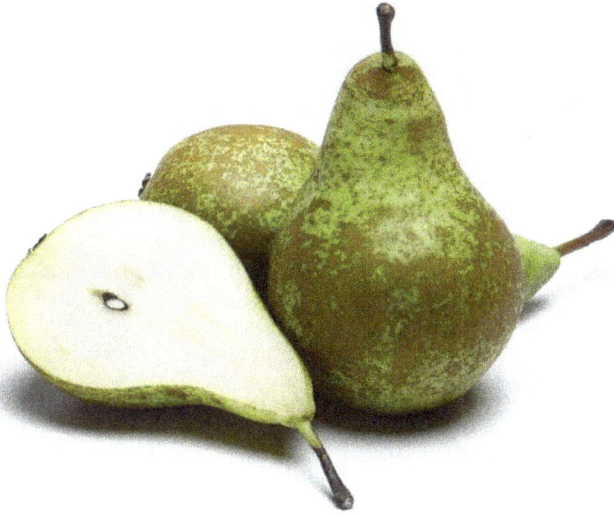

Asian pear (*Pyrus pyrifolia*)

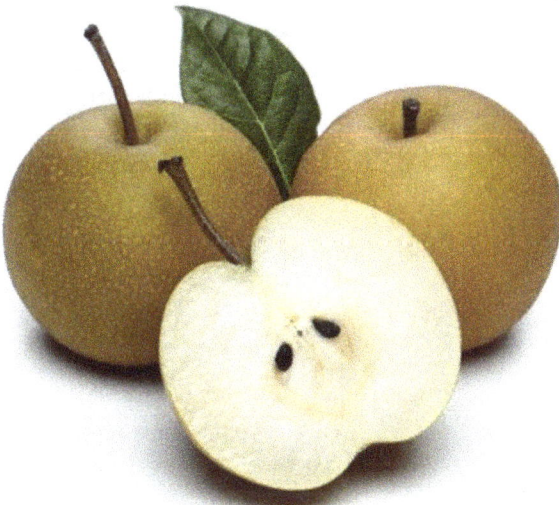

European pear (*Pyrus communis*)

**Figure 4.1**  Pictures showing Asian and European pears.

## 4.2  SYSTEMATIC CLASSIFICATION

| | | |
|---|---|---|
| Kingdom | – | Plantae |
| Division | – | Magnoliophyta |
| Class | – | Magnoliopsida |
| Order | _ | Rosales |
| Family | _ | Rosaceae |
| Sub-family | – | Amygdaloideae |
| Genus | – | *Pyrus* |

## 4.3 ORIGIN

Plants belonging to the *Pyrus* genus originated in central Asia. Later it was cultivated in other nearby countries also including India. In India, it was cultivated both in the eastern and western regions from the primary centre where it originated (Li et al. 2014). There were many wild species of pear which originated from Europe through Caucasus, Turkmenistan, Altai mountains, Siberia to China and Japan (Bunzel and Ralph 2006; Russell et al. 2009; Li et al. 2012). It grows in habitats like temperate regions of Europe and West Asia. More commonly it is harvested in the Northern Hemisphere in late summer to October. Its folk name is Bagu-goshaa or Naakh. It is good in pectin and in India it is grown in Punjab, Himachal Pradesh and Kashmir mainly. Its tree grows about 13 meters in height and has ovate leaves and white or rosy flowers (Kaur and Arya 2012). Scientific and common names of different species are given below (Hong et al. 2021):

| Scientific name | Other name |
|---|---|
| *Pyrus anatolica* | Turkey pear |
| *Pyrus bretschneideri* | Chinese white pear |
| *Pyrus clleryana* | Korean sun pear |
| *Pyrus communis* | European pear |
| *Pyrus malus* | Ussurian pear, Manchurian pear, Herbin pear |
| *Pyrus pashia* | Himalayan pear, Afghan pear |
| *Pyrus pyrifolia* | Asian pear, nakh |
| *Pyrus sinkiagenesis* | Xinjiang pear |
| *Pyrus amygdaliformis* | Almond-leaved pear |
| *Pyrus armeniacifolia* | Apricot-leaved pear |
| *Pyrus bourgaeana* | Iberian pear |
| *Pyrus nivalis* | Snow pear |
| *Pyrus syriace* | Syrian pear |

## 4.4 TRADITIONAL USES

In ancient times in Korea, pears were used as a medicine and also as a fruit since the Samhan period (300 BCE–300 CE). Its other uses were to relieve fever, quench thirst and suppress cough (Yang 2018). It was also considered as useful in conditions like dysarthria. It was also used against decomposition of burn wounds, relieving pain and enhancing urination and defecation. In addition to these effects, pears were believed to calm dyspnea and mental conditions. Moreover, pears were believed to have a moisturizing effect over lungs, have a cooling effect over the heart, facilitate sputum removal and detoxification alcohol poisoning. Their flowers were used to clean dirt over the face. The bark of the pear tree, especially its decoction, was used to fight against diseases commonly caused during winters. The leaves of the pear tree were used to treat scrotal hernia while pounded leaf extract was used to treat mushroom poisoning (Hong et al. 2021).

There are around 26 primary species of pears having more than 5,000 cultivars around the globe. Despite being distributed widely around the world, all species belonging to the genus *Pyrus* are able to undergo interspecific hybridization. *Pyrus* species are mainly divided into three groups as species having small fruit with two carpels, those having large fruit with five carpels and their hybrids with three or four carpels. It was reported that Asian pear species are small fruited species and are five in number, mainly distributed in China, Japan and Korea, where it was for ornamental purpose or as rootstocks. On the other hand, *P. communis* originated in Europe. Some Asian and European pear species are given as follows:

## Asian pear species

*P. calleryana* Decne

*P. koehnei* C.K.Schneid

*P. dimorphophylla* Makino

*P. betulaefolia* Bunge

## Medium-large fruited Asian pear species

*P. pashia* D.Don

*P. pyrifolia* Nakai

*P. hondoensis* Nakai and Kikuchi

*P. ussuriensis* Maxim

## West Asian species

*P. amygdaliformis* Vill

*P. elaegrifolia* Pall

*P. glabra* Boiss

*P. salicifolia* Pall

*P. syriaca* Boiss

*P. regelii* Rehd.

## European and North African species

*P. communis* L.

*P. spinosa* Forssk

*P. cordata* Desv.

*P. cossonii* Redher

*P. gharbiana* Trab

*P. mamorensis* Trab

*P. bourgaeana* Decne

*P. calleryana* Decne

Many volatile compounds are ester, alcohols, hydrocarbons, aldehyde, ketones, etc. These are produced during various metabolic processes, ripening, harvesting and other processing stages. Pear composition also varied with species, variety, treatments, etc. (Qin et al. 2012; Li et al. 2014). Among all these volatile compounds aldehydes are dominant in *P. bretshneideri* and *P. pyrifolia* and the second most abundant are alcohols and esters. *P. communis* is the species which has been most widely studied (Qin et al. 2012).

## 4.5 NUTRITIONAL COMPOSITION OF PEAR

The major components present in pear fruit are water which is about 80%, sugar and fructose which is about 15% and fibre which is about 2%. The concentration of these constituent components varies along the varieties of pear cultivars. Korean pear has been reported to be higher in water, sugar and potassium levels than the western pear cultivars. Also, the latter is found higher in fibre and calcium content than the former one (Lee et al. 2012). Research evidence also showed the presence of compounds like arbutin, oleanolic acid, rutin and ursolic acid in pear (Hong et al. 2021). In addition, vitamin C, malic acid and minerals like magnesium, potassium, calcium and iron favours pH of blood and ionic homeostasis as reported by research (Brahem et al. 2017).

### 4.5.1 Dietary Fibre

Pears are a great source of dietary fibre. Fibre is mainly of two kinds: Water soluble and water insoluble. Water soluble fibre includes mucilage, gums and pectin while the insoluble fibre consists of lignin, cellulose and different kinds of hemicelluloses. The dietary fibres present in foods treat many diseases like constipation, diabetes, cardiovascular diseases (CVDs), diverticulosis and obesity. The insoluble fibre content of pear is also highest among the fruits commonly consumed, which is 2.3 g/100 g. The dietary fibre content ranges from 3.16 g to 4.1 g per 100 g for a medium sized pear (130 g) that makes the pear a "good source" of dietary fibre as defined by the Foods Standard Australia New Zealand (FSANZ). Some of these fibres act as prebiotic for selectively enhancing the growth and activities of gut microflora which ultimately confers many beneficial health effects. Pear when mixed with sea buckthorn, plum carrot or beetroot containing insulin reported to stimulate the growth of *Lactobacillus* or *Enterococcus* (Ramnani et al. 2010; Roberfroid et al. 2011). The fibre like cellulose, hemicellulose which are insoluble fibres and soluble pectin and have laxative effects (Ramnani et al. 2010; Roberfroid et al. 2011; Kolniak-Ostek 2016a; Yang 2018).

### 4.5.2 Carbohydrates

Peers are unique in their carbohydrate composition. While other fruits contain glucose or sucrose as the major sugar, in pear, the predominant sugar is fructose. However, the sugar content of different species and cultivars of pear varies. Usually glucose is present in higher concentration in Asian pear varieties than in European pear varieties. Also, Asian pear varieties contain a lower fructose to glucose ratio than the latter. Other sugar components in pear are sorbitol, an alcohol sugar. Its concentration is generally higher than in other common fruits.

### 4.5.3 Glycaemic Index

It is used to determine how much blood sugar levels are raised by specific foods. Glycaemic index (GI) of pears ranges from 33 to 42 (Atkinson et al. 2008). The GI of pears and apples are comparable and is lower than other fruits which are most commonly consumed. GI is actually a relative ranking of food sugars on the basis of how they affect the glucose levels in the blood. GI values range from 0 to 100 with pure glucose arbitrarily given the value of 100. Its value below 55 is considered low and foods having GI values ranging from 56 to 69 and above

70 are considered moderate and high, respectively. Foods which are lower in GI value are more slowly digested, absorbed, and metabolized eventually leading to lower and slower elevation in the blood sugar level.

### 4.5.4 Phytochemicals

Various phytochemicals are present in pear. These are those substances present in plant foods that are beneficial for human health. However, nutrients are essential for normal human health and body functions but the phytonutrients or phytochemicals are not essential for life despite having many beneficial functions. It is evident from research that the presence of phytochemicals in various foods imparts many health benefits. These phytochemicals acts as antioxidants which play a major role in protecting the cells, proteins and DNA against the oxidative damage. Other phytochemicals include polyphenols that are flavonoids which are categorized into anthocyanins, triterpenes, glucosides, flavones and its related compounds (Brahem et al. 2017; Kolniak-Ostek et al. 2020). The primary flavonoid present in pear is cyanidin which is an anthocyanin and is specifically found in red skinned pears. Epicatechin present in pear is dominant after cyanidin that belongs to favan-3-ol category. Pears also contain many phenolic acids and are a good source of it. It specifically contains acids like chlorogenic, ferulic and citric and arbutin. Citric acid enhances the rate of iron absorption in the body, with 1 g of it having been reported to enhance the absorption of iron by 300%. Some pear varieties are reported to contain over 2 g/kg fresh pear. However, citric acid is present in higher concentrations than in apples which is about 84–168 mg/kg (Hudina and Stampar 2000). Ferulic acid present in pear is also reported to have several health benefits. It exhibits properties like anti-inflammatory, anti-atherogenic, and is also effective against problems like diabetes and ageing. It also imparts neuroprotective and hepatoprotective properties (Srinivasan et al. 2007; Zhao and Moghadasian 2008). Arbutin present in pears exhibits antioxidant, anti-hyperglycaemic and anti-hyperlipidemic effects. These polyphenol compounds are present in higher levels in leaves of the pear plant than in seeds. Similarly, its concentration is higher in seeds than in the peel of the pear fruit. Generally, the peel of the pear fruit is richer in phytochemicals than the pulp (Kolniak-Ostek and Oszmiański 2015; Pascoalino et al. 2021). The peel of the pear fruit is thick due to pectin and stone cells present in it along with a thick wall of cellulose and lignin (Yan et al. 2014; Lee et al. 2015). There may be a close relationship between the synthesis, transfer and deposition of lignin with that of stone cell formation.

Arbutin, a hydroquinone-β-D-glucopyranoside is present in pear and is recognized for its antioxidant, antibiotic, anti-hyperglycaemic, anti-hyperlipidemic and skin whitening properties (Eun et al. 2012; Cho et al. 2015; Öztürk et al. 2015). Its breakdown product is hydroquinone that is a potent skin bleaching agent, used for the purpose of incorporating fragrance in cosmetics. It is also used as a reducing agent and potent inhibitor against the polymerization reactions of melanin. Some research studies conducted in both *in vivo* and *in vitro* revealed that hydroquinone works as a mediator for immune function. One of the richest sources of natural arbutin is reported to be the peel of the Korean pear. It can also serve as a potent pear-specific intake biomarker (Deisinger 1996; Ulaszewska et al. 2018).

Chlorogenic acid is an abundant bioactive compound in pear after arbutin. It is a 5-O-caffeoylquinic acid present in the flesh and peel of pear fruit.

It exhibits biological functions like anti-inflammatory and antioxidant function. Mechanically, it causes reduction of TNF-α and downregulates IL-8 production in Caco-2 and RAW264.7 cells. It also inhibits inflammation *in vivo* by protecting nerve cells and enhancing wound healing of tissues (Hwang et al. 2014; Cho et al. 2015; Liang and Kitts 2015; Kolniak-Ostek 2016b; Naveed et al. 2018; Wang et al. 2021). It is also reported to increase NOS, COX and hyperpolarizing factor signalling pathways derived by endothelium which ultimately induces a direct endothelium-dependent vasodilation (Tom et al. 2016). Research evidence also provides that the chlorogenic acid also plays a vital role in protecting DNA against damage induced by ionizing radiations. This property of chlorogenic acid depicts its radio-protective property (Mun et al. 2018).

Caffeic acid is a polyphenol present in small quantities in the peel and flesh of pear. It is reported to have neuroprotective effects when used along with caffeine. It also enhances the production of collagen protein in the body. In the case of cancer of the colon cells (HCT 15), it reduces the membrane potential of cell mitochondria and generation of ROS and showed chemo-preventive potential (Jaganathan 2012; Magnani et al. 2014; Akomolafe et al. 2017; Sidoryk et al. 2018).

Flavonoids like quercetin and isorhamnetin and flavanols like epicatechin and pro-anthocyanidins are generally predominantly present in pears. Other flavonoids present in pears are quercetin 3-O-glucoside and catechol, a dulcisflavan (Kay et al. 2012; Kolniak-Ostek and Oszmiański 2015; Lee et al. 2015; Brahem et al. 2017). These compounds have effect over the fruit quality. They also play a major role in determining the colour of the fruit and resistance of plant against harmful things (Fischer et al. 2007; Öztürk et al. 2015; Kolniak-Ostek 2016b). Anthocyanidin aglycone, a constituent part of anthocyanins which is a water-soluble pigment, is mainly found among red skinned pear varieties (Veberic et al. 2015; Brahem et al. 2017). These flavonols have been reported to have diverse biological functions *in vitro* like modulation in enzymatic activity and decreased proliferation of the cells. They also act as potent antibiotic, antiallergic agents and have a strong effect against diarrhoea, ulcer, cancer and inflammation. They also act as a scavenger against free radical reactions (Estrela et al. 2017). Among all the flavonoids that are identified in the pear, the most dominant was arbutin and then catechin. Quercetin and epicatechin were present in lower concentrations than catechin (Li et al. 2012, 2014).

Malaxinic acid, a glucoside, is actually 4-(O-β-D- glucopyranosyl)-3-(3'-methyl-2'-butenyl) benzoic acid. It inhibits 21–26 kDa protein which induces cancer cell proliferation (Moon et al. 2017). Its other beneficial functions include inhibiting the growth of cells responsible for cancer such as BAEC, HT1080, HeLa and B16 and antioxidative defence in blood circulation (Lee et al. 2011a; Cho et al. 2015; Moon et al. 2017; Truong et al. 2017).

Triterpenoids, specifically ursolic acid, oleanolic acid and betulinic acid, had been reported in European pear cultivars. In it, these are present in higher concentrations in the peel than in its flesh (Kolniak-Ostek 2016b). Triterpenoids possess structural similarity with that of steroids. Research evidence showed that it inhibits aromatase responsible for converting androgens into estrogens. It also increases consumption of body energy that results into decreased obesity and enhanced tolerance towards glucose levels. It also possesses antioxidant property along with antitumour, antidiabetic, anti-inflammatory and antimicrobial properties. It is also crucial in the reduction of hepatic steatosis (Kunkel et al. 2012; Ayeleso et al. 2017). Structures of various phytochemicals present in pears are given Figure 4.2.

## 4.6 IDENTIFICATION AND CHARACTERIZATION

Fruits being a colourful and flavourful in one's diet, also serve as a source of energy, vitamins, minerals, dietary fibre and other nutrients which play a major role in determining their nutritive value (Chen et al. 2007). Arbutin (hydroquinone-β-D-glucopyranoside) is a popular skin whitening agent and has antibiotic properties also (Eun et al. 2012; Cho et al. 2015; Öztürk 2015). Its breakdown product is hydroquinone which is a potent skin bleaching agent and inhibits polymerization reactions of the melanin. It also mediates immune functions both *in vivo* and *in vitro* in animals (Eun et al. 2012). In oriental pears, arbutin was found in higher concentration in the peel which was three to five times greater than in the pulp. Therefore, its peel, especially that of Korean varieties, is among the potent sources of natural arbutin (Öztürk et al. 2015).

Ascorbic acid is present as a soluble antioxidant in pears. The other compounds are glutathione and tocopherol. Carotenoids are a natural isoprenoid pigment which is synthesized mostly in photosynthetic organisms. It is related to

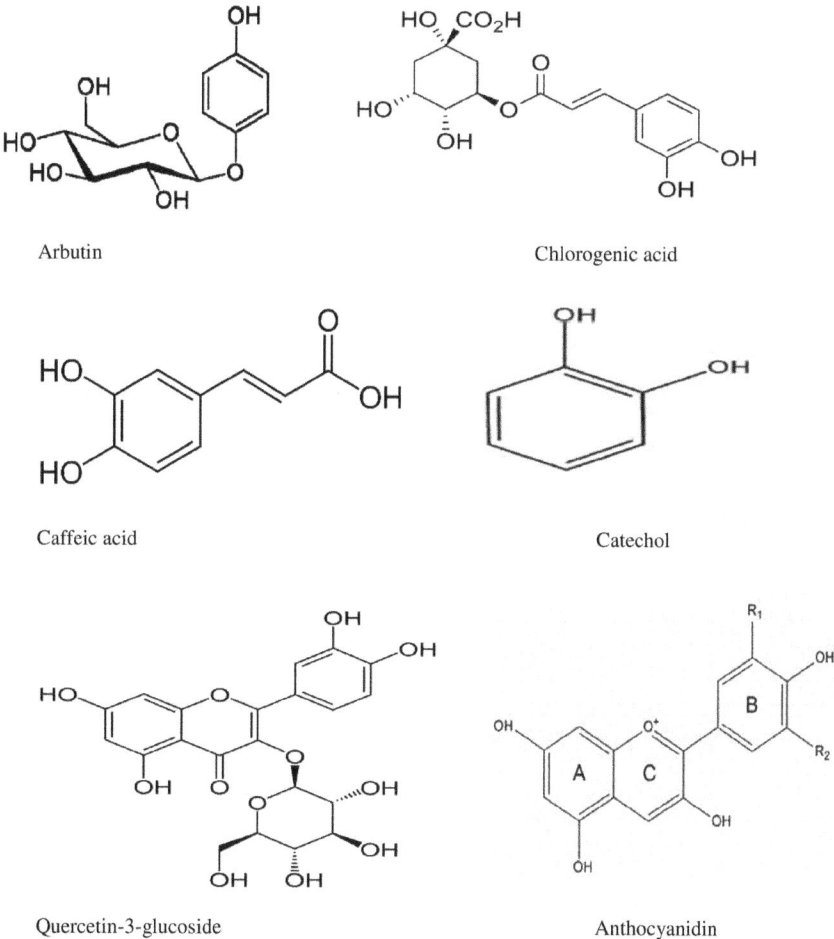

Arbutin

Chlorogenic acid

Caffeic acid

Catechol

Quercetin-3-glucoside

Anthocyanidin

**Figure 4.2** Structures of different phytochemicals present in pear. (*Continued*)

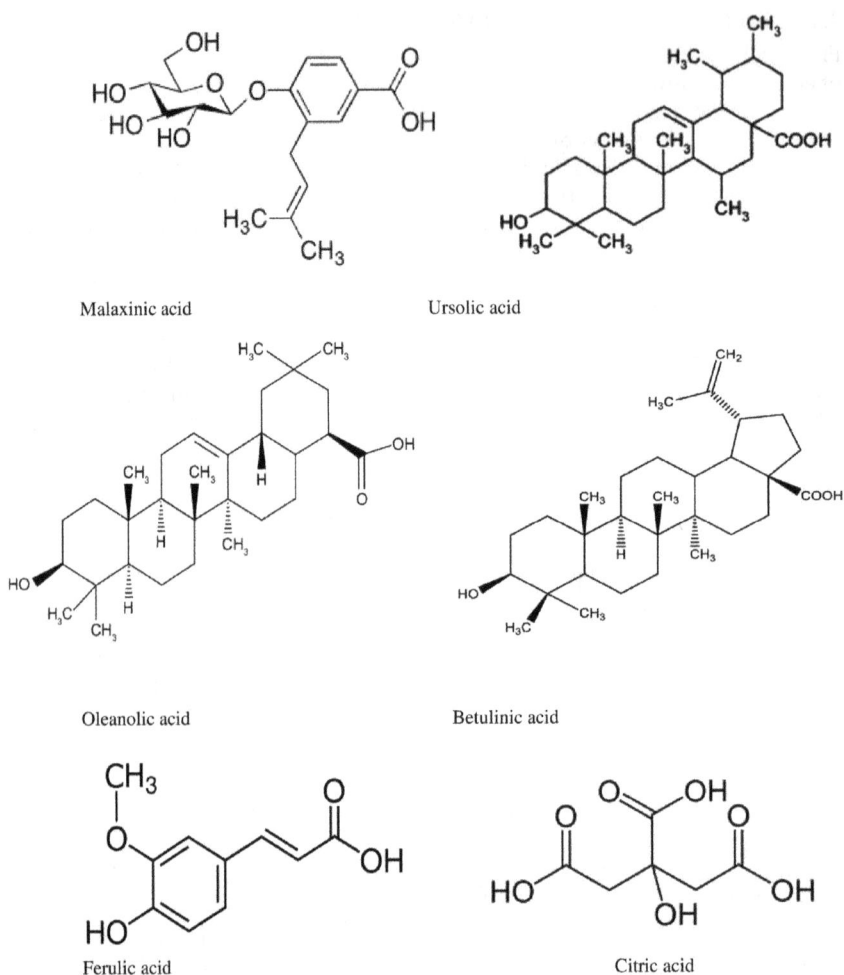

Malaxinic acid

Ursolic acid

Oleanolic acid

Betulinic acid

Ferulic acid

Citric acid

**Figure 4.2** (*Continued*)

provitamin-A, antioxidants, regulation of cell differentiation and proliferation, and immune function. It also stimulates cell to cell communication and acts as a modulator against the metabolism of carcinogens. Intake of carotenoids is related to the reduction in the risk of diseases like cancer, CVDs, cataract and macular degeneration. It was also reported to be correlated with improved immune function (Dias et al. 2009). However, low carotenoid intake has been reported to increase the risk of cancer, cataract, skin diseases and CVDs (Aust et al. 2001). Carotenoids that are dominant in pear are α- and β-carotenes, β-cryptoxanthin, lycopene, zeaxanthin and lutein. Levels of carotenoids present in a particular pear varies with its species, varieties, geographical area of cultivation and kind of harvesting. Major sugars, amino acids and organic acids present in pear include fructose, glucose and sucrose; asparagine and serine; and malic acid, citric acid, quinic acid and shikimic acid, respectively. Minerals present in pears include potassium that helps in controlling salt balance, calcium that helps in bone development and zinc which is required for normal immune functioning. Among these, potassium was dominant in pears which is followed by magnesium and calcium (Chen et al. 2007). The concentration of fibres is also significant in pear fruit. It is reported that the peel of the pear fruit contains higher levels of dietary fibre than its pulp (Leontowicz et al. 2003). Pears have high levels of dietary fibres among the common fruits that are eaten daily like apples and citrus fruits. The fibre present in pear fruit is much better in quality than other kinds of dietary fibre due to the existence of associated bioactive compounds (Barroca et al. 2006). Total phenolic, total flavonoids, total anthocyanin and total triterpene contents are considered to determine the nutritive value of foods. Table 4.1 shows different

## Table 4.1: Different Kinds of Compounds Present in Pear

| S. No. | Compound | Substituent | Source | Reference |
|---|---|---|---|---|
| A | | **Lupeol Ester** | | |
| 1 | Lup-20(29)-ene-3β-yl Eicosanoate | • $CO(CH_2)_{18}CH_3$=R1 <br> • $CH_3$=R2 | Pyrus serotine Rhed. | Tomosaka et al. (2001) |
| 2 | Lup-20(29)-ene-3β-yl Docosanoate | • $CO(CH_2)_{20}CH_3$=R1 <br> • $CH_3$=R2 | P. serotine Rhed. | Tomosaka et al. (2001) |
| 3 | Lup-20(29)-ene-3β-yl tetracosanoate | • $CO(CH_2)_{22}CH_3$=R1 <br> • $CH_3$=R2 | P. serotine Rhed. | Tomosaka et al. (2001) |
| 4 | Lup-20(29)-ene-3β-yl hexacosanoate | • $CO(CH_2)_{24}CH_3$=R1 <br> • $CH_3$=R2 | P. serotine Rhed. | Tomosaka et al. (2001) |
| 5 | Lup-20(29)-ene-3β-yl octacosanoate | • $CO(CH_2)_{26}CH_3$=R1 <br> • $CH_3$=R2 | P. serotine Rhed. | Tomosaka et al. (2001) |
| B | | **Phenolic Acid Esters** | | |
| 1 | Protocatechuoylcallerya nin-3-O-β-glucopyranoside | Glc=R | P. calleryana | Nassar et al. (2011) |
| 2 | 3'-Hydroxybenzyl-4-hydroxybenzoate-4'-O-β-glucopyranoside | H=R | P. calleryana | Nassar et al. (2011) |
| C | | **Polyphenols** | | |
| 1 | Chlorogenic acid | OH=R | Leaf of Pyrus sp. | Sioud and Luh (1966) |
| 2 | Ferulic acid | • $OCH_3$=R <br> • H=R' | P. bretschneideri Rehd. | Li et al. (2012b) |
| 3 | Caffeic acid | • OH=R <br> • H=R' | P. bretschneideri Rehd. | Li et al. (2012b) |
| 5 | P-Coumaroylquinic acid | H=R | Leaf of Pyrus sp. | Sioud and Luh (1966) |
| 6 | Arbutin | Glc=R | Pyrus cv. Kiefffer | Durkee et al. (1968) |
| 7 | Catechin | • R1=R3=OH <br> • H=R2 <br> • H=R4 | P. communis L. cv. Bartlett | Sioud and Luh (1966) |
| 8 | Leucocyanidin | • HO=R1 <br> • H=R2 <br> • HO=R3 <br> • HO=R4 | P. communis L. cv. Bartlett | Sioud and Luh (1966) |
| 9 | Epicatechin | • H=R1 <br> • R2=R3=OH <br> • H=R4 | P. communis L. cv. Bartlett | Sioud and Luh (1966) |

(Continued)

## Table 4.1: Different Kinds of Compounds Present in Pear (*Continued*)

| S. No. | Compound | Substituent | Source | Reference |
|---|---|---|---|---|
| 10 | Quercitrin | • R1=R2=R5=OH<br>• H=R3Rham-O=R4 | *P. communis* L. | Sioud and Luh (1966); Li et al. (2012a) |
| 11 | Quercetin | • R2=R4=R5=O<br>• R1=R3=H | *P. bretscneideri* Rehd. | Sioud and Luh (1966); Li et al. (2012a) |
| 12 | Isoquercitrin | • R1=R2=OH<br>• R3=H<br>• R4=O-gluA<br>• OH=R5 | *P. communis* L. | Sioud and Luh (1966) |
| 13 | Quercetin-7-O-xyloside | • R1=R3=H<br>• R2=R4=OH<br>• R5=O-xyloside | *P. communis* L. cvs. Bosc, D'Anjou and Bartlett | Oleszek et al. (1994) |
| 14 | Isoquercetin-3-O-glucoside | R4=O-glu | *P. communis* L. cv. Bon Chretien | Nortjé and Koeppen (1965) |
| 15 | Isoquercetin-3-O-malonyl glucoside | R4=O-malonyl glucoside | *P. communis* | Oleszek et al. (1994) |
| 16 | Isoquercetin-3-O-rutinoside | R4=O-rutinoside | *P. communis* | Oleszek et al. (1994) |
| 17 | Isorhamnetin-3-O-glucoside | • H=R1<br>• R2=OH<br>• R3=OCH$_3$ | *P. communis* cv. L. Bon Chretien | Nortjé and Koeppen (1965) |
| 18 | Isorhamnetin-3-O-rhamnoglucoside | • H=R1<br>• HO=R2<br>• R3=OCH$_3$<br>• R4=O- Rha<br>• HO=R5 | *P. communis* cv. Chretien L. Bon | Nortjé and Koeppen (1965) |
| 19 | Isorhamnetin-3-O-rhamnogalactoside | • H=R1<br>• HO=R2<br>• R3=OCH$_3$<br>• R4=O-Rha-Gal<br>• HO=R5 | *P. communis* cv. Chretien L. Bon | Nortjé and Koeppen (1965) |
| 20 | Isorhamnetin-3-O-rutinoside | • H=R1<br>• HO=R2<br>• R3=OCH$_3$<br>• R4=O-rutinoside<br>• HO=R5 | *P. communis* | Oleszek et al. (1994) |
| 21 | Isorhamnetin-3-O-galactorhamnoside | • H=R1<br>• HO=R2<br>• R3=OCH$_3$<br>• R4=O-Gal-Rha<br>• HO=R5 | *P. communis* | Oleszek et al. (1994) |
| 22 | 2-O-(cis-coumaroyl) malic acid | R1=R2=H | *P. pyrifolia* Nakai | Lee et al. (2011b) |
| 23 | 2-O-(cis-coumaroyl) malic acid 1-methyl ester | • H=R1<br>• R2=CH | *P. pyrifolia* Nakai | Lee et al. (2011b) |
| C | | **Steroids** | | |
| 1 | Daucosterol | Glu=R | *P. bretschneideri* Rehd.; *P. communis* L. | Zuo and Liu (1997) |

(*Continued*)

## Table 4.1: Different Kinds of Compounds Present in Pear (*Continued*)

| S. No. | Compound | Substituent | Source | Reference |
|--------|----------|-------------|--------|-----------|
| 2 | β-Sitosterol | H=R | *P. bretschneideri* Rehd.; *P. communis* L. | Zuo and Liu (1997) |
| **D** | | **Triterpenes** | | |
| 1 | Ursolic acid | • R1=R2=H<br>• R3=COOH<br>• R4=β-OH | *P. bretschneideri* Rehd. | Huang et al. (2010); Li et al. (2012a) |
| 2 | α-Amyrin | • R1=R2=H<br>• R3=CH$_3$<br>• R4=β-OH | *P. bretschneideri* Rehd. | Li et al. (2012a) |
| 3 | Tormentic acid | • R1=-OH<br>• HO=R2<br>• R3=COOH<br>• R4=β-OH | *P. pashia* | Zhao et al. (2013) |
| 4 | Euscaphic acid | • R1=-OH<br>• HO=R2<br>• R3=COOH<br>• R4=α-OH | *P. pashia* | Zhao et al. (2013) |
| 5 | Oleanolic acid | H=R | *P. bretschneideri* Rehd. | Huang et al. (2010); Li et al. (2012a) |
| 6 | Lupeol | • H=R1<br>• R2=CH$_3$ | *P. communis* L. | Zuo and Liu (1997) |
| 7 | Betulin | • H=R1<br>• R2=CH$_2$OH | *P. communis* L. | Zuo and Liu (1997) |
| 8 | Betulinic acid | • H=R1<br>• R2=COOH | *P. communis* L. | Zuo and Liu (1997) |
| **E** | | **Others** | | |
| 1 | Ditubyl phthalate | R=CH$_2$CH$_3$ | *P. bretschneideri* Rehd. | Li et al. (2012a) |
| 2 | Disobutyl phthalate | R-(CH$_3$)$_2$ | *P. bretschneideri* Rehd. | Li et al. (2012a) |

kinds of compounds present in pear. Figure 4.3 shows the different kinds of compounds identified in pear fruit.

Different parts of pear such as pear skin, flower and other parts of pear tree contain different kinds of phenolic compounds such as p-coumaroylmalic acid, derivatives of vanillic acid, catechin, p-coumaroylquinic acid, epicatechin, pro-anthocyanidins, cyanidin, isorhamnetin, kaempferol, 3-O-galactoside of quercetin and some non-glycosylated flavones and flavonols (Lin and Harnly 2008). Pear peel is reported to have much higher and more varieties of phenolic compounds than pear flesh. Phenolic compounds of pear peels of *Pyrus* species were analysed through a standardized profiling method. This method was based on the use of liquid chromatographic techniques with a diode array and ionization or mass spectrometric detection. About thirty-four flavonoid compounds were identified along with 19 hydroxyl-cinnamates, arbutin and chlorogenic acid (Lin and Harnly 2008).

Identification of bioactive compounds present in pear fruit was also done and it was obtained that the seeds of eight kinds of pear (*P. communis* L.) cultivars

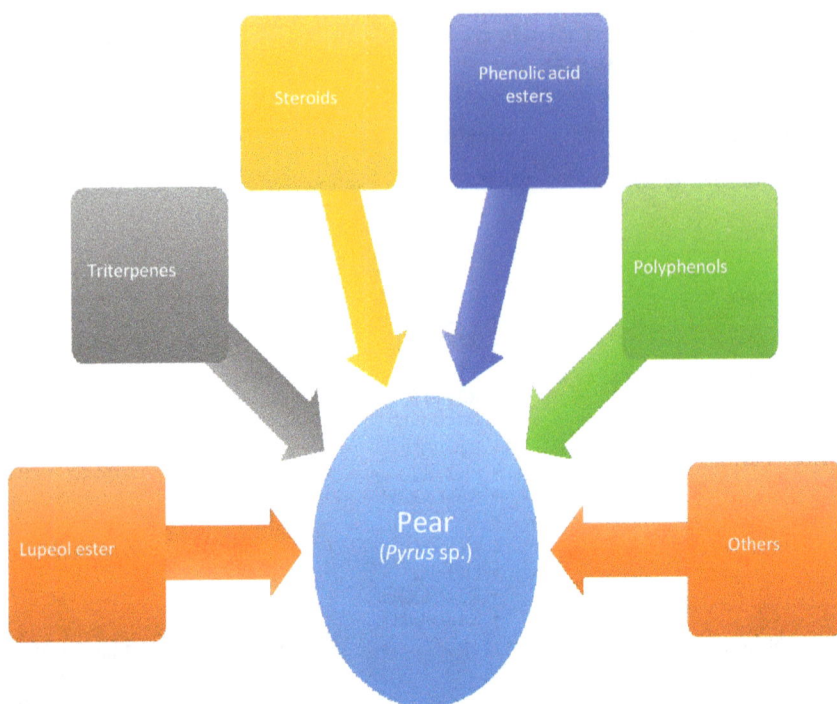

**Figure 4.3** Different kinds of compounds identified in pear fruit.

contain lipophilic bioactive compounds. The main tocohromanol present in all the pear cultivars that were studied was γ-tocopherol. Some compounds present in pears are considered as potential allies since these have great ability to fight against various degenerative diseases. These are tocotrienol and tocopherol homologues which are lipophilic bioactive compounds (Aggarwal et al. 2010). Phytosterols have desirable effects over human health; for instance they help in lowering the cholesterol levels in blood serum (Chen et al. 2008). The compound squalene possesses antioxidant activity that helps to protect the mammary epithelial cells against oxidative DNA damage by causing reduction in the reactive oxygen species levels (Warleta et al. 2010). It is actually a 3-O-carbon isoprenoid which is a precursor of vitamin D, cholesterol and many steroid hormones. HPLC and spectrophotometric method were used for the characterization tocopherol of oils and carotenoids present in the seeds of the pear, respectively. Unsaturated fatty acids were dominant in it. The main fatty acids found in the pear seed oil were palmitic acid, stearic acid, oleic acid and linoleic acid. In the pear kept under study, four tocopherol and two tocotrienol homologues were identified. The tocochromanol dominant in it was γ-tocochromanol while α-tocochromanols and δ-tocochromanols were present in lower quantities than γ tocochromanol. The sterols identified in pear seed oils were campesterol, β-sitosterol, avenasterol, cholesterol, gramisterol, stigmasterol and citrostadienol. However, β-sitosterol was the predominant one among all these in each cultivar (Gornas et al. 2014; Pugejeva et al. 2014). The content of bioactive molecules in pear seed oils was reported to be significantly affected by the cultivar (Gornas et al. 2015). Another study (Jiang et al. 2019) provided that levels of vitamin C and other bioactive compounds were higher in Asian pears. Tocochromanols are lipophilic having vitamin E activity and are identified using HPLC and UPLC techniques. Studies reported that higher levels of γ-tocochromanol intake is associated with lowered risk of prostate cancer and chronic diseases (Wright et al. 2007; Aggarwal et al. 2010). The highest content of γ-tocochromanol was reported in seeds of the pear cultivars "Williams Bon Chretien" and lowest in "Latgale" (Reiland and Slavin 2015). Noryje and Koeppen isolated and identified flavonols glycosides in pear. However, the presence of flavonols glycoside in *Pyrus* species was reported by Wagenbreth (1959). The glycosides such as kaempferol and quercetin were identified in leaves of *P. communis*. The presence of epigenin and luteolin glycosides were also reported later in the leaves of certain *Pyrus* species. Phenolic compounds in pear are generally higher in its peel as compared to its levels in the flesh. These are secondary metabolites of plants and give unique stringent taste to it. These are also responsible for colour changes in the fruit. They also play a crucial role in browning reactions and flavour changes. Their content also varies across different cultivars of pear. Major phenolic compounds detected in pear peel and flesh are arbutin and chlorogenic acid while those detected in minor quantities are rutin hydrate and rutin tri-hydrate (Spanos and Wrolstad 1990; Tanrıöven and Eksi 2005). These phenolic compounds also contribute to plant defence mechanism and human metabolic activities. They exhibit antioxidative, antimutagenic and anti-carcinogenic activities (Ramandthan and Das 1992; Tomas-Lorente et al. 1992). They also have protective effects against cancer, cataract, bacteria, fungus and CVDs (Weidenböerger et al. 1990; Tomas-Lorente et al. 1992). Most commonly occurring phenolic acids present in pears are chlorogenic acid, arbutin and epicatechin (Spanos and Wrolstad 1990). Chlorogenic acid acts as a potent antioxidant and chemo-preventive agent. It helps in the functioning of the immune system and reduces the toxic effects of chemothcrapy drugs (Morton et al. 2000; Kris-Etherton et al. 2002).

Different parts of the pear such as peel, flower bud, leaf bud, young fruit and flesh of fruit contain variable amounts of phenolic compound that can be determined using HPLC methods. But generally, their content is much higher and varied in the peel than their levels in the flesh of pear fruit (Galvis-Sanchez et al. 2003; Cui et al. 2005; Lin and Harnly 2008). The major phenolic acids present in pear are arbutin and chlorogenic acid in peel and flesh of the fruit, but the concentration of arbutin is higher than the latter in most of the pear fruits. The other phenolic acids present in pear are epicatechin, catechin, caffeic acid, coumaric acid and rutin trihydrate. The concentration of caffeic acid is generally higher in the peel than in the flesh of the pear fruit. Similarly, catechin and epicatechin were dominant in the peel than in the flesh (Öztürk et al. 2014).

Vitamin C, vitamin E and vitamin B-complex are higher than protein and fat in pears. Pears are also very good source of dietary fibre, copper and potassium. However, when pears are eaten along with the peel, they serve as an extraordinary source of dietary fibre. The fact is that the content of arbutin and chlorogenic acid were higher than rutin hydrate (quercetin-3-rutinoside hydrate) and rutin trihydrate (quercetin-3-rutinoside-trihydrate) in the peel and flesh of the pear fruit (Escarpa and Gonzalez 2000; Galvis-Sanchez et al. 2003; Cui et al. 2005; Lin and Harnly 2008; Öztürk et al. 2014). The polyphenols and triterpenes present in pear exhibit great antioxidant and anti-inflammatory properties. Furthermore, the plant extracts rich in polyphenols were found to have inhibitory effects against $\alpha$-glucosidase and $\alpha$-amylase. They also possess antidiabetic activity by inhibiting $\alpha$-glucosidase activity (Lee and Kader 2000; Cui et al. 2005; Lin and Harnly 2008).

Pear pomace ethanol (PPE) extract was identified for improving the effects of insulin sensitivity via activation of insulin signalling pathway in T3 cells and high fat diet fed animals. It was obtained that PPE extract had improved the sensitivity of insulin and concluded that it improves high fat diet-induced insulin resistance (*in vivo*) through the activation of insulin signalling pathway in T3 cells *in vitro* (Öztürk et al. 2015).

Phenolic compounds are compounds known for their biological activity that strengthen the organism and prevent diseases. They have strong antioxidant and anti-inflammatory effects (Hider et al. 2001; Sun et al. 2002; Scalbert et al. 2000; Gharras 2009; Pandey and Rizvi 2009). They also possess strong antiviral (Likhitwitayawuid et al. 2005; Chavez et al. 2006), antimicrobial (Cushnie and Lamb 2005; Nohynek et al. 2006), anti-mutagenic and anticancer properties (Lopez-Lazaro 2002; Kandaswami et al. 2005; Lakhanpal and Rai 2007; Boots et al. 2008; Pastore et al. 2009). Many studies revealed that there exists a strong correlation between the consumption of phenolic compounds such as quercetin glycosides rich foods and a reduced risk of developing neurodegenerative and CVDs (Spencer 2010; Weichselbaum et al. 2010; Dajas 2012; Gonzalez-Vallinas et al. 2013). For their identification HPLC and spectrophotometric techniques were employed. In addition to its antioxidant and anti-inflammatory activities (Zhang et al. 2010; Sato et al. 2011) chlorogenic acid was reported to lower the risk of type 2 diabetes mellitus, improve cardiac and vascular functions and inhibit carcinogenic processes (Stefanska et al. 2012; Thomas and Pfeiffer 2012; Cinkilic et al. 2013; Kanno et al. 2013). The compounds like quercetin glycosides prevent angiotensis-converting enzyme, thus having an antihypertensive effect (Balasuriya and Rupasinghe 2012). Moreover, the highest content of flavonols and chlorogenic acid was found in "Concordia" and "Grabova" cultivars, respectively (Liaudanskas et al. 2017).

Chlorogenic acid was reported to be present in higher concentrations as 106.7–247.5 mg/00 g in fresh immature Korean pears (Cho et al. 2015). Results of many studies provided that chlorogenic acid reduces TNF-$\alpha$ and downregulates IL-8 production in Carco-2 cells and RAW267.7 cells. It also helps in the protection of neurons and healing of wounds *in vivo* and also inhibits inflammation (Hwang et al. 2014; Liang and Kitts 2015). It was also reported that it raises NOS, COX and endothelium-derived hyperpolarizing factor signalling pathways thus inducing a direct endothelium-dependent vasodilation (Tom et al. 2016). It was identified that intake of chlorogenic acid up to 6 months (330 mg/100 mL of water) significantly improves the cognitive functions, verbal memory, complex attention, executive function and motor domains of the central nervous system (Kato et al. 2018). It is also believed to have radio-protective effects (Mun et al. 2018). Caffeic acid is present in pear flesh and peel in minor amounts (56.2 mg/kg) (Eun et al. 2012; Öztürk et al. 2015). It also favours apoptosis, ROS generation and reduction in the potential of mitochondrial membrane of the cells and showed chemo-preventive potential in cancer cells of the colon such as HCT 15 cells (Jaganathan 2012).

Korean pears increase the synthesis of ATP in the cells, thus enhancing the growth of hepatocytes (Yoon et al. 2006). Pear extracts also enhance cell proliferation, synthesis of DNA in hepatocytes and suppress hepatic lipid peroxidation (You et al. 2017). Fresh weighed immature Korean pear contains about 182.5–368.9 mg/100 g of flavonoids (Cho et al. 2015). A study (Brahem et al. 2017) reported that epicatechin was predominant as terminal and extension units among flesh and peel of European and Tunisian pears. The predominant phytochemical present in Korean pear is malaxinic acid whose concentration decreases as the fruit matures. A typical immature Korean pear contains about 0.46–5.86 mg/100 g of fresh weight (Lee et al. 2013; Cho et al. 2015). It also inhibits cancer cells growth such as BAEC, HT1080, HeLa and B16/BL6 (Lee et al. 2011a, 2017; Cho et al. 2015; Truong et al. 2017).

Among oriental pears, arbutin in present in concentrated amounts in the peel of the pear fruit (1.20 mg/g fresh weight). This was three to five times higher than the arbutin content in the pulp of the pear fruit (Cui et al. 2005; Yim and Nam 2016). It was also reported that Korean pears are the richest in arbutin among all (Deisinger 1996; Ulaszewska et al. 2018).

The cellulose nanofibres of Japanese pear reduces inflammation by suppressing the fibroses or butyrate-mediated inhibition of NF-kB in inflammatory bowel disease (Azuma et al. 2014). Pear vinegar suppresses the myeloperoxidase-mediated activation of inflammatory cells and decreases the serum concentration of IL-6 (Cho et al. 2018). Arbutin present in different parts of the pear has anti-inflammatory effects on pro-inflammatory cytokines, such as IL-1β, TNF-α and MCP-1 (Li et al. 2014; Migas and Krauze-Baranowska 2015).

It was reported in a study that pear, when mixed with carrot or plum or beetroot along with insulin stimulates the growth of *Lactobacillus/Enterococcus* (Ramnani et al. 2010). Intake of apples in combination with pears lowers the chances of occurrence of type 2 diabetes mellitus up to 18% (Guo et al. 2017). Extracts of immature Asian and Yaguang pear have significant effects over the reduction of fasting glucose levels than diabetic controls in rats, which is supposed to be related to the inhibition of α-glucosidase (Wang et al. 2015; Ci et al. 2018). When twenty-two different fruit juices were compared, it was obtained that juice extracted from Chinese white pear was high in the activity against the inhibition of α-glucosidase *in vitro* (He et al. 2017). Pears are supposed to reduce triglycerides, total cholesterol and low-density lipoprotein levels while increasing high-density cholesterol (Velmurugan and Bhargava 2013). However, the peel of the pear has more hypolipidemic properties than pulp (19.4% for total cholesterol, 14.6% for triglycerides and 33.3% for low-density lipoprotein) which is due to the higher content of catechin in peel than in pulp (Hong et al. 2021).

Pear components prevent carcinogenesis of aromatic hydrocarbons. The benzo pyrene, an aromatic hydrocarbon, induces carcinogenesis by two mechanisms by making DNA-adducts and producing ROS (Clementino et al. 2017; David and Gooderham 2018). Specifically, Korean pear inhibits lung cancer in mice (males) (Yang et al. 2005). Korean pears stimulate the digestion of polycyclic aromatic hydrocarbons, mainly their excretion. Lipid peroxidation and mitochondrial stress were also reduced in the people consuming Korean pear (Yang 2006). Since nitrites are widely used in the food processing operations especially in case of meat, there are more chances of their interaction with amines, thus producing strong carcinogenic compounds like nitrosamines. Therefore, they act as an anti-carcinogenic due to their nitrite scavenging activity.

Moreover, Asian pears were reported to exhibit greater scavenging activity against nitrite than in other plants such as onions (50%) or kiwis (75.3%), which is 80.7 to 86.7%, generally (Min et al. 2013; Kim et al. 2014). When mice were treated with pectin of Asian pear, the sensitivity of tracheal smooth muscle to the electric field stimulation and acetylcholine was reduced up to significant levels. Serum allergen-specific lgE was reduced up to 70% (Lee et al. 2004). It was reported that the chlorogenic acid present in pear improves function of blood vessels and protection of endothelial cells to the oxidative damage induced by HOCL by raising the nitric oxide production and induction of Hmox-1 (Jiang et al. 2016).

## 4.7 HEALTH BENEFITS OF PEAR

There are many health benefits of pear. Their constituent components play different roles in maintaining the functioning of different body organs and affect the health conditions related to them.

### 4.7.1 Cardio Protection

CVDs are still among the most prominent reason of deaths in human beings. Other ill heart conditions that are affecting the heath of people across the globe include ischaemic heart disease, stroke and coronary heart disease (CHD). Chlorogenic acid present in pear has been reported to enhance the functioning of blood vessels. It also shields endothelial cells against the damage caused by alleviating nitric acid production along with the induction of Hmox-1 (Hong et al. 2021). Research evidence also provides that if apples and pears are eaten in good amounts, it reduces the risk of heart stroke in human beings. Various compounds present in pears like fibre and polyphenols exhibit synergistic effect which may ultimately reduce several risk factors associated with cardiovascular diseases such as pressure of the blood, body weight, lipid profile, inflammation and oxidative stress of the cells (Larsson et al. 2013). The other major contributor to CVDs includes abnormal plasma lipid concentration. Pear constituents favour the development of safe anti-hyperlipidemic compounds. Its anti-lipidemic effects are studied generally, in relation to its hyperglycaemic status reason being the more common incidence of hyperlipidemia among diabetic patients.

### 4.7.2 Hepatic Protection

Pears act as a hepatoprotective food along with diminishing effects over alcohol hangover symptoms. The metabolic pathway of alcohol in the human body is well known. The enzymes crucial for the metabolism of alcohol in the body are alcohol dehydrogenase and aldehyde dehydrogenase that enhance hangover severity. Its metabolism primarily occurs in the liver where enzyme alcohol dehydrogenase metabolizes it into acetaldehyde. This acetaldehyde is a potent toxic metabolite which raises lipid peroxidation reactions in the liver and enhances oxidative stress (Lee et al. 2013; Zhang et al. 2016; Kim et al. 2018). The acetaldehyde thus produced is then further acted upon by aldehyde dehydrogenase which in turn produces acetate. The acetate thus produced is eliminated by the kidney in the end. Drinking alcohol leads to conditions like headache, diarrhoea, fatigue, dizziness and difficulty in concentrating. This may lead to loss of activeness in daily life.

### 4.7.3 Anti-Obesity Effects

Overweight people are generally recommended to change their lifestyle and modify eating habits. They are suggested to include those foods in their diet that generally impart good satiety value but are less dense in energy. These may include foods rich in dietary fibre that have less calorific value. Many research studies favour the consumption of pears as a food to fight against obesity by reducing the calorie intake and promotion of exercise. Pear fibres help in the weight management since they are less energy dense (0.64 kcal/g) and have good amounts of dietary fibre (De-Oliveira et al. 2008; Nieman et al. 2015; Sharma et al.

2018). It reduces the cortisol levels by 22% immediately post exercise, ultimately favouring speedy recovery from strenuous exercises (Hong et al. 2021).

### 4.7.4 Anti-Carcinogenic Effects

Research showed that pears possess anti-mutagenic and anti-carcinogenic properties. They can inhibit the carcinogenesis of various polycyclic hydrocarbons including benzoprene having two primary carcinogenic mechanisms and formation of DNA-adducts. In addition, pears also inhibit the production of ROS (Clementino et al. 2017; David and Gooderham 2018). Korean pears inhibit cancer by mediating AME for polycyclic aromatic hydrocarbons, reduction of ROS, nitrite scavenging and antioxidant properties due to phenolic acids. In pears the acids like chlorogenic and malaxinic exhibit anti-carcinogenic properties such as inhibiting the proliferation reactions of breast and liver cancer cells (He and Liu 2008; Roleira et al. 2015).

### 4.7.5 Antidiabetic Effects

Recently conducted research studies showed that pears exhibit antidiabetic effects. This is owed to the antihyperlipidemic properties of pears (Koch and Deo 2016; Guo et al. 2017). The beneficial properties of pear towards the reduction of type 2 diabetes mellitus have also been well-established in many research studies conducted *in vivo* and *in vitro*, which also provides the evidence for a strong relation between the increased intake of pear and improvement in type 2 diabetes mellitus (Hong et al. 2021). Control over the level of lipids is more crucial in diabetic patients since they are at higher risk of CVDs. This antihyperlipidemic property of pear is related to its glycaemic index levels. The enzymes α-amylase and α-glucosidase have a critical role in the mediation of hyperglycaemia. These promote digestion and metabolism of sugars obtained from the diet taken. These possess pharmacological applications for treating hyperglycaemia (Barbosa et al. 2013; Sarkar et al. 2015). By inhibiting α-amylase and α-glucosidase, pears serve as an alternative in regulating postprandial hyper-glycaemia without causing any significant side effects. The inhibitory activities of these enzymes present in pear were also validated by many *in vitro* and *in vivo* research studies.

### 4.7.6 Anti-Inflammatory Effects

Pears also help in fighting against the diseases related to the gastrointestinal system such as inflammatory bowel disease, colitis, Crohn's disease and gastric ulcer disease. It can be considered as nature's digestive powerhouse. Studies reported that it possesses a wide spectrum of anti-inflammatory properties by suppressing immune responses due to the presence of different kinds of compounds present in it (Hong et al. 2021). The malabsorption of fermentable oligosaccharides, disaccharides and monosaccharides results in gastrointestinal conditions like irritable bowel syndrome. These compounds primarily include honey and high fructose corn syrup, polyols like sorbitol found in fruits and certain artificial sweetened fruits, fructose found in fruits and fructans like insulin found in wheat and onions. A medium pear provides about 7 g (approx.) of sorbitol. Pears contain an excess of fructose content that is the highest of any fruit (3–8 g/100 g) (Shepherd and Gibson 2006). High anthocyanin and flavonol intake have anti-inflammatory effects as reported in many research studies. It reduces acute inflammation, oxidative stress and cytokines. Also, flavonols such as catechin, epicatechin, etc., when taken in higher amounts, reduce biomarkers of oxidative stress. The latter includes myeloperoxidase, LPL-A2 and isoprostanes, which is an index of creatinine (Hong et al. 2021).

### 4.7.7 Respiratory Protection

The fact that pear helps to fight against allergic and ill respiratory conditions is supported by many research studies. The Asian pear is recognized for its role in lung cleaning and phlegm dissipation. Higher intake of pear along with apples is strongly associated with reduced incidence of bronchial hyper-reactivity, asthma and chronic pulmonary obstructive pulmonary disease (Hosseini et al. 2017; Kaluza et al. 2017). The unique combination of phytochemicals like polyphenols and flavonoids in pears plays a key role in treating allergic inflammatory and respiratory diseases. The flavonoids (rutin and quercetin) down-regulate the activation of mast cell activation, thus playing an important role in the treatment of allergic diseases (Park et al. 2008). Allergic diseases like rhinitis and eczema could get cured by the antioxidants present in the pear which reduces the inflammation by the protection of tissues from oxidative stress. Rhinitis is a condition of prolonged runny or blocked nose or sneezing without a cold and eczema is the condition of dry skin along with itchy and scaling skin.

### 4.7.8 Skin-Lightening Effects

In cosmetology, most of the people desire to have a fairer skin tone along with reduced aging effects such as wrinkles. The property of pears imparting skin-lightening effects is due to the presence of phytochemicals such as arbutin present in quality amounts in it. This effect is correlated to the tyrosinase inhibition. Tyrosinase plays a crucial role in the generation of generating dark pigments particularly melanin (Eun et al. 2012; Seo et al. 2012). Another phenolic compound present in pear is protocatechuic acid which is also a potent anti-melanogenic and skin-whitening agent. It suppresses the melanogenic in the skin by inhibiting tyrosinase and hindering the expression of other enzymes related to melanogenesis (Truong et al. 2017).

### 4.7.9 Metabolic Health Markers

Pears act as a potent metabolic health marker by contributing towards a healthy metabolic profile due to compounds like anthocyanins, chlorogenic acid, ferulic acid and soluble fibre (Srinivasan et al. 2007; Zhao and Moghadasian 2008; Min et al. 2013; Guo et al. 2017). Many metabolic abnormalities conditions exist like dyslipidaemia, i.e., elevated concentration of total cholesterol, triglycerides, low density lipoprotein cholesterol and high density lipoprotein cholesterol, hypertension, chronic inflammation and abnormal glucose metabolism. These metabolic abnormalities have a crucial role in several ill health conditions like heart-related diseases, type 2 diabetes mellitus, cancer and dementia. Different kinds of compounds are present in pears. These can be categorized under different groups as polyphenols, lupeol ester, triterpenes, phenolic acid esters, steroids and others that include phthalate. Table 4.2 shows bioactive compounds in pear (ancient and modern cultivars).

Pear has juicy and delicious taste and is used for the production of juice, wine, puree and jams and jellies. In countries like China, Japan and Korea pear was used as a traditional remedy for eliminating constipation and cough, and also to reduce alcohol toxicity in ancient times. It's the fifth important temperate species after banana, orange, apple and grapes. It is produced most in China followed by Italy, United States Argentina, Spain, Turkey and South Africa. Some other Asian countries such as India, Japan and Korea have kept pear production ranging from 0.20 to 0.45 m during 2002–2011 (Lee et al. 2012).

## Table 4.2: Bioactive Compounds in Pear (Ancient and Modern Cultivars)

### Ancient Cultivars

| Cultivars | Aroma Compounds | Reference |
|---|---|---|
| "Yali" pear (*P. bertschneideri* Reld) | Hexanoic acid, ethyl ester, acetic acid, hexanal, butanoic acid and farnesene | Chen et al. (2006b) |
| "Bartlett" pear | Ethyl(E,Z)-2,4-decadienoate and ethyl(E,E)-2,4-decadienoate | Jennings and Sevenants (1964) |
| "La France" pear (*P. communis* L.) | Ethyl acetate, propyl acetate, butyl acetate and hexyl acetate | Shiota (1990) |
| "Le Conte" pear | Ethyl butanoate, ethyl hexanoate, hexyl acetate and ethyl-2-methyl butanoate | Omaima et al. (2010) |
| Asian pear (*P. serotina*) | Ethyl-2-methylbutanoate, ethyl hexanoate, ethyl butanoate, ethyl-2-methylpropanoate, hexyl acetate, ethyl heptanoate, hexanal, ethyl pentanoate and ethyl propanoate | Takeoka et al. (1992) |
| "Kuerle" fragrant pear | Ethanol, hexanal, ethyl acetate, ethyl propionate, ethyl butanoate, ethyl-2-methylbutanoate, ethylhexanoate, hexyl acetate, ethyl octanoate, octyl acetate and ethyl (E,Z)-2,4-decadienoate | Chen et al. (2006a) |

### Modern Cultivars

| Cultivars | Aroma Compounds | Reference |
|---|---|---|
| "Packham's Triumph" pear | Hexyl acetate, butyl acetate and pentyl acetate | Takeoka et al (1992) |
| *P. ussuriensis* | Esters of ethyl acetate, ethyl butanoate, ethyl-2-methyl butanoate, ethyl octanoate and ethyl hexanoate; aldehydes of hexanal and 2-hexanal | Qin et al. (2012) |
| "Pingxiangli" pear | Esters, hexanal, ethyl butanoate, ethyl-2-methylbutanoate, ethyl hexanoate and hexyl acetate | Li et al. (2014) |

Various nutritional components identified in pears are sugars, organic acids, amino acids, vitamins, volatile, phosphorous, iron, potassium, calcium, magnesium, etc. Studies provide that different pear varieties exhibit varied nutritional compositions and have a wide range of taste and flavour. European pear (*P. communis)* is rich in calorie and sugar content while Asian pear (*P. pyrifolia* and *P. bretschneideri*) usually provides higher water content and lower levels of sugar and starch. Asian pear is consumed commonly for its health imparting benefits and European pear is consumed for its good taste.

Major organic acids present in it include malic and citric acid (Sha et al. 2011). Composition of glucose, fructose and sucrose are crucial in determining the sweetness of these fruits. Many phytonutrients like hydroxycinamic acids (chlorogenic acid, gentisic acid, syringic acid and vanellic acid), hydroxycinnamic acids (coumaric acid, ferulic acid and 5-caffeoylquinic acid), hydroxyquinones (arbutin) and flavonols (catechin and epicatechin), flavonols (quercetin, isorhamnetin, kaempferol) are present. Other compounds present in pears are anthocyanins which are responsible for antioxidant and anti-inflammatory effects and colouring of pear and its products and carotenoids (β-carotene, lutein and zeaxanthin) which are one of the important phytonutrients in pears (Lee et al. 2011b; Li et al. 2014). Table 4.3 summarizes the pharmacological applications of pear.

## Table 4.3: Pharmacological Applications of Pear

| Function | Method Used in the Study | Compounds Responsible | Mechanism of Action |
|---|---|---|---|
| Antidiabetic and hypoglycaemic activity | *In vivo* and *in vitro* studies | High fibre content | By lowering the blood glucose levels |
| Anti-obesity | *In vivo* | High fibre content | • By lowering low density lipoprotein and triglycerides and accelerating fat metabolism • By reducing the calorie intake due to high fibre content |
| Alcohol detoxification and hepatoprotection | Human, *in vivo* and *in vitro* studies | | By alleviating alcohol dehydrogenase and aldehyde dehydrogenase levels, lowering blood alcohol and acetaldehyde and blocking lipid accumulation in hepatocytes |
| Anti-inflammatory | *In vivo* | Anthocyanins, triterpenoids and flavonols such as ursolic acid, α-amyrin and quercetin | • By preventing fibrosis and inhibition of NFkB (nuclear factor kappa-light-chain-enhancer of activated β-cells) • By alleviating the number of MPO-mediated inflammatory cells and lowering serum levels of serum interleukin-6 |
| Antiallergic | *In vivo* | Rutin and quercetin | • Acts as anti-asthmatic agent by suppressing allergic asthma through the reduction of serum specific IgE levels i.e., immunoglobin E and inflammatory signs • By reducing mast cell activation and histamine release |
| Bronchodilatory and anti-asthma | *In vivo* and *in vitro* studies | Phytochemicals like polyphenols and flavonoids | By blocking $Ca^2$ channels in trachea muscle cells and by ACE inhibition. |
| Hypolipidemic | *In vivo* and *in vitro* studies | Catechin | By raising high density cholesterol and lowering plasma low density lipoprotein, triglycerides and cholesterol |
| Skin-lightening | *In vivo* | Phytochemicals such as arbutin and protocatechuic acid | By preventing formation of cellular melanin and expression of melanogenesis and its related enzymes |
| Anti-carcinogenic Reduces chances of lung cancer, oral cancer and breast cancer | *In vitro* | Chlorogenic acid and malaxinic acid | By favouring rapid excretion of polycyclic aromatic hydrocarbons |
| Antioxidant activity | *In vivo* | Vitamin C and other phenolic acids | By scavenging free radicals |
| Cardio protective | *In vivo* | Chlorogenic acid, fibre and polyphenols | By reducing the prevalence of stroke and increased production of nitric oxide and induction of Hmox-1 |

*(Continued)*

## Table 4.3: Pharmacological Applications of Pear (*Continued*)

| Function | Method Used in the Study | Compounds Responsible | Mechanism of Action |
|---|---|---|---|
| Improves gastro intestinal health and prevents gastric lesions | *In vivo* | Phenolic acids (chlorogenic acid, ferulic acid) and soluble fibres | By improving the metabolism of food components and inhibiting myeloperoxidase activation of inflammatory cells such as leucocytes |

## 4.8 CONCLUSION

Pear is consumed widely around the globe. It possesses great nutraceutical properties. In this chapter, a holistic view of different health benefits of pear components was provided. It also gives an overview of the recent research done on bioactive compounds of pear fruit. These compounds have been identified using different techniques predicting the beneficial effects of these. However, the evaluation of the role played by different factors affecting the concentration, efficacy and potency of the different bioactive compounds in the pear fruit is also important. Moreover, most of the research done till date was focused on cultivars being cultivated traditionally in ancient times, which shows the need of further research focusing more on newly emerged cultivars which might include hybrid varieties. Future research must be conducted considering these points which will further help in elucidating and validating the nutraceutical value of pear components.

## REFERENCES

Aggarwal, B. B., C. Sundaram, S. Prasad, and R. Kannappan. 2010. "Tocotrienols, the vitamin E of the 21st century: Its potential against cancer and other chronic diseases." *Biochemical Pharmacology* 80: 1613 1631.

Akomolafe, S., A. Akinyemi, O. Ogunsuyi, S. Oyeleye, G. Oboh, and O. Adeoyo. 2017. "Effect of caffeine, caffeic acid and their various combinations on enzymes of cholinergic, monoaminergic and purinergic systems critical to neurodegeneration in rat brain—*in vitro*." *Neurotoxicology* 62: 6–13.

Atkinson, F., K. Foster-Powell, and J. Brand-Miller. 2008. "International tables of glycemic index and glycemic load values." *Diabetes Care 31*: 12–19.

Aust, O., H. Sies, W. Stahl, and M. C. Polidori. 2001. "Analysis of lipophilic antioxidants in human serum and tissues: Tocopherols and carotenoids." *Journal of Chromatography 936*: 83–93.

Ayeleso, T., M. Matumba, and E. Mukwevho. 2017. "Oleanolic acid and its derivatives: Biological activities and therapeutic potential in chronic diseases." *Molecules 22(11)*: 1915–1924.

Azuma, K., T. Osaki, S. Ifuku, H. Saimoto, M. Morimoto, O. Takashima, T. Tsuka, T. Imagawa, Y. Okamoto, and S. Minami. 2014. "Anti-inflammatory effects of cellulose nanofiber made from pear in inflammatory bowel disease model." *Bioactive Carbohydrates and Dietary Fibre 3(1)*: 1–10.

Balasuriya, N., and H. P. V. Rupasinghe. 2012. "Antihypertensive properties of flavonoid-rich apple peel extract." *Food Chemistry 135(4)*: 2320–2325.

Barbosa, A. C. L., D. Sarkar, M. D. S. Pinto, C. Ankolekar, D. Greene, and K. Shetty. 2013. "Type 2 diabetes relevant bioactive potential of freshly harvested and long-term stored pears using *in vitro* assay models." *Journal of Food Biochemistry 37(6): 677–686.*

Barroca, M. J., R. P. F. Guine, A. Pinto, F. M. Gonçalves, and D. M. S. Ferreira. 2006. "Chemical and microbiological characterization of Portuguese varieties of pears." *Food and Bioproducts Processing 84*: 109–111.

Boots, A. W., L. C. Wilms, E. L. R. Swennen, J. C. S. Kleinjans, A. Bast, and G. R. M. M Haenen. 2008. "*In vitro* and ex vivo anti-inflammatory activity of quercetin in healthy volunteers." *Nutrition Journal 24(8): 703–710.*

Brahem, M., C. M. G. C. Renard, S. Eder, M. Loonis, R. Ouni, M. Mars, and C. L. Bourvellec. 2017. "Characterization and quantification of fruit phenolic compounds of European and Tunisian pear cultivars." *Food Research International 95*: 125–133.

Bunzel, M., and J. Ralph. 2006. "NMR characterization of lignins isolated from fruit and vegetable insoluble dietary fiber." *Journal of Agricultural and Food Chemistry 54*: 8352–8361.

Chavez, J. H., P. C. Leal, and R. A. Yunes. 2006. "Evaluation of antiviral activity of phenolic compounds and derivatives against rabies virus." *Veterinary Microbiology 116(3): 53–59.*

Chen, Z. Y., R. Jiao, and K. Y. Ma. 2008. "Cholesterol-lowering nutraceuticals and functional foods." *Journal of Agricultural and Food Chemistry 56*: 8761–8773.

Chen, J., Z. Wang, J. Wu, Q. Wang, and X. Hu. 2007. "Chemical compositional characterization of eight pear cultivars grown in China." *Food Chemistry 104(1): 268–275.*

Chen, J. L., J. H. Wu, Q. Wang, H. Deng, and X. S. Hu. 2006a. "Changes in the volatile compounds and chemical and physical properties of Kuerle fragrant pear *(Pyrus serotina* Reld) during storage." *Journal of Agricultural and Food Chemistry 54*: 8842–8847.

Chen, J. L., S. J. Yan, Z. S. Feng, L. X. Xiao, and X. S. Hu. 2006b. "Changes in the volatile compounds and chemical and physical properties of Yali pear *(Pyrus bertschneideri* Reld) during storage." *Food Chemistry 97*: 248–255.

Cho, J., S. Lee, E. H. Kim, H. R. Yun, H.Y. Jeong, Y. G. Lee, W. Kim, and J. Moon. 2015. "Change in chemical constituents and free radical-scavenging activity during pear *(Pyrus pyrifolia)* cultivar fruit development." *Bioscience, Biotechnology and Biochemistry 79(2): 260–270.*

Cho, K., A. Parveen, M. C. Kang, L. Subedi, J. H. Lee, S. Y. Park, M. R. Jin, H. Yoon, Y. K. Son, and Y. Kim. 2018. "*Pyrus ussuriensis* Maxim. leaves extract ameliorates DNCB-induced atopic dermatitis-like symptoms in NC/Nga mice." *Phytomedicine 48*: 76–83.

Ci, Z., C. Jiang, Y. Cui, and M. Kojima. 2018. "Suppressive effect of polyphenols from immature pear fruits on blood glucose levels." *Journal of Food and Nutrition Research 6(7):* 445–449.

Cinkilic, N., S. K. Cetintas, and T. Zorlu. 2013. "Radioprotection by two phenolic compounds: Chlorogenic and quinic acid, on X-ray induced DNA damage in human blood lymphocytes *in vitro.*" *Food and Chemical Toxicology 53:* 359–363.

Clementino, M., X. Shi, and Z. Zhang. 2017. "Prevention of polyphenols against carcinogenesis induced by environmental carcinogens." *Journal of Environmental Pathology, Toxicology, and Oncology 36(1):* 87–98.

Cui, T., K. Nakamura, L. Ma, J. Li, and H. Kayahara. 2005. "Analyses of arbutin and chlorogenic acid, the major phenolic constituents in oriental pear." *Journal of Agricultural and Food Chemistry 53(10):* 3882–3887.

Cushnie, T. P., and A. J. Lamb. 2005. "Antimicrobial activity of flavonoids." *International Journal of Antimicrobial Agents 26(5):* 343–356.

Dajas, F. 2012. "Life or death: Neuroprotective and anticancer effects of quercetin." *Journal of Ethnopharmacology 143(2):* 383–396.

David, R. M., and N. Gooderham. 2018. "Mechanistic evidence that benzo [a] pyrene promotes an inflammatory microenvironment that drives the metastatic potential of human mammary cells." *Archives of Toxicology 92:* 3223–3239.

Deisinger, P. J. 1996. "Human exposure to naturally occurring hydroquinone." *Journal of Toxicology and Environmental Health 47(1):* 31–46.

De-Oliveira, M., R. Sichieri, and R. Mozzer. 2008. "A low-energy-dense diet adding fruit reduces weight and energy intake in women." *Appetite 51(2):* 291–295.

Dias, M. G., F. C. Camoes, and L. Oliveira. 2009. "Carotenoids in traditional Portuguese fruits and vegetables." *Food Chemistry 113:* 808–815.

Durkee, A. B., F. B. Johnston, P. A. Thivierge, and P. A. Poapst. 1968. "Arbutin and a related glucoside in immature pear fruit." *Journal of Food Science 33(5):* 461–463.

Escarpa, A., and M. C. Gonzalez. 2000. "Evaluation of high-performance liquid chromatography for determination of phenolic compounds in pear horticultural cultivars." *Chromatographia 51(2):* 37–43.

Estrela, J. M., S. Mena, E. Obrador, M. Benlloch, G. Castellano, and R. Salvador. 2017. "Polyphenolic phytochemicals in cancer prevention and therapy: Bioavailability versus bioefficacy." *Journal of Medicinal Chemistry 60(23):* 9413–9436.

Eun, J., J. Eo, and B. Lee. 2012. "Functional compounds and biological activity of Asian pear." *Food Science and Industry 45(1):* 60–69.

Fischer, T. C., C. Gosch, J. Pfeiffer, H. Halbwirth, C. Halle, and K. Stich. 2007. "Flavonoid genes of pear (*Pyrus communis*)." *Trees 21(5):* 521–529.

Galvis-Sanchez, A., A. Gil-lzquierdo, and M. I. Gil. 2003. "Comparative study of six pear cultivars in terms of their phenolic and vitamin C contents and antioxidant capacity." *Journal of Science, Food and Agriculture 83*: 995–1003.

Gharras, H. E. 2009. "Polyphenols: Food sources, properties and applications—A review." *International Journal of Food Science & Technology 44(12): 2512–2518.*

Gonzalez-Vallinas, M., M. Gonzalez-Castej, A. Rodrıguez-Casado, and A. Ramırez–Molina. 2013. "Dietary phytochemicals in cancer prevention and therapy: A complementary approach with promising perspectives." *Nutrition Reviews 71(9): 585–599.*

Gornas, P., I. Misina, B. Lace, G. Lacis, and D. Seglina. 2015. "Tocochromanols composition in seeds recovered from different pear cultivars: RP-HPLC/FLD and RP-UPLC-ESI/MSn study." *Food Science and Technology 62*: 104–107.

Gornas, P., M. Rudzinska, and D. Segliṇa. 2014. "Lipophilic composition of eleven apple seed oils: A promising source of unconventional oil from industry by-products." *Industrial Crops and Products 60*: 86–91.

Guo, X., B. Yang, J. Tang, J. Jiang, and D. Li. 2017. "Apple & pear consumption and type 2 diabetes mellitus risk: A meta-analysis of prospective cohort studies." *Food and Function 8(3): 927–934.*

He, X., and R. H. Liu. 2008. "Phytochemicals of apple peels: Isolation, structure elucidation, and their antiproliferative and antioxidant activities." *Journal of Agricultural and Food Chemistry 56(21): 9905–9910.*

He, M., J. Zeng, L. Zhai, Y. Liu, H. Wu, and R. Zhang. 2017. "Effect of *in vitro* simulated gastrointestinal digestion on polyphenol and polysaccharide content and their biological activities among 22 fruit juices." *Food Research International 102*: 156–162.

Hider, R. C., Z. D. Liu, and H. H. Khodr. 2001. "Metal chelation of polyphenols." *Methods in Enzymology 335*: 190–203.

Hong, S. Y., E. Lansky, S. S. Kang, and M. Yang. 2021. "A review of pears (*Pyrus* spp.), ancient functional food for modern times." *BMC Complementary Medicine and Therapies 21(219): 2–14.*

Hosseini, B., B. S. Berthon, P. Wark, and L. G. Wood. 2017. "Effects of fruit and vegetable consumption on risk of asthma, wheezing and immune responses: A systematic review and meta-analysis." *Nutrients 9(4): 341–352.*

Huang, L. J., W. Y. Gao, X. Li, W. S. Zhao, Q. Huang, and C. X. Liu. 2010. "Evaluation of the *in vivo* antiinflammatory effects of extracts from *Pyrus bretschneideri* Rehd." *Journal of Agricultural and Food Chemistry 58(16):* 8983–8987.

Hudina M., and F. Ŝtampar. 2000. "Sugars and organic acids contents of European *Pyrus comminus* L. and Asian *Pyrus serotina* r Rehd. pear cultivars. *Acta Alimentaria 29(3): 217–230.* https://doi.org/10.1556/aalim.29.2000.3.2

Hwang, S. J., Y. Kim, Y. Park, H. Lee, and K. Kim. 2014. "Anti-inflammatory effects of chlorogenic acid in lipopolysaccharide-stimulated RAW 264.7 cells." *Inflammation Research* 63(1): 81–90.

Jaganathan, S.K. 2012. "Growth inhibition by caffeic acid, one of the phenolic constituents of honey, in HCT 15 colon cancer cells." *The Scientific World Journal* 2012: 372345.

Jennings, W. G., and M. R. Sevenants. 1964. "Volatile esters of Bartlett pear. III. a." *Journal of Food Science* 29: 158–163.

Jiang, R., J. M. Hodgson, E. Mas, K. D. Croft, and N. C. Ward. 2016. "Chlorogenic acid improves ex vivo vessel function and protects endothelial cells against HOCl-induced oxidative damage, via increased production of nitric oxide and induction of Hmox-1." *Journal of Nutritional Biochemistry* 27: 53–60.

Jiang, G., K. Lee, K. Ameer, and J. Eun. 2019. "Comparison of freeze-drying and hot air-drying on Asian pear (*Pyrus pyrifolia* Nakai 'Niitaka') powder: Changes in bio-accessibility, antioxidant activity, and bioactive and volatile compounds." *Journal of Food Science and Technology* 56(6): 2836–2844.

Kaluza, J., S. C. Larsson, N. Orsini, A. Linden, and A. Wolk. 2017. "Fruit and vegetable consumption and risk of COPD: A prospective cohort study of men." *Thorax* 72(6): 500–509.

Kandaswami, C., L. T. Lee, and P. P. Lee. 2005. "The antitumor activities of flavonoids." *In vivo* 19(5): 895–909.

Kanno, Y., R. Watanabe, H. Zempo, M. Ogawa, J. Suzuki, and M. Isobe. 2013. "Chlorogenic acid attenuates ventricular remodeling after myocardial infarction in mice." *International Heart Journal* 54(3): 176–180.

Kato, M., R. Ochiai, K. Kozuma, H. Sato, and Y. Katsuragi. 2018. "Effect of chlorogenic acid intake on cognitive function in the elderly: A pilot study." *Evidence-Based Complementary and Alternative Medicine* 2(1): 84–89.

Kaur, R., and V. Arya. 2012. "Ethnomedicinal and phytochemical perspectives of *Pyrus communis* Linn." *Journal of Pharmacognosy and Phytochemistry* 1(2): 14–19.

Kay, C. D., L. Hooper, P. A. Kroon, E. B. Rimm, and A. Cassidy. 2012. "Relative impact of flavonoid composition, dose and structure on vascular function: A systematic review of randomised controlled trials of flavonoid-rich food products." *Molecular Nutrition & Food Research* 56(11):1605–1616. doi: 10.1002/mnfr.201200363.

Kim, M., S. Lim, J. Kim, D. Choe, J. Kim, and M. Kang. 2018. "Effect of mixed fruit and vegetable juice on alcohol hangovers in healthy adults." *Preventive Nutrition and Food Science* 23(1): 1–7.

Kim, D., G. Shin, Y. Lee, J. S. Lee, J. Cho, S. Baik, and O. Lee. 2014. "Assessment and comparison of the antioxidant activities and nitrite scavenging activity of commonly consumed beverages in Korea." *Food Chemistry* 151: 58–64.

Koch, E. R., and P. Deo. 2016. "Nutritional supplements modulate fluorescent protein bound advanced glycation endproducts and digestive enzymes related to type 2 diabetes mellitus." *BMC Complementary Medicine 16(1)*: 338–346.

Kolniak-Ostek, J. 2016a. "Chemical composition and antioxidant capacity of different anatomical parts of pear (*Pyrus communis* L.)." *Food Chemistry 203*: 491–497.

Kolniak-Ostek, J. 2016b. "Identification and quantification of polyphenolic compounds in ten pear cultivars by UPLC-PDA-Q/TOF-MS." *Journal of Food Composition and Analysis 49*: 65–77.

Kolniak-Ostek, J., D. Klopotowska, K. P. Rutkowski, A. Skorupinska, and D. E. Kruczynska. 2020. "Bioactive compounds and health-promoting properties of pears (*Pyrus communis* L.) fruits." *Molecules 25(19)*: 44–49.

Kolniak-Ostek, J., and J. Oszmiański. 2015. "Characterization of phenolic compounds in different anatomical pear (*Pyrus communis* L.) parts by ultra-performance liquid chromatography photodiode detector-quadrupole/time of flight-mass spectrometry (UPLC-PDA-Q/TOF-MS)." *International Journal of Mass Spectrometry 392*:154–163.

Kris-Etherton, P. M., K. D. Hecker, A. Bonanome, S. M. Coval, A. E. Binkoski, K. F. Hilpert, A. E. Griel, and T. D. Etherton. 2002. "Bioactive compounds in foods: Their role in the prevention of cardiovascular disease and cancer." *American Journal of Medicine 113(324)*: 71–88.

Kunkel, S. D., C. J. Elmore, K. S. Bongers, S. M. Ebert, D. K. Fox, and M. C. Dyle. 2012. "Ursolic acid increases skeletal muscle and brown fat and decreases diet-induced obesity, glucose intolerance and fatty liver disease." *PLoS One 7(6)*: 393–412.

Lakhanpal, P., and D. K. Rai. 2007. "Quercetin: A versatile flavonoid." *Internet Journal of Medical Update 2(2)*: 22–37.

Larsson, S. C., J. Virtamo, and A. Wolk. 2013. "Total and specific fruit and vegetable consumption and risk of stroke: A prospective study." *Atherosclerosis 227(1)*: 147–152.

Lee, S., J. Cho, H. Y. Jeong, D. E. Jeong, D. Kim, and S. Cho. 2015. "Comparison of bioactive compound contents and *in vitro* and ex vivo antioxidative activities between peel and flesh of pear (*Pyrus pyrifolia* Nakai)." *Food Science and Biotechnology 24(1)*: 207–216.

Lee, K. H., J. Y. Cho, H. J. Lee, Y. K. Ma, J. Kwon, S. H. Park, S. H. Lee, J. A. Cho, W. S. Kim, K. H. Park, and J. H. Moon. 2011a. "Hydroxycinnamoylmalic acids and their methyl esters from pear (*Pyrus pyrifolia* Nakai) fruit peel." *Journal of Agricultural and Food Chemistry 59*: 10124–10128.

Lee, K. H., J. Cho, H. J. Lee, K. Y. Park, Y. Ma, and S. Lee. 2011b. "Isolation and identification of phenolic compounds from an Asian pear (*Pyrus pyrifolia* Nakai) fruit peel." *Food Science and Biotechnology 20(6)*: 1539–1545.

Lee, Y. G., J. Cho, J. Park, S. Lee, W. Kim, and K. Park. 2013. "Large-scale isolation of highly pure malaxinic acid from immature pear (*Pyrus pyrifolia* Nakai) fruit." *Food Science and Biotechnology 22(6):* 1539–1545.

Lee, H., T. Isse, T. Kawamoto, H. Woo, A. K. Kim, and J. Y. Park. 2012. "Effects and action mechanisms of Korean pear (*Pyrus pyrifolia* cv. Shingo) on alcohol detoxification." *Phytotherapy Research 26(11):* 1753–1758.

Lee, H. J., H. Y. Jeong, M. R. Jin, H. J. Lee, J. Cho, and J. Moon. 2017. "Metabolism and antioxidant effect of malaxinic acid and its corresponding aglycone in rat blood plasma." *Free Radical Biology and Medicine 110:* 399–407.

Lee, S. K., and A. A. Kader. 2000. "Preharvest and postharvest factors influencing vitamin C content of horticultural crops." *Postharvest Biology and Technology 20:* 207–220.

Lee, J. C., S. C. Pak, S. H. Lee, C. S. Na, S. C. Lim, C. H. Song, Y. H. Bai, and C. H. Jang. 2004. "Asian pear pectin administration during pre-sensitization inhibits allergic response to ovalbumin in BALB/c mice." *Journal of Alternative and Complementary Medicine 10(3):* 527–534.

Leontowicz, M., S. Gorinstein, H. Leontowicz, R. Krzeminski, A. Lojek, E. Katrich, M. Cíz, O. Martin-Belloso, R. Soliva-Fortuny, R. Haruenkit, and S. Trakhtenberg. 2003. "Apple and pear peel and pulp and their influence on plasma lipids and antioxidant potentials in rats fed cholesterol-containing diets." *Journal of Agricultural and Food Chemistry 51:* 5780–5785.

Li, X., T. T. Wang, B. Zhou, W. Y. Gao, J. G. Cao, and L. Q. Huang. 2014. "Chemical composition and antioxidant and anti-inflammatory potential of peels and flesh from 10 different pear varieties (*Pyrus* spp.)." *Food Chemistry 152:* 531–538.

Li, X., J. Y. Zhang, W. Y. Gao, and H. Y. Wang. 2012a. "Study on chemical composition, anti-inflammatory and antimicrobial activities of extracts from Chinese pear fruit (*Pyrus bretschneideri* Rehd.)." *Food and Chemical Toxicology 50:* 3673–3679.

Li, X., J. Y. Zhang, W. Y. Gao, H. Y. Wang, J. G. Cao, and L. Q. Huang. 2012b. "Chemical composition and anti-inflammatory and antioxidant activities of either pear cultivars." *Journal of Agricultural and Food Chemistry 60:* 8738–8744.

Liang, N. D., and D. Kitts. 2015. "Role of chlorogenic acids in controlling oxidative and inflammatory stress conditions." *Nutrients 8:* 16–22.

Liaudanskas, M., K. Zymone, J. Viskelis, A. Klevinskas, and V. Janulis. 2017. "Determination of the phenolic composition and antioxidant activity of pear extracts." *Journal of Chemistry 5:* 2–9.

Likhitwitayawuid, K., B. Supudompol, B. Sritularak, V. Lipipun, K. Rapp, and R. F. Schinazi. 2005. "Phenolics with anti-HSV and anti-HIV activities from *Artocarpus gomezianus*, *Mallotus pallidus*, and *Triphasia trifolia*." *Pharmaceutical Biology 43(8):* 651–657.

Lin, L., and J. M. Harnly. 2008. "Phenolic compounds and chromatographic profiles of pear skins (*Pyrus* spp.)." *Journal of Agricultural and Food Chemistry 56*: 9094–9101.

Lopez-Lazaro, M. 2002. "Flavonoids as anticancer agents: Structure–activity relationship study." *Current Medicinal Chemistry – Anticancer Agents 2(6)* 691–714.

Magnani, C., V. L. B. Isaac, M. A. Correa, and H. R. N. Salgado. 2014. "Caffeic acid: A review of its potential use in medications and cosmetics." *Analytical Methods 6(10):* 3203–3210.

Migas, P., and M. Krauze-Baranowska. 2015. "The significance of arbutin and its derivatives in therapy and cosmetics." *Phytochemistry Letters 13*: 35–40.

Min, T. S., M. J. Park, J. H. Moon, W. S. Kim, S. H. Lee, Y. D. Cho, and S. H. Park. 2013. "Bio-active substances and physiological activity of pears." *Journal of Applied Biological Chemistry 56(2):* 83–87.

Moon, J., J. Cho, S. Lee, and W. Kim. 2017. "Development and application of functional resource using pear." *Horticultural Science and Technology 35*: 36–37.

Morton, L. W., A. Caccetta, A. A. C. Rima, I. B. Puddey, and K. D. Croft. 2000. "Chemistry and biological effects of dietary phenolic compounds: Relevance to cardiovascular disease." *Clinical Experimental Pharmacology Physiology 27*: 152–159.

Mun, G., S. Kim, E. Choi, C. S. Kim, and Y. Lee. 2018. "Pharmacology of natural radioprotectors." *Archives of Pharmacal Research 41(11):* 1033–1050.

Nassar, M. I., T. K. Mohamed, and S. A. El-Toumy. 2011. "Phenolic metabolites from *Pyrus calleryana* and evaluation of its free radical scavenging activity." *Carbohydrate Research 346*: 64–66.

Naveed, M., V. Hejazi, M. Abbas, A. A. Kamboh, G. J. Khan, and M. Shumzaid. 2018. "Chlorogenic acid (CGA): A pharmacological review and call for further research." *Biomedicine & Pharmacotherapy 97*: 67–74.

Nieman, L. K., B. M. Biller, J. W. Findling, M. H. Murad, J. Newell-Price, M. O. Savage, and A. Tabarin. 2015. "Treatment of Cushing's syndrome: An endocrine society clinical practice guideline." *Journal of Clinical Endocrinology & Metabolism 100(8):* 2807–2831.

Nohynek, L. J., L. L. Alakomi, and M. P. Kahkonen. 2006. "Berry phenolics: Antimicrobial properties and mechanisms of action against severe human pathogens." *Nutrition and Cancer 54(1):* 18–32.

Nortjé, B. K., and B. H. Koeppen. 1965. "The flavonol glycosides in the fruit of *Pyrus communis* L. Cultivar bon Chréstien." *Biochemical Journal 97*: 209–213.

Oleszek, W., M. J. Amiot, and S. Y. Aubert. 1994. "Identification of some phenolics in pear fruit." *Journal of Agricultural and Food Chemistry 42*: 1261–1265.

Omaima, M., H. A. Hamouda, and M. A. Abd-El-Mageed. 2010. "Effect of calcium and some antioxidants treatments on storability of Le *conte* pear fruits and its volatile components." *Nature and Science 8(5):* 109–126.

Öztürk, A., L. Demirsoy, H. Demirsoy, A. Asan, and O. Gul. 2014. "Phenolic compounds and chemical characteristics of pears (Pyrus communis L.)." *International Journal of Food Properties* 4: 1–34.

Öztürk, A., L. Demirsoy, H. Demirsoy, A. Asan, and O. Gul. 2015. "Phenolic compounds and chemical characteristics of Pears *(Pyrus communis L.)." International Journal of Food Properties* 18(3): 536–546. doi: 10.1080/10942912.2013.835821.

Pandey, K. B., and S. I. Rizvi. 2009. "Plant polyphenols as dietary antioxidants in human health and disease." *Oxidative Medicine and Cellular Longevity* 2(5): 270–278.

Park, H., S. Lee, H. Son, S. Park, M. Kim, and E. Choi. 2008. "Flavonoids inhibit histamine release and expression of pro-inflammatory cytokines in mast cells." *Archives of Pharmacal Research* 31(10): 1303–1311.

Pascoalino, L. A., F. S. Reis, M. A. Prieto, J. C. M. Barreira, C. F. R. Ferreira, and L. Barros. 2021. "Valorization of bio-residues from the processing of main Portuguese fruit crops: From discarded waste to health promoting compounds." *Molecules* 26(9): 2624.

Pastore, S., S. Potapovich, and V. Kostyuk. 2009. "Plant polyphenols effectively protect HaCaT cells from ultraviolet C-triggered necrosis and suppress inflammatory chemokine expression." *Annals of the New York Academy of Sciences* 1171: 305–313.

Qin, G., S. Tao, Y. Cao, J. Wu, H. Zhang, W. Huang, and S. Zhang. 2012. "Evaluation of the volatile profile of 33 *Pyrus ussuriensis* cultivars by HS-SPME with GC–MS." *Food Chemistry* 134, 2367–2382.

Ramandthan, L., and N. P. Das. 1992. "Studies on the control of lipid oxidation in ground fish by some polyphenolic natural products." *Journal of Agricultural and Food Chemistry* 40: 17–21.

Ramnani, P., E. Gaudier, M. Bingham, P. Bruggen, K. M. Tuohy, and G. R. Gibson. 2010. "Prebiotic effect of fruit and vegetable shots containing Jerusalem artichoke inulin: A human intervention study." *British Journal of Nutrition* 104(2): 233–240.

Reiland, H., and J. Slavin. 2015. "Systematic review of pears and health." *Food and Nutrition* 50(6): 301–305. doi: 10.1097/NT.0000000000000112.

Roleira, F. M., E. J. Tavares-da-Silva, C. L. Varela, S. C. Costa, T. Silva, and J. Garrido. 2015. "Plant derived and dietary phenolic antioxidants: Anticancer properties." *Food Chemistry* 183: 235–258.

Roberfroid, M., G.R. Gobson, L. Hoyles, A.L. McCartney, R. Rastall, I. Rowland, D. Wolvers, B. Watzl, H. Szajewska, B. Stahl, et al. 2011. "Prebiotic effects: Metabolic and health benefits." *British Journal of Nutrition* 104: S1–S63.

Russell, W. R., A. Labat, L. Scobbie, G. J. Duncan, and G. Duthie. 2009. "Phenolic acid content of fruits commonly consumed and locally produced in Scotland." *Food Chemistry* 115: 100–104.

Sarkar, D., C. Ankolekar, M. Pinto, and K. Shetty. 2015. "Dietary functional benefits of Bartlett and Starkrimson pears for potential management of hyperglycemia, hypertension and ulcer bacteria helicobacter pylori while supporting beneficial probiotic bacterial response." *Food Research International* 69: 80–90.

Sato, Y., S. Itagaki, and T. Kurokawa. 2011. "*In vitro* and *in vivo* antioxidant properties of chlorogenic acid and caffeic acid." *International Journal of Pharmaceutics 403(2):* 136–138.

Scalbert, A., I. T. Johnson, and M. Saltmarsh. 2000. "Polyphenols: Antioxidants and beyond." *American Journal of Clinical Nutrition 81(1):* 215–217.

Seo, D., J. Jung, J. Lee, E. Jeon, W. Kim, and C. Park. 2012. "Biotechnological production of arbutins (alpha- and beta-arbutins), skin-lightening agents, and their derivatives." *Applied Microbiology and Biotechnology 95(6):* 1417–1425.

Sha, S. F., J. C. Li, J. Wu, and S. L. Zhang. 2011. "Characteristics of organic acids in the fruit of different pear species." *African Journal of Agricultural Research 6(10):* 2403–2410.

Sharma, K., S. Kang, D. Gong, S. Oh, E. Park, and M. Oak. 2018. "Combination of *Garcinia cambogia* extract and pear pomace extract additively suppresses adipogenesis and enhances lipolysis in 3T3-L1 cells." *Pharmacognosy Magazine 14(54):* 220–226.

Shepherd, S. J., and P. R. Gibson. 2006. "Fructose malabsorption and symptoms of irritable bowel syndrome: Guidelines for effective dietary management." *Journal of the American Dietetic Association 106(10):* 1631–1639.

Shiota, H. 1990. "Changes in the volatile composition of La France pear during maturation." *Journal of Agricultural and Food Chemistry* 52: 421–429.

Sidoryk, K., A. Jaromin, N. Filipczak, P. Cmoch, and M. Cybulski. 2018. "Synthesis and antioxidant activity of caffeic acid derivatives." *Molecules* 23: 219–226.

Sioud, F. B., and B. S. Luh. 1966. "Polyphenolic compounds in pear puree." *Food Technology 535:* 183.

Spanos, G. A., and R. E. Wrolstad. 1990. "Influence of variety, maturity, processing and storage on the phenol composition of pear juice." *Journal of Agricultural and Food Chemistry* 38: 817–824.

Spencer, J. P. E. 2010. "The impact of fruit flavonoids on memory and cognition." *British Journal of Nutrition 104(3):* 40–47.

Srinivasan, M., A. Sudheer, and V. Menon. 2007. "Ferulic acid: Therapeutic potential through its antioxidant property." *Journal of Clinical Biochemistry and Nutrition 40(2):* 92–100.

Stefanska, B., H. Karlic, F. Varga, K. Fabianowska-Majewska, and A. G. Haslberger. 2012. "Epigenetic mechanisms in anticancer actions of bioactive food components—The implications in cancer prevention." *British Journal of Pharmacology 167(2): 279–297.*

Sun, J., Y. F. Chu, X. Wu, and R. H. Liu. 2002. "Antioxidant and antiproliferative activities of common fruits." *Journal of Agricultural and Food Chemistry 50(25):* 7449–7454.

Takeoka, G. R., R. G. Buttery, and R. A. Flath. 1992. "Volatile constituents of Asian pear (*Pyrus serotina*)." *Journal of Agricultural and Food Chemistry 40:* 1925–1929.

Tanrıöven, D., and A. Eksi. 2005. "Phenolic compounds in pear juice from different cultivars." *Food Chemistry 93: 89–93.*

Thomas, T., and A. F. Pfeiffer. 2012. "Foods for the prevention of diabetes: How do they work?" *Metabolism Research and Reviews 28(1): 25–49.*

Tom, E. N. L., C. Girard-Thernier, and C. Demougeot. 2016. "The Janus face of chlorogenic acid on vascular reactivity: A study on rat isolated vessels." *Phytomedicine 23(10): 1037–1042.*

Tomas-Lorente, F., C. Garcia-Viguera, F. Ferreres, and F. A. Tomas-Barberan. 1992. "Phenolic compounds analysis in the determination of fruit jam genuineness." *Journal of Agricultural and Food Chemistry 40: 1800–1804.*

Tomosaka, H., H. Koshino, and T. Tajika. 2001. "Lupeol esters from the Twig bark of Japanese pear (*Pyrus serotina* Rhed.) cv. Shinko." *Bioscience, Biotechnology, and Biochemistry 65(5): 1198–1201.*

Truong, X. T., S. Park, Y. Lee, H. Y. Jeong, J. Moon, and T. Jeon. 2017. "Protocatechuic acid from pear inhibits melanogenesis in melanoma cells." *International Journal of Molecular Science 18(08): 1809–1818.*

Ulaszewska, M., N. Vázquez-Manjarrez, M. Garcia-Aloy, R. Llorach, F. Mattivi, and L. O. Dragsted. 2018. "Food intake biomarkers for apple, pear, and stone fruit." *Genes and Nutrition 13(1): 29–36.*

Veberic, R., A. Slatnar, J. Bizjak, F. Stampar, and M. Mikulic-Petkovsek. 2015. "Anthocyanin composition of different wild and cultivated berry species." *LWT – Food Science and Technology 60(1): 509–517.*

Velmurugan, C., and A. Bhargava. 2013. "Antidiabetic and hypolipidemic activity of fruits of *Pyrus communis* L. in hyperglycemic rats." *Asian Journal of Pharmaceutical and Clinical Research 6(5): 108–111.*

Wagenbreth, A. 1959. "Das Vorkommen zweier Flavonoidgarnituren in der Gattung *Pyrus*." *Flora 147: 164–166.*

Wang, Z., C. J. Barrow, F. R. Dunshea, and H. A. R. Suleria. 2021. "A comparative investigation on phenolic composition, characterization and antioxidant potentials of five different Australian grown pear varieties." *Antioxidants 10(2): 151–159.*

Wang, T., X. Li, B. Zhou, H. Li, J. Zeng, and W. Gao. 2015. "Antidiabetic activity in type 2 diabetic mice and α-glucosidase inhibitory, antioxidant and anti-inflammatory potential of chemically profiled pear peel and pulp extracts (*Pyrus* spp.)." *Journal of Functional Foods 13*: 276–288.

Warleta, F., M. Campos, Y. Allouche, C. Sanchez-Quesada, J. Ruiz-Mora, G. Beltran, and J. J. Gaforio. 2010. "Squalene protects against oxidative DNA damage in MCF10A human mammary epithelial cells but not in MCF7 and MDA-MB-231 human breast cancer cells." *Food and Chemical Toxicology 48*: 1092–1100.

Weichselbaum, E., L. Wyness, and S. Stanner. 2010. "Apple polyphenols and cardiovascular disease—A review of the evidence." *Nutrition Bulletin 35(2):* 92–101.

Weidenböerger, M., H. Hindorf, H. C. Jha, and P. Tsotsonos. 1990. "Antifungal activity of flavonoids against storage fungi the genus *Aspergillus*." *Phytochemistry 29*: 1103–1105.

Wright, M. E., S. J. Weinstein, K. A. Lawson, D. Albanes, A. F. Subar, and L. B. Dixon. 2007. "Supplemental and dietary vitamin E intakes and risk of prostate cancer in a large prospective study." *Cancer Epidemiology Biomarkers and Prevention 16*: 1128–1135.

Yan, C., M. Yin, N. Zhang, Q. Jin, Z. Fang, and Y. Lin. 2014. "Stone cell distribution and lignin structure in various pear varieties." *Scientia Horticulturae 174*: 142–152.

Yang, M. 2006. "Functional study of Korean pears." *Korean Journal of Horticultural Science and Technology 24*: 50–56.

Yang, M. 2018. "Detoxification of pears." In *Daily Consumption of Korean Pears for Health*, pp. 55–67. Edited by Pear Research Institute, National Institute of Horticultural and Herbal Science: Rural Development Administration.

Yang, M., C. Park, D. Kim, and H. Jeong. 2005. "Antimutagenic and anticarcinogenic effects of Korean pears." *Cancer Prevention Research 10(2):* 124–127.

Yim, S., and S. Nam. 2016. "Physiochemical, nutritional and functional characterization of 10 different pear cultivars (*Pyrus* spp.)." *Journal of Applied Botany and Food Quality 89*: 73–81.

Yoon, B., K. Kim, and S. Park. 2006. "Effects of pear extracts cultured under conventional and environment-friendly conditions on cell proliferation in rat hepatocytes." *Applied Biological Chemistry 49(3):* 233–237.

You, M., J. Rhyu, and H. Kim. 2017. "Pear pomace water extract suppresses hepatic lipid peroxidation and protects against liver damage in rats fed a high fat/cholesterol diet." *Food Science and Biotechnology 26(3):* 801–806.

Zhang, X., H. Huang, and T. Yang. 2010. "Chlorogenic acid protects mice against lipopolysaccharide-induced acute lung injury." *Injury 41(7):* 746–752.

Zhang, Y., F. Wang, Y. Zhou, Y. Li, T. Zhou, and J. Zheng. 2016. "Effects of 20 selected fruits on ethanol metabolism: Potential health benefits and harmful impacts." *International Journal of Environmental Research and Public Health 13(4):* 399–406.

Zhao, M., L. Cai, J. M. He, T. P. Yin, Y. C. Sui, M. T. Luo, and Z. T. Ding. 2013. "Chemical constituents from the branches and leaves of *Pyrus pashia.*" *Chinese Journal of Chemistry 33:* 1284–1290.

Zhao, Z., and M. Moghadasian. 2008. "Chemistry, natural sources, dietary intake and pharmacokinetic properties of ferulic acid: A review." *Food Chemistry 109:* 691–702.

Zuo, K. X., and J. K. Liu. 1997. "Studies on the chemical constituents of *Pyrus communis.*" *Acta Botanica Sinica 29(1):* 84–87.

# 5 Mango

*Varun Kumar, Amarjeet Kumar, and Deependra Rajoriya*

## CONTENTS

## 5.1 INTRODUCTION

Mango (*Mangifera indica* L.), family Anacardiaceae, is a fruit plant grown widely in the tropical and subtropical countries of the world. Mango is one of the most important commercial crops worldwide in terms of production, marketing, and consumption. Mango trees thrive in tropical and subtropical regions, are evergreen, grow to a height of around 18 meters, and produce fruit 4–6 years after planting. It is pleasant in taste, aroma, and rich in nutrition (Ibarra-Garza et al., 2015). Mango production is second to bananas in terms of quantity and value among internationally traded tropical fruits, and fifth in terms of overall production among major fruit crops worldwide (Tjiptono et al., 1984; Yaacob and Subhadrabandhu, 1995). Mango production is expected to reach around 26 million tons per year worldwide (FAO, 2007). The world production of mango is estimated at 42 million tons per year; India is the largest producer of mango with 1,525,000 tons per year, followed by China, Kenya, Thailand, Indonesia, Pakistan, and Mexico. Mexico is the largest exporter with 287,771 tons per year (FAOSTAD, 2015). It is known as the "King of Fruits" due to its chemical composition, and it is the world's second most traded tropical fruit and fifth in total production (FAOSTAD, 2015). Mango, whether fresh or processed, is a nutritionally and satiating alternative for a balanced diet. Figure 5.1 shows how it can be divided into three parts: Pulp (Mesocarp), peel (Epicarp), and seed kernel (Endocarp). It is considered to be high in bioactive compounds (BaCs), which have potential nutritional and health-promoting properties. It has been recommended that

DOI: 10.1201/9781003259213-5

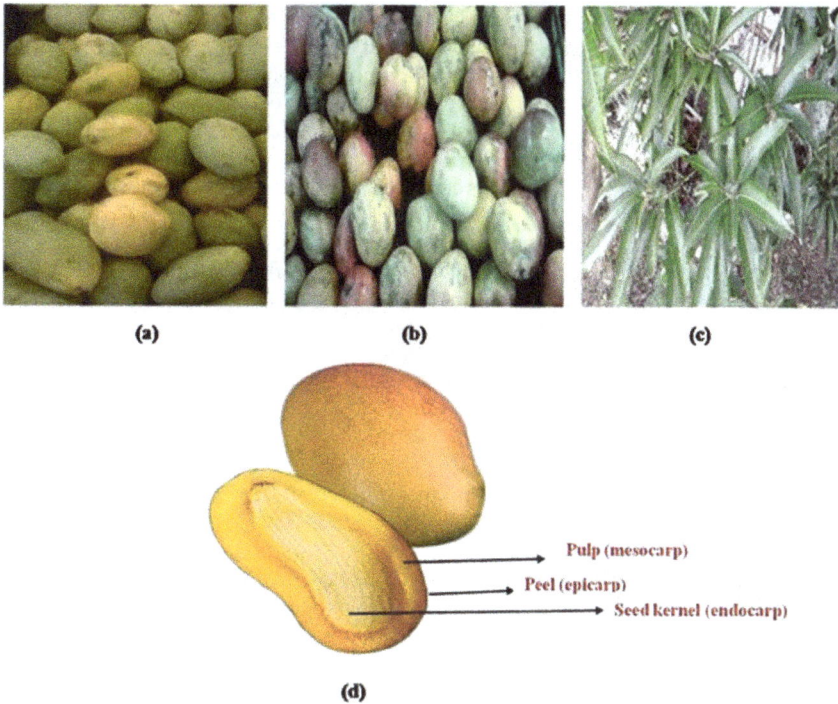

**Figure 5.1** *M. indica* (mango) fruits (a, b, d) and leaves (c). (From Ediriweera et al., 2017.)

the consumption of fruits and vegetables around 400 g/day could reduce the risk of chronic diseases such as cardiovascular disease, diabetes, and obesity (World Health Organization, 2003). As a result, it is a major fruit that is rich in functionality and nutraceutical properties, including xanthones and polyphenols, which can defend us from various types of diseases (Berardini et al., 2005). This chapter's goal is to provide the latest investigated information on the content and accessibility of various BaCs originating from different parts of mango such as peel, seed, and kernel so that researchers and/or other health experts can more accurately assess the dietary intake of these BaCs, investigate their physiological functions, and determine their links to health and disease. It is critical to have data on BaC food sources to determine dietary consumption. Furthermore, this information could be used to target mango consumption as part of a broader dietary management strategy for a variety of diseases and disorders, as well as increase consumer preference for mango.

## 5.2 TAXONOMY AND BOTANICAL DESCRIPTION

*Mangifera* is a genus in the Anacardiaceae family that contains approximately 69 different species, with *M. indica* (mango) being the most common (Mukherjee, 1972; Slippers et al., 2005). Mango is an annual plant broad canopy tree with a height range of 8–40 m. (Litz, 2009). Mango's bark is thick, brown-gray, and crudely ruptured (Nandwani, 2013). The leaves range in length from 15 to 45 cm

(Nandwani, 2013). The length of the leaf petiole varies from 1–10 cm (Nandwani, 2013). The leaf of mango comes in various shapes and sizes (lanceolate, linear-oblong, ovate-lanceolate, oval, roundish-oblong, and oblong) (Figure 5.1) (Nandwani, 2013). A few mango cultivars have red, green, and yellow leaves, along with bright upper leaf surfaces (Nandwani, 2013; Huda et al., 2015). Male and hermaphrodite flowers grow in the same panicle as mango flowers, which can be 6–8 mm in diameter. In inflorescences, there are approximately 4,500–5,000 tiny petals with red/purple spots on the petals (Nandwani, 2013; Huda et al., 2015).

Even though inflorescences have a large number of flowers, only a few will develop into fruits. The flowering period lasts from January to April, and the majority of the petals are subsessile and have a pleasant aroma. Mango fruit (Figure 5.1) is a drupe of various shapes, sizes, and colors. The extract of fruit can be yellow, orange, red, or green. The fruit seeds are oval or elongated in shape, among a stiff endocarp protected in a woody fiber (Sivakumar et al., 2011).

## 5.3 NUTRITIONAL COMPOSITION

Mango pulp's nutritional makeup is mainly determined through variety/type, site as well as the climate of the production area, along with the maturity of fruits (Abbasi et al., 2015; Maldonado-Celis et al., 2019). The nutritional value of mango is shown in Table 5.1. The nutritional composition of mango pulp are high in carbohydrates (16%–18%), proteins, fat, and dietary fiber, in addition to organic acids (Lemmens et al., 2013). It is also rich in ascorbic acid and retinol as well as minerals such as calcium, iron, and phosphorus. Mango pulp gives a lot of energy: 100 g of fresh pulp delivers 60–190 kcal. Mango pulp includes 75%–85% water in addition to the other important nutritional ingredients (Table 5.1).

### 5.3.1 Macronutrients

Mango has different kinds of carbohydrates depending on their maturation level. Unripe mango contains starch and pectin, but ripe one contains sugars (fructose, glucose, and sucrose). Starch is transformed into glucose and fructose throughout the ripening process. Many species, including Alphonso (Reddy and Reddy, 2005; Yashoda et al., 2006), Deshahari (Kalra et al., 1983), and Tommy Atkins, show a rise in monosaccharide and disaccharide concentration content in the mature fruit (Tasneem, 2004). Pectin contains gelling properties, which is necessary for the firmness of the fruit; concentration reduces as the fruit ripens, producing a sweeter, and smoother fleshy tissue (Bello-Pérez et al., 2007; Dar et al., 2016). The most important sugars, which are glucose, fructose, and sucrose, occur in the stages of maturation and ripening of mango (Reddy and Reddy, 2005; Dar et al., 2016; US Department of Agriculture, 2020). Mango fruit has a modest protein content (0.5%–5.5%) when compared to carbohydrates (Table 5.1). Mango protein concentration varies depending on the place of production. Mango grown in Peru, for example, has the highest protein content, while that grown in Columbia has the lowest. The amount of component amino acids varies depending upon the maturation stage of fruits, the area, and the species (Tharanathan et al., 2006).

### 5.3.2 Micronutrients

#### 5.3.2.1 Vitamins and Minerals

Mango pulp comprises vital micronutrients such as vitamins and minerals according to the USDA 2006 database. Vitamins A and C are greater in comparison to vitamins E, K, and B (Vallarino and Osorio, 2019). The quantity of vitamin C differs; hence, regular mango eating might meet the need for dietary intake of vitamins C and A (World Health Organization, 2003). Vitamin C is

## Table 5.1: Nutritional Information of *M. indica* (Mango) Peel, Pulp, and Seed Kernel

| Compound (100/g) | Peel | Pulp | Seed Kernel |
| --- | --- | --- | --- |
| Water (g) | 72.5 | 83.46 | 9.1 |
| Energy (kcal) | 454 | 60 | 327 |
| Carbohydrate(g) | 28.2 | 14.98 | 18.2 |
| Protein (g) | 3.6 | 0.82 | 6.61 |
| Total lipid (fat) (g) | 2.2 | 0.38 | 9.4 |
| Total sugars(g) | 25 | 19.64 | 70 |
| Dietary fiber (g) | 40–72.5 | 1.6 | 2.8 |
| **Minerals (mg) (100/g)** | **Peel** | **Pulp** | **Seed Kernel** |
| Calcium (Ca) | 150 | 11 | 450 |
| Iron (Fe) | 40.6 | 0.16 | 11.9 |
| Magnesium (Mg) | 100 | 10 | 100 |
| Phosphorus(P) | – | 14 | 140 |
| Potassium (K) | 75 | 168 | 365 |
| Sodium (Na) | 50 | 1 | 150 |
| Zinc (Zn) | 1.74 | 0.09 | 1.1 |
| Copper (Cu) | 10.4 | 0.04–0.32 | – |
| Selenium (Se) | – | 0–0.6 | – |
| **Vitamins (100/g)** | **Peel** | **Pulp** | **Seed Kernel** |
| Vitamin C (mg) | 18–257 | 36.4 | 17 |
| Thiamine (mg) | – | 0.028 | 0.08 |
| Riboflavin (mg) | – | 0.038 | 0.13 |
| Niacin (mg) | – | 0.669 | 0.19 |
| Pantothenic acid (mg) | – | 0.119 | 0.12 |
| Folate (µg) | – | 43 | – |
| Vitamin A (µg) | 100 | 54 | – |
| Vitamin E (mg) | 0.25–59 | 0.9 | 1.3 |
| **Organic Acids (%) (100/g)** | **Peel** | **Pulp** | **Seed Kernel** |
| The citric acid | – | 0.7 | – |
| Metallic acid | – | 0.5 | – |

*Source:* From Lebaka et al. (2021).

needed for collagen tissue renewal, iron assimilation, and scurvy anticipation (Diplock et al., 1998). The antioxidant properties, immunity, visual benefits, antitumor, and anti-cardiovascular disease impacts of vitamin A and its metabolites have increased interest (Shenai, 1999). Because vitamin A concentrations range from 1,000 to 6,000 IU, one mango fruit delivers 10%–13% of the recommended daily allowance (RDA). Mango eating is the most straightforward method for preventing vitamin A insufficiency (Muoki et al., 2009; Matheyambath et al., 2016). Mango pulp has lower vitamin E and K contents than vitamin A. As the fruit ripens, their numbers grow as well. In contrast, Indian varieties such as deshahari have small vitamin E content in mature fruit (Singh et al., 2011). Mango pulp provides about 1.3 mg of active form α-tocopherol of vitamin E (Robles-Sánchez et al., 2009). The concentrations of vitamin C and E in mango fruit have an inverse connection (Mène-Saffrané, 2018). In the fresh fruit pulp, the vitamin B-complex level varies as the fruit matures (Dar et al., 2016). Mango pulp might be an excellent supply of elemental elements, which are required for many metabolic activities. It is also an excellent source of minerals, such as sodium, copper, iron, calcium, manganese, zinc, selenium, phosphorus, and boron (Table 5.1).

## 5.4 CHEMISTRY OF BIOACTIVE COMPOUNDS

*Mangiferin* is a well-known polyphenolic compound with diverse bioactive attributes that have been widely investigated (Ichiki et al., 1998). Amounts of various polyphenols in mango vary depending on the part and variety (Ma et al., 2011). Polyphenols (flavonoids, xanthones, and phenolic acids) are the most common types of compounds in mango (Berardini et al., 2005). The main polyphenolic compounds found in mango are mangiferin, gallic acid, catechins, quercetin, kaempferol, protocatechuic acid, ellagic acids, propyl, and methyl gallate, rhamnetin, and anthocyanins (Nayan et al., 2018). Abdalla et al. (2007) discovered the polyphenolic content of mango by analyzing the many polyphenolic components. Among the bioactive components discovered in the mango seed kernel are tannin, gallic acid, coumarin, caffeic acid, vanillin, mangiferin, ferulic acid, cinnamic acid, and unknown compounds (Masibo and He, 2009). The total phenolic content of the mango kernel was determined to be 112 mg/GAE/100 g. According to Palafox-Carlos et al. (2012), mango peels have a high concentration of polyphenols, carotenoids, and dietary fiber. These polyphenols include mangiferin pentoxide, quercetin, syringic acid, and ellagic acid (Ajila et al., 2007). Figure 5.2. showing the structures of some common BaCs of M. indica (mango).

### 5.4.1 Tannins and Derivatives Compounds

Kabuki et al. (2000) found that an ethanolic extract from mango kernels has antibacterial activity against bacterial species, as well as food-borne diseases. The extract was discovered to be primarily composed of polyphenols, although the antimicrobial compounds were not identified. Subsequently, it was discovered that mango kernel extracts have a high concentration of hydrolyzable tannins, and the antibacterial activity was related to the existence of gallotannins (Kabuki et al., 2000; Berardini et al., 2004). Tian et al. (2013) reported that gallotannins isolated from the *Galla chinensis* plant, which belongs to the Anacardiaceae family, have antibacterial properties. *Galla chinensis* extracts demonstrated remarkable broad-spectrum antimicrobial properties against three Gram-negative (*Escherichia coli*, Shielladysenteriae, *Salmonella* Typhimurium) and three Gram-positive (*Bacillus subtilis, Staphylococcus aureus, Bacillus cereus*) bacteria species. Other studies have discovered that gallotannins through the *Galla chinensis* plant and extracts have antimicrobial properties (Aruoma, 1998; Zhu et al., 2002; Lima et al., 2006).

### 5.4.2 Mangiferin

Mangiferin is referred to as a "super antioxidant" since it is considered to be a simpler antioxidant except for the natural source of an antioxidant such as ascorbic acid and tocopherol. It is contained in the xanthone which has antioxidant properties. Mango kernel isolates were subsequently found to contain a high level of C-glucosyl xanthones, which have good thermal stability (Sanchez et al., 2000; Luo et al., 2012). It defends the mango kernel against a variety of stressors (both static and dynamic), including pathogenic microflora (Muruganandan et al., 2005). It is a pharmacologically active phytochemical used to treat several immunodeficiency disorders in Indian pharmacology (Scartezzini and Speroni, 2000).

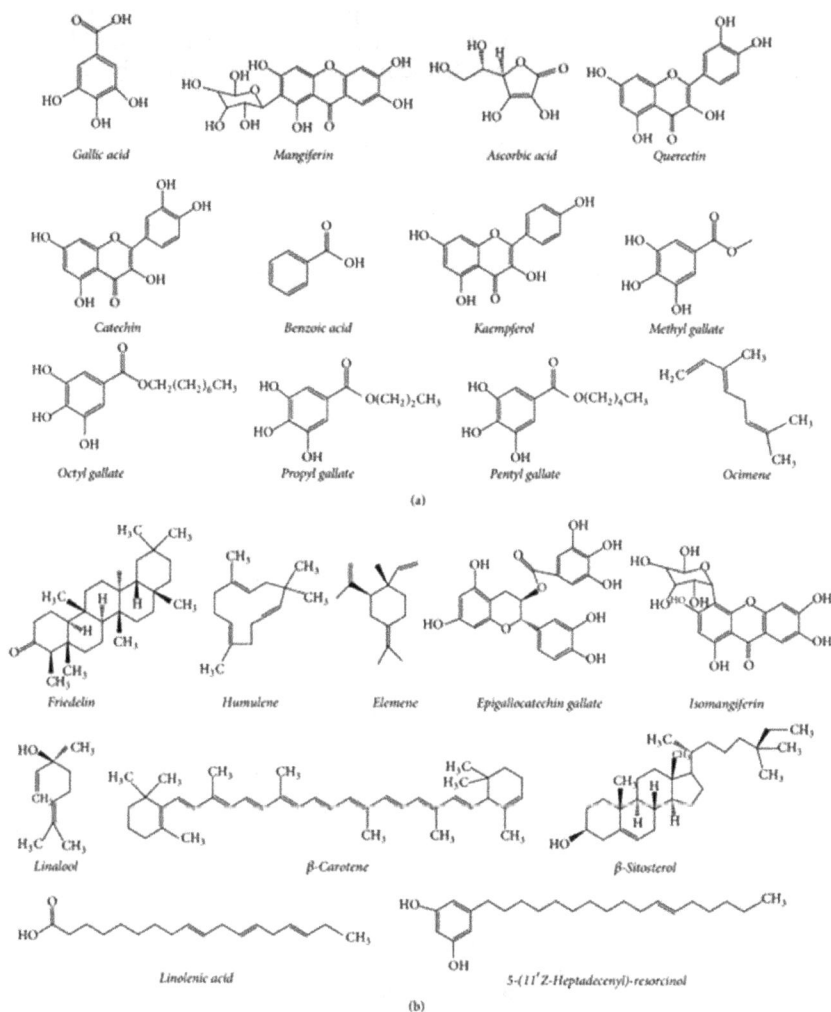

**Figure 5.2** Structures of some common BaCs of *M. indica* (mango). (From Ediriweera et al., 2017.)

### 5.4.3 Flavonoids

A mainly prevalent form of polyphenol is flavonoids, which are categorized into six classes based on their amount of oxidation. Such categories consist of flavones, isoflavones, flavanones, flavonols, anthocyanins, and proanthocyanins. Proanthocyanidins are primarily accountable for the astringency of plant-based foods (Santos et al., 2003). Mango have few antagonistic flavonoids which include quercetin, isoquerecetin fisetin, astragalin, and epicatechin (Rozema et al., 2002).

### 5.4.4 Quercetin

Quercetin is classified as a coloring composite since it imparts color to flowers, fruits, and vegetables. Quercetin rutinoside (rutin) and similar glycosides have been identified from the mango peels (Schieber et al., 2000; Berardini et al., 2005;

Tunchaiyaphum et al., 2013).The mango major glycosides are reported such as quercetin-3-galactoside, quercetin 3-glucoside, and quercetin-3-arabinoside. Other flavonol glycosides were only found in trace amounts, although quercetin aglycon was discovered.

### 5.4.5 Anthocyanins

Humans should consume approximately 200 mg/dL of anthocyanins per day (Duthie et al., 2000). The anthocyanin concentration is also affected by the quantity of ripeness of the mango fruit. The concentration of anthocyanin of ripe mango was 360–565 mg/100 g, compared to 203–326 mg/100 g in unripe mango, with a unique anthocyanin 7-Omethylcyanidin 3-O-D-galactopyranoside also discovered.

### 5.4.6 Acids Phenolics

Mango contains a huge amount of phenolic acids, but the most abundant are acid, carboxylic acid, 3,4-dihydroxybenzoic acid, acid propyl ester, acid methyl ester, and carboxylic acid propyl ester (Raṣtraelli et al., 2002). Polyol are esterified glucose structures. The oxidation of galloyl residues in ellagitannins produces these phenolic acids biosynthetically (Scalbert and Williamson, 2000). Hydrolyzable tannins are phenolic acid derivatives that occur in smaller amounts than dense tannins. The application as additives in foods and their products, gallotannins are usually recommended as safe agents. The digestive processes of tannins produce acids or ellagic acid units (Scalbert and Williamson, 2000).

### 5.4.7 Gallic Acid and Derivatives

Gallic acid and its derivatives occur as gallotannins and ellagitannins in both free and bound morphemes with tannins. The acid's structure includes hydroxyl and acid groups, and the compound can combine through other forms of ester, also known as gallic acid. Because acid does not form a compound with protein, it does not have an astringent taste. After six hydrolyzable tannins, gallic acid was determined as the key polyphenolic molecule available in mango (Kim et al., 2007). Depending on the extraction method, the number of acids varied in the mango kernel (Soong and Barlow, 2004).

### 5.4.8 Carotenoids

M. indica carotenoids are synthesized in mango fruits in excessive amounts as the fruit ripens (Vazquez-Caicedo et al., 2005). According to Godoy and Rodriguez-Amaya (1989), β-carotene is the dominant carotenoid in mango, accounting for 48%–84% of the total carotenoid content, and the presence of 16 other carotenoids in ripe mango, including neo-β-carotene, mono-epoxy-β-carotene, auroxanthin, and zeaxanthin (Klaui and Bauernfeind, 1981). Chen et al. (2004) have investigated the enhancement of carotenoid concentration in the mango peel which is rich in vitamin A activity and antioxidant properties. Varakumar et al. (2011) investigated identical results but added that the high vitamin A capacity and antioxidant properties were due to the appearance of a large amount of β-carotene content.

### 5.5 MECHANISM OF BIOACTIVE COMPOUNDS FOR ANTIMICROBIAL ACTIVITY

According to Ajila and Prasada Rao (2013), the significant antioxidant potential of mango fiber is attributable to confined phenolic. Antimicrobial activities of mango fruit extract may be related to leakage of bacterial cell 258 with lowering membrane permeability (Lambert et al., 2001; Oussalah et al., 2006). The bacterial cell wall has two ends: A non-polar hydrophobic end and a polar, hydrophilic end (Cristani et al., 2007). The hydrophobic end of the membrane interacts with an aliphatic side chain, while the hydrophilic end interacts with the hydrophobic benzene formula and phenols polar side which is found in the mango kernel. The structure of the membrane changes when the permeability of the membrane decreases, preventing substrates from entering the cell (Cristani et al., 2007). Tannins in mango extract are formed by constant complexes through proteins and a few carbohydrates in the microbial cell wall (Chung et al., 1998). The permeability of the cell wall causes the breakdown of the proton pump, a decrease in membrane potential, ATP pool scarcity, and ion loss (Di Pasqua et al., 2006; Turina et al., 2006). Tannin in mango extract alters the structural arrangement of different types of fatty acids, phospholipids layers, and polysaccharides when passing through the cytoplasmic membrane and cell membrane (Burt, 2004; Longbottom et al., 2004). It can also disrupt cell composition by coagulating cytoplasm (Burt, 2004). The effect of quercetin on the bacterial membrane might prevent toxins from being secreted. It can bind toxins discharged into the environment as well as inhibit trans-membrane activity outside the cell wall (Ultee et al., 2000; De Souza et al., 2010; Akthar et al., 2014). The antimicrobial effect of the mango fruit extract might be explained by a protest on bacterial degradation caused by suppression of iron, organic processes, a lack of necessary substrates for bacterial development, or blocking of extracellular bacterial enzymes (Cushnie and Lamb, 2005; Raybaudi-Massilia et al., 2009). Phenolic chemicals can donate protons and transfer electrons (Pietta, 2000). Ingestion of the mango kernel extract reduces intestinal morbidity by enhancing sodium chloride and water reabsorption (Sairam et al., 2003; Raybaudi-Massilia et al., 2009). Mango fruit has natural antibacterial characteristics because of the occurrence of numerous phytochemicals which are shown more effective against Gram-positive bacteria than Gram-negative bacteria (Kabuki et al., 2000). Using dietary dosages of methanolic extract of the mango kernel has been shown in many studies to increase antibacterial activity and system strength (Sahu et al., 2007). The system activation and microbicidal activity of the kernel extract of mango may be a latent mechanism for regulating infectious illnesses (David and Diemert, 2006). It was discovered that a more concentrated dosage of kernel extract was required for efficient mangiferin action against Gram-negative and Gram-positive bacteria (Stoilova et al., 2008). In a comparative experimental investigation, Sairam et al. (2003) found that magnesium sulfate causes diarrhea in mice, and purgative in mice is typically administered with aqueous and methanolic extracts of a mango kernel. These extracts demonstrated anti-diarrheal efficacy equivalent to that of the high-quality medication loperamide. Using a mixture of kernel oil and extract at varying doses, the overall bacterial count was decreased throughout this experiment. The oxidative stability of sunflower-seed oil rose and was enhanced as a result of this mixture. According to the findings, mango kernel oil and extract might be used as a usual antioxidant and antibacterial agent. The mythical use of mango for the improvement of the current ways to heal bacterial diseases was also confirmed in this investigation. Antimicrobial properties of methanol and ethanol extract from the mango kernel against entrusting fungus, acid uric bacteria, Gram-positive, and Gram-negative were examined by Amgad et al. (2012). The usual inhibitory zones varied from 5 to 18 mm in vitro antibacterial activities of ethanol and methanol extracts of the mango kernel. *Mycobacterium smegmatis* has the best inhibitory zone (18 mm). The ethanolic and methanolic extracts of mango kernels, on the other hand, showed good inhibitory activity against all of the strains tested. Diterpenoids isolated from several *Scutellaria* plants showed high bactericidal efficacy against Gram-positive bacteria, as well as inhibiting the growth of *Mycobacterium tuberculosis* (Kurek et al., 2011; Garcia et al., 2012). Rakholiya et al. (2013) compared the antibacterial potential of mango wastes. The findings of the experiment revealed that mature mango seed kernels and peels were more resistant to infections than unripe mango seed kernels and peels. The antibacterial power of the mango seed was likewise shown to be greater than that of the mango peel. El-Hawary and Rabeh (2014) investigated the antimicrobial and antifungal effectiveness of three mango cultivars: Zebdeya, Hindili, and cobaneya. Antimicrobial, antifungal, immunostimulant, and anti-carcinogenic activities were also assessed. This cultivar also showed significant antifungal activity against *Candida albicans*; however, none of the cultivars showed antifungal activity against *Aspergillus flavus*. It was also shown that the peel volatile oils of mango cobaneya and *Mangifera* zebdeya exhibited significant immunostimulant effect, as indicated by a low macrophage movement indicator. The antitumor ability of mango peel essential oils was investigated in vitro aligned with HCT-11,6, HepG2 neoplastic, and MCF-7 cell lines. The biofilm of *Enterococcus faecalis* within the channel produces discomfort and is removed by ordinary irritants with no infection to the body. Subbiya et al. (2013) studied plant materials with the least amount of side effects for passage treatment. Across the dentinal biofilm of *Enterococcus faecalis*, the antibacterial impending of mango kernel extract was assessed and associated with usual irritants. Extracts and common irritants were used to perform both microdilution and agar diffusioperiodod over *E. faecalis* planktonic cells. Three weeks was the period of the study. The application of mango kernel extract against an *E. faecalis* passage biofilm resulted in a major decrease in colony-forming units and antibacterial activity equivalent to that of 5% NaOCl. The mango peel ethanolic extract was shown to have the best antifungal efficacy. Mango peel extracts not only have antibacterial properties, but they also help antibiotics work better. In this context, research was done to assess *S. aureus* antibiotic resistance to norfloxacin, erythromycin, and tetracycline (De Oliveira et al., 2011).

## 5.6 HEALTH BENEFITS AND REGULATORY MECHANISMS IN VARIOUS CHRONIC DISEASES

The entire mango tree has long been used as a traditional Indian medicine system to treat a variety of diseases and distress. Mangiferin, quercetin, catechins, and kaempferol are essential BaCs found in all parts of the mango tree. In current history, various researchers have investigated ethnopharmacological and pharmacological for efficacies of different BaCs of mango. This scientific proof highlights the significance of mango by-products in the treatment of various chronic diseases, such as hypertension, diabetes, asthma, cancer, and pulmonary and gastrointestinal hemorrhage, with higher efficacy and reduced side effects (Figure 5.3; Ediriweera et al., 2017). Approximately 500 scientific papers on the occurrence, chemical synthesis, structure, and therapeutic nature of mangiferin have been published to date. The vast majority of investigation originates in Bangladesh and India. Iran, Brazil, and Nigeria also contribute to the therapeutic effects of mango. Ramesh et al. (2011) investigated the antidiabetic effects of a mango seed kernel alcoholic extract. The mango seed kernel extract was compared to tolbutamide. In contrast to the control group, the results demonstrated that mango seed kernel extract had a significant effect on hypoglycemia in normal rats after 3 hours after medication administration. In diabetic rats induced by naloxonexone, the mango

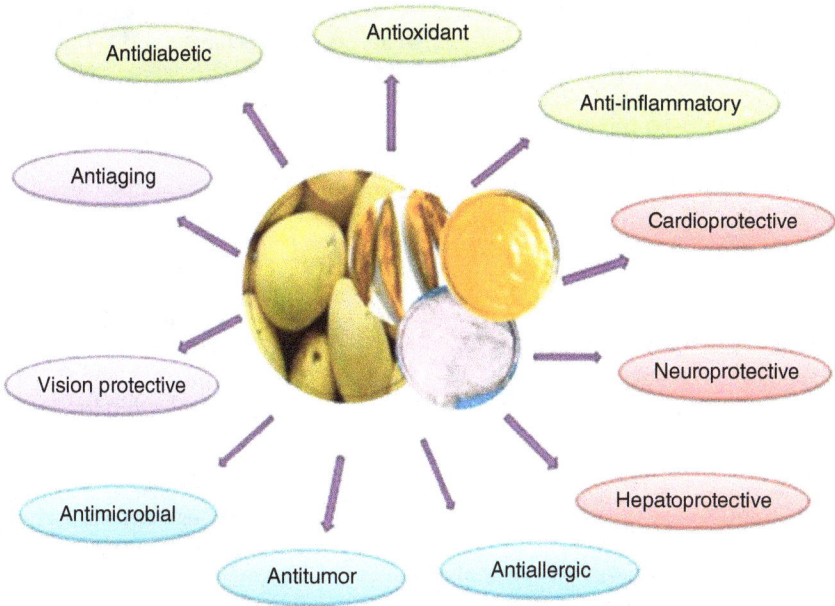

**Figure 5.3** Health benefits of BaCs in *M. indica* (mango). (From Lebaka et al., 2021.)

seed kernel extract significantly increased in levels. It was shown that mango seed kernel extract increases insulin assembly in the pancreas of Wistar rats and has a substantial effect with naloxone-induced diabetes. Tewtrakul et al. (2008) did a comparative research to assess the antiallergic and antibacterial capabilities of several Thai crops. The antiallergic and antibacterial activity of the mango seed was shown to be the highest, followed by the banana peel. As a result of these findings, mango waste (seed and peel) appears to have great beneficial capacity as well as might be employed as nutraceuticals to treat allergic and bacterial illnesses. The presence of a bioactive component, gall tannin, gives mango kernel oil qualities including immunomodulatory, anti-inflammatory, and antioxidative (Berardini et al., 2004). Abdullah et al. (2014) investigated the anti-carcinogenic effect of ethanolic mango kernel extract (MDA-MB-231 and MCF-7). The extract enhances cytotoxicity in MCF-7 and MDA-MB-231 cells, respectively, according to the results of this investigation. For additional validation of the cytotoxic activity properties, neutral red uptake, the antiproliferative, and lactate dehydrogenase tests were utilized. As a result, researchers discovered that mango kernel extract is more cytotoxic to estrogens and constructive carcinogenic cell lines than standard breast cells. Lamson and Brignall (2001) investigated cancer utilizing mango kernel extract as a treatment. To conclude the efficiency of mango kernel extract on immunological responses, Sahu et al. (2007) conducted a similar control as well as a randomized study on fish model. The results showed that mango kernel extract was easier to use for immunological responses linked to serum protein, superoxide generation, albumin, and fish survival. Following the findings, it was demonstrated that extract increases the capacity of fish to fight pathogenic infection and strengthens the antibody production. Due to the presence of the bioactive component "ellagic acid," mango kernel extracts have a wide range of physiological properties which have capacity to suppress DNA interaction, DNA adduct formation, and mutagenic activity in N-nitrosobenzyl methylamine and N-nitrosodiethylamine-induced lung carcinogenesis. It also has antiviral and antioxidant properties, as well as the ability to boost the activity of detoxification enzymes (Rashmeet et al., 2006). Masibo and He (2008) proposed that a little amount of ellagitannins (ellagic acid derivatives) in the human diet, rather than a large amount of pure ellagic acid, offers an effective target physiological function. Anthocynins have also been demonstrated as effective treatment of oxidative stress-related disorders such as cardiovascular disease and tumor (Duthie et al., 2000; Lazze et al., 2003). The efficacy of quercetin, mangiferin, and aglycone derivative of mangiferin, norathyriol were identified to boost the transitivity of peroxisome proliferator-activated receptors (Roberts-Thomson et al., 2008). According to Peng and Kuo (2003), quercetin is involved in the protection of Caco-2 cells from lipid peroxidation through peroxide and $Fe^{2+}$. Molina et al. (2003) describe the effect of quercetin on mouse liver for reduction of lipid oxidation and demonstrate the slow lipid oxidation by boosting glutathione levels; hence, quercetin in durians protects the liver from oxidative damage.

Quercetin works as an antihistamine and anti-inflammatory by functioning as an antioxidant (Nakaishi, 2000; Sanchez et al., 2000; Andreu et al., 2005a; Augustyniak et al., 2005). It is reported that the primary polyphenols in mango kernel extracts (mangiferin and catechin) prevent activation-induced necrobiosis (Hernandez et al., 2007). Because this reaction produces hydroxyl radicals, these mango kernel polyphenols may respond through $H_2O_2$ and block the Fentonon reaction among $Fe^{2+}$ and $H_2O_2$. Human T cells are protected by the reduction hydroxyloxal radicals. Mangiferin protected against radiation-induced disease and death, according to Jagetia and Baliga (2005). Mangiferin is thought to lower blood sugar levels by preventing glucose absorption from the gut. Mangiferin has both pancreatic and extra-pancreatic pathways to modulate diabetic applications, according to Muruganandan et al. (2005). Because of its multiple effects, the efficacy of mangiferin might be improved. Mangiferin also has antihyperlipidemic properties, lowering total cholesterol, triglycerides, and LDL levels in diabetic rats while raising HDL levels. Mangiferin possesses antifungal activity against *Thermoascus aurantiacus*, baker's yeast, *Trichoderma reesei*, and *A. flavus*, according to Singh et al. (2012). During one study, the therapeutic impact of mango peel and meat extracts containing bioactive molecules mangifein and quercetin phenolic substance were detected and studies on endothelial cell movement accountable for blood vessel development. The presence of mangiferin in mango extract has been shown to have health processes potential against disorders related to the poor creation of the newest blood capillaries (Daud et al., 2010). Mangiferin is a unique phenol that has been examined broadly for nutraceutical and medicinal capabilities in the treatment of degenerative illnesses such as cardiovascular disease and cancer. For maximum antioxidative action, the synergy of the various mango polyphenols is essential. Because of the presence of mangiferin, which is accountable for an antioxidant, mango extracts have hypoglycemic effects (Saleh and El-Ansari, 1975). Streptozotocin-induced diabetic rats were fed a diet enriched with mango peel powder during a trial. In comparison to the control group, the inclusion of mango peel powder resulted in a substantial increase in high-density lipoprotein (HDL) and a decrease in blood sugar, urine sugar, total cholesterol (TC), triglycerides, and lipid peroxidation (Gondi et al., 2015).

Mango peel extracts have been shown in many investigations to have anti-proliferative properties (dose dependent) against neoplastic cell lines. Scientists and academics had linked the mango peel's phenolic and flavonoid content to its possible health benefits (Kim et al., 2010). The scientific community is becoming more interested in the bioactive components (phytochemicals) found in fertilizer because of their potential to prevent and control a variety of microbial infectious diseases. Mango fruit wastes offer great curative and prevention potential against a variety of illnesses, particularly in terms of preventing the spread of infectious disease-causing microorganisms. However, the isolation and usage of potential compounds from mango fruit waste must be improved. Furthermore, pre-clinical research suggests that kernel isolate might be a viable substitute for antibiotics in terms of cost-effectiveness, adverse effects, and innate way of therapy. These pre-clinical experiments might be carried out in-depth through in vivo research investigations to determine the potency of each bioactive ingredient in mango fruit.

## 5.7 CONCLUSION

According to this review, several portions of mango trees, including the bark, leaves, fruit pulp, peel, and stone, are high in BaCs, as well as carotenoids, polyphenols, amino acids, carbohydrates, proteins, minerals, and dietary fiber. The concentrations of such chemicals differ depending on the mango genotype and growth conditions. These compounds have the potential to find a use in functional foods, medications, and commercial items. The synergy between both the numerous BaCs and ROS scavenging precursors resulted in the overall antioxidant activity (AoA) of mango fruit. Mango BaCs could be used in rational drug design and the discovery of metabolic pathway antagonists again for treatment of a wide range of illnesses and immune disorders. The evidence revealed here is a great resource for using and consuming mango products in human and animal nutrition. This, too, demonstrates BaC's therapeutic significance and possible application in the development of natural protective factors against pests, illnesses, and environmental stresses by the build-up of allergenic compounds and scavenging ROS compounds.

## REFERENCES

Abbasi, A. M., Guo, X., Fu, X., Zhou, L., Chen, Y., Zhu, Y., Yan, H., Liu, R. H. (2015). Comparative assessment of phenolic content and in vitro antioxidant capacity in the pulp and peel of mango cultivars. *International Journal of Molecular Sciences*, 16, 13507–13527.

Abdalla, A. E., Darwish, S. M., Ayad, E. H., El-Hamahmy, R. M. (2007). Egyptian mango by-product 1. Compositional quality of mango seed kernel. *Food Chemistry*, 103(4), 1134–1140.

Abdullah, A. S. H., Mohammed, A. S., Abdullah, R., Mirghani, M. E. S., Qubaisi, M. A. (2014). Cytotoxic effects of *Mangifera indica* L. kernel extract on human breast cancer (MCF-7 and MDA-MB-231 cell lines) and bioactive constituents in the crude extract. *BMC Complementary and Alternative Medicine, 14*, 1–10.

Ajila, C. M., Naidu, K. A., Bhat, S. G. and Prasada Rao, U. J. S. (2007). Bio-active compounds and antioxidant potential of mango peel extract. *Food Chemistry, 105*, 982–988.

Ajila, C. M., Prasada Rao, U. J. S. (2013). Mango peel dietary fibre: Composition and associated bound phenolics. *Journal of Functional Food, 5*, 444–450.

Akthar, M. S., Degaga, B., Azam, T. (2014). Antimicrobial activity of essential oils extracted from medicinal plants against the pathogenic microorganisms: A review. *Biological Sciences and Pharmaceutical Research, 2*, 001–007.

Amgad, A., Gied, A. E., Martin, R. P., Mahmoud, I. M., Abdelkareem, A. M., Hakami, A. M. A., et al. (2012). Antimicrobial activities of seed extracts of mango (*Mangifera indica* L.). *Advances in Microbiology, 2*, 571–576.

Andreu, G., Delgado, R., Velho, J., Curti, C., Vercesi, A. (2005a). Iron complexing activity of mangiferin, a naturally occurring glucosylxanthone, inhibits mitochondrial lipid peroxidation antioxidant activity. *Journal of Ethnopharmacology, 71*, 23–43.

Andreu, G., Delgado, R., Velho, J., Curti, C., Vercesi, A. (2005b). Iron complexing activity of mangiferin, a naturally occurring glucosylxanthone, inhibits mitochondrial lipid peroxidation induced by $Fe^{2+}$-citrate. *European Journal of Pharmacology, 513*, 47–55.

Aruoma, O. I. (1998). Free radicals, oxidative stress, and antioxidants in human health and diseases. *Journal of the American Oil Chemistry Society, 75*, 199–212.

Augustyniak, A., Waszkiewicz, E., Skrzydlewska, E. (2005). Preventive action of green tea from changes in the liver antioxidant abilities of different aged rats intoxicated with ethanol. *Nutrition, 2*, 925–932.

Bello-Pérez, L. A., García-Suárez, F., Agama-Acevedo, E. M. (2007). Indica carbohydrates. *Food, 1*, 36–40.

Berardini, N., Carle, R., Schieber, A. (2004). Characterization of gallotannins and benzophenone derivatives from mango (*Mangifera indica* L. cv. Tommy Atkins) peels, pulp and kernels by high-performance liquid chromatography/electrospray ionization mass spectrometry. *Rapid Communications in Mass Spectrometry, 18*, 2208–2216.

Berardini, N., Fezer, R., Conrad, J., Beifuss, U., Carle, R., Schieber, A. (2005). Screening of mango (*Mangifera indica* L.) cultivars for their contents of flavonol O-and xanthone C-glycosides, anthocyanins, and pectin. *Journal of Agricultural and Food Chemistry, 53*(5), 1563–1570.

Burt, S. (2004). Essential oils: Their antibacterial properties and potential applications in foods-A review. *International Journal of Food Microbiology, 94*, 223–253.

Chung, K. T., Lu, Z., Chou, M. W. (1998). Mechanism of inhibition of tannic acid and related compounds on the growth of intestinal bacteria. *Food and Chemical Toxicology, 36*, 1053–1060.

Cristani, M., D'Arrigo, M., Mandalari, G., Castelli, F., Sarpietro, M. G., Micieli, D., et al. (2007). Interaction of four monoterpenes contained in essential oils with model membranes: Implications for their antibacterial activity. *Journal of Agriculture and Food Chemistry*, 55, 6300–6308.

Cushnie, T. P. T., Lamb, A. J. (2005). Antimicrobial activity of flavonoids. *International Journal of Antimicrobial Agents*, 26, 343–356.

Dar, M. S., Oak, P., Chidley, H., Deshpande, A., Giri, A., Gupta, V. (2016). Nutrient and flavor content of mango (*Mangifera indica* L.) cultivars: An appurtenance to the list of staple foods. In *Nutritional Composition of Fruit Cultivars*; Elsevier: Amsterdam, The Netherlands, pp. 445–467.

Daud, N. H., Aung, C. S., Hewavitharana, A. K., Wilkinson, A. S., Pierson, J. T., Roberts-Thomson, S. J., Shaw, P. N., Monteith, G. R., Gidley M. J., Parat, M. O. (2010). Mango extracts and the mango component mangiferin promote endothelial cell migration. *Journal of Agriculture and Food Chemistry, 58,* 5181–5186.

David, J., Diemert, A. (2006). Diemert prevention and self-treatment of traveler's diarrhea. *Clinical Microbiology Reviews, 19,* 583–594.

de Oliveira, S. M. S., Falcão-Silva, V. S., Siqueira-Junior, J. P., Costa, M. J. C., de Melo Diniz, M. F. F. (2011). Modulation of drug resistance in *Staphylococcus aureus* by extract of mango (*Mangifera indica*) peel. *Revista Brasileira de Farmacognosia Brazilian Journal of Pharmacognosy, 21,* 190–193.

De Souza, E. L., De-Barros, J. C., De-Oliveira, C. E. V., Da-Conceicao, M. L. (2010). Influence of *Origanum vulgare* L. essential oil on enterotoxin production, membrane permeability and surface characteristics of *Staphylococcus aureus*. *International Journal of Food Microbiology, 137,* 308–311.

Di Pasqua, R., Hoskins, N., Betts, G., Mauriello, G. (2006). Changes in membrane fatty acids composition of microbial cells induced by addiction of thymol, carvacrol, limonene, cinnamaldehyde, and eugenol in the growing media. *Journal of Agricultural and Food Chemistry, 54,* 2745–2749.

Dietary Guidelines Advisory Committee. (2015). *Scientific Report of the 2015 Dietary Guidelines Advisory Committee: Advisory Report to the Secretary of Health and Human Services and the Secretary of Agriculture*; Dietary Guidelines Advisory Committee: Washington, DC.

Diplock, A., Charuleux, J. L., Crozier-Willi, G., Kok, F., Rice-Evans, C., Roberfroid, M., Stahl, W., Vina-Ribes, J. (1998). Functional food science and defence against reactive oxidative species. *British Journal of Nutrition, 80,* S77–S112.

Duthie, G. G., Duthie, S. J., Kyle, J. A. M. (2000). Plant polyphenols in cancer and heart disease: Implications as nutritional antioxidants. *Nutrition Research Reviews, 13,* 79–106.

Ediriweera, M. K., Tennekoon, K. H., Samarakoon, S. R. (2017). A review on ethnopharmacological applications, pharmacological activities, and bioactive compounds of *Mangifera indica* (*M. indica*). *Evidence-Based Complementary and Alternative Medicine*. DOI: 10.1155/2017/6949835.

El-Hawary, S. S., Rabeh, M. A. (2014). *Mangifera indica* peels: A common waste product with impressive immunostimulant, anticancer and antimicrobial potency. *Journal of Natural Sciences Research, 4*, 102–115.

FAO (2007). Food and Agriculture Organization of the United Nations. http://faostat.fao.org.

FAOSTAT. (2015). An Organization of the United Nations Food and Agricultural Organization of the United Nations. Retrieved from http://faostat.fao.org/site/339/default.aspx

Garcia, A., Bocanegra-Garcia, V., Palma-Nicolas, J. P., Rivera, G. (2012). Recent advances in antitubercular natural products. *European Journal of Medicinal Chemistry, 49*, 1–23.

Godoy, H. T., Rodriguez-Amaya, D. B. (1989). Carotenoid composition of commercial mangoes from Brazil. *Lebensmittel-Wissenschaft & Technologie, 22*, 100–103.

Gondi, M., Basha, S. A., Bhaskar, J. J, Salimath, P. V., Rao, U. J. (2015). Antidiabetic effect of dietary mango (*Mangifera indica* L.) peel in streptozotocin-induced diabetic rats. *Journal of the Science of Food and Agriculture, 95*, 991–999.

Hernandez, P. A., Rodriguez, P. C. A., Delgado, R. A., Walczak, H. (2007). Protective effect of *Mangifera indica* L. polyphenols on human T lymphocytes against activation-induced cell death. *Pharmacological Research, 55*, 167–73.

Huda, A. N., Salmah, M. R., Hassan, A. A., Hamdan, A., Razak, M. N. (2015). Pollination services of mango flower pollinators. *Journal of Insect Science, 15*(1).

Ibarra-Garza, I. P., Ramos-Parra, P. A., Hernández-Brenes, C., Jacobo-Velázquez, D. A. (2015). Effects of postharvest ripening on the nutraceutical and physicochemical properties of mango (*Mangifera indica* L. cv Keitt). *Postharvest Biology and Technology, 103*, 45–54.

Ibarretxe, G., Sanchez-Gomez, M. V., Campos-Esparza, M. R., Alberdi, E., Matute, C. (2006). Differential oxidative stress in oligodendrocytes and neurons after excitotoxic insults and protection by natural polyphenols. *Glia, 53*, 201–211.

Ichiki, H., Miura, T., Kubo, M., Ishihara, E., Komatsu, Y., Tanigawa, K., Okada, M. (1998). New antidiabetic compounds, mangiferin and its glucoside. *Biological and Pharmaceutical Bulletin, 21*(12), 1389–1390.

Jagetia, G. C., Baliga, M. S. (2005). Radioprotection by mangiferin in DBAxC57BL mice: A preliminary study. *Phytomedicine, 12*(3), 209–215. DOI: 10.1016/j.phymed.2003.08.003

Kabuki, T., Nakajima, H., Arai, M., Ueda, S., Kuwabara, Y., Dosako, S. (2000). Characterization of novel antimicrobial compounds from mango (*Mangifera indica* L.) kernel seeds. *Food Chemistry, 71*, 61–66.

Kalra, S., Tandon, D. (1983). Ripening-behaviour of "Dashehari" mango in relation to harvest period. *Scientia Horticulturae*, 1983, 19, 263—269. https://doi.org/10.1016/0304-4238(83)90073-0

Kim, Y., Brecht, K. J., Talcott, S. T. (2007). Antioxidant phytochemical and fruit quality changes in mango (*Mangifera indica* L.) following hot water immersion and controlled atmosphere storage. *Food Chemistry, 10*, 1016.

Kim, H., Moon, J. Y., Kim, H., Lee, D. S., Cho, M., Choi, H. K., Kimd, Y. S., Mosaddik, A., Cho, S. K. (2010). Antioxidant and antiproliferative activities of mango (*Mangifera indica* L.) Flesh and peel. *Food Chemistry, 121*, 429–436.

Klaui, H., Bauernfeind, J. C. (1981). Carotenoid as food colours. In *Carotenoids as Colorants and Vitamin A Precursors* (Bauernfeind J. C., ed.); Academic Press: New York, NY.

Kurek, A., Grudniak, A. M., Kraczkiewicz-Dowjat, A., Wolska, K. I. (2011). New antibacterial therapeutics and strategies. *Polish Journal of Microbiology, 60*, 3–12.

Lambert, R. J. W., Skandamis, P. N., Coote, P., Nychas, G. J. E, (2001). A study of the minimum inhibitory concentration and mode of action of oregano essential oil, thymol and carvacrol. *Journal of Applied Microbiology, 91*, 453–462.

Lamson, D., Brignall, M. (2001). Antioxidants and cancer. *III: Quercetin. Alternative Medicine Review, 5*, 196–209.

Lazze, M. C., Pizzala, R., Savio, M., Stivala, L. A., Prosperi, L., Bianchi, L. (2003). Anthocyanins protect against DNA damage induced by tert-butyl-hydroperoxide in rat smooth muscle and hepatoma cells. *Mutation Research, 535*, 103–115.

Lebaka, V. R., Wee, Y. J., Ye, W., Korivi, M. (2021). Nutritional composition and bioactive compounds in three different parts of mango fruit. *International Journal of Environmental Research and Public Health, 18*(2), 741.

Lemmens, L., Tchuenche, E. S., Van Loey, A. M., Hendrickx, M. E. (2013). Beta-carotene isomerisation in mango puree as influenced by thermal processing and high-pressure homogenisation. *European Food Research and Technology, 236*, 155–163.

Lima, Z. P., Severi, J. A., Pellizzon, C. H., Brito, A. R., Solis, P. N., Caceres, A., Giron, L. M., Vilegas, W., Hiruma-Lima, C. A. (2006). Can the aqueous decoction of mango flowers be used as an antiulcer agent? *Ethnopharm, 106*, 29–37.

Litz, R. E. (ed.). (2009). *The Mango: Botany, Production and Uses.* CABI Digital Library.

Longbottom, C. J., Carson, C. F., Hammer, K. A., Mee, B. J., Riley, T. V. (2004). Tolerance of *Pseudomonas aeruginosa* to *Melaleuca alternifolia* (Tea tree) oil. *Journal of Antimicrobial Chemotherapy, 54*, 386–392.

Luo, F., Lv, Q., Zhao, Y., Hu, G., Huang, G., Zhang, J., Sun, C., Li, X., Chen, K. (2012). Quantification and purification of mangiferin from Chinese *M. indica* (*Mangifera indica* L.) cultivars and its protective effect on human umbilical vein endothelial cells under $H_2O_2$-induced stress. *International Journal of Molecular Sciences, 13*, 11260–11274.

Ma, X., Wu, H., Liu, L., Yao, Q., Wang, S., Zhan, R., et al. (2011). Polyphenolic compounds and antioxidant properties in mango fruits. *Scientia Horticulturae, 129*(1), 102–107.

Maldonado-Celis, M. E., Yahia, E. M., Bedoya, R., Landázuri, P., Loango, N., Aguillón, J., Restrepo, B., Ospina, J. C. G. (2019). Chemical composition of mango (*Mangifera indica* L.) fruit: Nutritional and phytochemical compounds. *Frontiers in Plant Science, 10.*

Masibo, M., He, Q. (2008). Major mango polyphenols and their potential significance to human health. *Comprehensive Reviews on Food Science and Food Safety, 7*, 309–319.

Masibo, M., He, Q. (2009). Mango bio-active compounds and related nutraceutical properties: A review. *Food Reviews International, 25*, 346–370.

Matheyambath, A. C., Subramanian, J., Paliyath, G. (2016). Mangoes reference module in food science. In *Encyclopedia of Food and Health* (Paul, B. C., Told, F. F., eds.); Elsevier: Amsterdam, The Netherlands.

Mène-Saffrané, L. (2018). Vitamin E biosynthesis and its regulation in plants. *Antioxidants, 7*, 2.

Molina, M., Sanchez-Reus, I., Iglesias, I., Benedi, J. (2003). Quercetin, a flavonoid antioxidant, prevents and protects against ethanol-induced oxidative stress in mouse liver. *Biological and Pharmaceutical Bulletin, 26*, 1398–402.

Mukherjee, S. K. (1972). Origin of mango (*Mangifera indica*). *Economic Botany, 26*(3), 260–264.

Muoki, P. N., Makokha, A. O., Onyango, C. A., Ojijo, N. K. (2009). Potential contribution of mangoes to reduction of vitamin A deficiency in Kenya. *Ecology of Food and Nutrition, 48*, 482–498.

Muruganandan, S., Lal, J., Gupta, P. K. (2005). Immunotherapeutic effects of mangiferin mediated by the inhibition of oxidative stress to activated lymphocytes, neutrophils and macrophages. *Toxicology, 215*(1), 57–68.

Nakaishi, H. (2000). Effects of black current anthocyanoside intake on dark adaptation and VDT work-induced transient refractive alteration in healthy humans. *Alternative Medicine Review, 5*, 553–562.

Nandwani, D. (2013, June). Grafting of mango cultivars (*Mangifera indica* L.) in the US Virgin Islands. In *X International Mango Symposium, 1075*, 185–189.

Nayan, V., Onteru, S. K., Singh, D. (2018). *Mangifera indica* flower extract mediated biogenic green gold nanoparticles: Efficient nanocatalyst for reduction of 4-nitrophenol. *Environmental Progress & Sustainable Energy, 37*(1), 283–294.

Oussalah, M., Caillet, S., Lacroix, M. (2006). Mechanism of action of Spanish oregano, Chinese cinnamon, and savory essential oils against cell membranes and walls of *Escherichia coli* O157:H7 and *Listeria monocytogenes*. *Journal of Food Protection, 69*, 1046–1055.

Palafox-Carlos, H., Yahia, E., González-Aguilar, G. (2012). Identification and quantification of major phenolic compounds from mango (*Mangifera indica*, cv. Ataulfo) fruit by HPLC–DAD–MS/MS-ESI and their individual contribution to the antioxidant activity during ripening. *Food Chemistry, 135,* 105–111.

Peng, I., Kuo, S. (2003). Flavonoid structure affects inhibition of lipid peroxidation in Caco-2 intestinal cells at physiological conditions. *Journal of Nutrition, 133,* 2184–2187.

Pietta, P. G. (2000). Flavonoids as antioxidants. *Journal of Natural Products, 63,* 1035–1042.

Rakholiya, K., Kaneria, M., Desai, D., Chanda, S. (2013). Antimicrobial activity of decoction extracts of residual parts (seed and peels) of *Mangifera indica* L. var. Kesar against pathogenic and food spoilage microorganism. In *Microbial Pathogens and Strategies for Combating Them: Science, Technology and Education* (Méndez-Vilas, A., ed.); Formatex Research Center, Torremolinos-Malaga (Spain), pp. 850–856.

Ramesh, P. R., Parasuraman, S., Vijaya, C., Darwhekar, G., Devika, G. S. (2001). Antidiabetic effect of kernel seeds extract of *Mangifera indica* (Anacardiaceae). *International Journal of Pharma and Bio Science, 2,* 385–393.

Rashmeet, K., Reen, R. N., Stoner, G. D. (2006). Modulation of N-Nitrosomethylbenzylamin metabolism by black raspberries in the esophagus and liver of Fischer 344 rats. *Nutrition and Cancer, 54,* 47–57.

Raybaudi-Massilia, R. M., Mosqueda-Melgar, J., Soliva-Fortuny, R., Martin-Belloso, O. (2009). Control of pathogenic and spoilage microorganisms in fresh-cut fruits and fruit juices by traditional and alternative natural antimicrobials. *Comprehensive Reviews in Food Science and Food Safety, 8,* 157–180.

Reddy, L. V. (2005). *Production and Characterization of Wine Like Product from M. indica Fruits Mangifera indica* L.; Sri Venkateswara University: Tirupati, India.

Reddy, L., Reddy, O. V. S. (2005). Production and characterization of wine from mango fruit (*Mangifera indica* L.). *World Journal of Microbiology and Biotechnology, 21,* 1345–1350.

Roberts-Thomson, S. J., Wilkinson, A. S., Monteith, G. R., Shaw, P. N., Lin, C., Gidley, M. J. (2008). Effects of the mango components mangiferin and quercetin and the putative mangiferin metabolite norathyriol on the transactivation of peroxisome proliferator activated receptor isoforms. *Journal of Agriculture and Food Chemistry, 56,* 3037–3042.

Robles-Sánchez, R., Islas-Osuna, M., Astiazarán-García, H., Vázquez-Ortiz, F., Martín-Belloso, O., Gorinstein, S., GonzálezAguilar, G. (2009). Quality index, consumer acceptability, bioactive compounds, and antioxidant activity of fresh-cut "Ataulfo" mangoes (*Mangifera indica* L.) as affected by low-temperature storage. *Journal of Food Science, 74,* S126–S134.

Rozema, J., Bornman, J. F., Gaberscik, A., Haeder, D. P., Trost, T. (2002). The role of UV-B radiation in aquatic and terrestrial ecosystems-an experimental and functional analysis of the evolution of UV-absorbing compounds. *Journal of Photochemistry and Photobiology B: Biology, 66,* 2–12.

Sahu, S., Das, B. K., Pradhan, J., Mohapatra, B. C., Mishra, B. K., Sarangi, N. (2007). Effect of *Mangifera indica* kernel as a feed additive on immunity and resistance to *Aeromonas hydrophila* in *Labeorohita fingerlings. Fish and Shellfish Immunology, 23,* 109–118.

Sairam, K., Hemalatha, S., Kumar, A., Srinivasan, T., Ganesh, J., Shankar, M., et al. (2003). Evaluation of anti-diarrhoeal activity in seed extracts of *Mangifera indica. Journal of Ethnopharmacology, 84,* 11–15.

Saleh, N. A. M., El-Ansari, M. A. I. (1975). Polyphenolics of twenty local varieties of *Mangifera indica* L. *Planta Medica, 28,* 124–130.

Sanchez, G. M., Re, L., Giuliani, A., Nunez-Selles, A. J., Davison, G. P., Leon-Fernandez, O. (2000). Protective effects of *Mangifera indica* L. extract, mangiferin and selected antioxidants against TPA-induced biomolecules oxidation and peritoneal macrophage activation in mice. *Pharmacological Research, 42,* 565–573.

Santos, L. P., Aguirre, R. S., Fernandez, R. C., Robaina, M. D., Valle, L. G. (2003). Efectos del VIMANG sobre algunos marcadores de progresion de la infeccion por VIH-1 en pacientes cubanos. *Revista Cubana de Medicina Tropical, 55,* 115–118.

Scalbert, A., Williamson, G. (2000). Dietary intake and bioavailability of polyphenols. *Journal of Nutrition, 130*(8), 2073S–2085S. https://doi.org/10.1093/jn/130.8.2073S

Scartezzini, P., Speroni, E. (2000). Review on some plants of Indian traditional medicine with antioxidant activity. *Journal of Ethnopharmacology, 71,* 23–43.

Schieber, A., Ullrich, W., Carle, R. (2000). Characterization of polyphenols in mango puree concentrate by HPLC with diode array and mass spectrometric detection. *Innovative Food Science and Emerging Technologies, 1*(1), 161–166.

Shenai, J. P. (1999). Vitamin A supplementation in very low birth weight neonates: Rationale and evidence. *Pediatrics, 104,* 1369–1374.

Singh, R. K., Ali, S. A., Nath, P., Sane, V. A. (2011). Activation of ethylene-responsive p-hydroxyphenylpyruvate dioxygenase leads to increased tocopherol levels during ripening in mango. *Journal of Experimental Botany, 62,* 3375–3385.

Singh, O. P., Usha, K., Saboki, E., Srivastav, M., Dahuja, A. Singh, B. (2012). Enzymatic reactive oxygen species scavenging system in mango varieties resistant and susceptible to mango malformation. *Scientia Horticulturae, 138,* 81–89.

Sivakumar, D., Jiang, Y., Yahia, E. M. (2011). Maintaining mango (*Mangifera indica* L.) fruit quality during the export chain. *Food Research International, 44*(5), 1254–1263.

Slippers, B., Johnson, G. I., Crous, P. W., Coutinho, T. A., Wingfield, B. D., Wingfield, M. J. (2005). Phylogenetic and morphological re-evaluation of the *Botryosphaeria* species causing diseases of *Mangifera indica*. *Mycologia, 97*(1), 99–110.

Soong, Y.; Barlow, J. (2004). Antioxidant activity and phenolic content of selected fruit seeds. *Food Chemistry, 88,* 411–417.

Stoilova, I., Jirovetz, L. Stoyanova, A. (2008). Antioxidant activity of the polyphenol mangiferin. *EJEAF Chemistry, 7,* 2706–2716.

Subbiya, A., Mahalakshmi, K., Pushpangadan, S., Padmavathy, K., Vivekanandan, P., Sukumaran V. G. (2013). Antibacterial efficacy of *Mangifera indica* L. kernel and *Ocimum sanctum* L. leaves against *Enterococcus faecalis* dentinal biofilm. *Journal of Conservative Dentistry, 16,* 454–457.

Tasneem, A. Postharvest Treatments to Reduce Chilling Injury Symptoms in Stored Mangoes. Master's Thesis, McGill University, Ste-Anne-de-Bellevue, QC, Canada, 2004.

Tewtrakul, S., Itharat, A., Thammaratwasik, P., Ooraikul, B. (2008). Anti-allergic and antimicrobial activities of some Thai crops. *Songklanakarin Journal of Science and Technology, 30,* 467–473.

Tharanathan, R., Yashoda, H., Prabha, T. M. (2006). Indica (*Mangifera indica* L.) "The king of fruits"—An overview. *Food Reviews International, 22,* 95–123.

Tian, J., Zeng, X., Zeng, H., Feng, Z., Miao, X., Peng, X. (2013). Investigations on the antifungal effect of nerol against *Aspergillus flavus* causing food spoilage. *The Scientific World Journal, 2013,* 230795. https://doi.org/10.1155/2013/230795

Tjiptono, P., Lam, P. E., Mendoza, D. B., Kosiyachinda, S. Status of the mango industry in ASEAN In *Mango: Fruit Development, Postharvest Physiology and Marketing in ASEAN* (Mendoza, D. B., Wills, R. B. H., eds.); ASEAN Food Handling Bureau: Kuala Lumpur, Malaysia, 1984; 1–11.

Tunchaiyaphum, S., Eshtiaghi, M. N., Yoswathana, N. (2013). Extraction of bioactive compounds from mango peels using green technology. *International Journal of Chemical Engineering and Applications, 4,* 194–198.

Turina, A. V., Nolan, M. V., Zygadlo, J. A., Perillo, M. A. (2006). Natural terpenes: Self-assembly and membrane partitioning. *Biophysical Chemistry, 122,* 101–113.

Ultee, A., Kets, E. P., Alberda, M., Hoekstra, F. A., Smid, E. J. (2000). Adaptation of the food-borne pathogen *Bacillus cereus* to carvacrol. *Archive of Microbiology, 174,* 233–238.

US Department of Agriculture. USDA National Nutrient Database for Standard Reference, Release 1 April. Available online: https://ndb.nal.usda.gov/ndb (accessed on 15 June 2020).

USDA Nutritional Data Base for Standard Reference. http://www.nal.usda.gov/Fnic/Foodcomp/Data/Volume Release 19, 2006.

Vallarino, J. G., Osorio, S. (2019). Chapter 10: Organic acids. In *Postharvest Physiology and Biochemistry of Fruits and Vegetables* (Yahia, E., Carrillo-López, A., eds.); Elsevier: Amsterdam, The Netherlands, pp. 207–224.

Varakumar, S., Kumar, Y. S., Reddy, O. V. S. (2011). Carotenoid composition of mango (*Mangifera indica* L.) wine and its antioxidant activity. *Journal of Food Biochemistry, 35,* 1538–1547.

Vazquez-Caicedo, A. L., Sruamsiri, P., Carle, R. Neidhart, S. (2005). Accumulation of all-trans-b-carotene and its 9-cis and 13-cis stereoisomers during postharvest ripening of nine Thai mango cultivars. *Journal of Agricultural and Food Chemistry, 53,* 4827–4835.

World Health Organization. (2003). Report of a joint WHO/FAO expert consultation. In *Diet Nutrition and the Prevention of Chronic Diseases: WHO Technical Report Series*; WHO: Geneva, Switzerland.

Yaacob, O., Subhadrabandhu, S. (1995). *The Production of Economic Fruits in South-East Asia*; Oxford University Press: Kuala Lumpur, p. 419.

Yashoda, H. M., Prabha, T. N., Tharanathan, R. N. (2006). Mango ripening: Changes in cell wall constituents in relation to textural softening. *Journal of the Science of Food and Agriculture, 86,* 713–721.

Zhu, X. L., Chen, Q., Tang, R. Y. (2002). The inhibition of the aqueous extract of Chinese nutgall on five periodontal bacteria in vitro. *Chinese Journal of Conservative Dentistry, 12,* 255–257.

# 6 Pomegranate

*Tabussam Tufail, Huma Bader Ul Ain, Rabia Shabbir, Maha Hameed,
Farhan Saeed, Muhammad Afzaal, Anees Ahmed Khali, and
Ammar Ahmed Khan*

## CONTENTS

## 6.1 INTRODUCTION

Plants are a rich source of beneficial chemicals that are involved in thousands of secondary metabolic activities and do not indicate a metabolic path. Natural foods, such as botanical herbs, are the source of all of these herbal medicine items (Brielmann et al. 2006). Pomegranate contains valuable compounds. Pomegranate belongs to the Punicaceae plant and is also known as *Punica granatum* L. (Melgarejo-Sánchez et al. 2021). Pomegranate is a tree that attains 16 to 23 feet in height with multiple elliptic-shaped leaves about 3 inches long and 2 cm wide (Levin 2006). Fresh fruit purchases accounted for 9.3% of the average household spending in Spain in 2018 (MAPA 2019). Pomegranates may be gaining popularity as a result of a new scientific study that suggests they contain antibacterial, anticancer, cardioprotective, and anti-inflammatory effects. The herb can be used to treat diabetes, obesity, and increase aphrodisiac quality (Aviram and Rosenblat 2013).

It's a super fruit, a term that refers to fruits with high nutritional value and health-promoting qualities (Kumar and Neeraj 2018). Pomegranates have been used for medicinal purposes since antiquity, and pharmaceutical firms are now extracting bioactive components from the fruit to make capsules for nutritional supplements (Sidhu and Zafar 2012; Karimi et al. 2017). Pomegranates contain a variety of bioactive compounds, including alkaloids, ellagic acid, punicalagin, and other ellagitannins, as well as anthocyanins, flavonoids, tannins, and other phytochemicals, all of which may be beneficial to human health and disease prevention (Setiadhi et al. 2017). Cultivar, climate, growth method, storage conditions, and maturity all influence the bioactive profile (Kalaycıoğlu and Erim 2017; Fourati et al. 2020).

## 6.2 CULTIVATION

Both the Arabic and Hebrew names for pomegranate (rumman and rimmon) are said to mean "fruit of heaven," which lends credence to the fruit's popularity in these civilizations (Bhandari 2012). The Greeks, on the other hand, saw it as "fruit of the dead," providing support and upkeep to Hades' inhabitants (Lazongas 2017).

These two factors may indicate the incredible diversity of the pomegranate's prospective customer base. Pomegranate juice, in addition to being used as a fresh fruit or fruit juice, lends a unique flavor to many Middle Eastern cuisines, such as Iranian fessenjan (Ashton et al. 2006). These fruits were likely important to early desert explorers as a convenient source of water that was easy to carry and well-protected (Morton 1987).

The pomegranate is a sign of fertility and immortality, as well as riches, in Zoroastrianism (Al-Mutary and Abu-Taweel 2020). Pomegranates have long been connected with love, and they were one of Aphrodite's emblems (Abram 2009).

They're found throughout the world and have a vast genetic variety, as well as variances in phytochemical content (Melgarejo-Sánchez et al. 2021). The main production countries of pomegranates are India, Iran, Turkey, China, and the United States; however, India is the major pomegranate exporter in the world (Chandra et al. 2010). In Pakistan, pomegranate is still grown as a minor fruit: Baluchistan is the major producer of pomegranates and KPK and Punjab also produce pomegranates on a small scale (Aziz et al. 2020). It is also used as a popular fruit in Sri Lankan home gardens in dry and intermediate areas (Khan 2005).

## 6.3 VARIETIES

There are several kinds available, each of which is well-known for its flavor (Figure 6.1) (Levin 2006). Amongst the well-known are the following:

- *Bedana:* This fruit has delicate seeds that are white or brown in hue. The pulp is a pink-colored, delicious fruit that ranges in size from medium to giant (Lal et al. 2011).

- *Kandhar:* This has firm seeds with a pulp that is blood crimson in hue. This fruit is big and has a sour flavor (Chandra et al. 2010).

- *Alandi:* This fruit's seeds are extremely tough. It's a medium-sized fruit with a fleshy pink hue and a subacid pulp (Martinez et al. 2006).

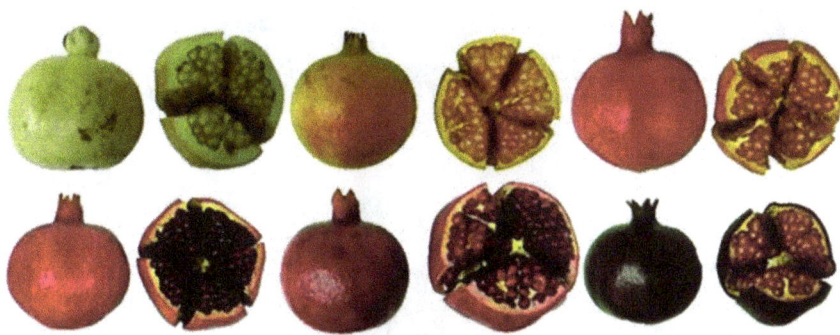

**Figure 6.1** Various varieties of pomegranate.

- *Dholki:* This fruit has a high commercial value. It contains firm seeds and a delicious white pulp. It has a lot of dark purple spots at the base. It is thought to be a classic plant.

- *Kabul:* This pomegranate cultivar is big, with a dark yellow skin and bitter flesh (Jalikop 2010).

- *Muscat Red:* The flesh is luscious, and the seeds are firm. This fruit has a thick covering and is generally modest in size.

- *Paper Shell:* This has a pleasant, sensational pulp with a fleshy covering, and the seeds are usually tender. It is usually round in form.

- *Poona:* The rind is grey to green in hue and frequently speckled. This fruit is big in size and has an orange to red color combination.

- *Spanish Ruby:* This fruit has an aromatic fragrant pulp with seeds that are usually delicate and brilliant in color. It comes in a variety of sizes, from medium to big.

- *Vellodu:* It's a medium-quality fruit with a pleasant flesh and big seeds.

## 6.4 NUTRIENTS IN POMEGRANATE

In addition to increased marketing of garden-fresh pomegranate fruit, a number of pomegranate-containing products have recently been introduced to the market and are extensively marketed for their health-promoting benefits (Kojadinovic et al. 2017). These products include pomegranate drinks; powdered and liquid polyphenolic extracts of pomegranate plant components such arils, blooms, leaves, and peel; pomegranate seed oil; and beauty care products using various pomegranate seed oil extracts (Yao and Xu 2021). Pomegranate has a number of medicinal chemicals that aid in the maintenance of homeostasis and the attainment of optimal health (Qu et al. 2012). Figure 6.2 shows the natural compounds present in pomegranate.

*Juice:* This is obtained by crushing the arils contains lignans, several organic acids such as gallic acid, alkaloids, ellagic acid, fatty acids, triterpenoids, flavonoids, phytosterols, and hydrolysable tannins (Aloqbi et al. 2016).

*Pericarp:* This includes tannins, flavonoids, ellagitannins, and punicalagins that can be hydrolyzed. Potassium and phosphorus were the first minerals

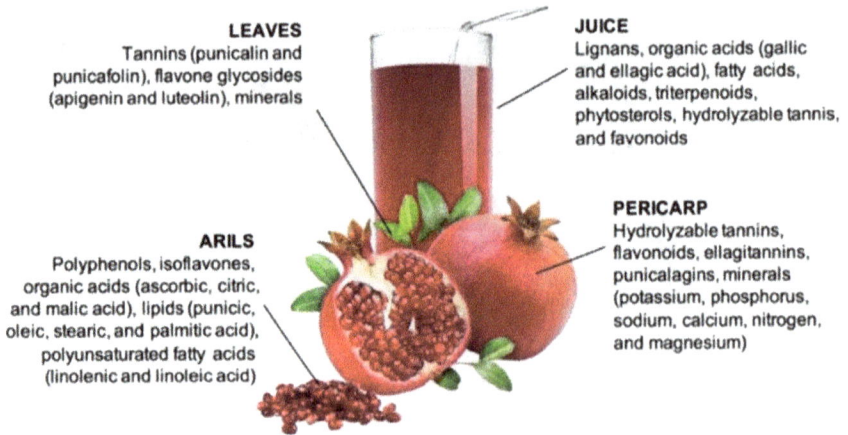

**LEAVES**
Tannins (punicalin and punicafolin), flavone glycosides (apigenin and luteolin), minerals

**JUICE**
Lignans, organic acids (gallic and ellagic acid), fatty acids, alkaloids, triterpenoids, phytosterols, hydrolyzable tannins, and favonoids

**ARILS**
Polyphenols, isoflavones, organic acids (ascorbic, citric, and malic acid), lipids (punicic, oleic, stearic, and palmitic acid), polyunsaturated fatty acids (linolenic and linoleic acid)

**PERICARP**
Hydrolyzable tannins, flavonoids, ellagitannins, punicalagins, minerals (potassium, phosphorus, sodium, calcium, nitrogen, and magnesium)

**Figure 6.2** The natural compounds of pomegranate.

separated from the pericarp, followed by sodium, calcium, magnesium, and nitrogen (Jalili et al. 2020).

*Seeds:* Polyphenols, isoflavones, and a number of substances with acidic properties are found in the seeds. They also have a high lipid content (punicic, oleic, stearic, and palmitic acid), as well as polyunsaturated fatty acids (linolenic and linoleic acid) (Madrigal-Carballo et al. 2009).

*Pomegranate leaves:* These contain a high amount of tannins, such as punicalin and punicafolin, as well as flavone glycosides like apigenin and luteolin. Minerals have been discovered in the leaves, just as they have in the pericarp (Farag et al. 2014).

A variety of factors influence the phytochemical profile including the cultivar, climate, growing practices, transformation, and product preservation (Li et al. 2015).

### 6.4.1 Macronutrients in Pomegranate

One pomegranate contains 234 calories, 4.7 grams of protein, 3.3 grams of fat, and 52.7 grams of carbohydrates (Alcaraz et al. 2017). Arils, or pomegranate seeds, are abundant in fiber, potassium, phosphorus, magnesium, and calcium. Seeds (10%) and arils (40%) make up the main component of the pomegranate fruit (50%) (Deshmukh et al. 2020). In arils, 85% water, 1.5% pectin, and 10% total sugars, organic acid, and bioactive substances are found (phenolics and flavonoids, primarily anthocyanins) (El Kar et al. 2011). The USDA provides nutritional statistics for a pomegranate with a diameter of 4 inches.

#### 6.4.1.1 Carbohydrates

The majority of calories in pomegranates come from carbohydrates. It has two types of carbohydrates (Mustafa et al. 2016). A medium-sized fruit has 21 grams of sugar and 6 grams of fiber, which is 21% of the daily recommended intake. In terms of carbs, sugars, and calories, the juice is different from the fruit. Pomegranate juice (one cup) includes 134 calories, 33 grams of carbohydrates, 31 grams of sugar, and 0 grams of fiber, according to USDA figures. Plain pomegranate juice has fewer calories, carbohydrates, and sugar than cocktails made with pomegranate juice. The glycemic load of pomegranate is calculated to be 18 (Brennand and Jorgenson 2020).

### 6.4.1.2 Proteins

Pomegranates have a low protein content. Three grams of protein are found in a medium-sized fruit. A bigger fruit can provide more than 5 grams of protein. Pomegranate juice, on the other hand, is nearly protein-free (0.4 grams per cup) (Elfalleh et al. 2011).

### 6.4.1.3 Fats

Pomegranate has a very low fat content. In a full fruit, saturated fat, polyunsaturated fat, and monounsaturated fat all amount to less than 1 gram. Unless you consume a substantial amount of this food, these modest amounts are unlikely to have a significant impact on your diet (Vroegrijk et al. 2011).

## 6.4.2 Micronutrients in Pomegranate
### 6.4.2.1 Vitamins and Minerals

Pomegranates are abundant in vitamins and minerals when eaten whole and fresh. On a 2,000-calorie diet, a medium-sized fruit contains 16 mg of vitamin C, or roughly 18% of the daily intake. Vitamin K, a fat-soluble vitamin that assists in blood-clotting activities in the body, is found in 28% of women and 21% of men who consume pomegranates on a daily basis. The recommended daily allowance (RDA) is the daily amount that covers virtually all healthy people's dietary needs (97%–98%). Pomegranates are also high in folate (15%), vitamin B6 (9%), copper (27%), thiamin (9%), and potassium (9%). Pomegranate juice still includes vitamin K, folate, and (some) copper, according to the USDA, but it has almost no vitamin C (Yilmaz et al. 2007).

## 6.5 BIOACTIVE COMPONENTS PRESENT IN POMEGRANATES

It is now well accepted that the biologically active compounds present in vegetables and fruits are responsible for their disease-prevention properties (Sood and Gupta 2015). Due to the presence of very beneficial physiologically active components such as phenolic acids, tannins, and flavonoids, pomegranate fruits have high nutritional value.

### 6.5.1 Phenolic Chemicals

Phenolic chemicals, which are found in a number of foods, including the pomegranate fruit, are one of the primary components responsible for a wide range of functional properties. Flavonoids are the most common and extensively dispersed category, with smaller simple molecules to highly polymerized combinations being found in nature. Phenolic acids, like their functional variants, have an aromatic structural ring connected to one or more hydrogenated substituents. Phenolic compounds are aromatic rings that have been hydroxylated, either directly or indirectly, with the hydroxy group connected to phenyl, substituted phenyl, or the aryl group (Ambigaipalan, et al. 2016).

### 6.5.2 Flavonoids

Flavonoids are compounds with 15 carbon atoms that have a low molecular weight. A three-carbon bridge connects two aromatic rings, which is commonly in the form of a heterocyclic ring (Ardekani et al. 2011).

### 6.5.3 Anthocyanins

Anthocyanins are the most plentiful and significant flavonoids found in pomegranate arils, from which juice is extracted. These pigments give the fruit and liquid their crimson color. Pomegranate juice contains a lot of anthocyanins (Zhang et al. 2011). The amount of hydroxylated clusters, the quality and type of linked sugars, as well as their form, the aromatic or aliphatic carboxylates attached to the sugar in the complex molecule, and the location of these connections are the key differences between them. The two types of phenolic acids contained in pomegranate juice are as follows:

1. *Hydroxybenzoic acids*, primarily ellagic and gallic acids, as well as ellagic acid

2. *Hydroxycinnamic acids*, most notably chlorogenic acid, caffeic acid, and p-coumaric acid

### 6.5.4 Tannins

Tannins are the high-molecular-weight phyto-polyphenols that are categorized into three biologically and chemically discrete groups: Proanthocyanidinsor condensed tannins (found in grapes, tea, cranberries), ETs or hydrolyzable tannins (found in strawberries, blueberries, raspberries), and the gallotannins (GTs). Pomegranate peel has an extraordinary concentration of hydrolyzable tannins, principally pedunculagin, punicalin, and punicalagin (Ismail et al. 2018). Their chemical structures differ from those of proanthocyanidins. Hydrolyzable tannins are esters of hexahydroxydiphenyl acetate and a polyol, often quinic acidor glucose. Pomegranate peel is comprised of hydroxybenzoic acids such as EA, gallagic, and EA glycosides in addition to the ETs. Anthocyanidins are comprised of the flavonoids such as luteolin, kaempferol, and quercetin.

## 6.6 HEALTH BENEFITS AND CHRONIC DISORDERS TARGETED BY POMEGRANATE

Excess production of Reactive Oxygen Species (ROS) exceeds the capacity of the endogenous antioxidant scavenging mechanism, leading to oxidative stress. This causes a variety of problems and illnesses because reactive oxygen species have negative effects on numerous molecules in the cell, resulting in consequences implicated in aging, cancer, diabetes mellitus, and other cardiovascular disorders (Kandylis and Kokkinomagoulos 2020). Medicinal plants, fruits, vegetables, and grains are said to be high in bioactive components including carotenoids, vitamins, phenolic compounds, and flavonoids, which protect against free radicals and oxidative stress. In vivo, there is an interacting network of antioxidant enzymes such as SOD and catalase that function as a defense mechanism for cells against oxidative stress (Zarfeshany et al. 2014). There are, however, nutritional sources of antioxidants such as vitamins C, A, and it E, as well as other endogenous compounds such as glutathione. Because of the numerous difficulties of oxidative stress caused by the detrimental effects of reactive oxygen species, there is a growing interest in natural substances with high antioxidant capabilities that can help avoid and treat some of these issues.

In addition to its historical benefits, it is used in a number of medical systems for a variety of ailments. Pomegranate components' combined action appears to be superior to that of single constituents. Several studies on the antioxidant, anti-carcinogenic, and anti-inflammatory properties of pomegranate constituents have been published in the last decade, with a focus on the treatment and prevention of cancer, cardiovascular disease, diabetes, dental problems, erectile dysfunction, bacterial infections and antibiotic resistance, and UV-induced skin damage (Sturgeon and Ronnenberg 2010). Possible applications include newborn brain ischemia, male infertility, and Alzheimer's disease. Obesity and arthritis are two conditions that affect people.

### 6.6.1 Cardiovascular Health

One of the most important risk factors for coronary heart disease is dyslipidemia. Pomegranates are strong in antioxidants such as anthocyanins and tannins, which may help prevent cholesterol accumulation in arteries and so protect the heart, which is marked by high levels of low-density lipoprotein cholesterol (LDL-C) and low levels of high-density lipoprotein cholesterol (HDL-C). Pomegranate fruit may help to reduce LDL levels in the body, which may protect the body against a stroke attack (Cao et al. 2015). Pomegranate leaf extract can reduce blood cholesterol in mice fed a high-lipid diet, according to the weight of rats. 400–800 mg of extract was administered over the course of 5 weeks. Rats that had been fed a high-fat diet and showed signs of obesity were chosen. The outcomes of this induction were considerable in terms of lowering total cholesterol and triglyceride levels in the body. Weight loss was accomplished, as was a reduction in fat absorption in the gut. Pomegranate leaf extract was discovered to reduce HDL levels in the body, implying that it has health benefits (Wang et al. 2010).

### 6.6.2 Diabetic Health

Diabetes is a common metabolic syndrome across the world, and its prevalence is also on the rise. Diabetes affects one out of every four people. One method of controlling diabetes mellitus is through nutrition, and the fruit of pomegranate plants and their derivatives can play a vital role in this. Much research has been conducted to investigate their antidiabetic efficacy. Katz et al. (2007), for example, investigated the hypoglycemic action of pomegranate blossoms, seeds, and juice (Banihani et al. 2013). This study shows that pomegranate blossoms and juice, by attaching to peroxisome proliferator-activated receptors and producing nitric oxide, may help avoid diabetes complications. The mechanisms underlying such benefits are mainly understood. Punicic acid (PA) is a conjugated linolenic acid that is a PUFAs (18:3 n-5). PA is also known as a "super CLnA," because its impact is stronger than that of a regular CLnA. Punicic acid (PA)—the primary component of pomegranate seed oil (PSO), which has potential therapeutic benefits in T2DM—is found mostly in the seeds of pomegranate fruit (Khajebishak et al. 2019).

### 6.6.3 Blood Pressure

Pomegranate juice has been shown to significantly lower systolic blood pressure. It contains potassium, which can help to reduce arterial stiffness and atherosclerosis. It improves blood flow to the heart and lowers the risk of a heart attack. Clinical researches have looked into the ability of pomegranate juice to improve endothelial function and blood pressure in the body (Asgary et al. 2017). Twenty-one hypertension patients were enlisted to see if the juicy component of the pomegranate may help them. They range in age from 30 to 67 years old. For 2 weeks, a group of 11 patients was given 150 mL of juice to drink at lunch or dinner. A second set of ten people received the same amount of water as the first. After the trial finished, the data showed a drop in systolic (p=0.002) and diastolic blood concentrations (0.038) in the juice drinkers. The level of endothelial adhesion molecule in the blood was also observed to be reduced (p = 0.008), which has curative implications for patients' endothelial functions and blood pressure profile.

### 6.6.4 Liver Health

If consumed consistently in hypercholesterolemia, obesity, and a diet heavy in fat, carbohydrates, and energy, pomegranate juice can help prevent non-alcoholic fatty liver disease. Kaur et al. (2006) investigated the hepatoprotective and antioxidant activity of pomegranate blossoms. The extract's efficiency was determined in vivo, and it was tested for its ability to protect against oxidative tissue damage at an acute level using an animal model, ferric nitrilotriacetate (Fe-NTA) produced hepatotoxicity in the animals (mice). These outcomes propose that the pomegranate blossoms have robust hepatoprotective and antioxidant properties, with the previous most likely being accountable for the latter (Ashoush et al. 2013).

### 6.6.5 Weight Loss

Pomegranates are high in antioxidants, polyphenols, and conjugated linolenic acid, all of which aid in fat burning and metabolism. Pomegranate juice might also help you lose weight. It's a healthier alternative to sugary drinks. Pomegranate juice is a low-calorie, nutritious alternative to all of the sugary beverages consumed on a regular basis (Sayed-Ahmed 2014). Pomegranates are high in fiber, which can bind excess fat and cholesterol in the body and ease its elimination, therefore preventing obesity. Pomegranate leaf stimulates fat and weight reduction to a great extent. If you buy pomegranate juice from a market, be sure there is no added sugar on the label. Added sugar contributes to weight gain. It is preferable to make fresh juice at home.

### 6.6.6 Cancer

By promoting consistent apoptosis in cancer cells, pomegranate extract has been associated with a drop in PC-3 carcinoma prostate cells. It also limits the spread of these dangerous cells to other parts of the body. Pomegranate juice has the ability to suppress cancerous cells in the human body. It can prevent blood from reaching tumors, causing them to shrink and finally die (Syed et al. 2007). Cancer cells in the breast and prostate exhibit significant evidence of degradation. It is well known that malignant cells that cause prostate cancer in adults can be inhibited. To analyze the influence of extract on cancer cells, scientists conducted a number of tests. Twenty-two people were given 8 oz. of pomegranate extract every day for 13 months. After that time period, conclusions were formed. The level of apoptosis of cancer cells in the serum was significantly reduced in an in vitro study. There was a 40% reduction in oxidative stress in serum. Anti-estrogenic properties are found in pomegranate extract. It can prevent breast cancer from starting by suppressing aromatase enzymes and cancer cell proliferation. Pomegranate extracts have a significant impact on hormone levels in the blood. Few studies have shown that endocrine breast cancer treatment has a reasonable impact in postmenopausal women with estrogen receptor positive MCF-7 breast tumors. Anticancer activities were tested in conjunction with tamoxifen at a concentration of 300 μg/mL. The growth of cancer cells is significantly halted.

### 6.6.7 Skin Health

Pomegranates are high in vitamin C, which is a great antioxidant for skin health. It slows the aging and wrinkle-forming process. Ellagitannins have been demonstrated in studies to suppress free radical production and protect against DNA breakage, skin burns, and depigmentation at concentrations ranging from 500 to 10,000 mg. It is believed that if we mix pomegranate peel powder with lemon juice and a tiny quantity of honey and apply it on our faces for a few minutes, we may eliminate dark circles around our eyes as well as treat pigmentation and sunburn (Ko et al. 2021).

### 6.6.8 Oral Health

Pomegranate includes chemicals, notably polyphenolic flavonoids, that may be regarded beneficial to oral cavity health, chiefly in terms of gingivitis development (Silvestro et al. 2009). Dental plaque and tooth loss are avoidable. Thanks to pomegranate seeds. It has antimicrobial properties that can be beneficial against oral bacteria. Gums' health can also be enhanced by their seeds. César de Souza Vasconcelos et al. (2003) found that a pomegranate extract gel used three times per day for 15 days was beneficial for individuals with candidiasis associated with denture stomatitis. Pomegranate extract mouthwash reduced aspartate aminotransferase saliva activity, an indication of cell damage that is elevated in periodontal disease patients (Nomura et al. 2006).

### 6.6.9 Gut Health

Pomegranates' influence on gut microbiota and possible usage as antibacterial agents are one of its most important health-related activities. The microbiota of the colon uses tannins, flavonols, anthocyanins, and phenolic and organic acid compounds in metabolic processes, but pomegranate seeds are also a good source of prebiotic fiber: "Fiber from the seeds contributes to gut health by serving as a prebiotic (food for probiotic, live, gut-friendly bacteria) and providing the necessary bulk to keep the bowel movement regular and optimize digestive health." Supplementation with pomegranate extract dramatically increased bacterial growth of *Bifidobacterium infantis* and *Bifidobacterium breve* (Bialonska et al. 2009).

### 6.6.10 Quality of Sperm

Pomegranate juice consumption increased epididymal sperm concentration, motility, spermatogenic cell density, the breadth of seminiferous tubules, and the thickness of the germinal cell layer in contrast to the control group; it also reduced the rate of aberrant sperm (Türk et al. 2008). Ellagic acid was protective against cyclosporine A-induced testicular and spermatozoal damage. Ellagic acid's antioxidant activity appears to be connected to a decrease in oxidative stress. Ellagic acid can therefore be taken alongside cyclosporine A to enhance its sperm quality in autoimmune diseases (Türk et al. 2016).

### 6.6.11 Bone Health

Later in life, joint inflammation can cause pain and edema. Pomegranate extract contains flavones that have anti-inflammatory properties and may help to reduce collagen-induced arthritis and painful joint swelling. Pomegranate seed oil extracts inhibit the enzyme's cyclooxygenases and lipoxygenases. Pomegranate juice inhibits these important inflammatory mediators by 23.8%, whereas seed oil reduces them by 75% (Spilmont et al. 2014). These extracts suppress matrix metalloproteinases, which are implicated in the degradation of the extracellular joint matrix in osteoarthritis patients. By limiting collagen breakdown, it protects joints from deterioration.

### 6.6.12 Antimicrobial Properties

Pomegranates have a large number of bioactive compounds that help to fight illnesses including diarrhea and ulcers. The parasitic and bacterial infections are reduced to the degree that it may protect against respiratory disorders and cancer. Because of their propensity to precipitate membrane proteins and block enzymes that promote cell lysis, elagic and gallic acids have been used as natural antibacterial agents against *Staphylococcus aureus* and *Escherichia coli* (Opara et al. 2009). Eighty percent of the inhibitory effects were demonstrated using this technique. Table 6.1 shows the antimicrobial activity of different parts of pomegranate fruit.

### 6.6.13 Anti-Inflammatory Properties

Inflammation and tenderness, the preliminary physiological guard system in the human body, may protect against impairment produced by somatic wounds, contaminants, and so on. This defensive system, which is also identified as short-term inflammation, has the capability to exterminate pathogenic microbes, eradicate irritants, and reserve customary physiological progressions. Long-term over-inflammation might effect in physiological dysfunctions such as asthma and autoimmune disorders like rheumatoid arthritis (Ismail et al. 2012). Rendering to Boussetta et al. (2009), the punicic acid, a conjugated fatty acid that is found in the oil of pomegranate seeds, possesses an in vivo anti-inflammatory influence via plummeting the neutrophil stimulation and the special effects of lipid peroxidation. Lee et al. (2019) explored four hydrolyzable tannins that were extracted from pomegranate through the technique of bioassay-guided fractionation: Punicalin, punicalagin, granatin B, and strictinin A. In vitro inquiries discovered that each of them had a dose-dependent and considerable inhibitory effect on the generation of nitric oxide (Lee et al. 2019).

### 6.6.14 Antiviral Properties

Pomegranate has the same antiviral action as vitamins E and C. Infections can be reduced by drinking juice on a regular basis, which improves the immune system's efficiency (Karimi et al. 2017). When investigated, the four primary polyphenols in pomegranate extracts (luteolin, EA, caffeic acid, and punicalagin) were found as the anti-influenza constituent, since it inhibited the replication of viral RNA. Pomegranate polyphenol extract has antiviral effects against influenza virus RNA replication. Punicalagin chemicals, which are found at a concentration of 40 µg/mL, have an inhibiting impact on viral RNA replication. Similarly, peel phenolics inhibit intracellular viral replication. Additionally, the pomegranate extract has microbiocidal effects against HIV-1 (Sundararajan et al. 2010).

### 6.6.15 Antioxidative Properties

One of prime reasons for food product superiority and satisfactoriness is oxidative corrosion. Revelation to the enzyme known as lipoxygenase, metal ions, heat, light, and ionizing radiation stimulate this method (Shabtay et al. 2008). As it comprises the loss of many vitamins and other important fatty acids, this category of oxidation considerably diminishes the nutritional value of a complete previously well-balanced meal. It also has an influence on the sensory value of the foodstuff, affecting the texture, color, or flavor, which curtails its shelf life and consequently can lead to customer dismissal. Researchers in the agro-food industry are emphasizing the need of discovering the antioxidant power of pomegranate ingredients to replace synthetic antioxidants, whose

## Table 6.1: Antimicrobial Activity of Different Parts of Pomegranate Fruit

| Plant Parts | Extracts | Strains of Bacteria | References |
|---|---|---|---|
| Arils | Water extracts | Bacillus megaterium<br>P. aeruginosa<br>S. aureus<br>Corynebacterium<br>Xerosis<br>Escherichia coli<br>Micrococcus luteus<br>Enterococcus faecalis | Duman et al. (2009) |
| Full (whole) fruit | Methanolic and aqueous extracts | S. typhi<br>Salmonella paratyphi<br>Salmonella typhimurium | Pasha et al. (2009) |
| Full (whole) fruit | Ethanolic and aqueous extracts | Different strains of Escherichia coli | Voravuthikunchai et al. (2004) |
| Full (whole) fruit | Ethanolic extracts | B. subtilis<br>P. aeruginosa | Nascimento et al. (2000) |
| Full (whole) fruit | Raw form extracts | E. coli<br>P. aeruginosa<br>Enterobact eraerogenes<br>Enteroccoccus faecalis<br>S. aureus | Salgado et al. (2009) |
| Full (whole) fruit | Water and ethanol extracts | Enterobacter sp.<br>Aeromonas sobria<br>Klebsiella pneumonia<br>Chryseobacterium sp. | Muangsan and Senamontee (2008) |
| Full (whole) fruit | Ethyl acetate extract | S. aureus<br>Methicillin-resistant | Parashar et al. (2009) |
| Peels | Aqueous extracts | S. aureus<br>Methicillin-resistant and Methicillin-sensitive | Gould et al. (2009) |
| Peels | Water, methanolic, ether, and choloroformic extracts | S. aureus<br>E. coli<br>L. monocytogenes<br>B. subtilis<br>Y. enterocolitica<br>P. aeruginosa<br>K. pneumoniae | Prashanth et al. (2001) |
| Peels | Butanol, hexane, and ethyl acetate | S. aureus<br>Methicillin-resistant | Machado et al. (2002) |
| Peels | Aqueous extracts | B. subtilis<br>S. aureus<br>E. coli<br>Proteus mirabilis<br>P. aeruginosa | McCarrell et al. (2008) |
| Peels | Water extracts | S. typhi | Perez and Anesini (1994) |
| Peels | Water extracts | P. aeruginosa | Kelly et al. (2009) |
| Arils and peels | Water extracts | P. aeruginosa<br>S. aureus | Opara et al. (2009) |
| Juices | Water extracts | Aeromonas hydrophila | Belal et al. (2009) |
| By-products | Water extracts | S. aureus<br>Pathogenic Clostridium | Bialonska et al. (2009) |

151

usage is becoming increasingly restricted owing to the secondary effects they may have. The antioxidant activity of apple juice, blueberry juice, black cherry juice, grape juice, cranberry juice, red wines, orange juice, and iced tea was shown to be at least 20% greater than any other, according to Rozenberg et al. (2016); however, pomegranate juice has high antioxidant activity. Table 6.2 shows antioxidant activity of pomegranate fruit.

## Table 6.2 Antioxidant Properties of Pomegranate Fruit

| Plant Parts | Analysis | Outcome | References |
|---|---|---|---|
| Leaf extract | DPPH | Pomegranate leaves 93.5% antioxidant enhancement | Lu et al. (2003) |
| Peels | Phosphomolybdenum complex | Ethyl acetate, methanol, and acetone revealed noticeable antioxidant ability, but the aquatic extract was the lowermost | Negi et al. (2003) |
| Peels, arils, EA extracts, and juice | DPPH | Worthy antioxidant property Stoutest from EA extracts of arils | Ricci et al. (2006) |
| Carpellary membrane, and pith | DPPH superoxide and free radicals | Strong lipid peroxidation inhibitory action in a liposome archetypal organization | Kulkarni et al. (2003) |
| Seeds, peel, and pulp | FRAP | Antioxidant action and may be the rich foundation of natural antioxidants | Guo et al. (2003) |
| Juices | DPPH | Antioxidant activity differed between cultivars and was proportional to the total phenolics in each juice type | Mousavinejad et al. (2009) |
| Peel of fruit | TEAC | Prodelphinid in strong antioxidants in aquatic phase | Plumb et al. (2002) |
| Peel of fruit | ABTS and DPPH radicals | Extraordinary free radical-scavenging influence | Okonogi et al. (2007) |
| Peel of fruit | ABTS and DPPH radicals | Strong antioxidant action | Rout et al. (2007) |
| Arils | TEAC and FRAP | Variations among cultivars were inordinate | Ozgen et al. (2008) |
| Seeds of fruit | FRAP | The extracts attained by various solvents showed numerous gradations of antioxidant action | Sadeghi et al. (2009) |
| Peel, seeds, and pulp | FRAP | Skin of the fruit had grander antioxidant action than seed and pulp | Haji Mahmoodi et al. (2008) |
| Flowers and juice | DPPH and FRAP | Both samples showed high antioxidant activity, due to the organic acids and anthocyanins which were present in the illustrations | Miguel et al. (2009) |
| Peels and seeds | FRAP | Peels presented very high level of total antioxidant but seeds had lesser capability | Surveswaran et al. (2007) |
| Leaves and fruits | ABTS and DPPH | Leaf and peel showed strong antioxidant activity | Zhang et al. (2008) |
| Juice or sour concentrate | Inhibition of peroxidation in linoleic acid system | Sour concentrate present higher antioxidant activity than juice | Orak (2009) |

## 6.7 THE SAFETY OF POMEGRANATE EXTRACT DIETARY SUPPLEMENTS

To make taking the bioactive polyphenols easier, pomegranate extracts, which include the primary antioxidants contained in pomegranates, have been molded into vegetal dietary supplements. Despite the fact that dietary supplements containing pomegranate extract are widely accessible, there has been little human research on their safety (Patel et al. 2008). Pomegranate, in various forms, has been shown to be safe to include into a healthy lifestyle in recent research studies. Giving rats two doses of pomegranate extract (0.4 and 1.2 mg/kg body weight) had no detrimental effects on food consumption, behavioral characteristics, weight growth, or physiological factors, according to Cuban research (Vidar et al. 2003). In a study conducted on human volunteers, Heber et al. (2007) looked at the safety of pomegranate extract dietary supplements. The purpose of the study was to see if 64 obese adults with high waistlines were safe. Each day, the patients were given one or two pomegranate extract capsules containing 710 mg (435 mg GAEs) or 1420 mg of pomegranate extract, respectively (870 mg of GAEs). The researchers concluded that none of the people tested at either location had any significant negative impacts. Rats were given higher dosages of pomegranate extract orally for 37 days in another trial. Any of the blood parameters evaluated in the trial rats showed no significant increases in noxiousness, which was corroborated by liver and kidney investigations (Cerda et al. 2003). Another research found no significant effects on blood chemistry, renal, liver, or cardiac functions in individuals with carotid artery stenosis who ingested pomegranate juice (121 mg/L EA equivalents) for up to three years (Aviram et al. 2004). Patel et al. (2008) discovered no toxicologically significant changes in clinical interpretations, ocular inspections, body masses, body weight, feed intakes, clinical pathology values, or structure weights after pomegranate extract treatment. There were no adverse effects discovered, and the blood chemistry and hematological indicators were all within normal laboratory ranges.

## 6.8 CONCLUSION

As a result of its supposed health benefits, pomegranate consumption has skyrocketed. The juice, skin, and seeds of the pomegranate are high in a range of high-value chemicals that may have physiological effects. Pomegranates are a nutritious and appealing fruit crop with a high bioactive profile. Pomegranate juice or extract, according to a growing body of data, may assist to avoid and even treat a range of illnesses, such as diabetes and cardiovascular disease; it may also help to prevent and halt the development of some carcinomas, as well as safeguard oral and skin health. There aren't a lot of negative impacts. Customers may benefit from the wide spectrum of health benefits of pomegranate by taking concentrated, low-cost pomegranate juice or standardized pomegranate extract capsules. Pomegranate has been examined extensively over the years and has a number of impressive medicinal properties, particularly in vitro and in vivo investigations. Because of its antioxidant properties, it is thought to be superior to green tea. This fruit's components have all been used in the food industry to prevent and treat illness. Even at 1,420 mg, pomegranate extract has no negative effects on the liver or other organs and can be taken as a natural supplement. However, in order to reap the benefits of this fruit and compete for its export on the world market, it is critical to encourage its production in both traditional and nontraditional ways at this time. More research and testing are needed to determine the benefits of pomegranate in treating diarrheal diseases and controlling fungal growth. The power of this fruit to combat diseases has the potential to revolutionize the food and medical industries.

## REFERENCES

Abbaspour, N., Hurrell, R., & Kelishadi, R. (2014). Review on iron and its importance for human health. *Journal of Research in Medical Sciences: The Official Journal of Isfahan University of Medical Sciences, 19*(2), 164.

Abram, M. (2009). The pomegranate: Sacred, secular, and sensuous symbol of ancient Israel. *Studia Antiqua, 7*(1), 4.

Alcaraz, F., Martínez, J. J., García, F., & Hernández, F. (2017, September). Mineral composition and sensory characteristics of twenty pomegranate cultivars. In *IV International Symposium on Pomegranate and Minor Mediterranean Fruits* 1254, 83–90.

Al-Mutary, M. G., & Abu-Taweel, G. M. (2020). Effects of pomegranate juice on the sexual behavior, fertility and protective activity against aluminum exposure in male mice. *Journal of King Saud University-Science, 32*(6), 2688–2695.

Aloqbi, A., Omar, U., Yousr, M., Grace, M., Lila, M. A., & Howell, N. (2016). Antioxidant activity of pomegranate juice and punicalagin. *Natural Science, 8*(06), 235.

Ambigaipalan, P., de Camargo, A. C., & Shahidi, F. (2016). Phenolic compounds of pomegranate by products (outer skin, mesocarp, divider membrane) and their antioxidant activities. *Journal of Agricultural and Food Chemistry, 64*(34), 6584–6604.

Ambigaipalan, P., de Camargo, A. C., & Shahidi, F. (2017). Identification of phenolic antioxidants and bioactives of pomegranate seeds following juice extraction using HPLC-DAD-ESI-MSn. *Food Chemistry, 221*, 1883–1894.

Anderson, J. W., Baird, P., Davis, R. H., Ferreri, S., Knudtson, M., Koraym, A., ... & Williams, C. L. (2009). Health benefits of dietary fiber. *Nutrition Reviews, 67*(4), 188–205.

Anderson, J. W., & Siesel, A. E. (1990). Hypocholesterolemic effects of oat products. *New Developments in Dietary Fiber*, 17–36.

Arai, S. (2002). Global view on functional foods: Asian perspectives. *British Journal of Nutrition, 88*(S2), S139–S143.

Ardekani, M. R. S., Hajimahmoodi, M., Oveisi, M. R., Sadeghi, N., Jannat, B., Ranjbar, A. M., ... & Moridi, T. (2011). Comparative antioxidant activity and total flavonoid content of Persian pomegranate (*Punica granatum* L.) cultivars. *Iranian Journal of Pharmaceutical Research: IJPR, 10*(3), 519.

Asgary, S., Keshvari, M., Sahebkar, A., & Sarrafzadegan, N. (2017). Pomegranate consumption and blood pressure: A review. *Current Pharmaceutical Design, 23*(7), 1042–1050.

Ashoush, I. S., El-Batawy, O. I., & El-Shourbagy, G. A. (2013). Antioxidant activity and hepatoprotective effect of pomegranate peel and whey powders in rats. *Annals of Agricultural Sciences, 58*(1), 27–32.

Ashton, R., Baer, B., & Silverstein, D. (2006). *The Incredible Pomegranate Plant & Fruit.* Tempe: Third Millennium Publishing.

Aviram, M., & Rosenblat, M. (2013). Pomegranate for your cardiovascular health. *Rambam Maimonides Medical Journal, 4*(2).

Aziz, S., Firdous, S., Rahman, H., Awan, S. I., Michael, V., & Meru, G. (2020). Genetic diversity among wild pomegranate (*Punica granatum*) in Azad Jammu and Kashmir region of Pakistan. *Electronic Journal of Biotechnology, 46*, 50–54.

Banihani, S., Swedan, S., & Alguraan, Z. (2013). Pomegranate and type 2 diabetes. *Nutrition Research, 33*(5), 341–348.

Bar-Ya'akov, I., Tian, L., Amir, R., & Holland, D. (2019). Primary metabolites, anthocyanins, and hydrolyzable tannins in the pomegranate fruit. *Frontiers in Plant Science, 10*, 620.

Basu, T. K., & Srichamroen, A. (2010). Health benefits of fenugreek (*Trigonella foenum-graecum leguminosse*). In *Bioactive Foods in Promoting Health* (pp. 425–435). Academic Press.

Bhandari, P. R. (2012). Pomegranate (*Punica granatum* L.). Ancient seeds for modern cure? Review of potential therapeutic applications. *International Journal of Nutrition, Pharmacology, Neurological Diseases, 2*(3), 171.

Bialonska, D., Kasimsetty, S. G., Schrader, K. K., & Ferreira, D. (2009). The effect of pomegranate (*Punica granatum* L.) by products and ellagitannins on the growth of human gut bacteria. *Journal of Agricultural and Food Chemistry, 57*(18), 8344–8349.

Bigliardi, B., & Galati, F. (2013). Innovation trends in the food industry: The case of functional foods. *Trends in Food Science & Technology, 31*(2), 118–129.

Blum, A., Monir, M., Wirsansky, I., & Ben-Arzi, S. (2005). The beneficial effects of tomatoes. *European Journal of Internal Medicine, 16*(6), 402–404.

Borek, C. (2001). Antioxidant health effects of aged garlic extract. *Journal of Nutrition, 131*(3), 1010S–1015S.

Brennand, C. P., & Jorgenson, S. (2020). Preserving Pomegranates.

Brielmann, H. L., Setzer, W. N., Kaufman, P. B., Kirakosyan, A., & Cseke, L. J. (2006). Phytochemicals: The chemical components of plants. *Natural Products From Plants, 2*, 1–49.

Bystrická, J., Kavalcová, P., Musilová, J., Vollmannová, A., Tóth, T., & Lenková, M. (2015). Carrot (*Daucus carota* L. ssp. sativus (Hoffm.) Arcang.) as source of antioxidants. *Acta Agriculturae Slovenica, 105*(2), 303–311.

Cabrera, C., Artacho, R., & Giménez, R. (2006). Beneficial effects of green tea—A review. *Journal of the American College of Nutrition, 25*(2), 79–99.

Cao, K., Xu, J., Pu, W., Dong, Z., Sun, L., Zang, W., ... & Liu, J. (2015). Punicalagin, an active component in pomegranate, ameliorates cardiac mitochondrial impairment in obese rats via AMPK activation. *Scientific Reports, 5*(1), 1–12.

Cardoso Carraro, J. C., Dantas, M. I. D. S., Espeschit, A. C. R., Martino, H. S. D., & Ribeiro, S. M. R. (2012). Flaxseed and human health: Reviewing benefits and adverse effects. *Food Reviews International, 28*(2), 203–230.

Caruso, A., Barbarossa, A., Tassone, A., Ceramella, J., Carocci, A., Catalano, A., ... & Sinicropi, M. S. (2020). Pomegranate: Nutraceutical with promising benefits on human health. *Applied Sciences, 10*(19), 6915.

César de Souza Vasconcelos, L., Sampaio, M. C. C., Sampaio, F. C., & Higino, J. S. (2003). Use of *Punica granatum* as an antifungal agent against candidosis associated with denture stomatitis. *Mycoses, 46*(5-6), 192–196.

Chandra, R., Babu, K. D., Jadhav, V. T., Jaime, A., & Silva, T. D. (2010). Origin, history and domestication of pomegranate. *Fruit, Vegetable and Cereal Science and Biotechnology, 2*, 1–6.

Das, L., Bhaumik, E., Raychaudhuri, U., & Chakraborty, R. (2012). Role of nutraceuticals in human health. *Journal of Food Science and Technology, 49*(2), 173–183.

Deshmukh, M. S., Kachave, T. R., & Kanase, P. M. (2020). Evaluation of macro and micro nutrient status of pomegranate orchards from Maharashtra region by soil and leaf analysis. *Journal of Pharmacognosy and Phytochemistry, 9*(1), 1378–1382.

Dillard, C. J., & German, J. B. (2000). Phytochemicals: Nutraceuticals and human health. *Journal of the Science of Food and Agriculture, 80*(12), 1744–1756.

DiNicolantonio, J. J., Bhutani, J., & O'Keefe, J. H. (2015). The health benefits of vitamin K. *Open Heart, 2*(1), e000300.

Dobrenova, F. V., Grabner-Kräuter, S., & Terlutter, R. (2015). Country-of-origin (COO) effects in the promotion of functional ingredients and functional foods. *European Management Journal, 33*(5), 314–321.

Duman, A. D., Ozgen, M., Dayisoylu, K. S., Erbil, N., & Durgac, C. (2009). Antimicrobial activity of six pomegranate (*Punica granatum* L.) varieties and their relation to some of their pomological and phytonutrient characteristics. *Molecules, 14*(5), 1808–1817.

El Kar, C., Ferchichi, A., Attia, F., & Bouajila, J. (2011). Pomegranate (*Punica granatum*) juices: Chemical composition, micronutrient cations, and antioxidant capacity. *Journal of Food Science, 76*(6), C795–C800.

Elfalleh, W., Tlili, N., Ying, M., Sheng-Hua, H., Ferchichi, A., & Nasri, N. (2011). Organoleptic quality, minerals, proteins and amino acids from two Tunisian commercial pomegranate fruits. *International Journal of Food Engineering, 7*(4).

El-Sheshtawy, H. S., Aiad, I., Osman, M. E., Abo-ELnasr, A. A., & Kobisy, A. S. (2016). Production of biosurfactants by *Bacillus licheniformis* and *Candida albicans* for application in microbial enhanced oil recovery. *Egyptian Journal of Petroleum, 25*(3), 293–298.

Espín, J. C., García-Conesa, M. T., & Tomás-Barberán, F. A. (2007). Nutraceuticals: Facts and fiction. *Phytochemistry, 68*(22–24), 2986–3008.

Farag, R. S., Abdel-Latif, M. S., Emam, S. S., & Tawfeek, L. S. (2014). Phytochemical screening and polyphenol constituents of pomegranate peels and leave juices. *Agricultural Soil Science, 1*(6), 86–93.

Fourati, M., Smaoui, S., Hlima, H. B., Elhadef, K., Braïek, O. B., Ennouri, K., ... & Mellouli, L. (2020). Bioactive compounds and pharmacological potential of pomegranate (*Punica granatum*) seeds-a review. *Plant Foods for Human Nutrition*, 1–10.

Gruenwald, J., Freder, J., & Armbruester, N. (2010). Cinnamon and health. *Critical Reviews in Food Science and Nutrition, 50*(9), 822–834.

Haug, A., Høstmark, A. T., & Harstad, O. M. (2007). Bovine milk in human nutrition–A review. *Lipids in Health and Disease, 6*(1), 1–16.

Hay, E., Lucariello, A., Contieri, M., Esposito, T., De Luca, A., Guerra, G., & Perna, A. (2019). Therapeutic effects of turmeric in several diseases: An overview. *Chemico-Biological Interactions, 310*, 108729.

Huang, W. Y., Cai, Y. Z., & Zhang, Y. (2009). Natural phenolic compounds from medicinal herbs and dietary plants: Potential use for cancer prevention. *Nutrition and Cancer, 62*(1), 1–20.

Ismail, T., Sestili, P., & Akhtar, S. (2012). Pomegranate peel and fruit extracts: A review of potential anti-inflammatory and anti-infective effects. *Journal of Ethnopharmacology, 143*(2), 397–405.

Jalikop, S. H. (2010). Pomegranate breeding. *Fruit, Vegetable and Cereal Science and Biotechnology, 4*(S2), 26–34.

Jalili, S., Tabatabee Naini, A., Ashrafi, M., & Aminlari, M. (2020). Antioxidant activity of pericarp extract from different varieties of pomegranate fruit. *Journal of Agricultural Science and Technology, 22*(1), 95–107.

Kalaycıoğlu, Z., & Erim, F. B. (2017). Total phenolic contents, antioxidant activities, and bioactive ingredients of juices from pomegranate cultivars worldwide. *Food Chemistry, 221*, 496–507.

Kandylis, P., & Kokkinomagoulos, E. (2020). Food applications and potential health benefits of pomegranate and its derivatives. *Foods, 9*(2), 122.

Karimi, M., Sadeghi, R., & Kokini, J. (2017). Pomegranate as a promising opportunity in medicine and nanotechnology. *Trends in Food Science & Technology, 69*, 59–73.

Katz, S. R., Newman, R. A., & Lansky, E. P. (2007). *Punica granatum*: Heuristic treatment for diabetes mellitus. *Journal of Medicinal Food, 10*(2), 213–217.

Kaur, G., Jabbar, Z., Athar, M., & Alam, M. S. (2006). *Punica granatum* (pomegranate) flower extract possesses potent antioxidant activity and abrogates Fe-NTA induced hepatotoxicity in mice. *Food and Chemical Toxicology, 44*(7), 984–993.

Kaur, S., & Das, M. (2011). Functional foods: An overview. *Food Science and Biotechnology, 20*(4), 861.

Khajebishak, Y., Payahoo, L., Alivand, M., & Alipour, B. (2019). Punicic acid: A potential compound of pomegranate seed oil in Type 2 diabetes mellitus management. *Journal of Cellular Physiology, 234*(3), 2112–2120.

Khan, A. (2005). A survey of nematodes of pomegranate in lower Sindh, Pakistan. *Sarhad Journal of Agriculture (Pakistan).*

Ko, K., Dadmohammadi, Y., & Abbaspourrad, A. (2021). Nutritional and bioactive components of pomegranate waste used in food and cosmetic applications: A review. *Foods, 10*(3), 657.

Kojadinovic, M. I., Arsic, A. C., Debeljak-Martacic, J. D., Konic-Ristic, A. I., Kardum, N. D., Popovic, T. B., & Glibetic, M. D. (2017). Consumption of pomegranate juice decreases blood lipid peroxidation and levels of arachidonic acid in women with metabolic syndrome. *Journal of the Science of Food and Agriculture, 97*(6), 1798–1804.

Lal, S., Ahmed, N., & Mir, J. I. (2011). Effect of different chemicals on fruit cracking in pomegranate under karewa condition of Kashmir Valley.

Lazongas, E. G. (2017). Side: The personification of the pomegranate. *Personification in the Greek World*, 99–109.

Leboy, P. S. (2006). Regulating bone growth and development with bone morphogenetic proteins. *Annals of the New York Academy of Sciences, 1068*(1), 14–18.

Lee, Y. S., Lai, Y. X., & Li, C. Y. (2019). Anti-inflammatory effects of punicalagin on LPS-activated microglia. *The FASEB Journal, 33*(S1), 542.13.

Levin, G. M. (2006). *Pomegranate* (pp. 1–130). Tempe: Third Millennium Publishing.

Li, X., Wasila, H., Liu, L., Yuan, T., Gao, Z., Zhao, B., & Ahmad, I. (2015). Physicochemical characteristics, polyphenol compositions and antioxidant potential of pomegranate juices from 10 Chinese cultivars and the environmental factors analysis. *Food Chemistry, 175*, 575–584.

Lv, X., Zhao, S., Ning, Z., Zeng, H., Shu, Y., Tao, O., ... & Liu, Y. (2015). Citrus fruits as a treasure trove of active natural metabolites that potentially provide benefits for human health. *Chemistry Central Journal, 9*(1), 1–14.

Madrigal-Carballo, S., Rodriguez, G., Krueger, C. G., Dreher, M., & Reed, J. D. (2009). Pomegranate (*Punica granatum*) supplements: Authenticity, antioxidant and polyphenol composition. *Journal of Functional Foods, 1*(3), 324–329.

Martinez, J. J., Melgarejo, P., Hernández, F., Salazar, D. M., & Martinez, R. (2006). Seed characterisation of five new pomegranate (*Punica granatum* L.) varieties. *Scientia Horticulturae, 110*(3), 241–246.

Maughan, R. J., King, D. S., & Lea, T. (2004). Dietary supplements. *Journal of Sports sciences, 22*(1), 95–113.

McKay, D. L., & Blumberg, J. B. (2006). A review of the bioactivity and potential health benefits of peppermint tea (*Mentha piperita* L.). *Phytotherapy Research: An International Journal Devoted to Pharmacological and Toxicological Evaluation of Natural Product Derivatives, 20*(8), 619–633.

Melgarejo-Sánchez, P., Núñez-Gómez, D., Martínez-Nicolás, J. J., Hernández, F., Legua, P., & Melgarejo, P. (2021). Pomegranate variety and pomegranate plant part, relevance from bioactive point of view: A review. *Bioresources and Bioprocessing, 8*(1), 1–29.

Messina, M. J. (1999). Legumes and soybeans: Overview of their nutritional profiles and health effects. *American Journal of Clinical Nutrition, 70*(3), 439s–450s.

Mustafa, S. M., Chua, L. S., El-Enshasy, H. A., Majid, F. A. A., & Malek, R. A. (2016). A review on fruit juice probiotication: Pomegranate. *Current Nutrition & Food Science, 12*(1), 4–11.

Morton, J. F. (1987). *Fruits of Warm Climates*. JF Morton.

Opara, L. U., Al-Ani, M. R., & Al-Shuaibi, Y. S. (2009). Physico-chemical properties, vitamin C content, and antimicrobial properties of pomegranate fruit (*Punica granatum* L.). *Food and Bioprocess Technology, 2*(3), 315–321.

Pandey, M., Verma, R. K., & Saraf, S. A. (2010). Nutraceuticals: New era of medicine and health. *Asian Journal of Pharmaceutical and Clinical Research, 3*(1), 11–15.

Partearroyo, T., Samaniego-Vaesken, M. D. L., Ruiz, E., Aranceta-Bartrina, J., Gil, Á., González-Gross, M., ... & Varela-Moreiras, G. (2020). Plate waste generated by Spanish households and out-of-home consumption: Results from the ANIBES study. *Nutrients, 12*(6), 1641.

Pasha, C. (2016). Screening of small peptides from various germinating seeds having antimicrobial activity. *IOSR Journal of Pharmacy and Biological Sciences (IOSR-JPBS).-2016*, (11 (1)), 52.

Patel, C., Dadhaniya, P., Hingorani, L., & Soni, M. G. (2008). Safety assessment of pomegranate fruit extract: Acute and subchronic toxicity studies. *Food and Chemical Toxicology, 46*(8), 2728–2735.

Pezzuto, J. M. (2008). Grapes and human health: A perspective. *Journal of Agricultural and Food Chemistry, 56*(16), 6777–6784.

Prakash, S., Kumar, M., Kumari, N., Thakur, M., Rathour, S., Pundir, A., ... & Mekhemar, M. (2021). Plant- based antioxidant extracts and compounds in the management of oral cancer. *Antioxidants, 10*(9), 1358.

Prior, R. L., Rogers, T. R., Khanal, R. C., Wilkes, S. E., Wu, X., & Howard, L. R. (2010). Urinary excretion of phenolic acids in rats fed cranberry. *Journal of Agricultural and Food Chemistry, 58*(7), 3940–3949.

Qu, W., Breksa III, A. P., Pan, Z., & Ma, H. (2012). Quantitative determination of major polyphenol constituents in pomegranate products. *Food Chemistry, 132*(3), 1585–1591.

Rahman, M. S. (2007). Allicin and other functional active components in garlic: Health benefits and bioavailability. *International Journal of Food Properties, 10*(2), 245–268.

Rautiainen, S., Manson, J. E., Lichtenstein, A. H., & Sesso, H. D. (2016). Dietary supplements and disease prevention—A global overview. *Nature Reviews Endocrinology, 12*(7), 407–420.

Reventlow, H. G. (2009). *History of Biblical Interpretation, Volume 1: From the Old Testament to Origen* (Vol. 50). Society of Biblical Lit.

Ross, S. M. (2009). Pomegranate: Its role in cardiovascular health. *Holistic Nursing Practice, 23*(3), 195–197.

Rozenberg, S., Body, J. J., Bruyere, O., Bergmann, P., Brandi, M. L., Cooper, C., ... & Reginster, J. Y. (2016). Effects of dairy products consumption on health: Benefits and beliefs—A commentary from the Belgian Bone Club and the European Society for Clinical and Economic Aspects of Osteoporosis, Osteoarthritis and Musculoskeletal Diseases. *Calcified Tissue International, 98*(1), 1–17.

Ruis, A. R. (2015). Pomegranate and the mediation of balance in early medicine. *Gastronomica: The Journal of Food and Culture, 15*(1), 22–33.

Sang, S., & Chu, Y. (2017). Whole grain oats, more than just a fiber: Role of unique phytochemicals. *Molecular Nutrition & Food Research, 61*(7), 1600715.

Sanlier, N., & Üstün, D. (2021). Egg consumption and health effects: A narrative review. *Journal of Food Science, 86*(10), 4250–4261.

Santini, A., Cammarata, S. M., Capone, G., Ianaro, A., Tenore, G. C., Pani, L., & Novellino, E. (2018). Nutraceuticals: Opening the debate for a regulatory framework. *British Journal of Clinical Pharmacology, 84*(4), 659–672.

Santoyo, G., Orozco-Mosqueda, M. D. C., & Govindappa, M. (2012). Mechanisms of biocontrol and plant growth-promoting activity in soil bacterial species of Bacillus and Pseudomonas: A review. *Biocontrol Science and Technology, 22*(8), 855–872.

Sayed-Ahmed, E. F. (2014). Evaluation of pomegranate peel fortified pan bread on body weight loss. *International Journal of Nutrition and Food Sciences, 3*(5), 411–420.

Setiadhi, R., Sufiawati, I., Zakiawati, D., Nur'aeny, N., Hidayat, W., & Firman, D. R. (2017). Evaluation of antibacterial activity and acute toxicity of pomegranate (*Punica granatum* L.) seed ethanolic extracts in Swiss Webster mice. *J Dentomaxillofacial Sci, 2*(2), 119–123.

Shabtay, A., Eitam, H., Tadmor, Y., Orlov, A., Meir, A., Weinberg, P., ... & Kerem, Z. (2008). Nutritive and antioxidative potential of fresh and stored pomegranate industrial by product as a novel beef cattle feed. *Journal of Agricultural and Food Chemistry, 56*(21), 10063–10070.

Shiban, M. S., Al-Otaibi, M. M., & Al-Zoreky, N. S. (2012). Antioxidant activity of pomegranate (*Punica granatum* L.) fruit peels. *Food and Nutrition Sciences, 2012.*

Sidhu, J. S., & Zafar, T. A. (2012). Super fruits: pomegranate, wolfberry, aronia (chokeberry), acai, noni, and amla. *Handbook of fruits and fruit processing,* 653–679.

Sood, A., & Gupta, M. (2015). Extraction process optimization for bioactive compounds in pomegranate peel. *Food Bioscience, 12,* 100–106.

Spilmont, M., Léotoing, L., Davicco, M. J., Lebecque, P., Mercier, S., Miot-Noirault, E., ... & Coxam, V. (2014). Pomegranate and its derivatives can improve bone health through decreased inflammation and oxidative stress in an animal model of postmenopausal osteoporosis. *European Journal of Nutrition, 53*(5), 1155–1164.

Sturgeon, S. R., & Ronnenberg, A. G. (2010). Pomegranate and breast cancer: Possible mechanisms of prevention. *Nutrition Reviews, 68*(2), 122–128.

Sundararajan, A., Ganapathy, R., Huan, L., Dunlap, J. R., Webby, R. J., Kotwal, G. J., & Sangster, M. Y. (2010). Influenza virus variation in susceptibility to inactivation by pomegranate polyphenols is determined by envelope glycoproteins. *Antiviral Research, 88*(1), 1–9.

Syed, D. N., Afaq, F., & Mukhtar, H. (2007, October). Pomegranate derived products for cancer chemoprevention. *Seminars in Cancer Biology, 17*(5), 377–385.

Türk, G., Sönmez, M., Aydin, M., Yüce, A., Gür, S., Yüksel, M., ... & Aksoy, H. (2008). Effects of pomegranate juice consumption on sperm quality, spermatogenic cell density, antioxidant activity and testosterone level in male rats. *Clinical Nutrition, 27*(2), 289–296.

Türk, G., Çeribaşı, S., Sönmez, M., Çiftçi, M., Yüce, A., Güvenç, M., ... & Aksakal, M. (2016). Ameliorating effect of pomegranate juice consumption on carbon tetrachloride-induced sperm damages, lipid peroxidation, and testicular apoptosis. *Toxicology and Industrial Health, 32*(1), 126–137.

Vroegrijk, I. O., van Diepen, J. A., van den Berg, S., Westbroek, I., Keizer, H., Gambelli, L., ... & Voshol, P. J. (2011). Pomegranate seed oil, a rich source of punicic acid, prevents diet-induced obesity and insulin resistance in mice. *Food and Chemical Toxicology, 49*(6), 1426–1430.

FRUITS AND THEIR ROLES IN NUTRACEUTICALS AND FUNCTIONAL FOODS

Walter, M., & Marchesan, E. (2011). Phenolic compounds and antioxidant activity of rice. *Brazilian Archives of Biology and Technology, 54*, 371–377.

Wang, R., Ding, Y., Liu, R., Xiang, L., & Du, L. (2010). Pomegranate: constituents, bioactivities and pharmacokinetics. *Fruit, Vegetable and Cereal Science and Biotechnology, 4*(2), 77–87.

Xiao, C. W. (2008). Health effects of soy protein and isoflavones in humans. *Journal of Nutrition, 138*(6), 1244S–1249S.

Yadav, R. P., & Tarun, G. (2017). Versatility of turmeric: A review the golden spice of life. *Journal of Pharmacognosy and Phytochemistry, 6*(1), 41–46.

Yao, Y., & Xu, B. (2021). New insights into chemical compositions and health promoting effects of edible oils from new resources. *Food Chemistry*, 130363.

Yilmaz, Y., Çelik, I., & Isik, F. (2007). Mineral composition and total phenolic content of pomegranate molasses. *Journal of Food Ag and Environment, 5*(3/4), 102.

Zarfeshany, A., Asgary, S., & Javanmard, S. H. (2014). Potent health effects of pomegranate. *Advanced Biomedical Research, 3*.

Zhang, L., Fu, Q., & Zhang, Y. (2011). Composition of anthocyanins in pomegranate flowers and their antioxidant activity. *Food Chemistry, 127*(4), 1444–1449.

# 7 Papaya

*Bharti Mittu, Abida Bhat, Mahaldeep Kaur, and Sandaldeep Kaur*

## CONTENTS

## 7.1 INTRODUCTION

Plant-based formulations are widely used in disease prevention and treatment and have been known since the ancient times. These products have been associated with various advantages over man-made drugs and are associated with fewer side effects and do not disrupt biochemical and physiological pathways. Papaya (*Carica papaya* L.) is a member of the Caricaceae family, used widely in disease treatment and management around the world, particularly in tropical and subtropical regions. *C. papaya* leaves, barks, roots, latex, fruit, flowers, and seeds are all used in folk medicine to treat a variety of diseases

DOI: 10.1201/9781003259213-7

(Jaiswal et al. 2010). The constituents that are rich in papaya pulp are vitamins (vitamin A, C, E, and B complex, pantothenic acid, and folate) and minerals (magnesium and potassium) (Vij and Prashar 2015). The antioxidant ability of papaya constituents led to the neutralization of generated free radicals thereby preventing the pathogenesis. Fiber is an important constituent that plays a role in cholesterol reduction. The primary source of proteinases such as papain, chymopapain, glycyl endopeptidase, and caricain are present in the latex of papaya (Anuar et al. 2008). The fruit contains papain, which aids digestion and is used to tenderize meat (Rahmani et al. 2014). Constituents of papaya aid in prevention and treatment of disease and modulate a variety of actions like anti-inflammatory, antitumor, hepatoprotective, and antioxidant activities. Other findings reported the anti-inflammatory activity of seeds of *C. papaya*. Previous literature reported the anthelmintic property of papaya latex against intestinal nematodes of mammalian hosts (Amazu et al. 2010; Khor et al. 2021). This chapter summarizes the nutritional, phytochemical constituents, and health benefits of papaya in the prevention and treatment of the disease.

## 7.2 OCCURRENCE

The papaya, *C. papaya* L., is a herbaceous tree belonging to the Caricaceae family (succulently soft-wooded). By the early 1500s, Europeans had discovered papaya in the Western Hemisphere tropics (Watts 1967), and it was quickly disseminated by various interests. All over the world, papaya is cultivated in tropical and subtropical climates, primarily for its melon-like flavor fruit.

## 7.3 CLASSIFICATION OF PAPAYA

Brassicales (also known as Capparales) is the order in which the Caricaceae are classified (Olson 2002). Recently, it has become widely accepted that the genus *Carica* L. contains only one species, *C. papaya*, and that the Caricaceae family includes six genera (Badillo 2000; Van Droogenbroeck et al. 2002, 2004; Manshardt and Wenslaff 1989; Behera et al. 2021).

### Classification of Papaya

| | |
|---|---|
| Domain | Flowering plant |
| Kingdom | Plantae |
| Phylum | Steptophyta |
| Class | Magnoliophyta |
| Order | Brassicales |
| Family | Caricaceae |
| Genus | *Carica* |
| Species | *Papaya* |

*Vasconcellea* (not "*Vasconcella*") highland papayas are found to be closest to the *C. papaya* (Badillo 2000; Van Droogen et al. 2002). Many *Vasconcellea* species have fruit that is edible (Scheldeman et al. 2002); commercial cultivation of Caricaceae is restricted to papaya, toronche, babaco, chamburo (ababai), and higacho. The chamburo, also known as mountain papaya, *V. cundinamarcensis* (also known as *V. pubescens*) is cultivated in America and also has edible fruits (Scheldeman et al. 2002; Vega-Gálvez et al. 2022).

Babaco (also known as *V. pentagona*) is generally grown in western South America (particularly Ecuador), and is grown in other parts of the world like South Africa, Italy, New Zealand, and Spain (Scheldeman et al. 2002; Villarreal et al. 2003). Babaco is thought to be an F1 hybrid (also called *V. heilbornii* but occasionally referred to as *V. heilbornii*) (Morales et al. 2004).

Higacho (or toronche in general) is a hybrid of *V. heilborniivar*. Chrysopetala (also known as *V. chrysopetala*) is also found in Ecuador, where it is commercially important (Rahmani et al. 2014; Patil et al. 2021; Vega-Gálvez et al. 2022).

## 7.4 NUTRITIONAL ATTRIBUTES OF THE PLANT

Kingdom plant is regarded as a source of current drugs because of its abundant production of various secondary metabolites and bioactive molecules. They exhibit prophylactic and therapeutic properties that boost immunity and safeguard life. Papaya (*C. papaya* Linn.) has long been recognized as a nutritious plant having medicinal properties. Each fragment of the papaya has its own nutraceutical properties, such as the stem, fruit, root, seed, latex, flower, leaf, and rinds. It is widely used in ethnomedicine for the treatment and prevention of diseases. It acts as a stimulant of appetite, helps in tenderization of meat, abortifacient, and vermifuge. A series of scientific attempts were made over decades to validate the nutraceutical ability of papaya (Kaliyaperumal et al. 2014; Dotto and Abihudi 2021).

This fruit is well-known throughout the world, with the maximum yield occurring in subtropical and tropical regions. The constituents that are rich in papaya pulp are vitamins (vitamin A, C, E, and B complex, pantothenic acid and folate) and minerals (magnesium and potassium). In addition, enzyme papain is present in papaya, which effectively increase the motility of the intestine and helps in the treatment of sports lesions, traumas, and allergies. Previous literature reported the existence of proteolytic enzymes such as chymopapain that has been associated with various antimicrobial activities such as antifungal, antibacterial, and antiviral. The seeds contain phenolic compounds such as glucosinolates, tocopherols, β-cryptoxanthin, benzyl isothiocyanate, carotenoids, and β-carotene. The oil extracted from the seed is primarily composed of palmitic, linoleic, and stearic acids and oleic fatty acid.

However, leaves are rich in fibers and polyphenolic compounds such as tocopherol, flavonoids, benzyl isothiocyanate, and saponins. Previous literature reported the protective effects of nutrients on illnesses related to the cardiovascular system such as heart attacks and strokes and in the prevention of damage due to free radicals. In addition, it helps in reducing the levels of cholesterol in the body and aids in treatment of diabetes. The pulp, leaves, and seeds have also been associated with antihypertensive, antioxidant, hypolipidemic, and hypoglycemic properties. The fruit is a rich source of beta-carotene (888 IU/100 g), which helps in protection from free radical damage, as well as aids in cardiovascular diseases and diabetes mellitus (types 1 and 2) (Rinnerthaler et al. 2015; Oche et al. 2017; Santana et al. 2019; Dotto and Abihudi 2021).

## 7.5 PHYTOCHEMICAL CONSTITUENTS OF PAPAYA

Constitutes of papaya vary in different parts of the plant, such as fruits, leaves, and seeds. Phytochemical examination of the leaves revealed the presence of saponins, cardiac glycosides, and alkaloid. The previous findings suggested that phenolic acids are the main compound present in the leaves of *C. papaya*; chlorogenic acid is present in trace amounts compared to coumarin and flavonoid compounds. It contains significant amounts of minerals, vitamins, and flavonoids. The ripe fruit is rich in vitamins A and C, as well as calcium. The pawpaw is also rich in vitamin C having varying amounts depending on maturity stage. The constituents of red-fleshed papaya and yellow-fleshed papaya differ. According to a previous study, in red-fleshed papaya the total lycopene content was significantly greater than that of yellow-fleshed fruit. The seeds of papaya have a variety of main ingredients, and these ingredients play an important role in prevention and treatment. A prior article stated that the seed is rich in crude fiber, proteins, lipids, as well as significant amounts of calcium and phosphorus. The presence of glucosinolates was also found in the seed (Azarkan et al. 2003; Fernandes et al. 2006; Thomás et al. 2009; Dotto and Abihudi 2021; Khor et al. 2021).

The flavor, nutritional value, and digestive properties of papaya fruit are highly valued all over the world. It contains the enzyme when the fruit is unripe. Papain is a cysteine protease (EC3.4.22.2) with a similar mechanism of action like pepsin in the gastric juices. Papain is extracted from the latex of unripe fruit. The active papain was found to be present in greater amounts in the green fruits. Three other cysteine proteases were extracted from the latex of papaya such as Chymopapain, Caricain (EC 3.4.22.30), and Papaya protease IV (EC 3.4.22.25) (Nagarathna et al. 2021).

### 7.5.1 Papain

Papain is a proteolytic enzyme belonging to the papain superfamily and plays an essential role in various biological processes of all living organisms. It has a wide range of proteolytic activity against proteins, short chain polypeptides, amino acid ester, and amide links and is widely used in nutraceutical and pharmaceutical industries. It breaks down the basic amino acid peptide bonds. It is a globular protein with a single chain having a molecular weight of 23406 DA and 212 amino acids connected by four disulphide bridges. It is stable and active in various harsh conditions, including high temperatures (Menard et al. 1990; Olmoss 2012).

### 7.6 BIOACTIVE COMPOUNDS PRESENT IN PAPAYA

Papaya, like any other fruit, contains different biologically active compounds such as carotenoids, vitamins, flavonoids, phenolics, and minerals (Vuong et al. 2015; Udomkun et al. 2016). Other parts of the papaya fruit that have shown to be rich in bioactive compounds are the leaves and seeds of the plant (Table 7.1). Papaya seeds contain proteins, glucosinolates, fiber, phenolics, flavonoids, and lipids, whereas the leaves of the plant contain flavonoids, tannins, alkaloids, saponins, phenolics, and steroids (Saeed et al. 2014). It has many beneficial health effects which are majorly attributed to the bioactive compounds present in it, making this a complete functional food (Santana et al. 2019). Extraction of these compounds from papaya fruit involves various extraction methods of which ultrasound-assisted and high hydrostatic pressure assisted extraction show efficient extraction and improved analysis (Siriamornpun et al. 2015). People consume papaya as fresh raw, as juice, in dried form, or in other industrial processed forms. Large amounts of papaya seeds and peel left as waste products, thus discarded. But the study indicates that papaya peel is a great source of bioactive components, which can be changed into a number of value-added products like dietary fibers, adsorbents, biomedicine, biomaterials, biofuels (Pathak et al. 2019).

Ultraviolet (UV-B and UV-C) radiations on papaya fruit induce synthesis of secondary metabolites in them with antioxidant properties apart of the temperature and stress (Storey 2019). Bioactive compounds have been associated with therapeutical properties against varied diseases that are present in different tissues of papaya and are consumed in different regions with diversified eating styles (Annegowda et al. 2014, Rivera-Pastrana et al. 2014). These bioactive compounds have medicinal value to act as an anticancer agent,

## Table 7.1: Nutritional Value Present in Seeds, Leaves, and Fruit of Papaya Plant in General Which May Vary According to Its Different Types of Origin

| Tissue Part | Bioactive Compound | Nutritional Content | Function |
|---|---|---|---|
| Seeds | β-Carotene | 888 μg/g | • Papaya seeds having therapeutical value are usually discarded<br>• These are a good source of unsaturated fatty acids, dietary fiber, minerals, photochemicals, phenolic compounds, and antioxidants |
| | Zinc | 6.17 mg/100 g | |
| | Phosphorus | 566.9 mg/100 g | |
| | Manganese | 3.10 mg/100 g | |
| | Copper | 1.09 mg/100 g | |
| | Magnesium | 332.5 mg/100 g | |
| | Iron | 5.80 mg/100 g | |
| | Vitamin C | 11.7 mg/100 g | |
| | Vitamin B2 | 0.05 mg/100 g | |
| | Vitamin B3 | 0.26 mg/100 g | |
| | Vitamin B1 | 0.05 mg/100 g | |
| | Fiber | 2.1 g/100 g | |
| | Flavonoids | 3.6% | |
| | Anthraquinones | 21.5% | |
| | Glycosides | 9.17% | |
| | Linolenic acid | 0.90% | |
| | Linoleic acid | 6.06% | |
| | Arachidic acid | 1.10% | |
| Leaves | Protein | 5.8 g/100 g | • Papaya leaves have many medicinal uses as they contain a rich source of bioactive compounds<br>• These have anticancer, anti-inflammatory, antioxidative, and antibacterial properties |
| | Ascorbic acid | 126.2 mg/100 g | |
| | Calcium | 366.1 mg/100 g | |
| | Magnesium | 32.4 mg/100 g | |
| | Zinc | 26.19 mg/kg | |
| | Iron | 29.17 mg/kg | |
| | Manganese | 7.92 mg/kg | |
| | Vitamin C | 68.59 mg/100 g | |
| | Vitamin E | 39.78 mg/100 g | |
| | Flavonoids | 899.53 mg/100 g | |
| | Saponins | 898.07 mg/100 g | |
| | Alkaloids | 1569.13 mg/100 g | |
| | Tannins | 310.50 mg/100 g | |
| Fruit | Protein | 0.6 g/100 g | • Papaya fruit is available throughout the season and is a good source of nutrition with low calorie intake |
| | Dietary fiber | 0.8 g/100 g | |
| | Beta-carotene | 888 IU/100 g | |
| | Potassium | 257 mg/100 g | |
| | Iron | 0.1 mg/100 g | |
| | Calcium | 24 mg/100 g | |
| | Magnesium | 10 mg/100 g | |
| | Potassium | 257 mg/100 g | |
| | Sodium | 3 mg/100 g | |
| | Lipids | 0.1 g/100 g | |
| | Carbohydrates | 7.2 g/100 g | |

*Sources:* From Udomkun et al. (2015); Fernandez et al. (2019); Sivasankari et al. (2019); Devanesan et al. (2021); Shaban et al. (2021).

antioxidant, anti-inflammatory, antiviral, antimicrobial, anti-angiogenic, and wound healing properties (Kushwaha et al. 2021). Papaya during its ripening stage emits volatile organic compounds (VOCs) used as non-invasive markers for determining the ripening stage and nutritional quality of which recent studies have shown methyl hexanoate, 3-carene, and longifolene as three markers with a valid correlation between the ripening stage and its nutritional value (Ugo et al. 2019). Bioactive compounds present in fruits affecting human health must be in an adequate dose concentration to avoid effects like cytotoxicity, embryotoxicity, and mutagenicity (Table 7.1).

Efficient extraction of bioactive compounds is also a challenging task which depends on selection of solvent, nature of solvent, time, temperature, pressure, and method of extraction. Storage and preserving the bioactive compounds in papaya can be attained by the drying, dehydration, and freeze-drying methods for a longer period of time (Annegowda et al. 2014; Santana et al. 2019).

## 7.7 STRUCTURAL CHARACTERIZATION OF BIOACTIVE COMPONENTS IN PAPAYA

### 7.7.1 GC-MS Analysis

Chear et al. (2016) used a hyphenated Agilent 6890N Network GC system coupled to an Agilent 5973i mass selective detector (Agilent Technologies, Germany) to determine the lipophilic constituents of C. *papaya* extracts. 10 mg/mL extract (in methanol) was separated on an HP-5MS column (30 m 0.25 mm, 0.25-m film thickness; Agilent Technologies, Waldbronn, Germany) with 1.2 mL/minute helium gas flow. The injection volume was 1 L with a splitless mode. The initial temperature of the column was set at 70°C for 2 minutes before gradually increasing to 280°C at a constant rate of 20°C per minute. The final temperature of 280°C was maintained in the column for another 20 minutes. The total duration of the run was 32.5 minutes. Electron impact ionization at 70 eV was used to acquire mass in the 40–550 m/z range. Spectral analysis was used to identify the compounds against the National Institute of Standards and Technology database, Gaithersburg, MD, USA (NIST 02). The detected compound's identity was determined by comparing the masses of their molecular ions, base ions, and fragment ions, as well as peak intensities with the database's reference standards discovered with a spectral matching quality of more than 90% were deemed acceptable (Chear et al. 2016; Khor et al. 2021). Figure 7.1(a) shows the total ion chromatograms (TIC) of (i) CPSC extract and (ii) CPSCE extract at a fixed concentration of 5 mg/mL, and Figure 7.1(b) shows the TIC chromatograms of conventional solvent extracts (i) CPHE extract, (ii) CPFD extract, and (iii) CPEE extract at a fixed concentration of 5 mg/mL. CPHE: C. *papaya* leaf hexane extract; CPFD: C. *papaya* leaf juice freeze-dried extract; CPEE: C. *papaya* leaf ethanol extract; CPSC: C. *papaya* leaf scCO$_2$ extract; CPSCE: C. *papaya* leaf scCO$_2$ extract with 5% ethanol.

### 7.7.2 HPLC Profiling of the Polar Extracts

For the analysis of CPL extracts, a simple high-performance liquid chromatography (HPLC) method was performed on an Agilent 1200 series HPLC system with a photodiode array detector (Agilent, Santa Clara, California, USA). A CPL sample stock solution was prepared at 500 g/mL in an 80:20 v/v methanol/water mixture and centrifuged to take out the particles that weren't dissolved. On an Eclipse, chromatographic separation was accomplished. C18 reversed phase column (4.6 mm 150 mm, 3.5 m) (Agilent Technologies, Santa Clara, California, USA) at a temperature of 30°C. The mobile phase used was a gradient of 0.1% formic acid in water (pH 2.65) and acetonitrile method with a flow rate of 1 mL/minute. Figure 7.2 shows the HPLC chromatogram of (a) CPEE extract, (b) CPFD extract, and (c) the rutin standard at 14.2 minutes (Khor et al. 2021).

### 7.7.3 Antioxidant Assay

#### 7.7.3.1 Scavenging Activity of DPPH

A prior study reported to assess the cocoa pod extracts' (CPEs') DPPH radical scavenging capacity of 1,1-diphenyl-2-picryl-hydrazyl (DPPH). The decolorization of the DPPH solution was used to determine the assay.

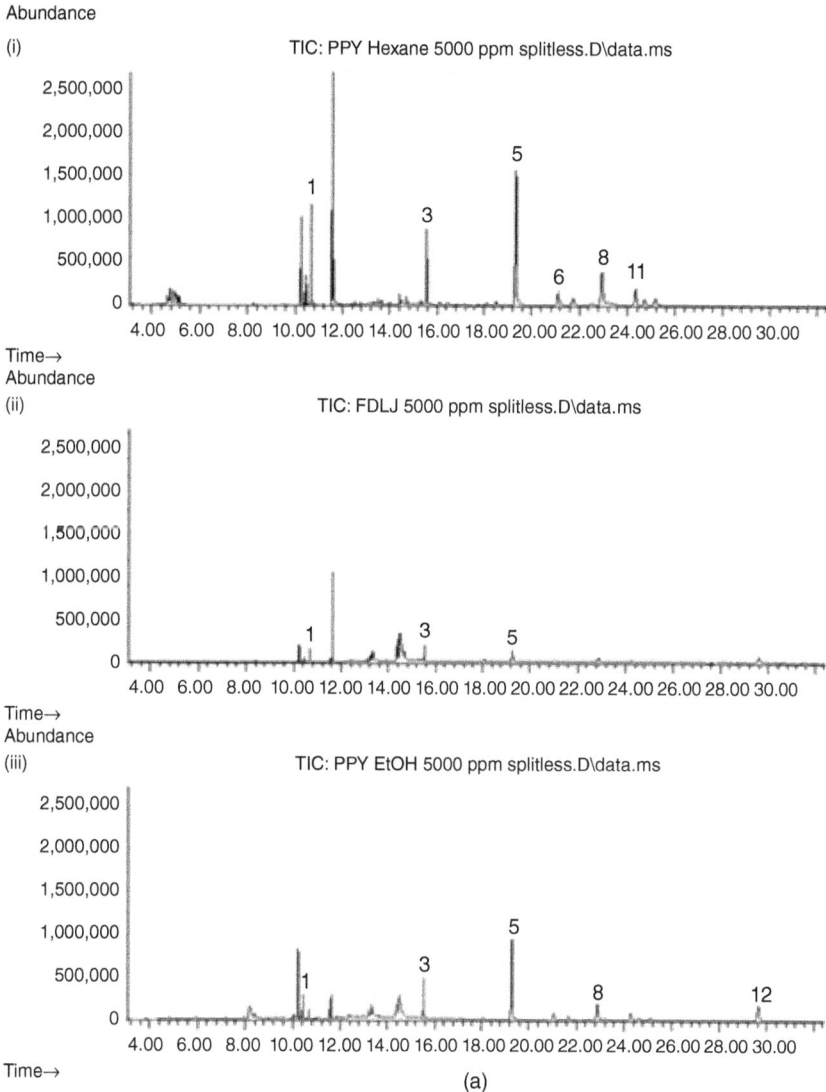

**Figure 7.1** (a) Total ion chromatograms (TIC) of (i) CPSC extract; (ii) CPSCE extract at a fixed concentration of 5 mg/mL. (*Continued*)

169

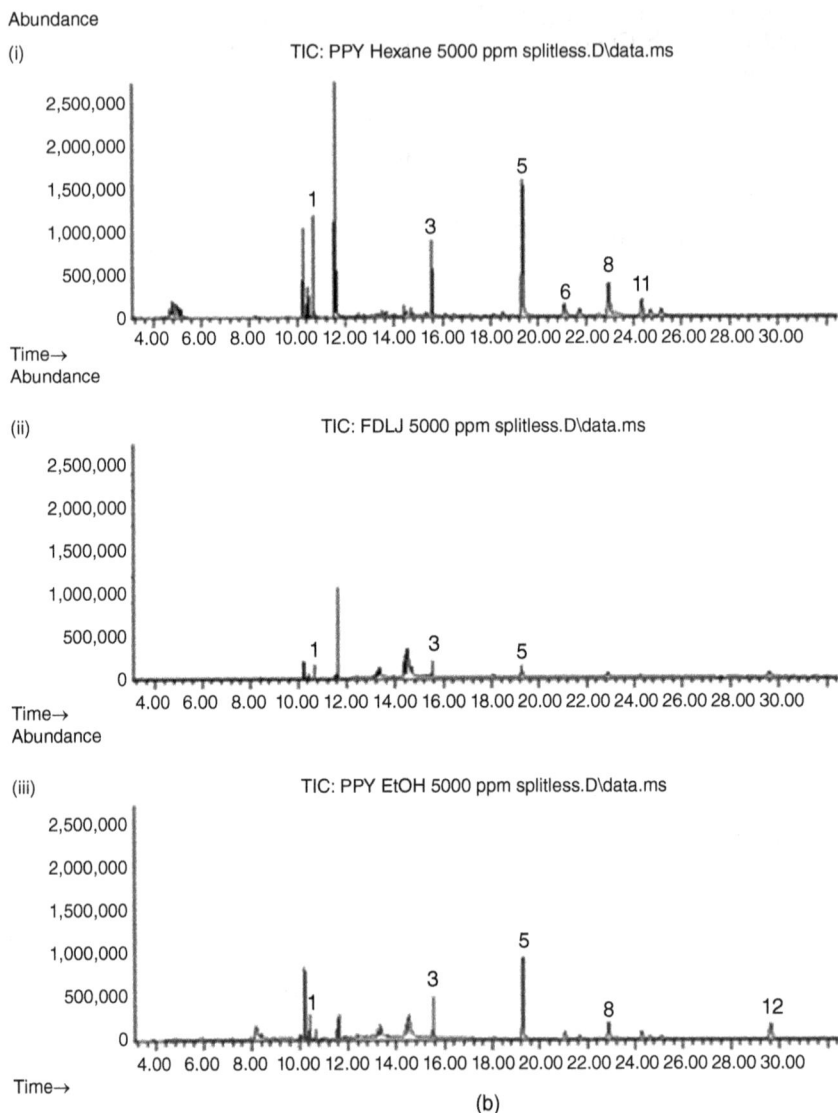

**Figure 7.1 (Continued)** (b) TIC chromatograms of conventional solvent extracts: (i) CPHE extract; (ii) CPFD extract; (iii) CPEE extract at a fixed concentration of 5 mg/ mL. CPHE: *C. papaya* leaf hexane extract; CPFD: *C. papaya* leaf juice freeze-dried extract; CPEE: *C. papaya* leaf ethanol extract; CPSC: *C. papaya* leaf scCO₂ extract; CPSCE: *C. papaya* leaf scCO₂ extract with 5% ethanol. (From Khor et al. 2021.)

Each contains ten microliters, and final concentrations ranging from 25 to 1,000 μg/mL and 25 to 200 μg/mL were added to a 96-well microtiter plate for the standard, followed by the addition of DPPH solution. The optical density of the solution was determined after 30 minutes of reaction in the dark measured at 517 nm (Brand-Williams et al. 1995).

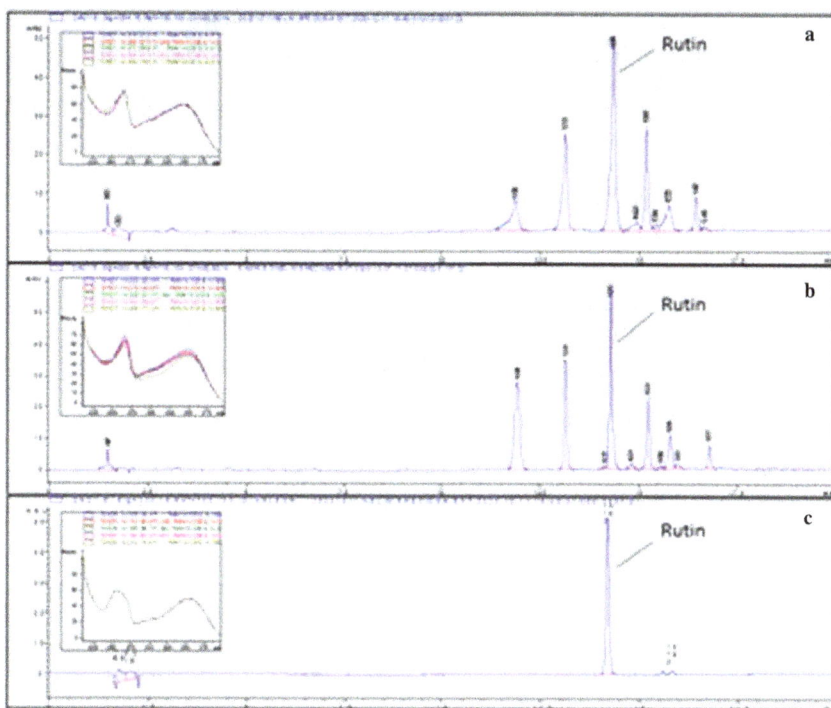

**Figure 7.2** HPLC chromatogram of (a) CPEE extract, (b) CPFD extract, and (c) the rutin standard at 14.2 minutes. (From Khor et al. 2021.)

### 7.7.3.2 Total Phenolic Content

The Folin–Ciocalteu method was used to evaluate the total phenolic content (TPC). In a 96-well flat bottom microplate, 20 L of 5 mg/mL CPEs in 25% (v/v) DMSO were mixed with 100 L of 1:4 diluted Folin–Ciocalteu reagent and vortex for 1 minute. After 2 minutes, 75 L of sodium carbonate solution (100 mg/mL) was added and the mixture was shaken at speed for 1 minute. After 2 hours, the absorbance was noted at 750 nm. The absorbance of the reaction mixture was performed with water instead of the extract and was subtracted from the absorbance of the reaction performed with CPE. As calibration standards, gallic acid (0.05–0.5 mg/mL) in 25% (v/v) DMSO were used. TPC was calculated as gallic acid equivalents (GAE) in milligrams per gram of CPE (mg GAE/g) (Chear et al. 2019; Khor et al. 2021).

### 7.7.3.3 Ferric-Reducing Antioxidant Power (FRAP)

The method of ferric-reducing antioxidant power (FRAP) of CPEs was measured as previously proposed. After 30 minutes, 280 L of freshly prepared FRAP reagent and 20 L of 1 mg/mL CPE in 5% DMSO were added to each well, and the absorbance was measured at = 593 nm. Fresh FRAP reagent was made by a combining sodium acetate buffer (300 mM, pH 3.6), a solution of TPTZ (10 mM) in 40 mM HCl, and 20 mM $FeCl_3.6H_2O$ in the ratio 10:1:1 (v/v/v).

Quantification of ferric-reducing antioxidant power of the extracts was used by plotting an analytical curve with varied concentrations of ascorbic acid (0.01–0.1 mg/mL). The results were mentioned in milligrams of ascorbic acid equivalents per g of CPE (mg AAE/g) (Bobo-García et al. 2015; Khor et al. 2021).

## 7.8 EXTRACTION METHOD AND ISOLATION METHODS

Papaya trees grown in a local fruit farm of Muar, Johor, Malaysia yielded 10 kg of fresh mature *C. papaya* leaves. To remove contaminants, the obtained leaves were rinsed with tap water. The material of the leaf was then divided into two parts: (a) Air-dried leaves were used for hexane (CPHE), ethanol (CPEE), and supercritical fluids (CPSC and CPSCE) extraction; and (b) Fresh leaves were used for leaf juice (CPFD) extraction. Prior to extraction procedures, the air-dried leaf material was kept in an airtight container and stored at 20°C (Boon et al. 2021).

### 7.8.1 Supercritical Fluid Extraction

The extraction of $scCO_2$ from air-dried CPL was carried out using Supercritical Fluid Preparative scale $CO_2$ extraction equipment (Taiwan Supercritical Technology) and extraction parameters. The $scCO_2$ extraction was carried out under the following conditions: Pressure 250 bar, temperature 35°C, extraction time of 3 h, and with or without 5% ethanol as a cosolvent. Extracts were stored at 20°C. CPSC and CPSCE extraction yields were 1.12% and 1.54%, respectively (Khaw et al. 2019). Figure 7.3. shows the extraction methods of bioactive components in Papaya.

#### 7.8.1.1 Maceration

In this process, 2 kg of air-dried CPL were extracted with hexane and ethanol, respectively, using the previously described procedures. All extracts were stored in a 20°C freezer until further analysis. Hexane and ethanol extraction yields were calculated approximately 5.2% and 15.6%, respectively (Khaw et al. 2020).

#### 7.8.1.2 Leaf Juice Extraction

In this process, 2 kg of fresh CPL were mixed with a juice extractor. The collected leaf juice was then filtered and freeze-dried to create the lyophilized leaf juice extract (CPFD). CPFD was stored at 20°C and the obtained extraction yield was about 14% (Boon et al. 2021).

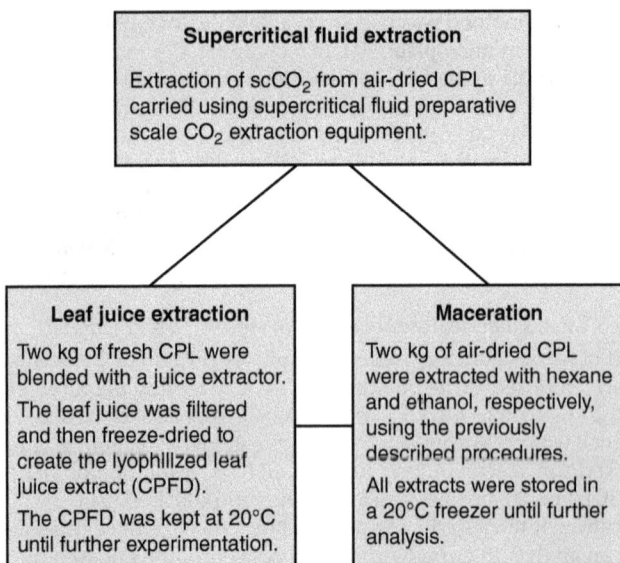

**Figure 7.3** Extraction methods of bioactive components in papaya.

## 7.9 APPLICATION OF THE ACTIVE INGREDIENTS

Papaya fruit contains valued ingredients that vary in different portions of the plant, such as fruits, leaves, and seeds. It contains saponins, cardiac glycosides, and alkaloids. A previous study confirmed the presence of phenolic acids in the leaves of C. papaya. It also contains chlorogenic acid in trace amounts. The ripe fruit is a rich source of vitamins A and C, flavonoids and coumarin compounds, and a variety of other minerals. The pawpaw is a rich source of vitamin C having varying amounts depending on maturity. The constituents of red-fleshed papaya and yellow-fleshed papaya differ markedly. According to a previous study, in red-fleshed papaya the total lycopene content was significantly higher than that of yellow-fleshed fruit. The seeds of papaya contain a variety of ingredients that play an important role in the treatment and prevention of disease. Previous literature stated that the seed is a good source of proteins, crude fiber, and lipids, as well as significant amounts of calcium and phosphorus; moreover, it also contains toxicants, such as glucosinolates (Rahmani and Aldebasi 2016).

## 7.10 HEALTH BENEFITS OF PAPAYA BIOACTIVE COMPOUNDS

Papaya plant parts have been traditionally utilized as a cure for different diseases due to their photochemical composition. Table 7.2 lists the therapeutic role of different parts of the papaya plant. Apart from diseases like diabetes, hypertension, malaria, dengue, and hypercholesterolemia, it is also now being explored for its anticancer potential (Kushwaha et al. 2021).

### Table 7.2: The Therapeutic Role of Different Parts of Papaya Plant

| Plant Part | Therapeutic Role | Bioactive Compound | Reference |
|---|---|---|---|
| Seeds | Liver disease | Phenolics, flavonoids, tannins, vitamin C, and triterpenoids | Nagarathna et al. (2021) |
| Stem straw | Antioxidant property | Hydrogen peroxide | Sivasankari et al. (2019) |
| Leaves | Cancer | Di-methyl flubendazole | Devanesan et al. (2021) |
| Leaves | Infectious diseases | Vitamin C, saponins, cystatin, and flavonoids | Alagendran et al. (2019) |
| Leaves | Antimicrobial | Saponins, flavonoids, alkaloids, and tannins | Attah et al. (2021) |
| Seeds | Antioxidant and antidiabetic | Hexadecanoic acid, methyl ester, 11-octadecenoic acid, methyl ester, n-hexadecanoic acid, oleochemicals-acid, and N,N-dimethyl | Reuben et al. (2021) |
| Leaves | Prostatic disease | Flavonoids, saponins, glycosides, alkaloids, and phenolics | Jin et al. (2020) |
| Unripe papaya | Cell death | Antioxidant compounds such as calcium, phosphate, and other bioactive agents | Oyebode et al. (2021) |
| Seeds | Antidepression | 9-Octadecenoic acid (Z)-methyl ester, hexadecanoic acid-methyl ester, and benzyl nitrile | Ardila et al. (2021) |
| Seeds | Prevention of nephrotoxicity and oxidative stress | 17-Octadecynoic acid, hexadecanoic acid methyl ester, 1,2-benzenedicarboxylic acid butyl 2-ethylhexyl ester | Kanadi et al. (2019) |

Papaya leaves presented a potent anti-angiogenic nature due to its constituents (lycopene, riboflavin, ascorbic acid, and quercetin) which showed docking interaction with VEGFR1 and VEGFR2 in one experimental study (Dotto and Abihudi 2021). The peel of the papaya is also a good source of bioactive compounds (carbohydrates, proteins, tannins, minerals, and vitamin A), which are otherwise mainly discarded, and are used in the cosmetic pharmaceutical industry for restoring/rebuilding damaged skin (Hall et al. 2018). Papaya seeds, being an unpalatable part of the fruit, are known for their antioxidant properties due to the presence of saponins, flavonoids, minerals, and alkaloids. In vitro antioxidant assays consisting of papaya seed extracts of hexane and ethyl acetate rich in saponins showed their inhibitory activity on α-amylase and glycosidase enzymes to reduce postprandial hyperglycemia in rat models (Islam et al. 2019). Various therapeutic drugs derived from plants such as berberine (*Berberis vulgaris*), bromelain (pineapple), taxol (Pacific yew), and papain (papaya) are widely used in different diseases due to the presence of effective compounds in their extracts producing responses against different biological pathways.

## 7.11 PHARMACOLOGICAL APPLICATIONS OF PLANTS
### 7.11.1 Anti-Inflammatory Activity

Plant cysteine proteinases have been shown in the literature to have anti-inflammatory properties. In a clinical study, the histological severity of inflammatory bowel disease was evaluated, and papain was found to be harmless and helpful for the treatment of chronic inflammatory and related diseases. Papaya seeds have also been revealed to have anti-inflammatory properties. When using the carrageenan method, the anti-inflammatory ability of the leaf extract including the reference drug was very poor. After carrageenan injection, the 100 mg/kg extract produced its maximum effect at 3 hours (2.7%), while the 200 mg/kg extract produced its effects at 3 hours (6.7%). After carrageenan administration, the indomethacin, which is a reference drug, caused a time-dependent reduction, with the effect being more pronounced at 3 hours (11.4%) (Salas et al. 2008; Amazu et al. 2010; Adedapo & Orherhe 2013; Dotto and Abihudi 2021).

### 7.11.2 Gastroprotective Activity

The leading causes of gastric ulcers and complications include numerous agents such as food ingredients, microorganisms, and drugs. Plant products have anti-ulcer properties, but the exact method is unknown. The anti-ulcerogenic activities of *C. papaya* extract on aspirin-induced ulcers in rats were determined, and the results indicated that *C. papaya* may exert its gastroprotective effect via free radical scavenging. A study was conducted to estimate the gastrointestinal effects of aqueous *C. papaya* seed extract on ethanol-induced gastric ulcers in male rats. The outcome revealed that the extract protected the gastric mucosa from the ethanol effect and extensively reduced gastric juice volume and acidity in a dose-dependent manner when compared to the control (Ologundudu et al. 2008; Okewumi and Oyeyemi 2012; Nagarathna et al. 2021).

### 7.11.3 Hepatoprotective Activity

Previous literature evaluated the hepatoprotective effects of *C. papaya* and vitamin E against carbon tetrachloride (CCL 4) which induces hepatotoxicity. The results confirmed that *C. papaya* and vitamin E provided important hepatoprotection against CCl4. Additional results confirmed that pretreatment with medium and maximum doses of *C. papaya* caused hepatotoxicity, but

*C. papaya* caused more significant changes in ALP levels than vitamin E. Another important study was conducted to investigate the antihepatotoxic activity of ethanol and aqueous extracts of *C. papaya*, and the results confirmed that ethanol and aqueous extracts of *C. papaya* demonstrated significant hepatoprotective activity against $CCl_4$-induced hepatotoxicity (Rajkapoor et al. 2002, Kantham 2009; Sadeque et al. 2012; Pandit et al. 2013; Dotto and Abihudi 2021)

### 7.11.4 Wound-Healing Activity

The main constituent of papaya latex is papain, a nonspecific cysteine proteinase capable of degrading a wide range of necrotic tissue substrates over a pH range of 3.0 to 12.0. This factor may have also contributed to faster wound healing, which was aided by the action of proteinases. Papain has antibacterial and antioxidant qualities connected to hydroxyl scavenging and iron chelating properties, as well as the ability to dislough necrotic tissue, prevent infection, and have antimicrobial and antioxidant activities associated to hydroxyl scavenging and iron chelating properties. They also show burn healing effects and minimize the risk of oxidative damage to tissue (Mahmood et al. 2005; Nayak et al. 2007; Tiwari et al. 2011; Dotto and Abihudi 2021; Nagarathna et al. 2021).

### 7.11.5 Anti-Fertility Activity

The anti-fertility properties of *C. papaya* were evaluated by providing different components of the fruit to adult and pregnant rats. Studies showed that the unripe fruit disrupted the estrous cycle and caused abortion. This outcome was overcome as the fruit grew stale or overripe. The chloroform extract of *C. papaya* seeds caused long-term azoospermia in langur monkeys. Papaya also has anti-implantation and abortifacient properties (Dosumu et al. 2008; Lakshman and Changamma 2013; Dotto and Abihudi 2021; Nagarathna et al. 2021).

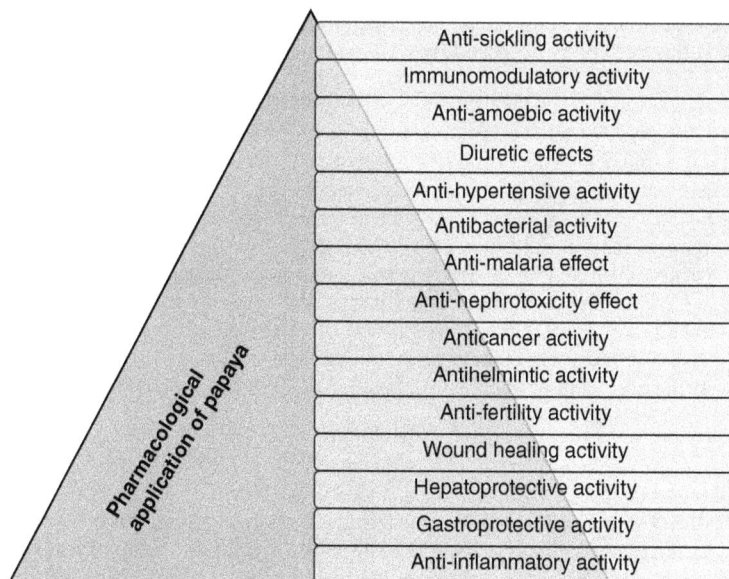

**Figure 7.4** Pharmacological applications of the plant.

### 7.11.6 Anthelmintic Activity

Papaya plants and its products have been used traditionally to treat infections caused by helminths. The presence of proteolytic enzymes in the papaya aids in the digestion of cuticles of nematodes. Moreover, the plant has also been used against nematodes in the gastrointestinal tract. In addition, *C. papaya* latex also digests the cuticle of ascari (Stepek et al. 2004; Dotto and Abihudi 2021; Nagarathna et al. 2021).

### 7.11.7 Anticancer Activity

Pharmaceutical formulations comprising various proteolytic enzymes (papain) were initially utilized as adjuvants in the treatment of malignant disorders despite a lack of understanding of their method of action. Experiments reveal that the activation of cytokine production by human peripheral blood mononuclear cells is related to the effects of polyenzyme preparations after oral administration. Papaya has been shown to be able to treat a variety of cancer cell lines in vitro. The papaya enzyme papain has anticancer properties. Papain breaks down fibrin and proteins in cancer cells into amino acids. It also includes lycopene, which is extremely reactive to oxygen and free radicals, in addition to papain. Breast, lung, colon, pancreas, prostate, and leukemia malignancies are all treated with isothiocyanate. These enzymes have the ability to stop both cancer cell development and growth (Rahmani et al. 2014; Dotto and Abihudi 2021; Nagarathna et al. 2021).

Plant ingredients or products serve a therapeutic role in the prevention and treatment of cancer. Papaya and its essential elements play a key function in cancer management in this regard. A significant study looked at the result of aqueous-extracted *C. papaya* leaf fraction on the development of various tumor cell lines and the antitumor effect of human lymphocytes, and the results revealed that the CP extract had growth inhibitory action on tumor cell lines derived from cervical carcinoma (Hela), breast adenocarcinoma (MCF-7), hepatocellular carcinoma (HepG2), lung adenocarcinoma (PC14), and pancreatic malignancies. In addition, T-cell lymphoma (Jurkat), plasma cell leukemia (ARH77), Burkitt's lymphoma a (Raji), and anaplastic large cell lymphoma (Raji) were all shown to be suppressed by CP extract (Karpas-299) (Otsuki et al. 2010).

### 7.11.8 Anti-Nephrotoxicity Effect

Experiments were conducted to determine the nephroprotective role of ethanolic extracts of papaya seed and pumpkin seed, and the results confirmed that ethanolic extracts of both types of seeds protected against cisplatin-induced nephrotoxicity, and antioxidant studies such as nitric oxide scavenging activity and lipid peroxidation in kidney also supported the nephroprotective activity of both types of seeds. The results of a study to assess the protective effect of *C. papaya* L. aqueous seed extract on gentamicin-induced hepatotoxicity and nephrotoxicity revealed that administration of aqueous extract prior to gentamicin exposure prevented severe biochemical changes as well as disruptions in liver and kidney structure (Debnath et al. 2010; Nale et al. 2012; Madinah et al. 2015).

### 7.11.9 Anti-Malaria Effect

Malaria is one of the world's most dangerous diseases. However, in order to control malaria and its complications, a safe and effective treatment method is essential. In this vista, numerous medicinal plants have confirmed their role in malaria control. According to the finding, concentrations of ethanol leaf extracts of 25, 50, 100, and 150 g/mL showed potential inhibitory efficacy against the CQ-sensitive strain with IC 50 values of 40.75%, 36.54%, 25.30%, and 18.0% and against the CQ-resistant strain with IC 50 values of 50.23%, 32.50%, 21.45%, and

23.12% against *P. falciparum* (Dawkins et al. 2003; Akujobi et al. 2010; Orhue and Momoh 2013; Nagarathna et al. 2021).

### 7.11.10 Antibacterial Activity

Bacteriostatic activity was discovered in the seeds of *C. papaya* against *Bacillus subtilis, Enterobacter cloacae, Escherichia coli, Salmonella typhi, Staphylococcus, Proteas vulgaris, Pseudomonas aeruginosa,* and *Klebsiella pneumonia*. The extract was more efficient against the gram-negative bacteria when compared to the gram-positive bacteria (Leite et al. 2005; Nagarathna et al. 2021).

### 7.11.11 Antihypertensive Activity

A papaya leaf decoction can be utilized as an antihypertensive medication. In a study on Agboville villagers, located 80 kilometers from Abidjan (West Africa), the papaya plant showed hypotensive effects when fed orally (Koffi et al. 2009; Nagarathna et al. 2021).

### 7.11.12 Diuretic Effects

According to previous findings, when *C. papaya* root extracts were administered orally to rats at a dose of 10 mg/kg, they showed considerably enhanced urine production, which was 74% of the effect of an equivalent dose of hydrochlorothiazide (Sripanidkulchai et al. 2001; Nagarathna et al. 2021).

### 7.11.13 Anti-Amoebic Activity

A cold macerated aqueous extract of matured papaya seeds has also been shown to have anti-amoebic activity against *Entamoeba histolytica* (Lohiya et al. 2002; Nagarathna et al. 2021).

### 7.11.14 Immunomodulatory Activity

Human eosinophils are stimulated to degranulate and produce a superoxide anion when exposed to papain. The E-64 inhibitors prevented papain activation, implying that protease activity is required to initiate the eosinophil response. A protein G linked receptor most likely regulates this action in eosinophils (Mojica-Henshaw et al. 2003; Nagarathna et al. 2021).

### 7.11.15 Anti-Sickling Activity

Sickle cell disease (SCD) is caused by a mutation in hemoglobin within red blood cells, in which a glutamic acid at position 6 is replaced by valine. The extract of unripe papaya fruit contains anti-sickling properties. According to another study, *C. papaya* leaf extract possesses potent anti-sickling activities that are dose-dependent. The aqueous root extract of papaya, when administered orally to rats at a dose of 10 mg/kg, causes a significant increase in urine production and has urinary electrolyte excretion profiles comparable to hydrochlorothiazide (Oduola et al. 2006; Wright et al. 2007; Imaga et al. 2009; Nagarathna et al. 2021).

### 7.11.16 Hypoglycemic and Hypolipidemic Activity

The study reported that oral treatment with 0.1 mg/kg/day glibenclamide and 100–400 mg/kg/day *C. papaya* aqueous seed extract induced important, balanced, and progressive hypoglycemic and hypolipidemic results (Indran et al. 2008; Khor and Wong 2014).

## 7.12 CLINICAL TRIALS

Bioactive compounds in *C. papaya* explored for their medicinal value treating diseases such as malaria, dengue, hypertension, constipation, hypercholesterolemia, and cancer gained the attention of researchers. At certain doses, different medicinal plants and their constituents help in the prevention and treatment of disease. High concentration dosing can cause complications and alter a variety of biological activities. The toxicity of CP leaf extracts on Sprague-Dawley rats was investigated in a study, and the results suggested that the leaf juice of *C. papaya* had no toxicity effect (Debnath et al. 2010). Another study was conducted on the acute and chronic oral toxicity of *C. papaya* aqueous and ethanol leaf extracts in Wistar rats, and the results showed that no deaths or signs of acute oral toxicity were recorded. Oral sub-acute and sub-chronic toxicity included hypoglycemia, hypolipidemia, and hyperglycemia, as well as increased AST and BUN in aqueous and ethanol extract experimentations, respectively (Halim et al. 2011; Tarkang et al. 2012). The first clinical trial (NCT03567798) in 2017 for management of thrombocytopenia in chemotherapeutic cancer patients showed the efficacy of papaya extract (Heung et al. 2021). Papain (proteolytic enzyme) from milky papaya latex is FDA approved for application in enzymatic debridement in burns, wounds, and ulcers. Various other valuable bioactive compounds isolated from different parts of *C. papaya* are under clinical studies for understanding their pharmacological effects (Adedapo & Orherhe 2013; Agada et al. 2020, 2021; Attah et al. 2021).

## 7.13 CONCLUSION
*C. papaya* is a nutraceutical plant with numerous pharmacological activities. The plant has numerous medicinal properties. It contains high concentrations of enzymes and vitamins. It is a rich source of phytochemicals such as vitamins, antioxidants, flavonoids, polyphenols, and several minerals, as well as some important enzymes such as papain, lycopene, isothiocyanate, and some proteolytic enzymes that help to treat health problems. As a result, regular consumption of papaya helps in improving the health by removing the free radicals in the body and enhancing the immune system against foreign pathogens. The current review covers classification of *C. papaya* and its notable pharmacological activity, medicinal properties, and biochemical constituents and extraction methods of bioactive compounds in the fruit.

## REFERENCES
Adedapo, A., & Orherhe, V. 2013. "Antinociceptive and anti-inflammatory studies of the aqueous leaf extract of *C. papaya* in laboratory animals." *Asian Journal of Experimental Biological Sciences* 4(1):89–96.

Agada, R., Thagriki, D., Lydia, D. E., Khusro, A., Alkahtani, J., Al Shaqha, M. M., Alwahibi, M. S., & Elshikh, M. S. 2021. "Antioxidant and antidiabetic activities of bioactive fractions of *Carica papaya* seeds extract." *Journal of King Saud University-Science* 33(2):101342.

Agada, R., Usman, W. A., Shehu, S., & Thagariki, D. 2020. "In vitro and in vivo inhibitory effects of *Carica papaya* seed on α-amylase and α-glucosidase enzymes." *Heliyon* 6(3):e03618.

Akujobi, C. N., Ofodeme, C. N., & Enweani, C. A. 2010. "Determination of antibacterial activity of *C. papaya* (pawpaw) extracts." *Nigerian Journal of Clinical Practice* 13(1):55–57.

Alagendran, S., Puspha, N., Valarmathi, M., Fernandez, G., Chitra, M., Sudha, P., Kiruthiga, D., & Jayakumar, D. 2019. "Spectrophotometric method of ascorbic acid in *Carica papaya* L. extracts: An in vitro study." *Journal of Pharmacognosy and Phytochemistry* 8(6): 119–123.

Amazu, L. U., Azikiwe, C. C. A., Njoku, C. J., Osuala, F. N., Nwosu, P. J. C., Ajugwo, A. O., & Enye, J. C. 2010. "Antiinflammatory activity of the methanolic extract of the seeds of C. papaya in experimental animals." *Asian Pacific Journal of Tropical Medicine* 3(11):884–886.

Annegowda, H. V., Bhat, R., Yeong, K. J., Liong, M. T., Karim, A. A., & Mansor, S. M. 2014. "Influence of drying treatments on polyphenolic contents and antioxidant properties of raw and ripe papaya (Carica papaya L.)." *International Journal of Food Properties* 17(2):283–292.

Anuar, N. S., Zahari, S. S., Taib, I. A., & Rahman, M. T. 2008. "Effect of green and ripe C. papaya epicarp extracts on wound healing and during pregnancy." *Food and Chemical Toxicology* 46(7):2384–2389.

Ardila, D., Nasution, A. N., Wardhani, F. M., & Ikhtiari, R. 2021. "Anti-depression potential of papaya seed extracts in Wistar rat models: A study on body weights, blood glucose, interleukin-6 and malondialdehyde levels with force swimming and tail suspension tests." *Jurnal Teknologi Laboratorium* 10(2): 101–111. https://doi.org/10.29238/teknolabjournal.v10i2.316

Attah, F., Moses, E., Abalaka, A. U., & Tayo, O. 2021. "In-vitro investigation on the therapeutic potential of *Carica papaya* leaf extract on some pathogenic bacteria." *South Asian Research Journal of Natural Products* 4(1):9–15.

Azarkan, M., El Moussaoui, A., Van Wuytswinkel, D., Dehon, G., & Looze, Y. 2003. "Fractionation and purification of the enzymes stored in the latex of *Carica papaya*." *Journal of Chromatography B* 790(1–2):229–238.

Badillo, V. M. 2000. "Vasconcella St.-Hil. (Caricaceae) con la rehabilitacion de este ultimo." *Ernstia* 10(2):74–79.

Behera, S. K., Rath, A. K., & Sethy, P. K. 2021. "Maturity status classification of papaya fruits based on machine learning and transfer learning approach." *Information Processing in Agriculture* 8(2):244–250.

Bobo-García, G., Davidov-Pardo, G., Arroqui, C., Vírseda, P., Marín-Arroyo, M. R., & Navarro, M. 2015. "Intra-laboratory validation of microplate methods for total phenolic content and antioxidant activity on polyphenolic extracts, and comparison with conventional spectrophotometric methods." *Journal of the Science of Food and Agriculture* 95(1):204–209.

Brand-Williams, W., Cuvelier, M. E., & Berset, C. L. W. T. 1995. "Use of a free radical method to evaluate antioxidant activity." *LWT – Food Science and Technology* 28(1):25–30.

Chear, N. J. Y., Fauzi, A. N., Khaw, K. Y., Choi, S. B., Yaacob, N. S., & Lai, C. S. 2019. "Free radical scavenging and cytotoxic properties of acylated and non-acylated kaempferol glycosides from *Stenochlaena palustris*: A perspective on their structure–activity relationships." *Pharmaceutical Chemistry Journal* 53(3):188–193.

Chear, N. J. Y., Khaw, K. Y., Murugaiyah, V., & Lai, C. S. 2016. "Cholinesterase inhibitory activity and chemical constituents of *Stenochlaena palustris* fronds at two different stages of maturity." *Journal of Food and Drug Analysis* 24(2):358–366.

Dawkins, G., Hewitt, H., Wint, Y., Obiefuna, P. C., & Wint, B. 2003. "Antibacterial effects of C. papaya fruit on common wound organisms." West Indian Medical Journal 52(4):290–292.

Debnath, S., Babre, N., Manjunath, Y. S., Mallareddy, V., Parameshwar, P., & Hariprasath, K. 2010. "Nephroprotective evaluation of ethanolic extract of the seeds of papaya and pumpkin fruit in cisplatin-induced nephrotoxicity." Journal of Pharmaceutical Science and Technology 2(6):241–246.

Devanesan, S., Jayamala, M., AlSalhi, M. S., Umamaheshwari, S., & Ranjitsingh, A. J. 2021. "Antimicrobial and Anticancer properties of Carica papaya leaves derived di-methyl flubendazole mediated silver nanoparticles." Journal of Infection and Public Health 14(5):577–587.

Dosumu, O. O., Akinola, O. B., Oremosu, A. A., Noronha, C. C., & Okanlawon, A. O. 2008. "Antifertility effects of the aqueous extract of C. papaya (Linn.) seeds on estrous cycle and ovulation of adult cyclic Sprague-Dawley rats." Nigerian Journal of Health and Biomedical Sciences 7(2):31–33.

Dotto, J. M., & Abihudi, S. A. 2021. "Nutraceutical value of Carica papaya: A review." Scientific African 13:e00933.

Fernandes, F. A., Rodrigues, S., Gaspareto, O. C., & Oliveira, E. L. 2006. "Optimization of osmotic dehydration of papaya followed by air-drying." Food Research International 39(4): 492–498.

Fernandez, G., Chitra, M., Sudha, P., Kiruthiga, D., & Jayakumar, D. 2019. "Spectrophotometric method of Ascorbic acid in Carica papaya L. extracts: An in vitro study." Journal of Pharmacognosy and Phytochemistry 8(6):119–123.

Halim, S. Z., Abdullah, N. R., Afzan, A., Rashid, B. A., Jantan, I., & Ismail, Z. 2011. "Acute toxicity study of C. papaya leaf extract in Sprague Dawley rats." Journal of Medicinal Plants Research 5(10):1867–1872.

Hall, R. M., Mayer, D. A., Mazzutti, S., & Ferreira, S. R. 2018. "Simulating large scale SFE applied to recover bioactive compounds from papaya seeds." Journal of Supercritical Fluids 140:302–309.

Heung, T. Y., Huong, J. Y., Chen, W. Y., Loh, Y. W., Khaw, K. Y., Goh, B. H., & Ong, Y. S. 2021. "Anticancer potential of Carica papaya through modulation of cancer hallmarks." Food Reviews International 6:1–9.

Imaga, N. O. A., Gbenle, G. O., Okochi, V. I., Akanbi, S. O., Edeoghon, S. O., Oigbochie, V., & Bamiro, S. B. 2009. "Antisickling property of C. papaya leaf extract." African Journal of Biochemistry Research 3(4):102–106.

Indran, M., Mahmood, A. A., & Kuppusamy, U. R. 2008. "Protective effect of C. papaya L leaf extract against alcohol induced acute gastric damage and blood oxidative stress in rats." West Indian Medical Journal 57(4):323–326.

Islam, M. Z., Saha, T., Monalisa, K., & Hoque, M. M. 2019. "Effect of starch edible coating on drying characteristics and antioxidant properties of papaya." Journal of Food Measurement and Characterization 13(4):2951–2960.

Jaiswal, P., Kumar, P., Singh, V. K., & Singh, D. K. 2010. "*C. papaya* Linn: A potential source for various health problems." *Journal of Pharmacy Research* 3(5):998–1003.

Jin, B. R., Ju, J. Y., Nugroho, A., Lee, M., & An, H. J. 2021. *Carica papaya* leaf extract inhibits prostatitis-associated prostatic hyperplasia via the TRAF6/TAK1/MEK/NF-κB pathway. Biomedicine & Pharmacotherapy, 135, 111197.

Kaliyaperumal, K., Kim, H. M., Jegajeevanram, K., Xavier, J., & Vijayalakshmi, J. 2014. "Papaya: A gifted nutraceutical plant—A critical review of recent human health research." *Tang Humanitas Medicine* 4(1):1–17.

Kanadi, M. A., Abdullahi, A. I., Idi, A., Muhammad, I. U., Mohammed, A., & Wudil, A. M. 2019. "Bioassay-guided fractionation of *Carica papaya* seed extracts against potassium bromate-induced nephrotoxicity detected fatty acid-rich compounds and prevents oxidative stress in rat's kidney." *International Journal of Advances in Nephrology Research* 2(1): 1–12.

Kantham, S. 2009. "Influence of *C. papaya* Linn extracts on paracetamol and thioacetamide induced hepatic damage in rats." *The Internet Journal of Pharmacology* 9(1):1–6.

Khaw, K. Y., Parat, M. O., Shaw, P. N., Nguyen, T. T., Pandey, S., Thurecht, K. J., & Falconer, J. R. 2019. "Factorial design-assisted supercritical carbon-dioxide extraction of cytotoxic active principles from *C. papaya* leaf juice." *Scientific Reports* 9(1):1–12.

Khaw, K. Y., Shaw, P. N., Parat, M. O., Pandey, S., & Falconer, J. R. 2020. "Compound identification and in vitro cytotoxicity of the supercritical carbon dioxide extract of papaya freeze-dried leaf juice." *Processes* 8(5):610.

Khor, B. K., Chear, N. J. Y., Azizi, J., & Khaw, K. Y. 2021. "Chemical composition, antioxidant and cytoprotective potentials of *C. papaya* leaf extracts: A comparison of supercritical fluid and conventional extraction methods." *Molecules* 26(5):1489.

Khor, E. S., & Wong, N. K. 2014. "Potential antioxidant and cytotoxic properties of secondary metabolite extracts from *C. papaya* fruits and seeds." *International Journal of Pharmacy and Pharmaceutical Sciences* 6(7):220–224.

Koffi, N., Solange, T. M., Emma, A. A., & Noel, Z. G. 2009. "Ethanobotanical study of plants used to treat arterial hypertension, in traditional medicine." *European Journal of Scientific Research* 1(1): 1–10.

Kushwaha, K., Saini, S. S., Waghmode, B., Gaid, M., Agrawal, P. K., Roy, P., & Sircar, D. 2021 "Volatile components in papaya fruits are the non-invasive biomarkers to monitor the ripening stage and the nutritional value." *European Food Research and Technology* 247(4):907–919.

Lakshman, J., & Changamma, C. 2013. "Antispermatogenic effect of *C. papaya* seed extract on steroidogenesis in albino rats." *International Journal of Pharmacy and Pharmaceutical Sciences* 5(1): 67–69.

Leite, A. A., Nardi, R. M., Nicoli, J. R., Chartone-Souza, E., & Nascimento, A. M. 2005. "*C. papaya* seed macerate as inhibitor of conjugative R plasmid transfer from *Salmonella typhimurium* to *Escherichia coli* in vitro and in the digestive tract of gnotobiotic mice." *Journal of General and Applied Microbiology* 51(1):21–26.

Lohiya, N. K., Manivannan, B., Mishra, P. K., Pathak, N., Sriram, S., Bhande, S. S., & Panneerdoss, S. 2002. "Chloroform extract of *C. papaya* seeds induces long-term reversible azoospermia in langur monkey." *Asian Journal of Andrology* 4(1):17–26.

Madinah, N., Nozmo, M., & Ezekiel, I. 2015. "The protective effects of aqueous extract of *C. papaya* seeds in paracetamol induced nephrotoxicity in male Wistar rats." *African Health Sciences* 15(2):598–605.

Mahmood, A. A., Sidik, K., & Salmah, I. 2005. "Wound healing activity of *C. papaya* L. aqueous leaf extract in rats." *International Journal of Molecular Medicine and Advance Sciences* 1(4):398–401.

Manshardt, R. M., & Wenslaff, T. F. 1989. "Interspecific hybridization of papaya with other *Carica* species." *Journal of the American Society for Horticultural Science (USA)* 114:689–694.

Menard, R., Khouri, H. E., Plouffe, C., Dupras, R., Ripoll, D., Vernet, T., & Storer, A. C. 1990. "A protein engineering study of the role of aspartate 158 in the catalytic mechanism of papain." *Biochemistry* 29(28):6706–6713.

Mojica-Henshaw, M. P., Francisco, A. D., De Guzman, F., & Tigno, X. T. 2003. "Possible immunomodulatory actions of *C. papaya* seed extract." *Clinical Hemorheology and Microcirculation* 29(3–4):219–229.

Morales, A., Medina, D., & Yaguachi, B. 2004. "Diversidad genética, filogenética y distribución geográfica del género *Vasconcellea* en Sur de Ecuador." *Lyonia* 7(2):15–27.

Nagarathna, S. B., Jain, S. K., Arun, H. R., Champawat, P. S., Mogra, R., & Maherchandani, J. K. 2021. "An overview of papaya: Phytochemical constituents and its therapeutic applications." *Pharma Innovation Journal* 10(9): 45–49.

Nale, L. P., More, P. R., More, B. K., Ghumare, B. C., Shendre, S. B., & Mote, C. S. 2012. "Protective effect of *C. papaya* L. seed extract in gentamicin induced hepatotoxicity and nephrotoxicity in rats." *International Journal of Pharmacy and Biological Sciences* 3(3):508–515.

Nayak, B. S., Pereira, L. P., & Maharaj, D. 2007. "Wound healing activity of *C. papaya* L. in experimentally induced diabetic rats." *Indian Journal of Experimental Biology* 45:739–743.

Oche, O., John, O., Chidi, E., Rebecca, S. M., & Vincent, U. A. 2017. "Chemical constituents and nutrient composition of *C. papaya* and *Vernonia amygdalina* leaf extracts." *Journal of Complementary and Alternative Medical Research* 2(1):5.

Oduola, T., Adeniyi, F. A. A., Ogunyemi, E. O., Bello, I. S., & Idowu, T. O. 2006. "Antisickling agent in an extract of unripe pawpaw (*Carica papaya*): Is it real?" *African Journal of Biotechnology* 5(20):1947–1949.

Okewumi, T. A., & Oyeyemi, A. W. 2012. "Gastro-protective activity of aqueous *C. papaya* seed extract on ethanol induced gastric ulcer in male rats." *African Journal of Biotechnology* 11(34):8612–8615.

Olmoss, A. 2012. "Papain, a plant enzyme of biological importance: A review." *American Journal of Biochemistry and Biotechnology* 8(2):99–104.

Ologundudu, A., Lawal, A. O., Ololade, I. A., Omonkhua, A. A., & Obi, F. O. 2008. "The anti-ulcerogenic activity of aqueous extract of *C. papaya* fruit on aspirin-induced ulcer in rats." *International Journal of Toxicology* 5(2).

Olson, M. E. 2002. "Intergeneric relationships within the Caricaceae-Moringaceae clade (Brassicales) and potential morphological synapomorphies of the clade and its families." *International Journal of Plant Sciences* 163(1):51–65.

Orhue, P. O., & Momoh, A. R. M. 2013. "Antibacterial activities of different solvent extracts of *C. papaya* fruit parts on some gram positive and gram negative organisms." *International Journal of Herbs and Pharmacological Research* 2(4):42–47.

Otsuki, N., Dang, N. H., Kumagai, E., Kondo, A., Iwata, S., & Morimoto, C. 2010. "Aqueous extract of *C. papaya* leaves exhibits antitumor activity and immunomodulatory effects." *Journal of Ethnopharmacology* 127(3):760–767.

Oyebode, O. T., Olowofolahan, A. O., & Olorunsogo, O. O. 2021. "Toxic effects of unripe *Carica papaya* (Linn) fruit extract on healthy rat liver mitochondria." *Traditional and Integrative Medicine* 6(2).

Pandit, A., Sachdeva, T., & Bafna, P. 2013. "Ameliorative effect of leaves of *C. papaya* in ethanol and antitubercular drug induced hepatotoxicity." *British Journal of Pharmaceutical Research* 3:648–661.

Pathak, P. D., Mandavgane, S. A., & Kulkarni, B. D. 2019. "Waste to wealth: A case study of papaya peel." *Waste and Biomass Valorization* 10(6):1755–1766.

Patil, B. L., Narayan, K. S., & Gopalkrishna, A. M. 2021. "Diversity profiling of seed associated endophytic microbiome in important species of Caricaceae family." *Microbiology Research* 12(4):779–792.

Rahmani, A. H., & Aldebasi, Y. H. 2016. "Potential role of *C. papaya* and their active constituents in the prevention and treatment of diseases." *International Journal of Pharmacy and Pharmaceutical Sciences* 8(1):11–15.

Rahmani, A. H., Aly, S. M., Ali, H., Babiker, A. Y., & Srikar, S. 2014. "Therapeutic effects of date fruits (*Phoenix dactylifera*) in the prevention of diseases via modulation of anti-inflammatory, antioxidant and antitumour activity." *International Journal of Clinical and Experimental Medicine* 7(3):483.

Rajkapoor, B., Jayakar, B., Kavimani, S., & Murugesh, N. 2002. "Effect of dried fruits of *C. papaya* LINN on hepatotoxicity." *Biological and Pharmaceutical Bulletin* 25(12):1645–1646.

Rinnerthaler, M., Bischof, J., Streubel, M. K., Trost, A., & Richter, K. 2015. "Oxidative stress in aging human skin." *Biomolecules* 5(2):545–589.

Rivera-Pastrana, D. M., Gardea, A. A., Yahia, E. M., Martínez-Téllez, M. A., & González-Aguilar, G. A. 2014. "Effect of UV-C irradiation and low temperature storage on bioactive compounds, antioxidant enzymes and radical scavenging activity of papaya fruit." *Journal of Food Science and Technology* 51(12):3821–3829.

Sadeque, M. Z., Begum, Z. A., Umar, B. U., Ferdous, A. H., Sultana, S., & Uddin, M. K. 2012. "Comparative efficacy of dried fruits of *C. papaya* Linn. and vitamin-E on preventing hepatotoxicity in rats." *Faridpur Medical College Journal* 7(1):29–32.

Saeed, F., Arshad, M. U., Pasha, I., Naz, R., Batool, R., Khan, A. A., Nasir, M. A., & Shafique, B. 2014. "Nutritional and phyto-therapeutic potential of papaya (*Carica papaya* Linn.): An overview." *International Journal of Food Properties* 17(7):1637–1653.

Salas, C. E., Gomes, M. T., Hernandez, M., & Lopes, M. T. 2008. "Plant cysteine proteinases: Evaluation of the pharmacological activity." *Phytochemistry* 69(12):2263–2269.

Santana, L. F., Inada, A. C., Espirito Santo, B. L., Filiú, W. F., Pott, A., Alves, F. M., Guimarães, R. D., Freitas, K. D., & Hiane, P. A. 2019. "Nutraceutical potential of *Carica papaya* in metabolic syndrome." *Nutrients* 11(7):1608.

Scheldeman, X., Van Damme, P., & Romero Motoche, J. 2002. "Highland papayas in southern Ecuador: Need for conservation actions." In *International Symposium on Tropical and Subtropical Fruits. International Society for Horticultural Science (ISHS)* 575:199–205

Shaban, N. Z., El-Kot, S. M., Awad, O. M., Hafez, A. M., & Fouad, G. M. 2021. "The antioxidant and anti-inflammatory effects of *Carica papaya* Linn. seeds extract on CCl4-induced liver injury in male rats." *BMC Complementary Medicine and Therapies* 21(1):1–5.

Siriamornpun, S., Ratseewo, J., Kaewseejan, N., & Meeso, N. 2015. "Effect of osmotic treatments and drying methods on bioactive compounds in papaya and tomato." *RSC Advances.* 5(24):18579–18587.

Sivasankari M., Poongothai A., Sudha M., Saranraj P., & Amala K. 2019. "Antioxidant properties of papayasayanam extract of *Carica papaya* stem straw." *Journal of Drug Delivery and Therapeutics* 9(4):123–125.

Sripanidkulchai, B., Wongpanich, V., Laupattarakasem, P., Suwansaksri, J., & Jirakulsomchok, D. 2001. "Diuretic effects of selected Thai indigenous medicinal plants in rats." *Journal of Ethnopharmacology* 75(2–3):185–190.

Stepek, G., Behnke, J. M., Buttle, D. J., & Duce, I. R. 2004. "Natural plant cysteine proteinases as anthelmintics?." *Trends in Parasitology* 20(7):322–327.

Storey, W. B. 2019. "*Carica papaya.*" In *CRC Handbook of Flowering*, pp. 147–157. CRC Press.

Tarkang, P., Agbor, G., Armelle, T., Tchokouaha, L. R., David, K., & Ngadena, Y. 2012. "Acute and chronic toxicity studies of the aqueous and ethanol leaf extracts of *Carica papaya* Linn in Wistar rats. *Journal of Natural Product and Plant Resources* 2:617–627.

Thomás, G. E., Rodolfo, H. G., Juan, M. D., Georgina, S. F., Luis, C. G., Ingrid, R. B., & Santiago, G. T. 2009. "Proteolytic activity in enzymatic extracts from *C. papaya* L. cv. Maradol harvest by-products." *Process Biochemistry* 44(1):77–82.

Tiwari, P., Kumar, K., Panik, R., Pandey, A., Pandey, A., & Sahu, P. K. 2011. "Evaluation of aqueous extract of Roots of *C. papaya* on wound healing activity in albino Rats." *Journal of Chemical and Pharmaceutical Research* 3(4):291–295.

Udomkun, P., Nagle, M., Argyropoulos, D., Mahayothee, B., Latif, S., & Müller, J. 2016. "Compositional and functional dynamics of dried papaya as affected by storage time and packaging material." *Food Chemistry* 196:712–719.

Udomkun, P., Nagle, M., Mahayothee, B., Nohr, D., Koza, A., & Müller, J. 2015. "Influence of air drying properties on non-enzymatic browning, major bioactive compounds and antioxidant capacity of osmotically pretreated papaya." *LWT – Food Science and Technology* 60(2):914–922.

Ugo, N. J., Ade, A. R., & Joy, A. T. 2019. "Nutrient composition of *Carica papaya* leaves extracts." *Journal of Food Science and Nutrition Research* 2(3):274–282.

Van Droogenbroeck, B., Breyne, P., Goetghebeur, P., Romeijn-Peeters, E., Kyndt, T., & Gheysen, G. 2002. "AFLP analysis of genetic relationships among papaya and its wild relatives (Caricaceae) from Ecuador." *Theoretical and Applied Genetics* 105(2):289–297.

Van Droogenbroeck, B., Kyndt, T., Maertens, I., Romeijn-Peeters, E., Scheldeman, X., Romero-Motochi, J. P., & Gheysen, G. 2004. "Phylogenetic analysis of the highland papayas (*Vasconcellea*) and allied genera (Caricaceae) using PCR-RFLP." *Theoretical and Applied Genetics* 108(8):1473–1486.

Vega-Gálvez, A., Uribe, E., Pastén, A., Vega, M., Poblete, J., Bilbao-Sainz, C., & Chiou, B. S. 2022. "Low-temperature vacuum drying as novel process to improve papaya (*Vasconcellea pubescens*) nutritional-functional properties" *Future Foods* 100117.

Vij, T., & Prashar, Y. 2015. "A review on medicinal properties of *C. papaya* Linn." *Asian Pacific Journal of Tropical Disease* 5(1):1–6.

Villarreal, L., Dhuique-Mayer, C., Dornier, M., Ruales, J., & Reynes, M. 2003. "Évaluation de l'intérêt du babaco (*Carica pentagona* Heilb.)." *Fruits* 58(1):39–52.

Vuong, Q. V., Hirun, S., Chuen, T. L., Goldsmith, C. D., Murchie, S., Bowyer, M. C., Phillips, P. A., & Scarlett, C. J. 2015. "Antioxidant and anticancer capacity of saponin-enriched *Carica papaya* leaf extracts." *International Journal of Food Science & Technology* 50(1):169–177.

Watts, D. 1967. "Sauer, Carl Ortwin. The early Spanish main. Berkeley, university of california press, 306." *Cahiers de Géographie du Québec* 11(24):590–591.

Wright, C. I., Van-Buren, L., Kroner, C. I., & Koning, M. M. G. 2007. "Herbal medicines as diuretics: A review of the scientific evidence." *Journal of Ethnopharmacology* 114(1):1–31.

# 8 Watermelon

*Breetha Ramaiyan and Jasmeet Kour*

## CONTENTS

## 8.1 INTRODUCTION

Watermelon is one of the most common fruits and can be found abundantly around the globe for its juicy and peculiar taste (Paris 2015). It comes under the family Cucurbitaceae with the genus name of *Citrullus* and is botanically called pepo. Its biomass is categorized into three major components as flesh, rind, and skin. Watermelon is enjoyed primarily in tropical regions for its cooling and thirst-quenching properties (Ho et al. 2017). The shape of the fruit is majorly observed to be elongated and has a pale green to dark green exocarp. The scientific name of watermelon is traced from both Greek and Latin roots. The *Citrullus* part was derived from a Greek word "citrus" and the *lanatus* part is Latin, which translates as being wooly, mentioning the small hairs on the stems and leaves of the plant (Rahman 2013). The origin of this annual plant is observed to be from southern Africa; whereas, for over 200 years it's been consumed by major populations from all over the world. Since the fruit holds up to 93% water, it is called "watermelon" whereas the melon term is used because of its shape and pulpiness (Dubey et al. 2021). This berry fruit is largely consumed in its fresh form as juices, cocktails, mocktails, and salads for its sweetness and the highest amount of water content. It's also available in a diverse range of food products as an ingredient including spray-dried watermelon powder, watermelon squash, watermelon candy, pickles, and cakes. The tender leaves and fruits from the watermelon family are cooked as green vegetables. The fruit flesh along with the maze is cooked as porridge and is served as valuable stock feed, especially during times of drought. Also, the hollowed fruit can be used as a decorative container for cooking, serving, or storing berries and cut fruits (Albala 2011). The pulp and seeds of the watermelon fruit are prepared and presented in different ways around the globe based on various cultures and geographical patterns. The quality of this fruit

DOI: 10.1201/9781003259213-8

depends on the sweetness and the sugar content, mainly due to a combination of sucrose, glucose, and fructose. Sucrose and glucose account for 20%–40% and fructose for 30%–50% of total sugars in a ripened fruit. Watermelon serves as a rich source of nutrients, vitamins, amino acids, phytochemicals, minerals, and nutraceuticals and thus possesses various therapeutic properties. All parts of this fruit, including the rind and the seeds, provide greater nutritional value and are used in conventional medicines for their adequate accessibility and affordability (Enemor et al. 2019).

The purpose of this chapter is to establish an overview of the phytochemical and the nutraceutical attributes of the watermelon fruit. Major emphasis is given in elaborating on the therapeutic attributes, including antioxidative, antidiabetic, anticancer, and anti-inflammatory properties of watermelon against various health conditions, with evidence-based research anticipating stimulating further research on less-explored aspects of watermelon.

## 8.2 SCIENTIFIC CLASSIFICATION OF WATERMELON

Scientific classification or taxonomy is the science of naming, describing, and classifying organisms and includes all plants, animals, and microorganisms of the world. The current taxonomic system has levels in its hierarchy, from lowest to highest; they are species, genus, family, order, class, phylum, and kingdom. The scientific classification of watermelon is represented in Table 8.1.

## 8.3 COMMON NAMES USED FOR WATERMELON WORLDWIDE

Apart from the scientific names, every fruit and vegetable has a local name based on the region, culture, diversity, and geographical differences. The common terms generally used for watermelon all around the world are listed in Table 8.2.

## 8.4 ORIGIN AND BOTANICAL DESCRIPTION

Primarily, watermelon is an annual herb. It is usually a prostrate or climbing plant with numerous herbaceous, rigid stems which can quickly grow up to 3–10 meters in length. The plant is monoecious, where the male and female flowers are found in the same plant with hairy and long flower stalks growing up to 50 mm long. The ovary is found to be ovoid in structure, pubescent, with three placentas and is present with numerous ovules. In male flowers, the pistil is absent with 3–4 stamens (Nickrent et al. 1988). The tender parts of the leaves are generally observed with disorganized woolen-like structured hairs; meanwhile,

### Table 8.1: Scientific Classification of Watermelon

| | |
|---|---|
| Kingdom | Plantae |
| Division | *Magnoliophyta* |
| Class | *Magnoliopsida* |
| Order | *Cucurbitales* |
| Family | *Cucurbitaceae* |
| Scientific name | *Citrullus lanatus* |
| Synonyms | *Citrullus vulgaris* |
| Genus | *Citrullus* |
| Species | *lanatus* |

*Source:* From Erhirhie and Ekene (2013).

## Table 8.2: Common Names Used for Watermelon Worldwide

| | |
|---|---|
| Afrikaans | Waatlemoen |
| Arabic | Battikh, Bateekh, Betteakh (Egypt) |
| Bengali | Taramuj |
| Bulgarian | Dinia |
| Chinese | Xi gua, Shi yong xi gua, Choei koa, Ts'ing teng koa, Han koa, Hia koa |
| Czech | Lubenice meloun |
| Danish | Vandmelon |
| Dutch | Watermeloen |
| English | Watermelon |
| Finnish | Vesimeloni, Arpuusi |
| French | Melon d'eau, Pastèque |
| German | Wassemelone, Wassermelone, Gewöhnliche Wassermelone, Wasserzitrulle, Wasser-melone |
| Greek | Karpusi, Karpouzia (Cyprus) |
| Gujarati | Tarabuucha |
| Hebrew | Avatiach, Avatiach pashut |
| Hindi | Kharbuza (kharmuja), Tarabuuza (Tarbooz, Tarbuj, Tarbuz, Tarmuj) |
| Hungarian | Görögdinnye |
| Indonesian | Semangka, Cimangko (Indonesia), Watesan (Java) |
| Italian | Anguria, Cocomero, Melone d'acqua, Pastecca |
| Japanese | Suika, Shokuyou suika |
| Korean | Su bak (Soo bahk) |
| Macedonian | Lubenica |
| Mandarin | Xigua |
| Marathi | Tarabuuja |
| Nepalese | Tarabuujaa (Tarbuja) |
| Persian | Raqqi |
| Philippines | Pakwan |
| Polish | Arbuz, Kawon |
| Portuguese | Melancia, Melância |
| Punjabi | Tarabuuja |
| Romanian | Pepene verde |
| Russian | Arbuz, Arbuz stolovyj |
| Serbian | Lubenitsa |
| Slovenian | Lubenice |
| Spanish | Sandía (Spain), Melón de agua (Cuba), Albudeca |
| Sundanese | Samangka |
| Swahili | Mango, Mtikiti |
| Swedish | Vattenmelon |
| Tamil | Kumati Palam |
| Thai | Taeng chin, Taeng moh, Matao |
| Turkish | Karpuz |
| Ukrainian | Karpuz |
| Vietnamese | Döa haáu |

*Source:* From Lim (2012).

the mature parts are hairless and non-fleecy in appearance. The leaves of this plant are firm and compact on both sides. The average dimensions of the leaves vary from 60–200 mm in length and 40–150 mm in breadth. These plants are habitually segmented into three lobes, and the middle lobe is the largest one. The leaf stalks are conventionally hairy and grow up to 150 mm long. The fruit of this plant is typically globose to oblong and sometimes ovoid, measuring 15–70 cm long and weighing 0.3–4 kg. The seeds of the fruit are flattened, yellow to brown colored, and elliptical in structure (Chakravarty 1990).

## 8.5 NUTRITIONAL COMPOSITION OF WATERMELON

Every part of watermelon has healthy prospects, including the rind, flesh, and seeds, contributing more significant amounts of dietary and soluble fiber. Watermelon is a rich source of numerous energy-providing vitamins, including A, B, and C. The fruit is primarily found abundant with water content up to 92% by weight. The flesh part of this fruit contains bitter cucurbitacins (Zamuz et al. 2021).

According to the USDA, 100 g edible portion of watermelon contains 91 g of water, 134 kg of energy, 0.6 g of protein, 0.4 g of fat, 8 mg calcium, 9 mg phosphorus, 0.17 mg iron, 0.08 mg thiamine, and observable traces of niacin, ascorbic acid, and riboflavin (Hussain et al. 2019). It includes natural protein content in the range of $10.2 \pm 1.1$ g/100 g and crude lipid up to $1.8 \pm 0.1$ g/100 g. The edible parts of the flesh contain crude protein with the range of $14.8 \pm 3.3$ g/100 g and crude lipid up to $4.6 \pm 0.6$ g/100 g. Palmitic acid is present as $241.2 \pm 43.1$ mg/100 g, along with omega-3 (linolenic acid, $250.5 \pm 51.7$ mg/100 g) and omega-6 (linoleic acid, $251.9 \pm 50.5$ mg/100 g). These are the most available fatty acids seen in watermelon. Ripened watermelon contains polysaccharides such as 23% hemicellulose, 20% cellulose, 10% lignin, and 13% pectin. The seeds of this fruit provide a preeminent source of energy and have no hydrocyanic acid, making it the most eligible feed for livestock (Cecchi and de Carolis 2021). The prospective health benefit of watermelon is because of its all-natural availability of an antioxidant known as lycopene. One potential amino acid, citrulline, is abundant in watermelon, a precursor to arginine. The seeds of the watermelon are flat brown in color and have much higher nutritional value than the flesh of the fruit. It has a nutty flavor and contains possible trace amounts of vitamin C, fats, and riboflavins (Erhirhie and Ekene 2013).

## 8.6 PRESERVATION OF WATERMELON

Watermelon has a pH ranging between 5.2 and 6.7, making it a perishable fruit naturally. The water activity of this fruit is commonly higher and varies from 0.97 and 0.99. Therefore, it's far more vulnerable to pathogenic microorganisms because of the gram-positive bacteria, which might be very sensitive to low acidity.

The preservation of watermelon is challenging because of its low acid nature. To prolong the shelf-life and enhance the utilization process, watermelon juice is processed into a range of diverse products, evaluating customer's requirements for healthy, nutritious, and convenient sustenance. Regardless, extreme processing conditions can result in a lack of nutrients and phytochemicals in watermelon. Studies discovered that fruits undergo various types of operations like peeling, size reduction, mixing, and heat treatment throughout processing. In the fruit juice manufacture, high-temperature short-time processing is typically carried out. Although this approach efficiently minimizes microorganisms and enzymes, it subverts the dietary and antioxidant potential of fruit extracts. Currently, several research studies are being carried out at the utilization of progressive processing technology that not often has an effect on low molecular weight components like color, aromatic compounds, minerals, nutrients, and antioxidants in the course of operation. Heat is suggested to negatively affect the quality parameters of watermelon due to its thermo-sensitive nature. Temperatures above 78°C are pronounced to have an unfavorable impact on color shift, divergence of particles, and modulation in flavor. As a result, alternative processing technology which might be price-efficient without compromising the quality of the product ought to be carried out in the course of processing.

Since watermelon grade parameters are effortlessly depleted with the aid of using heat treatment, nonthermal processing strategies have to be applied to reduce the degradation of quality. Compared to thermal technology, nonthermal processing efficiently keeps nutrients, flavor, and color. High-pressure processing and pulsed electric power fields are amongst processing strategies which could maintain the quality parameters. An assortment of ultrasound and mild heat, which is referred as thermosonication, is found to be extra efficient in enzymatic and microbial inactivation without influencing the juice quality. Heat processing transforms lycopene and β-carotene from transconfiguration cis isomers, making them more bioavailable.

## 8.7 ETHNOMEDICINAL REFERENCE

Ethnomedicine is the study or comparison of the conventional medicine established with their bioactive compounds in plants and animals and is anciently being practiced by various ethnic groups, especially those with little access to Western medicines.

Freshly reaped leaves are mentioned as motshatsha, whereas parched leaves are traditionally comprehended as Kgwaile in the indigenous South African Sepedi vocabulary. Motshatsha, a leaf vegetable recipe, is made by cooking untouched succulent leaves of the citron variant of watermelon along with mature tomatoes and added salt and is commonly consumed with starch staples, especially maize or sorghum porridge or gruel.

Watermelon has been used globally in traditional medicines. Ripened fruit in higher doses serves as a medic; the seeds from watermelon roots are all used for creating decoctions and are utilized in the remedy of urinary tract infections and bedwetting concerns. The fruit is considered to be a diuretic and is effective in the treatment of renal stones (Ikram et al. 2015). Studies from the 1980s show that watermelon consumption was suggested for hypertension, and preliminary research studies have been conducted on its antihypertensive activities. In the northern parts of Sudan, watermelon is used for burns, swellings, rheumatism, and as an excellent laxative. The rind of the fruit is recommended in specific cases of alcohol poisoning. For their high protein and fat content, seeds are also used in the improvement of infant nutrition (Hamzah et al. 2013).

## 8.8 PHYTOCHEMICAL COMPOSITION IN VARIOUS PARTS OF WATERMELON

Currently, there is high interest in bioactive compounds originating from natural foods around the globe. Every individual is becoming more conscious about incorporating a healthier lifestyle in the form of incorporating nutraceutical and functionally active compounds in their standard dietary routine. Figure 8.1 shows the phytochemical composition in various parts of watermelon.

Bioactive compounds derived from watermelon have beneficial effects on improving overall health. Watermelon is primarily a combination of hemicelluloses, celluloses, lignin, and pectin, with sugars, proteins, polyphenolics, citrulline, lycopene, and carotenoids tagged along (Zia et al. 2021). The rind is observed to hold many phytonutrients such as terpenoids, sterols,

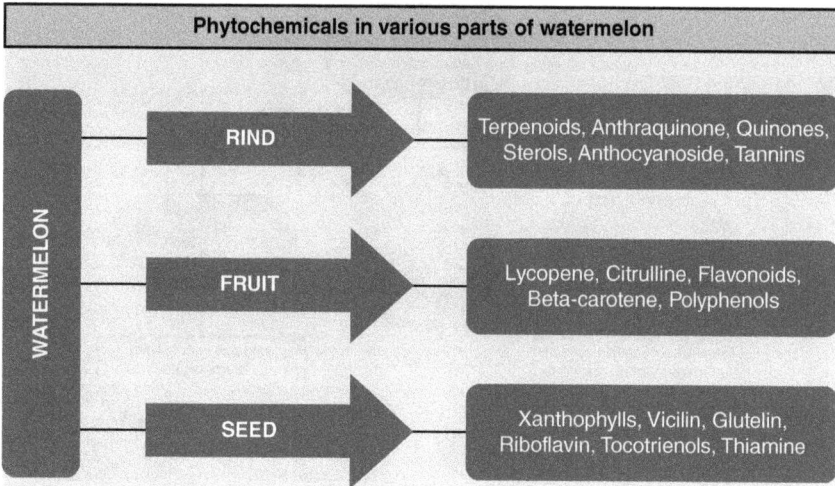

**Figure 8.1** Phytochemical composition in various parts of watermelon.

anthocyanoside, anthraquinone, tannins, and quinones. Nevertheless, the seeds provide phytochemicals like xanthophylls, riboflavin, vicilin, tocotrienols, glutelin, and thiamine.

Watermelon contains citrulline (24.7 mg/g), polyphenolic content (63.33 ± 1.455 mg TAE/g), (2.028 ± 0.061 mg RE/g) of flavonoids. The overall phenolic content in watermelon varies from 385 to 507 mg CAE/Kg. The functional compounds present in this fruit are alkaloids, phytates, tannins, oxalates, phenols, flavonoids, lycopene, citrulline, flavonoids, beta-carotene, polyphenols, and saponin (Zia et al. 2021).

## 8.9 BIOACTIVE PROPERTIES OF WATERMELON

Watermelon possesses considerable bioactive properties which are advantageous in enhancing the all-around physical health of an individual (Tarazona-Díaz et al. 2011). All the parts including the fruit, rind, and seeds are used in various basic and clinical research studies in understanding the role of the bioactive properties translated to human health. The role of watermelon in major lifestyle and metabolic diseases is discussed below.

### 8.9.1 Anti-Inflammatory Activity

Chronic low-grade inflammation is a condition resulting from the imbalance in pro-inflammatory and anti-inflammatory factors (Esser et al. 2014). Chronic inflammation promotes the inducement of gene mutations, inhibition of apoptosis, and the stimulation of cell proliferation and angiogenesis. Inflammation can also trigger non-genetic influences on gene expression that are associated with carcinogenesis. Watermelon and its extracts are proven to have anti-inflammatory properties. Figure 8.2 shows the anti-inflammatory properties of watermelon.

A study conducted with watermelon seed oil had shown anti-inflammatory activity against paw edema induced by carrageenan in a rat model (Deshmukh et al. 2015). Anti-inflammatory activity was compared with the standard diclofenac, and a significant reduction of edema was observed by watermelon seed oil when provided with the dosage of 100 mg/kg (Alka et al. 2018).

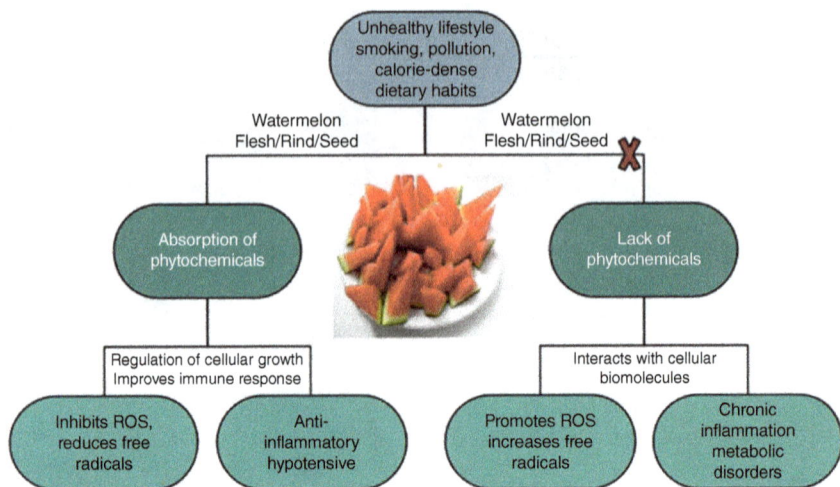

**Figure 8.2** Anti-inflammatory properties of watermelon.

Extract from watermelon is effectively used against inflammation and chronic pain caused due to inflammatory actions by inhibiting cyclooxygenase enzymes through anti-inflammatory and analgesic agents like Cucurbitacin and phytochemicals such as steroids in alkaloids and terpenoids. This was observed in a study by providing a methanolic extract of watermelon rinds to inflammation-induced rats. A reduction in rectal temperature post 4 hours of inflammation induction was noticed (Kumari et al. 2013).

Citrulline derived from natural sources like watermelon can be biologically available in greater amounts compared to synthetic sources of the same. In another study, citrulline extract from watermelon fruit is reported to decrease tumor necrosis factor-alpha (TNF-$\alpha$) production significantly in diabetic obese rats (Andersson 2003). Administration of watermelon extracts for 7 days is reported to reduce malonaldehyde with a significant increment in catalase, glutathione peroxidase, and superoxide dismutase activity in Wistar rats (Kolawole et al. 2019). It acts as a potential hydroxyl radical scavenger making it a natural antioxidant. On the other hand, vitamin C is known as a chain-breaking antioxidant that inhibits lipid peroxidation, and the ascorbate transportation in humans requires two types of SCVTs (sodium-dependent vitamin C transporters 1 and 2). Greater amounts of ascorbate are transported by SCVT1 in the liver, intestine, and kidney while SCVT2 transports the same in the brain and retinal cells (Ghanem et al. 2021). Conclusively, numerous studies advise that the regular consumption of vitamin C from watermelon can be beneficial as synthetic antioxidant supplements. Hence, watermelon is observed to increase antioxidative enzymes and anti-inflammatory agents preventing chronic low-grade inflammation. It regulates cellular growth and improves the immune response by counteracting inflammation and oxidative stress.

### 8.9.2 Anticancer Activity

Reactive oxygen species (ROS) are generated by cellular respiration as oxygen is reduced. It can be both advantageous and harmful; an unbalanced ROS system may promote oxidative stress and can lead to a series of pathological conditions such as cancer (Bergamini et al. 2004). In a biological system, various metabolic pathways are influenced by the dietary patterns and its active components and the regulation of gene expression leading to altering the molecular mechanism of carcinogenesis (Milner 2006). One of the best ingredients, lycopene is a beneficial phytonutrient in watermelon. It can be involved in the regulation of cancer growth by inhibiting the DNA mutation and functioning against the metastasis of the tumor. Considerable studies exist examining the effects of watermelon supplementation on DNA damage, inflammation, and cancer risk reduction (Holzapfel et al. 2013).

Among the different classes of cancers, colon cancer affect the human population majorly (Yoo et al. 2016). Colon cancer is basically caused when there is an altered balance in between the cellular multiplication and the automated cell death otherwise known as apoptosis. However, multiple investigations indicated that the appropriate alteration in regular dietary habits can intercept major types of colon cancers (Pou et al. 2012). The establishment of watermelon supplementation in rats infected with colon cancer is found to lower the cellular multiplication (Kaore and Kaore 2014). In addition, notable significant effects on apoptosis have not been distinguished. The tumoricidal attributes of the watermelon can be observed due to multiple components, but the most important one could be the availability of a generous amount of l-citrulline and its role involved in the generation of endothelial nitric oxide (NO) (Manivannan et al. 2020). On the other hand, the incorporation of watermelon fruit powder in the regular diets of male Sprague-Dawley rats instigated with colon cancer has lowered the health effects by ameliorating the emergence of deviating crypt foci via lowering the induced oxidative stress and inflammation to DNA (Jibril et al. 2022). Furthermore, an increment in the production of endogenous nitric oxide (eNOS) raised the chances of alleviating the ill effects of cancer, and the supplementation of watermelon has been beneficial in modulating the gene expressions relating to DNA repair enzymes leading to combat cancer naturally (Pan et al. 2009).

Meanwhile, in women, breast and cervical cancers are crucial types of cancers which affect them with a high fatality rate (Singh et al. 2011). A decoction from watermelon leaves is shown to provide the antiproliferative effects on breast and cervical cancer cell lines in a few investigations. Watermelon leaf extracts were experimented with against cervical cancer C33A, HeLa, and SiHa cell lines and breast adenocarcinoma MDA-MB-231 and MCF-7 cell lines. This is evidenced by the results of the in vitro MTT assay and the microscopic examination of the cell lines. The antiproliferative characteristics of watermelon leaf extracts are observed in both cancer cell lines in comparison with normal untreated cells. Nevertheless, the cervical cancer cell lines, specifically the C33A, exhibited increased sensitivity to the leaf extracts. Amidst the cancer cell lines study, the microscopic evaluation elucidated that there is a significant reduction in the cellular size of C33A, MCF-7, and MDA-MB-231 cell lines along with depletion of a number of cells as such (Sueakham et al. 2018).

Leukemia is a type of cancer caused due to the unusual multiplication of blood cells especially in the bone marrow (Khwaja et al. 2016). Multiple parts of watermelon are proven to have anticancer properties due to the availability of the indispensable pharmaceutically critical phytochemicals (Manivannan et al. 2020). The phytochemical "phytol," which is extracted from the sprouts of the watermelon fruit, is observed in inhibiting the unusual cell multiplication in mice models of human T-cell leukemia line Jurkat cell and human lung adenocarcinoma epithelial cell line A549—xenograft (Dash et al. 2020). In addition to that, the molecular mechanism supporting the phytol-mediated cell death or apoptosis included the initiation of intercellular reactive oxygen species via NADPH oxidase enzyme, which resulted in the detention of cell cycle patterns in the S-phase. The expressions of crucial proteins such as cyclin A, cyclin D, phosphatidylinositol-3-kinase (PI3K)/protein kinase b (Akt), and mitogen-activated protein kinase (MAPK) were downregulated and are resulted in the S-phase arrest. The protein cyclin A is essential for the genesis of DNA molecules and is involved in the development and advancement of S-phase in the cell cycle by binding to Cdk2 protein (Feitelson et al. 2015). Likewise, the evolution of G1 to S phase in the cell cycle is regulated by cyclin D; for example, the cyclin D phosphorylates the retinoblastoma tumor suppressor protein by docking instantly to Cdk4 or Cdk6. In addition, the results indicated that the modulation of cyclin A and D proteins was regulated by the reactive oxygen species which controlled the cell cycle in S-phase. Similarly, various studies have depicted the management of cyclin A and D genetic expressions adjudicated by the MAPKs and PI3K/Akt pathways (Leonardi et al. 2018). Both MAPKs and PI3K/Akt are implicated in multiple roles of cells such as cell proliferation, development, differentiation, extension, survival, maturation, and death or apoptosis. Nonetheless, the apoptosis process was not particularly interconnected to the phytol-induced mitotic catastrophe among the cancer cell lines. Similar remarks of non-apoptosis mediated cell death predominantly activated by the intercellular reactive oxygen species in cancer cell lines by phytochemicals have been registered. Across the board, the secondary metabolites observed in watermelon tissues can effectively lower the multiplication and maturation of cancer cells (Cardoso et al. 2018). Further investigations associated with the identification and extraction of the beneficial phytochemicals with effective anticancer prospects can help in the pursuit of drug development for various life-threatening cancer types (Wali et al. 2019). Habitual intake of watermelon revealed conceivable health advantages against numerous severe ailments. Most of the phytochemical components from watermelon are involved in diverse and complex metabolic networks. Hence, the molecular rationales by watermelon behind every disease should be considered, and the active compounds should be isolated and assessed individually gaining extensive knowledge on the same.

### 8.9.3 Antidiabetic Activity

Diabetes can be categorized into two types pivoting on etiopathogenesis. Type 1 diabetes is distinguished by the gradual destruction of pancreatic B cells due to the autoimmune reaction of the body directing to insulin deficiency. On the other hand, type 2 diabetes is the most typical condition of diabetes which involves gradual increments of insulin resistance. Urban and sedentary lifestyles along with calorie-dense dietary habits increase the diabetic population all around the globe (380 million individuals). This multifactorial metabolic condition prefers foods like watermelon in regulating glycemic index and beta-cell regeneration (Zia et al. 2021).

The well-known symptoms of non-insulin-dependent diabetes are the lowered level of synthesis and bioavailability of endothelial nitric oxide, and increased concentrations of glucose in blood plasma, free fatty acid levels, homocysteine, and methylarginines. Various studies recommend that the modulation of energy substrate oxidation, sensitivity to insulin, and hemodynamics are greatly controlled by nitric oxide in human systems (Levine et al. 2012). The synthesis of nitric oxide depends on L-arginine which functions as the forerunner and is converted by tetrahydrobiopterin (BH4)-dependent nitric oxide synthase enzyme. Based on the outcomes of numerous in vivo and in vitro experiments, it has been indicated that the dietary ingestion of L-arginine decreased the plasma levels of glucose in diabetic and obese rat models (Fu et al. 2005). In addition to that, L-arginine improved the vascular reactivity in animal prototypes and hyper-cholesterol patients (Mo et al. 1998).

A study conducted with obese diabetic mice kk-Ay for 9 weeks with the administration of citrulline (0.5 g/kg) has significantly reduced the serum insulin levels. Supplementation of crude extract of watermelon (7 days) in diabetic Wistar albino rats is observed in a significant reduction of blood glucose levels (Azizi et al. 2020). In another investigation, supplementation of watermelon rind was used for blood glucose levels past 4 weeks in diabetic rats. Watermelon rind is reported to improve the expression for endothelial nitric oxide synthase (eNOS) in comparison with the diabetic untreated group resulting in increased uptake of blood glucose into the tissues and inhibiting glycosylation of hemoglobin (Salehi et al. 2019). Several studies show the improved histological structure of the pancreas and elevated levels of insulin resulting in improved glucose metabolism with oral administration of crude watermelon or watermelon extracts. Diabetes-based neuronal abnormalities are attributed to the high intracellular glucose. The effect of lycopene was determined with special reference to its antioxidative and anti-inflammatory behavior on oxidative stress, cognitive function, and inflammation in streptozotocin (STZ) induced diabetic rats (Kuhad et al. 2008). During the ailment, acetyl cholinesterase activity, a biomarker of cholinergic dysfunction, increased in the cerebral cortex of diabetic rats about 1.8 fold. Moreover, a rise in thiobarbituric acid reactive substances was about twofold. It was concluded that lycopene has the ability to mitigate cognitive deficit, inflammation, and oxidative stress in diabetic rats. Diabetes induction influenced a significant elevation in serum glucose and lessening in body weight. Nevertheless, lycopene exhibited assuaging impact on diabetic rats by lowering serum glucose level up to 25%. Significant change in body weight was also controlled past 2 weeks of lycopene supplementation (Rauf et al. 2019).

### 8.9.4 Watermelon as a Sports Supplement

All sports events are classified into two categories: Aerobic and anaerobic workouts based on energy expenditure. Although the utilization of aerobic energy is quite dominant during any sports event, anaerobic energy is required for jumping, booting, attacking, pivoting, sprinting, changing in pace, and maintaining consistent forceful contractions (Foster et al. 2003). Sports athletes require specialized nutrients exclusively based on their body types and the types of sports they are involved in. This is usually different from normal dietary habits. Sports nutrients derived from natural sources are gaining interest in the global market (Arenas-Jal et al. 2020). They are recommended because there are no side effects with increased bioavailability facilitating the extra mile for athletes.

Watermelon serves as an excellent additive for sports enthusiasts in their daily dietary routine. It works as a pre-workout supplement. Citrulline is one of the major non-essential amino acid elements of the urea cycle tagged along with arginine and ornithine occurring in the liver. The bioavailability of citrulline in the watermelon is more significant compared to any pharmacological formulation (Hou et al. 2015). Citrulline from watermelon acts as a substrate of arginine. Arginine is the precursor for nitric oxide production by inducing isoform Nitric oxide synthase (iNOS). Nitric oxide enhances sports performance by improving vasodilatation, regulating blood flow, raising mitochondrial respiration, modulating glucose uptake and oxidation, and supporting minor contractile roles in skeletal muscle during all forms of energy expenditure (Collins et al. 2007). Creatine is primarily a nitrogenous organic acid generally found in the sarcoplasm of the muscles and helps in supplying energy to muscles from the kidney and liver. Creatine is reversibly phosphorylated to creatine phosphate by creatine kinase and stored in muscles as high energy phosphate, 98% in skeletal and heart muscles. In muscle, it gets converted to creatine phosphate. During muscle contraction, adenosine triphosphate (ATP) is regenerated by hydrolysis of creatine phosphate. This constant shuttling increases the supply of energy throughout the athletic performance. A study noticed that there was a reduction in the recuperation of pulse rate and muscle soreness post-consumption of 500 mL of watermelon juice (both natural or citrulline enriched) after 24 hours of physical training in athletes compared with placebo trials (Blohm et al. 2020). Numerous research studies demonstrated that watermelon possesses comprehensively nutritious phytonutrients. It serves as a favorable natural source for improving sports training by easing muscle exhaustion.

### 8.9.5 Cardiovascular Benefits of Watermelon

Cardiovascular diseases (CVD) are the result of a prolonged sedentary lifestyle and are registered as a foremost cause of mortality. Cardiac risk is advanced due to the regular consumption of a high cholesterol diet resulting in subacute chronic inflammation (Esposito and Giugliano 2006). Distinctively, low-density lipoprotein (LDL) cholesterol, serum amyloid A (SAA), and intercellular adhesion molecule (ICMA-1) are the threatening characteristics of CVD. This promotes atherosclerosis advancement and cardiovascular occurrences.

Hypercholesterolemia is a condition in which serum lipid level increases especially cholesterol and low-density lipoproteins (LDL) which further leads to atherosclerosis. Dietary lycopene exerts cardioprotective effects due to its high antioxidant property. Apart from lipid-lowering drug therapy, dietary interventions are promoted to attenuate hypercholesterolemia. The resulting data demonstrated that the rats fed on a hypercholesterolemic diet rendered a significant increase in serum total lipid level, total cholesterol, low and high-density lipoproteins, and reduced levels of glutathione peroxidase and malonaldehyde. On the contrary, a diet having lycopene mitigated the indications and symptoms of hypercholesterolemia (Naz et al. 2014). In another research study, the effect of lycopene was examined on macrophages. The derived outcomes displayed that macrophages enriched with lycopene beneficially repressed cellular cholesterol synthesis and ameliorated LDL receptor ability. This effect can result in enhancing the clearance of LDL from the plasma; thus, lycopene is recognized as a hypocholesterolemic agent (Palozza et al. 2010).

The watermelon is also helpful to lessen some other metabolic syndromes owing to vitamins A, B6, and C, magnesium, and potassium. Together with the above-mentioned nutrients, lycopene has health-promoting active components that are associated with a declined risk of cardiovascular disorders. CVD complications such as heart attacks, ischemic strokes, and atherosclerosis are encountered through the oxidation of low-density lipoprotein and the signs and symptoms of the same are subsided, followed by increased consumption of lycopene. Increased consumption of lycopene reduced the thickness of the internal layer of the blood vessels, resulting in the reduction of risk for myocardial infarction. Since the bioavailability of phytonutrients is more significant, a general intake of watermelon is more beneficial (Kohlmeier et al. 1997).

## 8.10 AGRO-BASED DERIVATES OF WATERMELON

In recent years, notable interest has been targeted on getting better significant additives from the "meals agro by-products" or "wasted by-products." Recycling them within the food chain in a greater monetary and sustainable way is an emerging challenge. Bioactive components found in food waste and by-products have been made available in the marketplace. Products have to go through a chain of techniques that can usually be manageable and low-cost effective (Helkar et al. 2016).

Meanwhile, the restoration of those compounds from the diverse plant matrices regularly calls for mixed approaches including biochemical, chemical, and physical treatments. Each technique is to make a certain selective extraction method for the transformation of those materials into meals and merchandise at a better cost.

The extraction strategies which can be presently used for the recovery of bioactive compounds from plant matrices are primarily based totally on the conventional strong-liquid extraction or Soxhlet extraction, which additionally constitutes the maximum ancient ones; whilst in current years, the unconventional extraction strategies consist of pressurized fluid extraction, supercritical fluid extraction, ultrasound-assisted extraction, microwave-assisted extraction, pulsed electric powered discipline extraction, and enzyme assisted extraction (Arias et al. 2022). However, it has to be borne in thoughts that those strategies can't be used indiscriminately and their preference relies upon diverse essential elements consisting of the kind of biomolecules and matrix, on scale processing (laboratory or business), and on the relationship among manufacturing costs and financial values of the compounds to be extracted. The business processing of watermelon commonly entails the separation of the preferred part of the fruit and the simultaneous generation of large quantities with the aid of using products, which can be especially constituted with the aid of using peel (30%–40%) and seeds (1%–2%) (Rico et al. 2020). Accordingly, the juice or pulp from watermelon is taken into consideration because it is the actual and safe portion to eat, while the rind and seeds are discarded as principal stable wastes. However, watermelon seeds are recognized to be particularly dietary; they may be an excellent source of numerous constituents, which include protein, B complex vitamins, minerals (i.e., magnesium, potassium, phosphorous, sodium, iron, zinc, manganese, and copper), and fatty acids, in addition to bioactive phytochemicals (Tabiri et al. 2016). Also, the watermelon rind incorporates citrulline. The seeds of watermelons are recognized to have financial benefits, mainly in international locations in which cultivation is on the increase. Overall, numerous studies found in literature turned into being targeted on special elements associated with watermelon by-products valorization, consisting of (a) the use of those by-products as uncooked components in the formulation of fortified food products, (b) the use of them as potential adsorbents for the elimination of heavy metals and dye, and (c) to offer new enriched practical extracts characterized with the aid of using health-promoting ingredients. Investigations confirmed that the incorporation of watermelon powder in baked desserts that are substituted with 5% flour and 10% with watermelon rinds retarded staling and hindered the lipid oxidation and unfastened fatty acid buildup throughout storage conditions (Innocent and Matenda 2018). The rind of the watermelon should be taken into consideration as a valuable waste product from which compounds with excessive organic and dietary cost consisting of citrulline can be derived. This compound, as pronounced with the aid of using several pieces of evidence, is of dietary and pharmacological significance and might be used as common ingredients or components for drinks and beverages. Reports evaluated a chemically protonated watermelon rind (PWR) as cost-effective and an adsorbent for the elimination of $Pb^{2+}$ and $Cu^{2+}$ ions from aqueous solution, demonstrating absorption of steel ions onto PWR, as a result selling its exploitation from aqueous solutions (Gupta et al. 2021). Similar findings report that the watermelon outer shell can be turned into an amazing and environmentally friendly and cost-effective biosorbent for the elimination of $Cu^{2+}$ from aqueous media. Overall, the authors advised to combine traditional extraction strategies (i.e., natural solvents), and autohydrolysis treatments (on strong residue) to be able to get better oligosaccharides, polyphenols, lignin, and cellulose.

## 8.11 CONCLUSION

As extensively described, watermelon incorporates a necessary matrix of bioactive compounds allotted within the flesh, the seeds, and the rind that have many beneficial consequences on human health. The rind and seeds constitute 60% of the watermelon, and that waste merchandise constitutes an antioxidant capacity in a few instances even better than that of the flesh (Banerjee et al. 2017). This is without a doubt proof that agricultural waste obtained from watermelon is well-suited for building up a sustainable economic system due to its diverse range of nutraceutical properties along with low cultivation prices and its adaptability to extreme climatic conditions throughout geographical patterns. Routine consumption of fruits and vegetables in a regular diet helps in imparting essential nutrients and enhances overall health status. The extensive availability of phytochemicals such as carotenoids, lycopene, anthocyanins, curcubitans, phenols, and flavonoids, along with vitamins and minerals, completes the preference of plant-based dietary habits. It reduces the hazards of a diverse range of threatening diseases such as cancer, cardiovascular diseases, neurodegenerative disorders, and aging-associated ailments. Watermelon is a proven and distinctive source of numerous phytochemicals proclaiming new age vitamins due to health pledging properties (Choudhary et al. 2015). The diversified qualities of watermelon have acquired the core attention of investigators in terms of digestion, bioavailability, and absorption. Watermelon encloses a multifarious amount of phytochemicals with required pharmaceutical significant prevalence, which are attributed to the generous occurrence of citrulline, lycopene, and polyphenols. Numerous pathological disorders and ailments along with their consequences on the biological system were encountered to be majorly reduced with the supplementation of watermelon and/or watermelon-based extracts (Kumar et al. 2021). The supplementation of watermelon extracts are ascertained to ameliorate the effects caused by those illnesses. Secondary metabolites derived from plant sources are observed to have nutraceutical potential. Various tissues of watermelon such as foliage, sprouts, nuts, rinds, and fruits serve as considerable conceivable medication targets involved in disorders such as diabetes, cancer, inflammation, and cardiovascular health. Even though watermelon turned into being the best supply of lycopene and citrulline amongst all end results, studies have discovered that as a minimum 85% of our nutritional lycopene is furnished with the aid of using tomato and primarily tomato-based merchandise; therefore, there may be a need to supply extra primarily watermelon-based products. Since watermelon demonstrates compatibility with the different end products, it may be used collectively with the ones to fabricate commodities that can be of additional commercial value. Research has indicated that the lycopene content of watermelon isn't absolutely depleted with the aid of using processing strategies (Zakynthinos and Varzakas 2016). Therefore, lycopene may be extracted from the watermelon for use in prescribed drugs and meal production as an ingredient. Monitoring the best attributes of watermelons throughout processing remains a continuous study to be able to produce excellent merchandise. Moving ahead, it's vital to decide the inner traits of watermelon as stricken by maturation and processing to be able to offer extensive information to food processing industries. Although, additional analyses dealing with the extraction of the active phytochemicals and studies of genetic regulatory mechanisms of the bioactive components in watermelon are demanded to increase the utilization of the phytochemicals in nutraceutical industries globally. Furthermore, the phytochemical and pharmacokinetic understanding of crucial secondary derivatives in watermelons can promote the drug designing process to tackle alarming conditions. In addition, being a wholesome functional food, the consumption of watermelon can avert the emergence of several disorders in humans. Watermelon also aids in keeping up the quality of life among the general population providing required energy and internal mechanisms benefiting a wide range of the sporting population. All things considered, the discovery of novel and innovative plant-based drugs with minimal to no side effects should be accelerated. The lacuna about the knowledge of plant-derived phytochemicals and their role in human health should be considered by aspiring researchers.

## REFERENCES

Albala, Ken, ed. *Food Cultures of the World Encyclopedia*, Vol. 2. ABC-CLIO, 2011.

Alka, Gupta; Singh Anamika; and Prasad Ranu. "A review on watermelon *Citrullus lanatus* medicinal seeds". *Journal of Pharmacognosy and Phytochemistry*, 7, no 3, 2018, 2222–2225.

Andersson, Annika K. "Role of inducible nitric oxide synthase and melatonin in regulation of β-cell sensitivity to cytokines," PhD diss, Acta Universitatis Upsaliensis, 2003.

Arenas-Jal, Marta; JM Suñé-Negre; Pilar Pérez-Lozano; and Encarna García-Montoya. "Trends in the food and sports nutrition industry: A review". *Critical Reviews in Food Science and Nutrition*, 60, no 14, 2020, 2405–2421. DOI:10.1080/10408398.2019.1643287

Arias, Ana; Gumersindo Feijoo; and Maria Teresa Moreira. "Exploring the potential of antioxidants from fruits and vegetables and strategies for their recovery". *Innovative Food Science & Emerging Technologies*, 2022, 102974. https://doi.org/10.1016/j.ifset.2022.102974

Azizi, Samaneh; Reza Mahdavi; Elnaz Vaghef-Mehrabany; Vahid Maleki; Nahid Karamzad; and Mehrangiz Ebrahimi-Mameghani. "Potential roles of citrulline and watermelon extract on metabolic and inflammatory variables in diabetes mellitus current evidence and future directions A systematic review". *Clinical and Experimental Pharmacology and Physiology*, 47, no 2, 2020, 187–198. DOI: 10.1111/1440-1681.13190

Banerjee, Jhumur; Ramkrishna Singh; R Vijayaraghavan; Douglas MacFarlane; Antonio F Patti; and Amit Arora. "Bioactives from fruit processing wastes Green approaches to valuable chemicals". *Food Chemistry*, 225, 2017, 10–22. DOI: 10.1016/j.foodchem.2016.12.093

Bergamini, Carlo; M Stefania Gambetti; Alessia Dondi; and Carlo Cervellati. "Oxygen reactive oxygen species and tissue damage". *Current Pharmaceutical Design*, 10, no 14, 2004, 1611–1626. DOI: 10.2174/1381612043384664

Blohm, Kara; Joshua Beidler; Phil Rosen; Jochen Kressler; and Mee Young Hong. "Effect of acute watermelon juice supplementation on post-submaximal exercise heart rate recovery blood lactate blood pressure blood glucose and muscle soreness in healthy non-athletic men and women". *International Journal of Food Sciences and Nutrition*, 71, no 4, 2020, 482–489. DOI: 10.1080/09637486.2019.1675604

Cardoso, Jean Carlos; Lee Tseng Sheng Gerald; and Jaime A Teixeira da Silva. "Micropropagation in the twenty-first century". *Plant Cell Culture Protocols*, 2018, 17–46.

Cecchi Teresa and Carla de Carolis. "Food processing industries food waste classification and handling target compounds". In *Bio-based Products from Food Sector Waste*, 17–78. Springer Cham, 2021. DOI: 10.1007/978-1-4939-8594-4_2

Chakravarty, HL. "The development of vegetable crops". *Biology and Utilization of the Cucurbitaceae*, 1990, 325.

Choudhary, BR; SM Haldhar; SK Maheshwari; R Bhargava; and SK Sharma. "Phytochemicals and antioxidants in watermelon *Citrullus lanatus* genotypes under hot arid region". 2015.

Collins, Julie K; Guoyao Wu; Penelope Perkins-Veazie; Karen Spears; P Larry Claypool; Robert A Baker; and Beverly A Clevidence. "Watermelon consumption increases plasma arginine concentrations in adults". *Nutrition*, 23, no 3, 2007, 261–266. DOI: 10.1016/j.nut.2007.01.005

Dash, Manoj Kumar; Namrata Joshi; and Yamini Bhusan Tripathi. "Identification of therapeutic targets for controlling COVID-19 pandemic by traditional system of Ayurvedic medicines: A systematic review". 2020.

Deshmukh, Chinmay D; Anurekha Jain; and Mukul S Tambe. "Phytochemical and pharmacological profile of *Citrullus lanatus* Thunb". *Biolife*, 3, no 2, 2015, 483–488. doi:10.17812/blj2015.32.18

Dubey, S; H Rajput; and K Batta. "Utilization of watermelon rind *Citrullus lanatus* in various food preparations: A Review". *Journal of Agricultural Science and Food Research*, 12, 2021, 318.

Enemor, VHA; CE Oguazu; AU Odiakosa; and SC Okafor. "Research article evaluation of the medicinal properties and possible nutrient composition of *Citrullus lanatus* watermelon seeds". *Research Journal of Medicinal Plant*, 13, no 4, 2019, 129–135. DOI: 10.3923/rjmp.2019.129.135

Erhirhie EO and NE Ekene. "Medicinal values on *Citrullus lanatus* watermelon pharmacological review". *International Journal of Research in Pharmaceutical and Biomedical Sciences*, 4, no 4, 2013, 1305–1312

Esposito Katherine and Dario Giugliano. "Diet and inflammation a link to metabolic and cardiovascular diseases". *European Heart Journal*, 27, no 1, 2006, 15–20. DOI: 10.1093/eurheartj/ehi605

Esser, Nathalie; Sylvie Legrand-Poels; Jacques Piette; André J Scheen; and Nicolas Paquot "Inflammation as a link between obesity metabolic syndrome and type 2 diabetes". *Diabetes Research and Clinical Practice*, 105, no 2, 2014, 141–150. DOI: 10.1016/j.diabres.2014.04.006

Feitelson, Mark A; Alla Arzumanyan; Rob J Kulathinal; Stacy W Blain; Randall F Holcombe; Jamal Mahajna; Maria Marino, et al. "Sustained proliferation in cancer mechanisms and novel therapeutic targets". In *Seminars in Cancer Biology*, 35, S25–S54. Academic Press, 2015. DOI: 10.1016/j.semcancer.2015.02.006

Foster, Carl; Jos J De Koning; Floor Hettinga; Joanne Lampen; Kerry L La Clair; Christopher Dodge; Maarten Bobbert; and John P Porcari. "Pattern of energy expenditure during simulated competition". *Medicine and Science in Sports and Exercise*, 35, no 5, 2003, 826–831. DOI: 10.1249/01.MSS.0000065001.17658.68

Fu, Wenjiang J; Tony E Haynes; Ripla Kohli; Jianbo Hu; Wenjuan Shi; Thomas E Spencer; Raymond J Carroll; Cynthia J Meininger; and Guoyao Wu. "Dietary L-arginine supplementation reduces fat mass in Zucker diabetic fatty rats". *Journal of Nutrition*, 135, no 4, 2005, 714–721. DOI: 10.1093/jn/135.4.714

Ghanem, Ali; Anna Maria Melzer; Esther Zaal; Laura Neises; Danny Baltissen; Omar Matar; Hannah Glennemeier-Marke, et al. "Ascorbate kills breast cancer cells by rewiring metabolism via redox imbalance and energy crisis". *Free Radical Biology and Medicine*, 163, 2021, 196–209. DOI: 10.1016/j.freeradbiomed.2020.12.012

Gupta, Archana; Vishal Sharma; Kashma Sharma; Vijay Kumar; Sonal Choudhary; Priyanka Mankotia; Brajesh Kumar, et al. "A review of adsorbents for heavy metal decontamination growing approach to wastewater treatment". *Materials*, 14, no 16, 2021, 4702. DOI: 10.3390/ma14164702

Hamzah, RU; AA Jigam; HA Makun; and EC Egwim. "Antioxidant properties of selected African vegetables fruits and mushrooms: A review". *Mycotoxin and Food Safety in Developing Countries London*, 2013, 203–249.

Helkar, P Bharat; Aksasha Kumar Sahoo; and NJ Patil. "Review food industry by-products used as a functional food ingredients". *International Journal of Waste Resources*, 6, no 3, 2016, 1–6. DOI: 10.4172/2252-5211.1000248

Ho, Lee-Hoon; Mohammad Moneruzzaman Khandaker; Joseph Bong; Choon Fah; and Thuan-Chew Tan. "Cultivation common diseases and potential nutraceutical values of watermelon". *Research Updates*, 2017, 71.

Holzapfel, Nina Pauline; Boris Michael Holzapfel; Simon Champ; Jesper Feldthusen; Judith Clements; and Dietmar Werner Hutmacher. "The potential role of lycopene for the prevention and therapy of prostate cancer from molecular mechanisms to clinical evidence". *International Journal of Molecular Sciences*, 14, no 7, 2013, 14620–14646. DOI: 10.3390/ijms140714620

Hou, Yongqing; Yulong Yin; and Guoyao Wu. "Dietary essentiality of 'nutritionally non-essential amino acids' for animals and humans". *Experimental Biology and Medicine*, 240, no 8, 2015, 997–1007. DOI: 10.1177/1535370215587913

Hussain, Shahid; Zed Rengel; Muhammad Qaswar; Mamoona Amir; and Muhammad Zafar-ul-Hye. "Arsenic and heavy metal cadmium lead mercury and nickel contamination in plant-based foods". In *Plant and Human Health*, Volume 2, pp. 447–490. Springer, Cham, 2019. DOI: 10.1007/978-3-030-03344-6_20

Ikram, Emmy Hainida Khairul; Roger Stanley; Michael Netzel; and Kent Fanning. "Phytochemicals of papaya and its traditional health and culinary uses—A review". *Journal of Food Composition and Analysis*, 41, 2015, 201–211. https://doi.org/10.1016/j.jfca.2015.02.010

Innocent K and RT Matenda. "Postharvest technology and value addition of watermelons *Citrullus lanatus*: An overview". *Journal of Postharvest Technology*, 6, no 2, 2018, 75–83.

Jibril, Muhammad Mustapha Azizah; Haji-Hamid Faridah; Abas Jeeven; Karrupan Abdulkarim Sabo Mohammed; Ahmad Haniff Jaafar; Mohd Sabri Pak Dek; and Nurul Shazini Ramli. "Watermelon *Citrullus lanatus* leaf extract attenuates biochemical and histological parameters in high-fat diet/ streptozotocin-induced diabetic rats". *Journal of Food Biochemistry*, 2022, e14058. DOI: 10.1111/jfbc.14058

Kaore, Shilpa N; and Navinchandra M Kaore. "Citrulline pharmacological perspectives and role as a biomarker in diseases and toxicities". In *Biomarkers in Toxicology*, pp. 883–905. Academic Press, 2014. https://doi.org/10.1016/ B978-0-12-404630-6.00053-1

Khwaja, Asim Magnus Bjorkholm; Rosemary E Gale; Ross L Levine; Craig T Jordan; Gerhard Ehninger; Clara D Bloomfield, et al. "Acute myeloid leukaemia". *Nature Reviews Disease Primers* 2, no 1, 2016, 1–22. DOI: 10.1038/ nrdp.2016.10

Kohlmeier, Lenore; Jeremy D Kark; Enrique Gomez-Gracia; Blaise C Martin; Susan E Steck; Alwine FM Kardinaal; Jetmund Ringstad, et al. "Lycopene and myocardial infarction risk in the EURAMIC Study". *American Journal of Epidemiology*, 146, no 8, 1997, 618–626. DOI: 10.1093/oxfordjournals.aje.a009327

Kolawole, Tolunigba; Ologhaguo Adienbo; and Victor Dapper. "Ameliorative effects of hydromethanolic extract of *Citrullus lanatus* watermelon rind on semen parameters reproductive hormones and testicular oxidative status following nicotine administration in male Wistar rats". *Nigerian Journal of Physiological Sciences*, 34, no 1, 2019, 83–90.

Kuhad, Anurag; Richa Sethi; and Kanwaljit Chopra. "Lycopene attenuates diabetes-associated cognitive decline in rats". *Life Sciences*, 83, no 3–4, 2008, 128–134. DOI: 10.1016/j.lfs.2008.05.013

Kumar, Manoj; Maharishi Tomar; Jayashree Potkule; Reetu Verma; Sneh Punia; Archana Mahapatra; Tarun Belwal, et al. "Advances in the plant protein extraction mechanism and recommendations". *Food Hydrocolloids*, 115, 2021, 106595. https://doi.org/10.1016/j.foodhyd.2021.106595

Kumari, Amrita; Juhi Rao; Jyoti Kumari; Neha Sharma; Pankaj Jain; Vivek Dave; and Swapnil Sharma. "Analgesic activity of aqueous extract of *Citrullus lanatus* peels". *Advances in Pharmacology and Pharmacy*, 1, no 3, 2013, 135–138. DOI: 10.13189/app.2013.010303

Leonardi, Giulia C; Luca Falzone; Rossella Salemi; Antonino Zanghì; Demetrios A Spandidos; James A Mccubrey; Saverio Candido; and Massimo Libra. "Cutaneous melanoma from pathogenesis to therapy". *International Journal of Oncology*, 52, no 4, 2018, 1071–1080. DOI: 10.3892/ijo.2018.4287

Levine, Arlene Bradley; David Punihaole; and T Barry Levine. "Characterization of the role of nitric oxide and its clinical applications". *Cardiology*, 122, no 1, 2012, 55–68. DOI: 10.1159/000338150

Lim, T. K. "*Citrullus lanatus*." In *Edible Medicinal and Non-Medicinal Plants*, Volume 2, pp. 179–190. Springer, Dordrecht, 2012. DOI 10.1007/978-94-007-1764-0_29.

Manivannan, Abinaya; Eun-Su Lee; Koeun Han; Hye-Eun Lee; and Do-Sun Kim. "Versatile nutraceutical potentials of watermelon—A modest fruit loaded with pharmaceutically valuable phytochemicals". *Molecules*, 25, no 22, 2020, 5258. DOI: 10.3390/molecules25225258

Milner, John A. "Diet and cancer facts and controversies". *Nutrition and Cancer*, 56, no 2, 2006, 216–224. DOI: 10.1207/s15327914nc5602_13

Mo, Wa; Ashok K Singh; Jose AL Arruda; and George Dunea. "Role of nitric oxide in cocaine-induced acute hypertension". *American Journal of Hypertension*, 11, no 6, 1998, 708–714. DOI: 10.1016/s0895-7061(98)00041-7

Naz, Ambreen; Masood Sadiq Butt; Muhammad Tauseef Sultan; Mir Muhammad Nasir Qayyum; and Rai Shahid Niaz. "Watermelon lycopene and allied health claims". *EXCLI Journal*, 13, 2014, 650.

Nickrent, Daniel L; W Hardy Eshbaugh; and Thomas K Wilson. The vascular flora of Andros Island Bahamas Dubuque IA Kendall/Hunt, 1988.

Palozza, Paola; Nadia Parrone; Rossella E Simone; and Assunta Catalano. "Lycopene in atherosclerosis prevention an integrated scheme of the potential mechanisms of action from cell culture studies". *Archives of Biochemistry and Biophysics*, 504, no 1, 2010 26–33. DOI: 10.1016/j.abb.2010.06.031

Pan, Min-Hsiung; Ching-Shu Lai; Slavik Dushenkov; and Chi-Tang Ho. "Modulation of inflammatory genes by natural dietary bioactive compounds". *Journal of Agricultural and Food Chemistry*, 57, no 11, 2009, 4467–4477. DOI: 10.1021/jf900612n

Paris, Harry S. "Origin and emergence of the sweet dessert watermelon *Citrullus lanatus*". *Annals of Botany*, 116, no 2, 2015, 133–148. DOI: 10.1093/aob/mcv077

Pou, Sonia Alejandra; María del Pilar Díaz; and Alberto Rubén Osella. "Applying multilevel model to the relationship of dietary patterns and colorectal cancer an ongoing case–control study in Córdoba Argentina". *European Journal of Nutrition*, 51 no 6, 2012, 755–764. DOI: 10.1007/s00394-011-0255-7

Rahman Bushra. "Phytochemical investigation of *Citrullus lanatus* watermelon rind", PhD diss, East West University, 2013.

Rauf, Abdur; Muhammad Imran; Tareq Abu-Izneid; Seema Patel; Xiandao Pan; Saima Naz; Ana Sanches Silva; Farhan Saeed; and Hafiz Ansar Rasul Suleria "Proanthocyanidins: A comprehensive review". *Biomedicine & Pharmacotherapy*, 116, 2019, 108999. DOI: 10.1016/j.biopha.2019.108999

Rico, Xiana; Beatriz Gullón; José Luis Alonso; and Remedios Yáñez. "Recovery of high value-added compounds from pineapple melon watermelon and pumpkin processing by-products: An overview". *Food Research International*. 132, 2020, 109086. DOI: 10.1016/j.foodres.2020.109086

Salehi, Bahare; Athar Ata; Nanjangud V Anil Kumar; Farukh Sharopov; Karina Ramírez-Alarcón; Ana Ruiz-Ortega; Seyed Abdulmajid Ayatollahi, et al. "Antidiabetic potential of medicinal plants and their active components". *Biomolecules*, 9, no 10, 2019, 551. DOI: 10.3390/biom9100551

Singh, Gopal K; Shanita D Williams; Mohammad Siahpush; and Aaron Mulhollen. "Socioeconomic rural-urban and racial inequalities in US cancer mortality part I—All cancers and lung cancer and part II—Colorectal prostate breast and cervical cancers". *Journal of Cancer Epidemiology*, 2011, 2011. DOI: 10.1155/2011/107497

Sueakham, Thidarat; Chalita Chantaramanee; and Panata Iawsipo. "Anti-proliferative effect of Thai watermelon leaf extracts on cervical and breast cancer cells". *NU International Journal of Science*, 15, 2018, 89–95.

Tabiri, Betty; Jacob K Agbenorhevi; Faustina D Wireko-Manu; and Elsa I Ompouma. "Watermelon seeds as food nutrient composition phytochemicals and antioxidant activity". *International Journal of Nutrition and Food Sciences*, 5, no 2, 2016, 139–144. DOI: 10.11648/j.ijnfs.20160502.18

Tarazona-Díaz Martha Patricia; Joana Viegas; Margarida Moldao-Martins; and Encarna Aguayo "Bioactive compounds from flesh and by-product of fresh-cut watermelon cultivars". *Journal of the Science of Food and Agriculture*, 91, no 5, 2011, 805–812. DOI: 10.1002/jsfa.4250

Wali, Adil Farooq; Sabhiya Majid; Shabhat Rasool; Samar Bassam Shehada; Shahad Khalid Abdulkareem; Aimen Firdous; Saba Beigh, et al. "Natural products against cancer: Review on phytochemicals from marine sources in preventing cancer". *Saudi Pharmaceutical Journal*. 27, no 6, 2019, 767–777. DOI: 10.1016/j.jsps.2019.04.013

Yoo, So Young; Seo Young Bang; Su-Nam Jeong; Dae Hwan Kang; and Jeong Heo. "A cancer-favoring oncolytic vaccinia virus shows enhanced suppression of stem-cell like colon cancer". *Oncotarget*, 7, no 13, 2016, 16479. DOI: 10.18632/oncotarget.7660

Zakynthinos G and T Varzakas. "Carotenoids from plants to food industry" *Current Research in Nutrition and Food Science*, 4, special issue, 2016, 38.

Zamuz, Sol; Paulo ES Munekata; Beatriz Gullón; Gabriele Rocchetti; Domenico Montesano; and José M Lorenzo. "*Citrullus lanatus* as source of bioactive components: An up-to-date review". *Trends in Food Science & Technology*. 111, 2021, 208–222. https://doi.org/10.1016/j.tifs.2021.03.002

Zia, Sania; Moazzam Rafiq Khan; Muhammad Asim Shabbir; and Rana Muhammad Aadil. "An update on functional nutraceutical and industrial applications of watermelon by-products A comprehensive review". *Trends in Food Science & Technology*, 114, 2021, 275–291. https://doi.org/10.1016/j.tifs.2021.05.039.

# 9 Pineapple

Shiv Kumar, Sugandha Sharma, Rahul Mehra, Poonam Baniwal,
Rekha Kaushik, and Sheetal Thakur

## CONTENTS

## 9.1 INTRODUCTION

The most sweet and fleshy product of a tree is fruit which may have seeds or can be eaten wholly as food. Pineapple is a fruit which is loved by most of people. Pineapple belongs to the family of *Ananas comosus,* Bromeliaceae (Table 9.1). It is a fiery plant with a height and width of 1–2 m (Sufian et al. 2020). It is cultivated in the tropical and coastal regions. It is cultivated on land which is 2,250,000 acres and its production is increasing continuously (Banik et al. 2011). It is one of the most essential fruit crops in the universe. Because of the excellent taste and flavor, it is called the queen of the fruitlet. Pineapple is known as the third tropical fruit after banana and citrus in the world (Kumar and Joshi 2013). It has vibrant tropical flavor, exceptional juiciness, and immense health benefits. In Malaysia, pineapple is also identified as nanas because they are used for many purposes in different variations (Laftah and Rahaman 2015). They can be used in red green pineapple for commercial uses. They mostly prefer Morris and Sarawak pineapple. It is comprised of major and minor elements (Asim et al. 2017). It contains proteolytic enzymes which are a bioactive compound (Kashyap et al. 2022). Pineapple is the richest source of cysteine proteases and bromelain which is there in its different parts (Sibaly and Jeetah 2017). Commercially, bromelain has been utilized in many food industries, cosmetics, and dietary supplements.

DOI: 10.1201/9781003259213-9

## Table 9.1: Scientific Classification of Pineapple

| | |
|---|---|
| Division | Magnoliophyta |
| Class | Liliopsida |
| Order | Bromeliales |
| Family | Bromeliaceae |
| Genus | *Ananas Mill* |
| Species | *Comosus* (L.) Merr |

*Source:* From Arun et al. (2015).

Pineapple contains the desired amount of carbohydrates, vitamin C, calcium, potassium, water, crude fiber and different minerals (Daud et al. 2014). It helps in maintaining the ideal body weight, proper nutrition, and good digestive system. Pineapple has a low quantity of sodium and fat. It contains 10–25 mg of vitamins (Yusof et al. 2012). Pineapple composition is mainly seen in the edible portion. It contains approximately 81.2% to 86.2% moisture, total solids of 13–19%, of which monosaccharides are the foremost components. Carbohydrates contain 85% of total solids and 2–3% of the organic acid and citric acid which makes up the fiber (Yusof et al. 2015). The pulp has much less nitrogenous compounds, ash content, and lipids (0.1%). Mature fruits have a protein digesting enzyme, 14% sugar, citric acid, bromelain, and good amount of malic acid, vitamins B and A (Asim et al. 2015). Pineapple is also considered as the medical diet for some of the diseases. Bromelain helps in the digestion of protein as it breaks down the complex protein into the simple amino acids when taken with meals (Jawaid and Khalil 2011). Pineapple can be served or consumed cooked, fresh and juiced and can also be preserved. Green pineapple can be used for the preparation of pickles. Syrup, squash, candy, and jelly are prepared from pineapple. From pineapple, vinegar, citric acid, alcohol, and calcium citrate can be produced (Devi et al. 2011). To maintain good personal health, the pineapple can be used as nutritional fruit. The pineapple can be consumed as raw or fresh pineapple juice (Cherian et al. 2011). The ripe fruits which are on the field are best for eating purpose but it is essential to remove the eyes, rind, crown and core. Pineapples are utilized as juiced, canned, and fresh (Rahman 2011). It can be used in a variety of food variants like jam, fruit salad, dessert, candy, ice cream, and in supplements to meat dishes. It can be consumed in the form of salads, desserts, puddings, as a garnish, cake, cooked in pies, and made into preserves and sauces. Pineapple can also be utilized in the various meat dishes and curries (Sharma et al. 2016a). Pineapple has bioactive compounds, nutritional value, physiochemical composition, and the health benefits. This chapter covers the health element of pineapple bioactive compounds as a treatment for various chronic disorders (Prabhu et al. 2021).

### 9.2 HISTORY

Pineapple was first discovered by Columbus and his mates in 1493 as it is an American plant. Pineapple was known all over South America in tropical as well as in coastal regions (Murthy and Yogesh 2014). De Oviedo was a government officer in Spanish who arrived in America and wrote documents about the pineapple varieties and also added the varieties of Indies. The plant "pineapple" was named as it looks like a pine cone (Ashraf et al. 2011). The native word Tupi was anana for the fruit which means excellent fruit. This is the common word in many languages. The pineapple was seen in stamped decorations and was an old sign for welcome (Barrett and Lloyd 2012). Pineapple was imported from the Caribbean in the 17th century due to its rareness and exotic features. Pineapple was considered a symbol for the wealthy family in America (Delian et al. 2012). The Portuguese introduced this fruit in whole tropical regions and the east and south coasts of Africa, China, Java, south India, Madagascar, Philippines, and Malaysia. Nowadays, pineapple plant varieties are available in medicinal, edible, and industrial applications (Kaparapu et al. 2020). Say for example, bromelain enzyme helps in respiration as it is extracted from its leaves. A combination of pineapple juice and salad is a dominant cleaner for boat decks. Pineapple dehydrated waste material is used as feed for chickens, pigs, cattle, and so forth (Pandey 2014).

### 9.2.1 Pineapple Characteristics and Physiology

Pineapple is highly known as an exotic fruit because of its juiciness, flavor, and aroma. There are many varieties of pineapple as it depends on the various shapes, colors, flavor, and sizes (Sharma 2015). Pineapple is medium in size than other tropical fruits which include various fruitlets. It leads to the maturation process from the top to the bottom part of the fruit (Banks et al. 2013). Pineapple is a non-climacteric fruits so the quality of the fruit changes. It does not change uniformly. It changes at the different levels of maturity (Ali et al. 2020).Indicators of maturity in pineapple are evaluated on the basis of chemical, physical, and physicochemical characteristics of the fruit with morphological and flavor characteristics. The postharvest handling and management affect the shelf life and quality of pineapple (Abu Bakar et al. 2013). In Malaysia, different varieties of pineapples are cultivated. The utilization of pineapple waste is high in the market in term of post-handling of the process of pineapple (Adiani et al. 2020). After planting, the pineapple tree bears the fruit up to 15 months to 2 years. After planting, the first three initial months are the important steps for the blossoming of fruit and ripening of the plant until it becomes sensitive to the cloud cover and temperature. The requirements of the crop are a 20°C and 30°C optimum temperature with proper sunlight and higher precipitation for pineapple growth (Amuah et al. 2019). The period of harvesting is one other important principle to assess the quality of pineapple that affects the chemical composition of the fruit. The maturity stage along with the different diseases and pests are the key points investigated in growing pineapples (De Ancos et al. 2016). The peel color depends on the harvesting time when it turns from green to yellow by semi-mechanized or manual harvesting. According to the standard sizes and shapes, pineapples are graded. There are several indicators like mechanical defects or different conditions which will affect the quality of food. The quality of food is said to be good when it is free from the serious defects (Antoniolli et al. 2012). Consequently, the harvesting decision is judged in terms of quality of fruit that depends on the maximum shelf life and post-harvest storage. The selected pineapples are then packed and transported which depends on the maturity, size, shape, and many other factors dependent on the condition of the fruit after harvest (Angel et al. 2015). Before the process of packaging, several steps are done like waxing, washing, drying, and fungicide treatment. After these processes, the pineapple precooled at 13°C to 15°C which depends on the dimension of the fruit for 12 hours (Aragón et al. 2012). Precooling is an essential process as it avoids the growth of microbes and stops the enzymatic degradation. The fruit is analyzed for the control of quality before it is packed and it is sealed until the period of shipment (Asim et al. 2015). During storage, the temperature should be between 8°C and 10°C in which packed fruits in cold storage room are loaded on pallets. The fruit should be stored at 85% to 95% relative humidity with a 10°C to 15°C temperature up to 1 month regarding the pineapple shelf life (Ali et al. 2020). Low temperature should be recommended for the storage of the fruit. The symptoms of chilling injury like quality deterioration, flesh and peel darkening, and imperfect fruit color progression will occur if the temperature is below 8°C. During the yield production, the internal quality characteristics mostly depend on the postharvest handling and storage condition (Campos et al. 2020). Pineapple has different varieties with different composition values and maturity stages. Today more than 100 varieties of pineapple exist, but only 6 to 8 pineapple varieties are produced commercially. Smooth Cayenne is the main variety of pineapple including more than 70% of cultivated pineapples around the world (Cannon and Ho 2018). Now it has been replaced by the MD2 which has been produced by the Smooth Cayenne hybridization. The MD2 has a longer lifespan, high sugar content and is more aromatic as likened to the other variations of pineapple. Morris is another variety of pineapple which is originated from the Queen Variety as it has a high resistance to disease and pest (Chaudhary et al. 2019). It is responsible for good flavor as it has deep yellow flesh, high sugar, and a spongy texture. This variety is mainly distributed in the native markets and exported as a yield fresh. The size, aroma, appearance, and skin color are the chief aspects which determine the quality of pineapple. Fresh consumption of the fruits depends on the type of variety and the maturity levels which are the internal attributes (Chiet et al. 2014).

### 9.2.2 Food Processing Industry

Fruits contain proteins, minerals, vitamins, and dietary fibers. There is a requirement to do the processing of fruits as to increase the shelf life and storage as they are perishable in nature (Dittakan et al. 2018). Fruit processing is done in many ways like drying, canning, new ingredient creation, and freezing so as to increase the value in the fruits.

There are many forms of processed fruits (Figure 9.1).

- Fresh pre-prepared which contains fruit salads as they have a short storage life because they include many ingredients like flavorings and sauces.

- Canned, such as canned peaches, apricots, mixed fruits, pineapple, and pears.

- Frozen items that contain frozen berries, pineapple, and mangoes which have a long convenience, easy storage, shelf life.

- Dried that contains dried apples, prunes, and apricots who have a shorter time period than fresh fruits.

- Juices that contain fresh fruit (Jain et al. 2022).

The fruit processing layout was proposed by the Central Food Technological Research Institute, Mysore, for the production of fruit juices. The process is done in four steps (Figure 9.2). In the first step, matured and fully ripe fruits

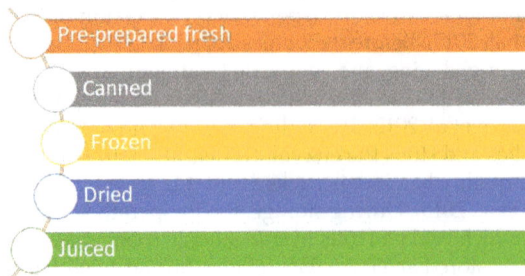

**Figure 9.1** Many forms of processed fruits. (From Dolhaji et al. 2018.)

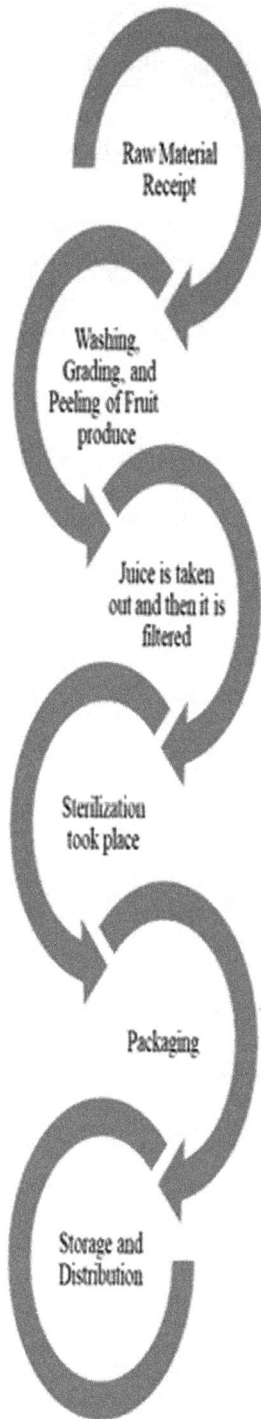

**Figure 9.2** Layout of the process of fruit processing. (From Soloman et al. 2016.)

are washed, cleaned, graded, and peeled. Now, juice is taken out from the fruits. It is then filtered so that seeds and fibers can be removed (Adelakun and Taiwo 2020). Now, the extracted juice is processed then sterilized. Now preservatives are added and then it is bottled. The sugar syrup and preservatives are added in juice in squash. Now it is mixed well until an even solution is achieved and then it is bottled. It can be explained well through a flowchart (Figure 9.3).

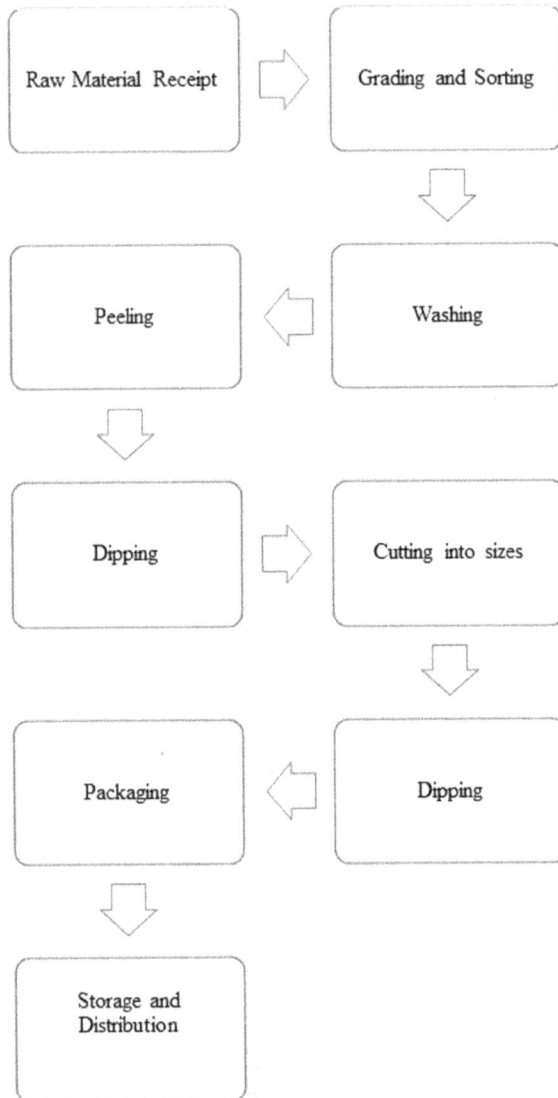

**Figure 9.3** Layout of the process of fruit processing of pineapple. (From Guimarães et al. 2016.)

There are many processes for the processing of pineapple (Guimarães et al. 2016).

- Firstly, the fresh cut and raw fruits are taken.

- Then sorting and grading for the wholesome fruit is done. After that fruit is kept till the fruit becomes yellow and achieves firmness at room temperature.

- When the fruit becomes firm then inspection is done and transferred into the washing tank.

- It is then chlorinated for five minutes at 200–500 ppm.

- After that, the skin is peeled with a sharp knife and fruit is cut into two halves lengthwise.

- After cutting, seeds are taken out with a spoon and underneath the tissue trim the seeds.

- Now packaging is done in which portions are kept in the boxes with cover in 5°C to allow it to store in a cool storage area.

- At the end, boxes are prepared for distribution to the consumer.

### 9.2.3 Nutritive Value of Pineapple

Macro- and micronutrients are found in the pineapple which makes it a nutritionally and valuably rich product. Due to the environmental condition and clone growth, there is variation in the nutrients and phytochemicals in pineapple (Hossain and Rahman 2011). The evaluation for this fruit composition is done by the researchers over the past years.

### 9.2.4 Macronutrients

Some authors say that macronutrients are those nutrients that provide the energy and some define that they are required in large amounts. Macronutrients include proteins, fats, and alcohol. However, some authors exclude the alcohol and include the dietary fiber and water (Ikram et al. 2020). Lipids and protein have low contribution in the pineapple fruit. The main source of energy in foods are carbohydrates. It provides 40% to 80% around total energy (Ismail et al. 2018). Types of carbohydrates also play a crucial role in the human health. Therefore, carbohydrates are very essential in our diet. Pineapple contains 80% of carbohydrates (Kargutkar and Brijesh 2018). Glucose, fructose, and sucrose are the sugars that are found in the pineapple. Sucrose is found in higher levels as compared to the other monosaccharides (Khalid et al. 2016). The sugars play a crucial role in the pineapple quality as to maintain the flavor quality and commercial acceptability. Pineapple is a fruit which is non-climacteric, so its sugar level depends on the time of harvest. The second carbohydrate found in pineapple is dietary fiber which leads to the few calories in the body (Lasekan and Abbas 2012). High dietary fruits like pineapple are highly suggested so as to prevent and reduce the problems of obesity. It also leads to other benefits such as quick intestinal transit, inhibition of some diseases like promotion of satiety and diverticulitis (Lasekan 2016).

### 9.2.5 Micronutrients

Micronutrients are those that are required in a low amount in the diet. They comprise minerals and vitamins which are the whole group of nutrients (Lasekan and Hussein 2018). Minerals are the inorganic compounds required in small amounts which are essential for life. Vitamins are the substances which enable the growth of human life and health present in the food (Leneveu-Jenvrin et al. 2020). Abundant health organizations have recommended the proper intake of micronutrients along with macronutrients in the diet around the world. As per the United States Food and Drug Administration (FDA), micro- and macronutrients are a good source as each food serving contains 10%–19% adequate intake or RDA for every nutrient (Lobo and Yahia 2017). Pineapples are excellent mineral (sodium and potassium) and vitamin sources (vitamin C, riboflavin, and thiamine). Some authors say that antioxidants which are the cluster of non-toxic mixtures are the micronutrients (Lorenzoni et al. 2012). Antioxidant micronutrients are defined as those which neutralize the oxidative stress and are involved in the many metabolic processes in the human body. Minerals (selenium and zinc) and vitamins (C, A, and E) are the foremost antioxidant micronutrients (Phoophuangpairoj and Srikun 2014). Nevertheless, phenolic mixtures are the main antioxidant complexes in the human diet because of its abundance and variety of plant origins in foods (Luengwilai et al. 2018).

## 9.3 ROLE OF PINEAPPLE IN FUNCTIONAL FOODS AND NUTRACEUTICALS

### 9.3.1 Important Functional Ingredients in Pineapple

This fruit has exceptional vibrant flavor, vast health benefits, and juiciness (Baniwal et al. 2021). It is the tank of minerals, antioxidants, and vitamins (Figure 9.4).

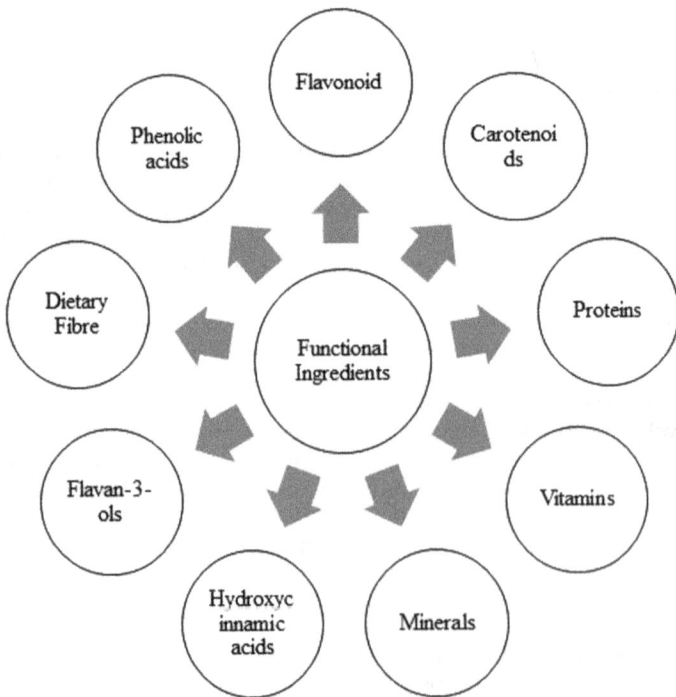

**Figure 9.4** Important functional ingredients in pineapple. (From Najeeb et al. 2021.)

A proteolytic enzyme (bromelain) which is sulfur-containing in pineapple helps in the digestion process. Pineapple is a natural anti-inflammatory and digestive aid fruit. It contains the phenolic substances in large amounts (Pino 2013). Pineapple is rich in fiber so it is very effective in curative irregular bowel movements and constipation. In any of the conditions like motion sickness, morning sickness, and nausea, pineapple juice is very effective (Prado and Spinacé 2019). It is full of macro- and micronutrients that are very necessary for the growth and development of physique. Fresh pineapple is also used to cure chest congestion, diphtheria, and bronchitis (Priyadarshani et al. 2019).

### 9.3.1.1 Polyphenols

- *Flavonid:* In pineapple, Myricetin was the abundant polyphenol found in it.

- *Flavan-3-ols:* A little Epicatechin is found in pineapple pulp and core. Basically hydro-phenolic compounds, i.e. flavan-3-ols are found in pineapple peel (Reinhardt et al. 2018). Higher amounts of Catechin and Epicatechin are observed in the dry fruit extract.

- *Phenolic acids:* In pineapple, Gallic acid was observed as a main polyphenol (Prabhu et al. 2021).
  - *Proteins:* Bromelain is found in fresh pineapples.
  - *Vitamins:* Vitamin B1, vitamin B6, and vitamin C are found in pineapple.
  - *Minerals:* The trace mineral Manganese is found in pineapple which is an important cofactor in many enzymes in antioxidant defenses and energy production Rahim et al. 2019). Calcium and potassium are also found in the pineapple. Manganese plays an important role in the growth of tissues and bones (Rahim et al. 2014).

### 9.3.2 Functional Ingredients with Its Properties

The functional ingredients are mostly the macro- and micronutrients and polyphenols which people can consume from pineapple (Table 9.2). These ingredients are taken regularly into the body (Neto et al. 2013).

### 9.3.2.1 Polyphenols

Polyphenols are naturally present in vegetables and fruits as they have groups of antioxidants (Kumar et al. 2018). They mainly consist of flavonoids that include isoflavones, flavones, flavonones, flavanols, anthocyanins, flavonols, and non-flavonoid polyphenols that include stilbenes, lignans, and phenolic acids (Sharma et al. 2016b). Direct quenching or scavenging of free oxygen radicals and enzyme inhibition that are used in oxidation are characterization of the mechanism of antioxidant activity of polyphenols (Fong and Hing 2016).

### 9.3.3 Pineapple as a Nutraceutical Source

Pineapple is a nutraceutical source which gives many beneficial health effects. It has the medicinal properties which have beneficial effects to the human body (Kumar et al. 2016). The fruits can decrease chronic diseases and promote well-being. These fruits are required on a daily basis. The fruits have a number of nutraceuticals which are very necessary for human health (Olaiya et al. 2016). Some fruits have strong antioxidant properties as well as rich nutraceutical properties like apple, banana, bael, custard apple, citrus, grape, guava, Indian blackberry, lemon, mango, mangosteen, papaya, pomegranate, pineapple, and sweet orange. These are the well-known sources of nutraceuticals (Shinde et al. 2014).

## Table 9.2: Functional Ingredients with Its Properties

| Functional Ingredients | | Properties | References |
|---|---|---|---|
| **Flavonoids** | | | |
| Flavonols | Myricetin | • Inhibit the oxidation of low density lipoprotein<br>• Reduce atherosclerosis<br>• Reduce cardiovascular disease<br>• Colon cancer inhibition | (Siti Rashima et al. 2019; Siti Roha et al. 2013) |
| Flavan-3-ols | Catechin | • Work as antitumor in stomach, liver duodenum, lungs, esophagus, and pancreas<br>• Prevent chronic inflammation which is related with carcinogenesis<br>• Reduce the making of nitrite<br>• Reduce cardiovascular disease<br>• Inhibit the low density lipoprotein oxidation<br>• Prevent the nitrosation | (Basumatary et al. 2021; Steingass et al. 2016) |
| | Epicatechin | • Decrease the diabetes<br>• Attenuation of heart health | (Steingass et al. 2014) |
| Carotenoids | β-carotene | • Inhibit cancer in mammary gland endometrium and lungs, colon, and liver<br>• Protect cornea against UV-induced erythema | (Steingass et al. 2020) |
| **Phenolic Acids** | | | |
| Hydroxybenzoic acid | Gallic acid | • Reduce hypertension, dyslipidemia, and atherosclerosis | (Steingass et al. 2015) |
| Hydroxycinnamic acid | Chlorogenic acid | • Prevent the hardening from arteries<br>• Prevent colon cancer | (Vollmer et al. 2020) |
| | Ferulic acid | • Protect from tumor<br>• Prevent degeneration of bone<br>• Protect from the symptoms of menopause | (Wei et al. 2014) |
| Dietary fibers | Hemi-cellulose, pectin | • Maintain bowel movement<br>• Lower the levels of cholesterol<br>• Control blood sugar levels | (Wei et al. 2011) |
| Proteins | Bromelain | • Act as anti-inflammatory<br>• Speed up recovery from surgery and injuries<br>• Remove the plaque from arterial walls<br>• Reduce blood clotting | (Yoyponsan et al. 2019 ; Zdrojewicz et al. 2018) |
| Vitamins | C, A, B1, B2, B3 | • Maintain healthy vision<br>• Improve immune functions<br>• Maintain bone health<br>• Regulate calcium and phosphorus by cell integrity | (Zhang et al. 2012 ; Zheng et al. 2012) |
| Minerals | K, Ca, P, Fe, Mn, Mg | • Decrease the danger of stroke and high BP<br>• Help in RBC production<br>• Prevent muscle cramps<br>• Proper functioning of tissues and cells | (Chaudhari et al. 2017 ; Singh and Sinha 2012) |

### 9.3.4 Disease Management with Nutraceuticals

Pineapple creates water residue in the form of pulp and peels. In these residues, phenolic compounds are present, which impart the nutraceutical properties in the fruit (Borkar et al. 2015). These properties, which are related to biology like antimutagenicity, antitumor, and antiaging activities, and not aggravating allergy activity, have been considered as both natural and synthetic antioxidants. Special consideration is highlighted on the bioactive compounds extracted from residual and expensive sources (McClements et al. 2015). In fruit residues, different phenolics are present which have antioxidant properties. Nutraceuticals and biopreservatives are there in the fruit residues. In pineapple, flavonols are present, which have anticancer, antioxidative, anti-inflammatory, and antiviral properties (Malla et al. 2013). It inhibits the human platelet aggregation and effect on capillary fragility. These antioxidants protect the cells from free radicals which inhibit the cancer and mutation because they act as a scavenging role (Malla et al. 2013). They protect against hydroxyl radicals, peroxy radicals, and superoxide anion which are the reactive oxygen species. Antioxidants act in various ways which include scavenging of free radicals, decomposition of peroxides, and forming complexes of redox-catalytic metal ions (Baker et al. 2012). There is a strong relation between a diet rich in fruits and vegetables and an increase in life expectancy and a decrease in the risk of cancer. The presence of phenolic acid in pineapple is responsible for antimutagenicity (Pal et al. 2014). Phenolic complexes reduce the low-density lipoprotein (LDL) oxidation as these compounds have hydroxyl groups shown in many of the research studies. These hydroxyl groups reduce the atherogenesis and prevent the LDL (Verma and Mishra 2016). Nutraceuticals also protect against cardiovascular diseases. Phenol based nutraceutical and functional food help to fight against CVD. Nutraceuticals found in pineapple also help in the prevention and cure of neurodegenerative disorders (Kannappan et al. 2011). It also helps to prevent metabolic disorders like obesity and diabetes.

## 9.4 BIOACTIVE COMPOUNDS FOUND IN PINEAPPLE

The compounds which are found in food in small constituents are called bioactive compounds. They are extra nutritional constituents (Gupta et al. 2014). These compounds are linked with the human body to give a positive effect on the well-being particularly on cardiovascular diseases, cancer, and aging. These compounds have a free radical scavenging ability and antioxidant properties (Manosroi et al. 2014). Many bioactive compounds are introduced. They are grouped on the bases of their chemical structure and function like flavonoids, glucosinolates, carotenoids, DF, monoterpenes, phytosterols, and ascorbic acid which is an active molecule. In pineapple pulp, the main bioactive compounds found are ascorbic acid, carotenoids, and PC which have antioxidant properties (Parashar et al. 2014). The important sources of bound phenolics and DF are pineapple by-products such as shells. Furthermore, pineapple is the richest source of bromelain, a medicinal drug which is a group of compounds, i.e. proteinase and many bioactive compounds (Praveen et al. 2014).

### 9.4.1 Ascorbic Acid

Pineapple contains a high level of vitamin C, which is also called ascorbic acid. Pineapple has antioxidants which are naturally water soluble and inhibit the development of major clinical conditions (Figure 9.5).

### 9.4.2 Phenolic Acid

Phenolic acid compounds are found in pineapple as the bioactive compounds essential for our health benefits (Figure 9.6). Phenolic compounds in pineapple depend on the variety, maturity, growing conditions as well as the environmental factors (Shinde et al. 2014).

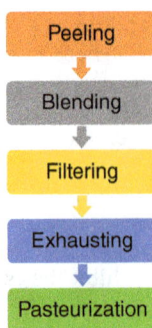

**Figure 9.5** Flowchart of different operations in pineapple.

The phenolic compounds content in pineapple is higher in residue as compared to flesh. In many studies it was shown that phenolic complexes have a parallel correlation with the antioxidant activities found in pineapple (Rajat et al. 2012).

### 9.4.3 Carotenoids

The most widespread pigments are carotenoids found in the pineapple as it contains the lipophilic and pro-vitamin A antioxidants (Figure 9.7). The carotenoid compounds contain the number of epoxide group which are found in pineapple (Figure 9.8).

### 9.4.4 Dietary Fiber

Non-starch polysaccharides are called dietary fiber (Mehra et al. 2020). Dietary fiber is the carbohydrate polymers which are not hydrolyzed by enzymes as

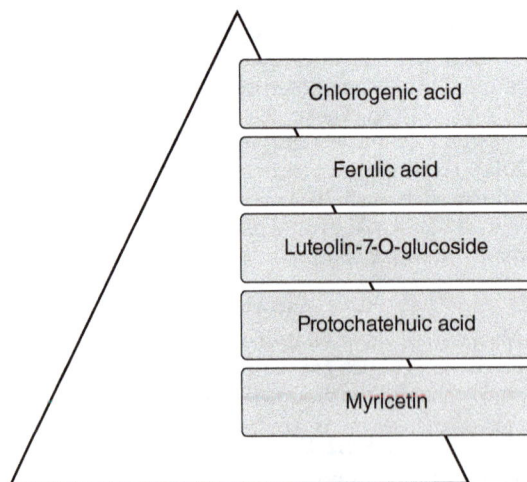

**Figure 9.6** Varieties of phenolic compounds found in pineapple. (From Shinde et al. 2014.)

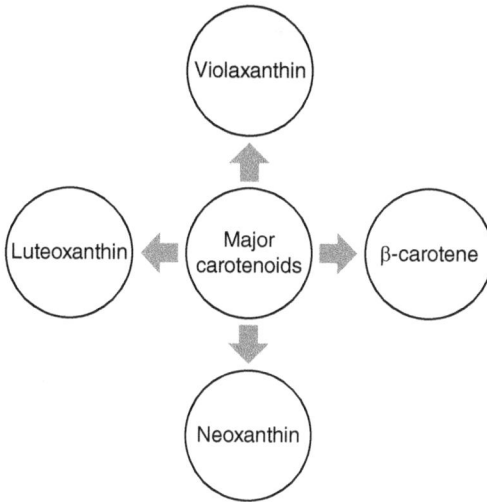

**Figure 9.7** Major carotenoids found in pineapple. (From Stephen 2013.)

they have 10 or more monomeric units (Figure 9.9). In the small intestine, these enzymes are found. The amount of dietary fiber found in pineapple depends on the variety of pineapple and its part (Ajit 2012). Dietary fiber is divided into two parts, i.e. water soluble and water insoluble depending on the solubility which has beneficial effects in the prevention of several diseases like diabetes and cardiovascular diseases (Smarta 2012).

Pineapple and its by-products are good sources of dietary fibers. By-products found in dietary fibers are used as an ingredient for functional and nutraceutical food products (Dall'Asta et al. 2012). High preservation of white color, colorants, high resistance to traction, and salt vapor are the natural properties found in the dietary fibers which are considered as the most favorable conditions in the food industry (Freitas et al. 2015).

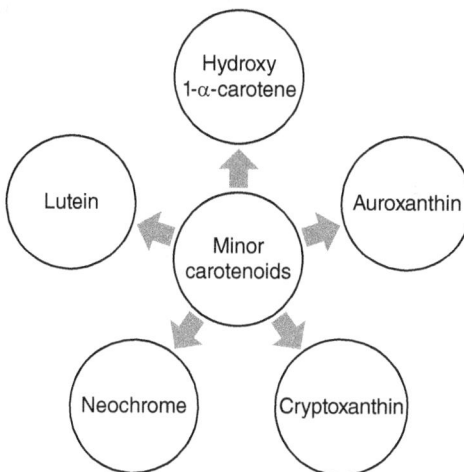

**Figure 9.8** Minor carotenoids found in pineapple. (From Patil 2011.)

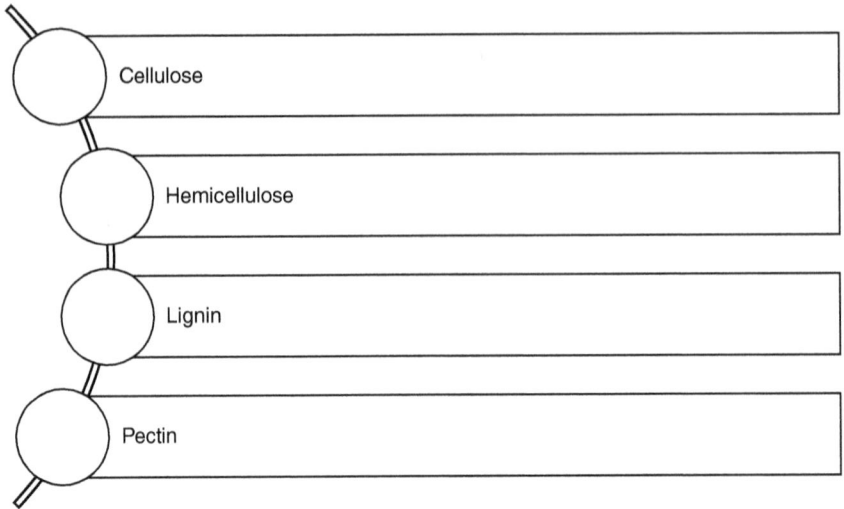

**Figure 9.9** Dietary fiber found in pineapple fiber. (From Çelik et al. 2015.)

### 9.4.5 Antioxidant Dietary Fibers

It is a natural product which combines the technological effect with beneficial health along with the natural antioxidants (Fu et al. 2011). In many studies it was seen that the parts of pineapple are the main source of dietary fiber which is associated with the phenolics that lead to the antioxidant activity (Figure 9.10).

Antioxidants are very beneficial for the health of the human. They protect from various diseases like diabetes, cardiovascular diseases, neurodegenerative diseases, regulation of insulin levels in blood, some types of cancer, and hypertension (Lu et al. 2014).

### 9.4.6 Bromelain

Bromelain is the proteolytic enzyme. This bioactive ingredient is the richest source found in pineapple found in many of the studies (Quirós-Sauceda et al. 2014). It is the complex combination of protease and non-protease compounds

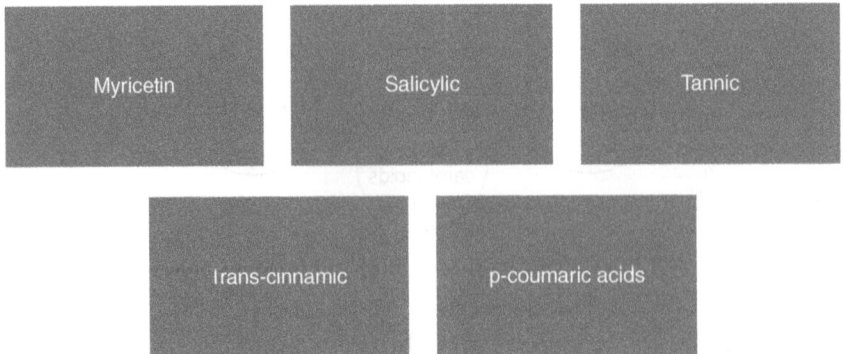

**Figure 9.10** Phenolic compound identified in the dietary fiber. (From Isuwan 2014.)

along with the other substances in small quantities. A free sulfhydryl group of proteolytic enzymes is necessary for proper enzymatic activity (da Silva et al. 2014). In the stem, bromelain is the present which is called stem bromelain. Bromelain is also present in fruit along with the pineapple by-product which is present in small quantities (Soares et al. 2012).

## 9.5 TRADITIONAL AND HEALTH BENEFITS OF PINEAPPLE
### 9.5.1 Traditional Uses

In several native cultures, pineapples are used as a medicinal plant. The fruit and roots of pineapple are eaten or applied as digestive and anti-inflammatory (Tuohy et al. 2012). In Tripura, it was traditionally utilized as an antiparasitic agent. Since 1876, bromelain has been known chemically. It is highly found in the pineapple stems and acts as a therapeutic compound (Sepúlveda et al. 2018). The fruit and roots of pineapple are eaten or applied as a proteolytic enzyme. In Tripura, pineapple is used as a vermifuge agent (Jirapornvaree et al. 2017). In some cultures, pineapple is associated with the welcome purpose. It is also used in woodworking as carved decorations. Pineapple is also used as a gift when meeting a person for the first time (Zakaria et al. 2021).

### 9.5.2 Health Uses

Many studies have proved that an adequate amount of nutrient intake is very essential for the human health (Figure 9.11). Pineapple was considered as the most effective bioactive component for health purpose (Zaki et al. 2017). The fruit is important as a diuretic, in the removal of intestinal worms as well as a contraceptive. Pineapple is used to boost the fat excretion as well as to increase the appetite for the nourishment in food (Meena et al. 2021). It acts as a proteolytic enzyme because of the bromelain which protect the soft tissues from inflammation. While its primary usage is as an anti-inflammatory, researchers have also shown that it has anticancer and antibacterial properties.

Pineapple is a good source of vitamins and micronutrients which are crucial for daily intake. Pineapple is incorporated in the diet as it has low calories (Roda and Lambri 2019). Pineapple is the richest source of vitamin C. Vitamin C keeps the cells healthy and acts as an antioxidant which fights against free radicals (Li and Komarek 2017). It delays osteoblast aging and monitors diabetic progression. Thiamine content present in pineapple also plays an essential part in monitoring the function of the nervous system (Nasri et al. 2014). Pineapple is important for those persons who suffer from the difficulty of the nervous system as it reduces the glucose metabolic level, red blood cell production as well as in diabetes (Selani et al. 2014). Pineapple is the richest source in dietary fiber as it

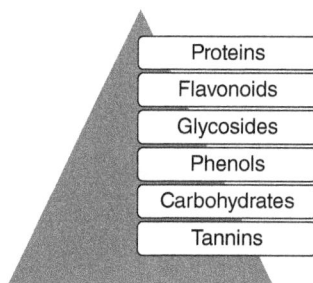

**Figure 9.11** Components in pineapple extract. (From Meena et al. 2021.)

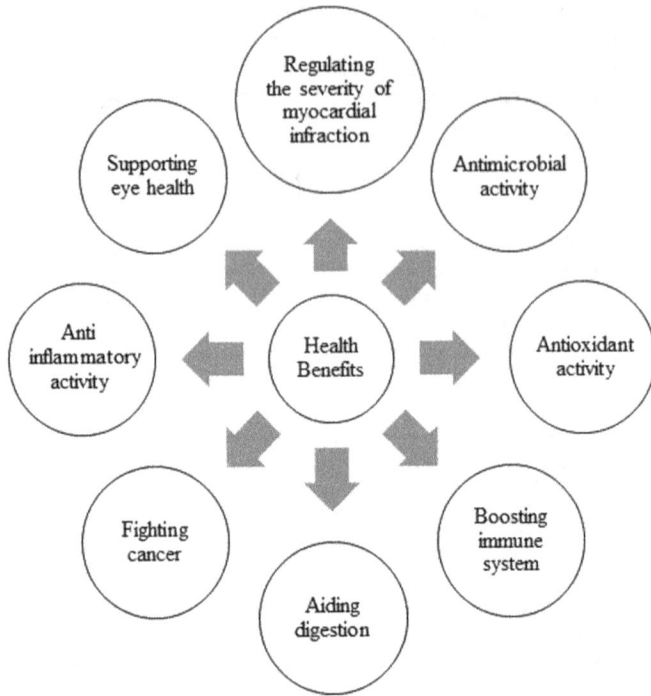

**Figure 9.12** Health benefits in pineapple.

heals the bowel movements and gastrointestinal function as well as constipation (Figure 9.12). Many researchers proved that dietary fiber is essential to reduce (Ackom and Tano-Debrah 2012)

- Colon cancer risk
- Cerebro-vascular risk
- Symptoms of diabetes and diarrhea

It was well-known that malic acid helps in preserving dental plaque formation, oral health as well as enhancing immunity present in pineapple. One of the trace elements found in pineapple is manganese which is very important for energy production (Devi et al. 2016). It controls blood glucose, alleviation of skeletal defects, insulin resistance, and type 2 diabetes. The trace elements include transferases and ligases which permit the effect of enzymes in oxidation and fight against the free radicals so as to degrade the cholesterol (Achumi et al. 2018). Many authors say that pineapple is very important for strengthening bone growth and for regulating emotional stability in adults. Pineapple is the richest source in bromelain which is a complex bioactive compound. It helps in the improvement of digestion, acts as an antioxidant and cardioprotective agent in the view of nutrients' components (Amaravathi et al. 2014). Bromelain is also used for the recovery of the following (Okeke et al. 2015):

- Sinusitis
- Pneumonia

- Bacterial infections
- Parasitic gastrointestinal infections, bronchitis
- Fights against the intestinal parasites such as nematodes and tapeworms

It is commonly used in treating the patient who are suffering from (Biswas et al. 2016).

- Thrombophlebitis so as to settle the edema, inflammation and skin infection
- Regulating the severity of myocardial infarction

## 9.6 CONCLUSION

It is the one of the most essential fruit crops in the universe. The pineapple can be consumed as raw or fresh pineapple juice. Pineapple is also considered as part of a medical diet for some of the diseases. The pineapple can be used as nutritional fruit. Macro- and micronutrients are found in the pineapple which make it a nutritionally and valuably rich product. This fruit has exceptionally vibrant flavor, vast health benefits, and juiciness. It is the tank of minerals, antioxidants and vitamins. A proteolytic enzyme (bromelain), which is sulfur-containing in pineapple, helps in the digestion process. Bioactive compounds are present in pineapple and have a positive effect on the well-being, particularly on cardiovascular diseases, cancer, and delaying the aging process. The ripe fruits which are on the field are best for eating purposes, but it is essential to remove the eyes, rind, crown, and core. Pineapples are utilized as juice, canned food, and fresh fruit. It can be used in a variety of food variants like jam, fruit salad, dessert, candy, ice cream, and as a supplement to meat dishes. It can be consumed in the form of salads, desserts, puddings, as a garnish, cake, cooked in pies, and made into preserves and sauces. Pineapple can also be utilized in various meal dishes and curries.

## REFERENCES

Abu Bakar, B. H., Ishak, A. J., Shamsuddin, R., & Wan Hassan, W. Z. (2013). Ripeness level classification for pineapple using RGB and HSI colour maps. *Journal of Theoretical & Applied Information Technology, 57*(3), 587–593.

Achumi, L. V., Peter, E. R. S., & Das, A. (2018). Studies on preparation of gummy candy using pineapple juice and carrot juice. *International Journal of Chemical Studies, 6*(5), 1015–1018.

Ackom, N. B., & Tano-Debrah, K. (2012). Processing pineapple pulp into dietary fibre supplement. *African Journal of Food, Agriculture, Nutrition and Development, 12*(6), 6823–6834.

Adelakun, O. E., & Taiwo, O. T. (2020). Physico-chemical and organoleptic evaluation of drink produced from pineapple (*Ananas comosus*) and tigernut (*Cyperus esculentus*). *Asian Food Science Journal, 14*(2), 1–8.

Adiani, V., Gupta, S., & Variyar, P. S. (2020). Microbial quality assessment of minimally processed pineapple using GCMS and FTIR in tandem with chemometrics. *Scientific Reports, 10*(1), 1–9.

Ajit, S. (2012). Nutraceuticals—Critical supplement for building a healthy India. *Ernst and Young, FICCI Task Force on Nutraceuticals,* 1–80.

Ali, M. M., Hashim, N., Abd Aziz, S., & Lasekan, O. (2020). Pineapple (*Ananas comosus*): A comprehensive review of nutritional values, volatile compounds, health benefits, and potential food products. *Food Research International, 137*, 109675.

Amaravathi, T., Vennila, P., Hemalatha, G., & Parimalam, P. (2014). Spiced pineapple ready-to-serve beverages. *Indian Journal of Science and Technology, 7*(11), 1831.

Amuah, C. L., Teye, E., Lamptey, F. P., Nyandey, K., Opoku-Ansah, J., & Adueming, P. O. W. (2019). Feasibility study of the use of handheld NIR spectrometer for simultaneous authentication and quantification of quality parameters in intact pineapple fruits. *Journal of Spectroscopy, 2019* 1–9.

Angel, L., Lizcano, S., & Viola, J. (2015, September). Assessing the state of maturation of the pineapple in its perolera variety using computer vision techniques. In *2015 20th Symposium on Signal Processing, Images and Computer Vision (STSIVA)* (pp. 1–6). IEEE.

Antoniolli, L. R., Benedetti, B. C., Souza Filho, M. D. S. M. D., Garruti, D. D. S., & Borges, M. D. F. (2012). Shelf life of minimally processed pineapples treated with ascorbic and citric acids. *Bragantia, 71*, 447–453.

Aragón, C., Carvalho, L., González, J., Escalona, M., & Amancio, S. (2012). The physiology of ex vitro pineapple (*Ananas comosus* L. Merr. var MD-2) as CAM or C3 is regulated by the environmental conditions. *Plant Cell Reports, 31*(4), 757–769.

Arun, K. B., Persia, F., Aswathy, P. S., Chandran, J., Sajeev, M. S., Jayamurthy, P., & Nisha, P. (2015). Plantain peel-a potential source of antioxidant dietary fibre for developing functional cookies. *Journal of Food Science and Technology, 52*(10), 6355–6364.

Ashraf, C. M., Iqbal, S., & Ahmed, D. (2011). Nutritional and physicochemical studies on fruit pulp, seed and shell of indigenous *Prunus persica*. *Journal of Medicinal Plants Research, 5*(16), 3917–3921.

Asim, M., Abdan, K., Jawaid, M., Nasir, M., Dashtizadeh, Z., Ishak, M. R., & Hoque, M. E. (2015). A review on pineapple leaves fibre and its composites. *International Journal of Polymer Science, 2015*, 1–16.

Asim, M., Jawaid, M., Abdan, K., & Ishak, M. R. (2017, December). Dimensional stability of pineapple leaf fibre reinforced phenolic composites. In *AIP Conference Proceedings* (vol. 1901, no. 1, p. 030016). AIP Publishing LLC.

Baker, V., Brady, B., & Veling, M. (2012). Regulatory environment for nutraceuticals and functional foods. National Research Council Canada Publications Archive, 11-6536.

Banik, S., Nag, D., & Debnath, S. (2011). Utilization of pineapple leaf agro-waste for extraction of fibre and the residual biomass for vermicomposting. *Indian Journal of Fibre and Textile Research* 36(2), pp. 172–177

Baniwal, P., Mehra, R., Kumar, N., Sharma, S., & Kumar, S. (2021). Cereals: Functional constituents and its health benefits. *Pharma Innovation Journal, 10*(2), 343–349.

Banks, J. M., Herman, C. T., & Bailey, R. C. (2013). Bromelain decreases neutrophil interactions with P-selectin, but not E-selectin, in vitro by proteolytic cleavage of P-selectin glycoprotein ligand-1. *PLoS One, 8*(11), e78988.

Barrett, D. M., & Lloyd, B. (2012). Advanced preservation methods and nutrient retention in fruits and vegetables. *Journal of the Science of Food and Agriculture, 92*(1), 7–22.

Basumatary, I. B., Mukherjee, A., Katiyar, V., Kumar, S., & Dutta, J. (2021). Chitosan-based antimicrobial coating for improving postharvest shelf life of pineapple. *Coatings, 11*(11), 1366.

Biswas, S., Masih, D., Singh, M., & Sonkar, C. (2016). Development and quality evaluation of Aloe vera and pineapple juice blended beverage. *International Research Journal of Engineering and Technology, 3*(10), 214–220.

Borkar, N., Saurabh, S. S., Rathore, K. S., Pandit, A., & Khandelwal, K. R. (2015). An insight on nutraceuticals. *PharmaTutor, 3*(8), 13–23.

Campos, D. A., Ribeiro, T. B., Teixeira, J. A., Pastrana, L., & Pintado, M. M. (2020). Integral valorization of pineapple (*Ananas comosus* L.) by-products through a green chemistry approach towards added value ingredients. *Foods, 9*(1), 60.

Cannon, R. J., & Ho, C. T. (2018). Volatile sulfur compounds in tropical fruits. *Journal of Food and Drug Analysis, 26*(2), 445–468.

Çelik, E. E., Gökmen, V., & Skibsted, L. H. (2015). Synergism between soluble and dietary fiber bound antioxidants. *Journal of Agricultural and Food Chemistry, 63*(8), 2338–2343.

Chaudhari, S. P., Powar, P. V., & Pratapwar, M. N. (2017). Nutraceuticals: A review. *World Journal of Pharmacy and Pharmaceutical Sciences, 6*, 681–739.

Chaudhary, V., Kumar, V., Vaishali, S., Sing, K., Kumar, R., & Kumar, V. (2019). Pineapple (*Ananas comosus*) product processing a review. *Journal of Pharmacognosy and Phytochemistry, 8*(3), 4642–4652.

Cherian, B. M., Leão, A. L., de Souza, S. F., Costa, L. M. M., de Olyveira, G. M., Kottaisamy, M., ... & Thomas, S. (2011). Cellulose nanocomposites with nanofibres isolated from pineapple leaf fibers for medical applications. *Carbohydrate Polymers, 86*(4), 1790–1798.

Chiet, C. H., Zulkifli, R. M., Hidayat, T., & Yaakob, H. (2014, March). Bioactive compounds and antioxidant activity analysis of Malaysian pineapple cultivars. In *AIP Conference Proceedings* (vol. 1589, no. 1, pp. 398–399). American Institute of Physics.

da Silva, L. M. R., De Figueiredo, E. A. T., Ricardo, N. M. P. S., Vieira, I. G. P., De Figueiredo, R. W., Brasil, I. M., & Gomes, C. L. (2014). Quantification of bioactive compounds in pulps and by-products of tropical fruits from Brazil. *Food Chemistry, 143*, 398–404.

Dall'Asta, M., Calani, L., Tedeschi, M., Jechiu, L., Brighenti, F., & Del Rio, D. (2012). Identification of microbial metabolites derived from in vitro fecal fermentation of different polyphenolic food sources. *Nutrition, 28*(2), 197–203.

Daud, Z., Hatta, M. Z. M., Kassim, A. S. M., Awang, H., & Aripin, A. M. (2014). Exploring of agro waste (pineapple leaf, corn stalk, and Napier grass) by chemical composition and morphological study. *BioResources, 9*(1), 872–880.

De Ancos, B., Sánchez-Moreno, C., & González-Aguilar, G. A. (2016). Pineapple composition and nutrition. *Handbook of Pineapple Technology,* 221–239.

Delian, E., Chira, L., Dumitru, L., Bădulescu, L., Chira, A., & Petcuci, A. (2012). Mineral content of nectarines fruits in relation to some fertilization practices. *Scientific Papers, Series B, Horticulture, 6,* 73–80.

Devi, L. U., Bhagawan, S. S., & Thomas, S. (2011). Dynamic mechanical properties of pineapple leaf fiber polyester composites. *Polymer Composites, 32*(11), 1741–1750.

Devi, L. K., Karoulia, S., & Chaudhary, N. (2016). Preparation of high dietary fibre cookies from pineapple (*Ananas comosus*) pomace. *International Journal of Science and Research, 5,* 1368–1372.

Dittakan, K., Theera-Ampornpunt, N., & Boodliam, P. (2018, November). Non-destructive grading of Pattavia pineapple using texture analysis. In *2018 21st International Symposium on Wireless Personal Multimedia Communications (WPMC)* (pp. 144–149). IEEE.

Dolhaji, N. H., Muhamad, I. I., Ya'Akub, H., & Abd Aziz, A. (2018). Evaluation of chilling injury and internal browning condition on quality attributes, phenolic content, and antioxidant capacity during sub-optimal cold storage of Malaysian cultivar pineapples. *Malaysian Journal of Fundamental and Applied Sciences, 14*(4), 456–461.

Fong, S. L., & Hing, L. K. (2016). Determination of physicochemical properties of osmo-dehydrofrozen pineapples. *Borneo Science, 14,* 71–84.

Freitas, A., Moldão-Martins, M., Costa, H. S., Albuquerque, T. G., Valente, A., & Sanches-Silva, A. (2015). Effect of UV-C radiation on bioactive compounds of pineapple (*Ananas comosus* L. Merr.) by-products. *Journal of the Science of Food and Agriculture, 95*(1), 44–52.

Fu, L., Xu, B. T., Xu, X. R., Gan, R. Y., Zhang, Y., Xia, E. Q., & Li, H. B. (2011). Antioxidant capacities and total phenolic contents of 62 fruits. *Food Chemistry, 129*(2), 345–350.

Guimarães, G. H. C., Silva, R. S., Madruga, M. S., Sousa, A. S. B., Brito, A. L., Lima, R. P., ... & Silva, S. M. (2016, June). Effect of plant-based coatings on the volatile profile of "Pérola" pineapple. In *VIII International Postharvest Symposium: Enhancing Supply Chain and Consumer Benefits-Ethical and Technological Issues 1194* (pp. 1519–1526).

Gupta, C., Sharma, G., & Chan, D. (2014). Resveratrol: A chemo-preventative agent with diverse applications. In Prakash D., Sharma G. (Eds.), *Phytochemicals of Nutraceutical Importance,* 47–60.

Hossain, M. A., & Rahman, S. M. (2011). Total phenolics, flavonoids and antioxidant activity of tropical fruit pineapple. *Food Research International*, 44(3), 672–676.

Ikram, M. M. M., Ridwani, S., Putri, S. P., & Fukusaki, E. (2020). GC-MS based metabolite profiling to monitor ripening-specific metabolites in pineapple (*Ananas comosus*). *Metabolites*, 10(4), 134.

Ismail, N. A. M., Abdullah, N., & Muhammad, N. (2018). Effect of microwave-assisted processing on quality characteristics of pineapple jam. *Journal of Advanced Research in Fluid Mechanics and Thermal Sciences*, 42(1), 24–30.

Isuwan, A. (2014). Agronomic traits and fruit quality of pineapple with different levels of chicken manure application. *Science, Engineering and Health Studies*, 67–73.

Jain, A., Mehra, R., Garhwal, R., Rafiq, S., Sharma, S., Singh, B., … & Kumar, H. (2022). Manufacturing and characterization of whey and stevia-based popsicles enriched with concentrated beetroot juice. *Journal of Food Science and Technology*, 1–9.

Jawaid, M. H. P. S., & Khalil, H. A. (2011). Cellulosic/synthetic fibre reinforced polymer hybrid composites: A review. *Carbohydrate Polymers*, 86(1), 1–18.

Jirapornvaree, I., Suppadit, T., & Popan, A. (2017). Use of pineapple waste for production of decomposable pots. *International Journal of Recycling of Organic Waste in Agriculture*, 6(4), 345–350.

Kannappan, R., Gupta, S. C., Kim, J. H., Reuter, S., & Aggarwal, B. B. (2011). Neuroprotection by spice-derived nutraceuticals: You are what you eat! *Molecular Neurobiology*, 44(2), 142–159.

Kaparapu, J., Pragada, P. M., & Geddada, M. N. R. (2020). Fruits and vegetables and its nutritional benefits. In *Functional Foods and Nutraceuticals*, 241–260. Springer, Cham.

Kargutkar, S., & Brijesh, S. (2018). Anti-inflammatory evaluation and characterization of leaf extract of *Ananas comosus*. *Inflammopharmacology*, 26(2), 469–477.

Kashyap, P., Kumar, S., Riar, C. S., Jindal, N., Baniwal, P., Guiné, R. P., … & Kumar, H. (2022). Recent advances in drumstick (*Moringa oleifera*) leaves bioactive compounds: Composition, health benefits, bioaccessibility, and dietary applications. *Antioxidants*, 11(2), 402.

Khalid, N., Suleria, H. A. R., & Ahmed, I. (2016). Pineapple juice. *Handbook of Functional Beverages and Human Health*, 489–500.

Kumar, P., & Joshi, L. (2013). Pollution caused by agricultural waste burning and possible alternate uses of crop stubble: A case study of Punjab. In *Knowledge Systems of Societies for Adaptation and Mitigation of Impacts of Climate Change*, 367–385. Springer, Berlin, Heidelberg.

Kumar, P., Kumar, N., & Omer, T. (2016). A review on nutraceutical "Critical supplement for building a healthy world". *World Journal of Pharmaceutical Sciences, 5*(3), 579–594.

Kumar, N., Neeraj, & Kumar, S. (2018). Functional properties of pomegranate (*Punica granatum* L.). *Pomegranate, 83,* 172.

Laftah, W. A., & Rahaman, W. A. W. A. (2015). Chemical pulping of waste pineapple leaves fiber for kraft paper production. *Journal of Materials Research and Technology, 4*(3), 254–261.

Lasekan, O. (2016). Flavor and aroma compounds of some exotic tropical fruits and berries: Biosynthetic pathways and metabolism. In *Postharvest Ripening Physiology of Crops,* 594–625. CRC Press.

Lasekan, O., & Abbas, K. A. (2012). Distinctive exotic flavor and aroma compounds of some exotic tropical fruits and berries: A review. *Critical Reviews in Food Science and Nutrition, 52*(8), 726–735.

Lasekan, O., & Hussein, F. K. (2018). Classification of different pineapple varieties grown in Malaysia based on volatile fingerprinting and sensory analysis. *Chemistry Central Journal, 12*(1), 1–12.

Leneveu-Jenvrin, C., Quentin, B., Assemat, S., Hoarau, M., Meile, J. C., & Remize, F. (2020). Changes of quality of minimally-processed pineapple (*Ananas comosus,* var."Queen Victoria") during cold storage: Fungi in the leading role. *Microorganisms, 8*(2), 185.

Li, Y. O., & Komarek, A. R. (2017). Dietary fibre basics: Health, nutrition, analysis, and applications. *Food Quality and Safety, 1*(1), 47–59.

Lobo, M. G., & Yahia, E. (2017). Biology and postharvest physiology of pineapple. *Handbook of Pineapple Technology: Production, Postharvest Science, Processing and Nutrition, 1,* 39–61.

Lorenzoni, A. S., Graebin, N. G., Martins, A. B., Fernandez-Lafuente, R., ZáchiaAyub, M. A., & Rodrigues, R. C. (2012). Optimization of pineapple flavour synthesis by esterification catalysed by immobilized lipase from Rhizomucormiehei. *Flavour and Fragrance Journal, 27*(2), 196–200.

Lu, X. H., Sun, D. Q., Wu, Q. S., Liu, S. H., & Sun, G. M. (2014). Physico-chemical properties, antioxidant activity and mineral contents of pineapple genotypes grown in China. *Molecules, 19*(6), 8518–8532.

Luengwilai, K., Beckles, D. M., Roessner, U., Dias, D. A., Lui, V., & Siriphanich, J. (2018). Identification of physiological changes and key metabolites coincident with postharvest internal browning of pineapple (*Ananas comosus* L.) fruit. *Postharvest Biology and Technology, 137,* 56–65.

Malla, S., Hobbs, J. E., & Sogah, E. K. (2013b). Functional foods and natural health products regulations in Canada and around the world: Nutrition labels and health claims. *Saskatoon, Saskatchewan, Canada: Report prepared for the Canadian Agricultural Innovation and Regulation Network,* 447–454.

Manosroi, A., Chankhampan, C., Pattamapun, K., Manosroi, W., & Manosroi, J. (2014). Antioxidant and gelatinolytic activities of papain from papaya latex and bromelain from pineapple fruits. *Chiang Mai Journal of Science*, 41(3), 635–648.

McClements, D. J., Zou, L., Zhang, R., Salvia-Trujillo, L., Kumosani, T., & Xiao, H. (2015). Enhancing nutraceutical performance using excipient foods: Designing food structures and compositions to increase bioavailability. *Comprehensive Reviews in Food Science and Food Safety*, 14(6), 824–847.

Meena, L., Sengar, A. S., Neog, R., & Sunil, C. K. (2021). Pineapple processing waste (PPW): Bioactive compounds, their extraction, and utilisation: A review. *Journal of Food Science and Technology*, 1–13.

Mehra, R., Kumar, H., Kumar, N., & Kaushik, R. (2020). Red rice conjugated with barley and rhododendron extracts for new variant of beer. *Journal of Food Science and Technology*, 57(11), 4152–4159.

Murthy, T. M. S., & Yogesh, M. S. (2014). An overview of food processing industry in India-challenges and opportunities. *Online International Interdisciplinary Research Journal*, 4(5), 187–193.

Najeeb, M. I., Sultan, M. T. H., Andou, Y., Shah, A. U. M., Eksiler, K., Jawaid, M., & Ariffin, A. H. (2021). Characterization of lignocellulosic biomass from Malaysian's Yankee pineapple AC6 toward composite application. *Journal of Natural Fibers*, 18(12), 2006–2018.

Nasri, H., Baradaran, A., Shirzad, H., & Rafieian-Kopaei, M. (2014). New concepts in nutraceuticals as alternative for pharmaceuticals. *International Journal of Preventive Medicine*, 5(12), 1487.

Neto, A. R. S., Araujo, M. A., Souza, F. V., Mattoso, L. H., & Marconcini, J. M. (2013). Characterization and comparative evaluation of thermal, structural, chemical, mechanical and morphological properties of six pineapple leaf fiber varieties for use in composites. *Industrial Crops and Products*, 43, 529–537.

Okeke, B. C., Agu, K. C., Uba, P. O., Awah, N. S., Anaukwu, C. G., Archibong, E. J., ... & Orji, M. U. (2015). Wine production from mixed fruits (pineapple and watermelon) using high alcohol tolerant yeast isolated from palm wine. *Universal Journal of Microbiology Research*, 3(4), 41–45.

Olaiya, C. O., Soetan, K. O., & Esan, A. M. (2016). The role of nutraceuticals, functional foods and value added food products in the prevention and treatment of chronic diseases. *African Journal of Food Science*, 10(10), 185–193.

Pal, A. K., Nagaich, U., Bharti, C., & Gulati, N. (2014). Formulation and evaluation of nutraceutical tablet using herbal drugs by direct compression method. *Journal of Drug Delivery and Therapeutics*, 4(2), 47–51.

Pandey, V. (2014). *Natural Antioxidants and Phyto-Chemicals in Plant Foods*. Satish Serial Publishing House.

Parashar, S., Sharma, H., & Garg, M. (2014). Antimicrobial and antioxidant activities of fruits and vegetable peels: A review. *Journal of Pharmacognosy and Phytochemistry*, 3(1).

Patil, C. S. (2011). Current trends and future prospective of nutraceuticals in health promotion. *BIOINFO Pharmaceutical Biotechnology, 1*(1), 1–7.

Phoophuangpairoj, R., & Srikun, N. (2014). Computerized recognition of pineapple grades using physicochemical properties and flicking sounds. *International Journal of Agricultural and Biological Engineering, 7*(3), 93–101.

Pino, J. A. (2013). Odour-active compounds in pineapple (*Ananas comosus* [L.] Merril cv. Red Spanish). *International Journal of Food Science & Technology, 48*(3), 564–570.

Prabhu, S., Molath, A., Choksi, H., Kumar, S., & Mehra, R. (2021). Classifications of polyphenols and their potential application in human health and diseases. *International Journal of Physiology, Nutrition and Physical Education, 6*, 293–301.

Prado, K. S., & Spinacé, M. A. (2019). Isolation and characterization of cellulose nanocrystals from pineapple crown waste and their potential uses. *International Journal of Biological Macromolecules, 122*, 410–416.

Praveen, N. C., Rajesh, A., Madan, M., Chaurasia, V. R., Hiremath, N. V., & Sharma, A. M. (2014). In vitro evaluation of antibacterial efficacy of pineapple extract (bromelain) on periodontal pathogens. *Journal of International Oral Health: JIOH, 6*(5), 96.

Priyadarshani, S. V. G. N., Cai, H., Zhou, Q., Liu, Y., Cheng, Y., Xiong, J., ... & Qin, Y. (2019). An efficient agrobacterium mediated transformation of pineapple with GFP-tagged protein allows easy, non-destructive screening of transgenic pineapple plants. *Biomolecules, 9*(10), 617.

Quirós-Sauceda, A. E., Ayala-Zavala, J. F., Sáyago-Ayerdi, S. G., Vélez-de La Rocha, R., Sañudo-Barajas, A., & González-Aguilar, G. A. (2014). Added dietary fiber reduces the antioxidant capacity of phenolic compounds extracted from tropical fruit. *Journal of Applied Botany and Food Quality, 87*, 227–233.

Rahim, H. A., Seng, C. K., & Rahim, R. A. (2014). Analysis for soluble solid contents in pineapples using NIR spectroscopy. *Jurnal Teknologi, 69*(8), 7–11.

Rahim, A., Adriani, M., Rahayu, P., Tjandrawinata, R. R., & Rachmawati, H. (2019). Green isolation and physical modification of pineapple stem waste starch as pharmaceutical excipient. *Drug Development and Industrial Pharmacy, 45*(6), 1029–1037.

Rahman, A. M. (2011). Study on modified pineapple leaf fibre. *Journal of Textile and Apparel, Technology and Management, 7*(2), 1–16.

Rajat, S., Manisha, S., Robin, S., & Sunil, K. (2012). Nutraceuticals: A review. *International Research Journal of Pharmacy, 3*(4), 95–99.

Reinhardt, D. H. R. C., Bartholomew, D. P., Souza, F. V. D., Carvalho, A. C. P. P. de, Pádua, T. R. P. de, Junghans, D. T., & Matos, A. P. de. (2018). Advances in pineapple plant propagation. *Revista Brasileira de Fruticultura, 40*(6), 1–22.

Roda, A., & Lambri, M. (2019). Food uses of pineapple waste and by-products: A review. *International Journal of Food Science & Technology, 54*(4), 1009–1017.

Selani, M. M., Brazaca, S. G. C., dos Santos Dias, C. T., Ratnayake, W. S., Flores, R. A., & Bianchini, A. (2014). Characterisation and potential application of pineapple pomace in an extruded product for fibre enhancement. *Food Chemistry, 163*, 23–30.

Sepúlveda, L., Romaní, A., Aguilar, C. N., & Teixeira, J. (2018). Valorization of pineapple waste for the extraction of bioactive compounds and glycosides using autohydrolysis. *Innovative Food Science & Emerging Technologies, 47*, 38–45.

Sharma S. P., & Brajbhushan. (2015). A study on nutritional efficacy of pineapple juice in the treatment of bronchial asthma. *International Journal of Scientific and Research Publications (IJSRP), 5*(1), 1–4.

Sharma, P., Ramchiary, M., Samyor, D., & Das, A. B. (2016a). Study on the phytochemical properties of pineapple fruit leather processed by extrusion cooking. *LWT – Food Science and Technology, 72*, 534–543.

Sharma, A., Singh, B. K., & Anand, N. (2016b). Fruit processing industry in India: A short review. *Cold Chain Logistics in Horticulture & Agriculture,* 1–17.

Shinde, N., Bangar, B., Deshmukh, S., & Kumbhar, P. (2014). Nutraceuticals: A Review on current status. *Research Journal of Pharmacy and Technology, 7*(1), 110–113.

Sibaly, S., & Jeetah, P. (2017). Production of paper from pineapple leaves. *Journal of Environmental Chemical Engineering, 5*(6), 5978–5986.

Singh, J., & Sinha, S. (2012). Classification, regulatory acts and applications of nutraceuticals for health. *International Journal of Pharma and Bio Sciences, 2*(1), 177–187.

Siti Rashima, R., Maizura, M., Wan Nur Hafzan, W. M., & Hazzeman, H. (2019). Physicochemical properties and sensory acceptability of pineapples of different varieties and stages of maturity. *Food Research, 5*, 491–500.

Siti Roha, A. M., Zainal, S., Noriham, A., & Nadzirah, K. Z. (2013). Determination of sugar content in pineapple waste variety N36. *International Food Research Journal, 20*(4), 1941–1943.

Smarta, R. B. (2012). Regulatory Perspective of Nutraceuticals in India, Interlink Marketing Consultancy Pvt. Ltd. Report, 1–12.

Soares, P. A., Vaz, A. F., Correia, M. T., Pessoa Jr, A., & Carneiro-da-Cunha, M. G. (2012). Purification of bromelain from pineapple wastes by ethanol precipitation. *Separation and Purification Technology, 98*, 389–395.

Soloman George, D., Razali, Z., & Somasundram, C. (2016). Physiochemical changes during growth and development of pineapple (*Ananas comosus* L. Merr. Cv. Sarawak). *Mdrsjrns, 18*(2), 491–503.

Steingass, C. B., Dell, C., Lieb, V., Mayer-Ullmann, B., Czerny, M., & Carle, R. (2016). Assignment of distinctive volatiles, descriptive sensory analysis and consumer preference of differently ripened and post-harvest handled pineapple (*Ananas comosus* [L.] Merr.) fruits. *European Food Research and Technology, 242*(1), 33–43.

Steingass, C. B., Grauwet, T., & Carle, R. (2014). Influence of harvest maturity and fruit logistics on pineapple (*Ananas comosus* [L.] Merr.) volatiles assessed by headspace solid phase microextraction and gas chromatography–mass spectrometry (HS-SPME-GC/MS). *Food Chemistry, 150,* 382–391.

Steingass, C. B., Jutzi, M., Müller, J., Carle, R., & Schmarr, H. G. (2015). Ripening-dependent metabolic changes in the volatiles of pineapple (*Ananas comosus* [L.] Merr.) fruit: II. Multivariate statistical profiling of pineapple aroma compounds based on comprehensive two-dimensional gas chromatography-mass spectrometry. *Analytical and Bioanalytical Chemistry, 407*(9), 2609–2624.

Steingass, C. B., Vollmer, K., Lux, P. E., Dell, C., Carle, R., & Schweiggert, R. M. (2020). HPLC-DAD-APCI-MSn analysis of the genuine carotenoid pattern of pineapple (*Ananas comosus* [L.] Merr.) infructescence. *Food Research International, 127,* 108709.

Stephen, D. (2013). Nutraceuticals: What are they and do they work? Kentucky Equine Research Inc. *Versailles, KY, 7*(4), 1–50.

Sufian, A. A. M., Othman, S. A., Hasrin, N. I., & Harun, S. N. I. (2020). Future of pineapple leaf paper: A review. *International Journal of Engineering Advanced Research, 1*(2), 1–6.

Tuohy, K. M., Conterno, L., Gasperotti, M., & Viola, R. (2012). Up-regulating the human intestinal microbiome using whole plant foods, polyphenols, and/or fiber. *Journal of Agricultural and Food Chemistry, 60*(36), 8776–8782.

Verma, G., & Mishra, M. K. (2016). A review on nutraceuticals: Classification and its role in various diseases. *International Journal of Pharmacy & Therapeutics, 7*(4), 152–160.

Vollmer, K., Chakraborty, S., Bhalerao, P. P., Carle, R., Frank, J., & Steingass, C. B. (2020). Effect of pulsed light treatment on natural microbiota, enzyme activity, and phytochemical composition of pineapple (*Ananas comosus* [L.] Merr.) juice. *Food and Bioprocess Technology, 13,* 1095–1109.

Wei, C. B., Ding, X. D., Liu, Y. G., Zhao, W. F., & Sun, G. M. (2014). Application of solid-phase microextraction for the analysis of aroma compounds from pineapple fruit. *Advanced Materials Research 988,* 397–406.

Wei, C. B., Liu, S. H., Liu, Y. G., Lv, L. L., Yang, W. X., & Sun, G. M. (2011). Characteristic aroma compounds from different pineapple parts. *Molecules, 16*(6), 5104–5112.

Yoyponsan, P., Thuengtung, S., Ogawa, Y., Naradisorn, M., & Sethal, S. (2019). Influence of harvest maturity and storage condition on changes on volatile compounds of "Phulae" pineapple fruit. *Journal of Food Science and Agricultural Technology (JFAT), 5,* 128–139.

Yusof, Y., Ahmad, M. R., Saidin, W., Mustapa, M. S., & Tahar, M. S. (2011). Producing Paper Using Pineapple Leaf Fiber. *Advanced Materials Research*, *383–390*, 3382–3386.

Yusof, Y., Yahya, S. A., & Adam, A. (2015). Novel technology for sustainable pineapple leaf fibers productions. *Procedia CIRP*, *26*, 756–760.

Zakaria, N. A., Rahman, R. A., Zaidel, D. N. A., Dailin, D. J., & Jusoh, M. (2021). Microwave-assisted extraction of pectin from pineapple peel. *Malaysian Journal of Fundamental and Applied Sciences*, *17*(1), 33–38.

Zaki, N. A. M., Rahman, N. A., Zamanhuri, N. A., & Hashib, S. A. (2017). Ascorbic acid content and proteolytic enzyme activity of microwave-dried pineapple stem and core. *Chemical Engineering Transactions*, *56*, 1369–1374.

Zdrojewicz, Z., Chorbinska, J., Biezynski, B., & Krajewski, P. (2018). Health-promoting properties of pineapple. *Pediatria I Medycyna Rodzinna-Paediatrics and Family Medicine*, *14*(2), 133–142.

Zhang, X., Shen, Y., Prinyawiwatkul, W., & Xu, Z. (2012). Volatile compounds in fresh-cut pineapple heated at different temperatures. *Journal of Food Processing and Preservation*, *36*(6), 567–573.

Zheng, L. Y., Sun, G. M., Liu, Y. G., Lv, L. L., Yang, W. X., Zhao, W. F., & Wei, C. B. (2012). Aroma volatile compounds from two fresh pineapple varieties in China. *International Journal of Molecular Sciences*, *13*(6), 7383–7392.

# 10 Banana

*Monika Choudhary and Amarjeet Kaur*

## CONTENTS

## 10.1 INTRODUCTION

Fruits are a good source of minerals, vitamins, fiber, and other bioactive compounds and are an essential part of a balanced and healthy diet. As per the recommendation of the World Health Organization (WHO), about 400 g of fruits and vegetables per capita per day must be consumed in diets. As consumption of fruits is not adequate in the diet, it leads to increased danger of chronic illnesses, poor health status, poor quality of life considered to be one of the risk factors related to increased mortality. Consuming fruits on a regular basis can lead to reduction in the incidences of cardiovascular problems, diabetes, gastrointestinal problems, and several types of cancer. Banana is a herbaceous plant belonging to the genus *Musa* and its family is Musaceae (Probojati et al. 2021), and is considered as one of the earliest crops grown since human agriculture started. The origin of the banana family ranges from India to Papua New Guinea including the Southeast Asian region (Arvanitoyannis and Mavromatis 2009; De Langhe et al. 2009). But this fruit was first domesticated by Papua New Guinea. Banana is the world's most leading fruit used everywhere. The name *Musa* is taken from the term "Mouz," an Arabic name. This word *Musa* was given to the banana plant to honor Antonia Musa (Roman physician) during the first century (Qamar and Shaikh 2018). There are more than 1,000 varieties of bananas that are produced worldwide. *Musa* Cavendish is considered as the most commercialized variety contributing about 45% of the global banana market. This variety has high production/yield per hectare and is less prone to injuries because of environmental factors.

Banana is grouped into four edible cultivars viz., *Eumusa, Rhodochlamys, Australimusa,* and *Callimusa*. The edible banana fruit is parthenocarpic; that is, it does not contain seeds. At present, there are diploid, triploid or tetraploid genome groups and their main genome groups are denoted as AA, AB, AAA, AAB, and ABB. Plantain belongs to *M. acuminata* (genome "A") and *M. balbisiana* (genome "B") species (Khawas et al. 2014). It is a variety of cultivated banana and also mentioned as a cooking type banana. Plantain is related to the AAB genome, whereas the commercially available export market Cavendish subgroup refers to the AAA genome (Qamar and Shaikh 2018). As cooking and dessert bananas contain a

DOI: 10.1201/9781003259213-10

good amount of nutrients, the fruit is the world's fourth leading agricultural crop (Campos et al. 2018). The countries exporting bananas usually export the Cavendish banana which is sweet and soft while the plantain bananas or the bananas used for cooking purposes possess firm and starchy fruit making them appropriate to be used as a vegetable for cooking (Sidhu and Zafar 2018). Due to mass cultivation and consumption of banana in the recent decades, it is the world's second largest fruit crop. The estimated gross production of banana is more than 139 million tons (FAO 2010a). India, China, Ecuador, Uganda, the Philippines, and Nigeria are the leading nations involved in banana and plantain production. Banana is considered as the most cost-effective, affordable, and readily available crop, with about 1,000 varieties of banana available throughout the world. These varieties vary in relation to their taste, color, flavor, and chemical composition and are consumed readily by people. In common, banana is said to be a dessert cultivar, while the plantain is considered to be a cooking cultivar (Oyeyinka and Afolayan 2020; Vu et al. 2018). This crop is principally grown for the fruit purpose but to a limited extent, for production of wine and some natural fibers (Khoozani et al. 2019).

This crop is mostly cultivated for its edible fruit. As a result, a significant amount of underutilized by-products and wastes are generated at the farms. To avoid these losses and prevent serious ecological damages, appropriate agriculture waste management practices must be adopted (Essien et al. 2005; Shah et al. 2005; Yabaya and Ado 2008). Although earlier people had been using this plant for food purposes only, now they have started to find out other possible ways of incorporating banana in their day-to-day life. Cultural diversification has expanded the use of banana by-products for wrapping clothes, foods and also in several ceremonial occasions (Kennedy 2009). Generally, modern agriculture has grouped and considered banana to be a cash crop or fruit crop commodity along with other crops like pineapple, sugarcane, oil palm, rice, and mangoes. These crops produce large quantity of cellulosic wastes identified as biomass or agricultural waste. To manage this massive amount of agricultural waste or biomass in an innovative method is a continuous and big challenge. But current trends favour the use of this available biomass for value addition to justify the requirements in the zones of food alternatives, fiber composites, renewable energy, textiles, and livestock feed (Rosentrater et al. 2009). Banana fruit contains nutrients in its pulp and peel having positive and valuable properties. Unripe banana consists of dietary fibers, indigestible compounds, and resistant starch. As the starch present in fruit degrades to sucrose and fructose as the fruit ripens, it results in reduction of starch content. Both banana pulp and peel contain carbohydrate, minerals (micro and macro), vitamins, and phenolic compounds.

However, approximately one–third of the banana that is produced is lost. One of the reasons for this loss is that banana is mostly consumed in the form of ripe bananas. But banana being a climacteric fruit, ripened bananas are more susceptible to mechanical injuries. Ripe fruit becomes perishable as the maturation process progresses making the storage and transportation a tedious process (Jiang et al. 2015). About 20% of banana is not found suitable for commercialization because of issues in size and appearance thus, increasing the loss (dos Santos Alves et al. 2016).

## 10.2 PRODUCTION AND GLOBAL MARKET

Banana is one of the plants that is grown almost in every country of the world. Banana has a harvested area of approximately 10 million hectares and is cultivated and produced by 130 countries ranging from tropical and subtropical regions, contributing to these nations' economies (Zhang et al. 2005). The fruit shows good growth and harvest at an altitude ranging up to 1,000 m and also in subtropics with even higher altitudes. As per the statistics of Food and Agriculture Organization,

2019, India is the major banana producing country with per annum production of about 30,460,000 tons, trailed by China and Indonesia. India at present is contributing its share of more than 25% of the world's total banana production (FAO 2010a).

Although India ranks top in the world's banana producers, only 0.04% is exported as the maximum of banana produced in the country is used in its own marketplace. Consequently, total export of banana from India is extremely small if associated to other important global banana exporting nations like Costa Rica, Ecuador, Colombia, and the Philippines. These countries share a contribution of more than 60% of the world's total exports of banana. The European Union and the United States are the top banana importing nations. African countries are the largest plantain-producing countries as plantain is one of the primary foods in that province. Uganda has an estimated production of about 9.6 million tons and is regarded as the foremost plantain producer country followed by Ghana and Rwanda. Banana production has usually been grouped into two types: The small-scale farmers being the majority that produce bananas primarily for self-consumption and for the local market whereas another group is involved in large plantations and companies that meet the needs of both national and international markets (FAO 2010a).

As per the statistics of FAO (2010b), 93.3 and 34.3 million tons of dessert bananas and plantains were produced, respectively, in 2010 which was quite high as compared to apples, oranges, and grapes with a total production of about 70, 69, and 68 million tons, respectively. But the total trade of this crop in the international market was even less than 20% of the total production and valued only about 7 billion Euros (Aurore et al. 2009). The common internationally used bananas for trading purpose are cultivated from AAA group varieties like "Cavendish," "Gros Michel," and "Grande Naine." Other well-known varieties which are endemic to a specific region include "Yangambi Km5, AAA", cultivated in East Africa, "Red banana, AAA" and "Mysore AAB" found in Southeast Asia as well as "Silk AAB" and "Bluggoe ABB" available although the tropical region (Ploetz et al. 2007). *Musa paradisica* L. (Musaceae) is being utilized in various countries for preventing and treating many health-related illnesses like diabetes, inflammation, dental plaque, diarrhea, etc. The increase in popularity of the banana is due to high pharmaceutical and nutraceutical value. Banana crop is unique as its every part, whether its fruit, pulp, seed, peel, flowers, leaves or bark, can be utilized (Arora et al. 2008; Jahan et al. 2010; Kumar 1992). Bananas are also considered to possess prebiotic properties as they contain 60%–80% of carbohydrates in the form of indigestible carbohydrates, i.e., cellulose, resistant starch, hemicelluloses, and lignin. These indigestible carbohydrates present in bananas act as a fuel for probiotic bacteria and thus promote production of probiotic substances which leads to prevention of pathogenic bacterial growth (Farees et al. 2017; Powthong et al. 2020).

## 10.3 SOURCE OF DIETARY NUTRIENTS

Banana pith from the pseudostem is consumed as a vegetable in many parts of the world including Sri Lanka, India, and Malaysia (Kennedy 2009; Subbaraya et al. 2006). It encompasses substantial value of sugar, minerals, and starch. Consumption of banana inflorescence as salad and vegetables is quite common in Southeast Asian countries since long times. Banana peels are rich in protein, total dietary fiber and lipids and fatty acids with content of about 8%–11%, 40%–50%, and 2.2%–10.9%, respectively) depending upon the genetic makeup of the fruit. The dietary fiber content is slightly on a higher side if compared with rice, barley, oats, and wheat brans (Emaga et al. 2008a; Sudha et al. 2007). The indigestible compound or resistant starch present in banana fruit is not absorbed in the small intestine and is taken to the large intestine for the digestion to occur. This distinctive property

## Table 10.1: Chemical Content of Banana Fruit (per 100 g)

| Parameter | Content |
|---|---|
| Energy | 371 kJ (89 kcal) |
| Moisture | 65.5–75.3 g |
| Protein | 0.9–4.9 g |
| Lipids | 0.3–2.9 g |
| Crude fiber | 1.6–2.9 g |
| Sugars | 23.9–43.8 g |
| Ash | 0.9–2.22 g |
| Pyridoxine | 0.40 g |
| Choline | 9.80 g |
| Pantothenic acid | 0.334 g |
| Vitamin C | 8.70 g |
| Riboflavin | 0.07 g |
| Niacin | 0.67 g |
| Vitamin B6 | 0.37 g |
| Folate | 20.00 µg |
| Vitamin A | 3.00 µg |
| Sodium | 1.00 g |
| Phosphorus | 22.00 g |
| Potassium | 358.00 g |
| Magnesium | 27.00 g |
| Zinc | 0.15 g |
| Calcium | 5.00 g |
| Iron | 0.26 g |

*Sources:* From Dotto et al. (2019); Kookal and Thimmaiah (2018); Mostafa (2021).

of banana makes it an ideal fruit for clients suffering from diabetes. Polyphenols, although present in less quantity in this fruit, function as good antioxidants and thus play their effective part in preventing metabolic degenerative ailments. Also, potassium is present in significant amount in the peels. Banana peels can be incorporated at a ratio of 10% in biscuits without affecting overall aroma, color, and taste of the product, making it suitable for the development of high dietary fiber and low-calorie food products (Joshi 2007). Banana fruit and its by-product possess many medicinal benefits. It aids in prevention of anemia as it stimulates the production of hemoglobin in the blood owing to having moderate levels of iron. Regulation of blood pressure is associated with the high content of potassium present in the fruit and its by-products (Leslie 1976). Chemical composition of banana fruit is presented in Table 10.1.

## 10.4 NUTRACEUTICALS AND BIOACTIVE COMPONENTS DERIVED FROM BANANA

Banana by-products contain many compounds that possess nutraceutical properties which can effectively and potentially be used by the pharmaceutical segment for commercializing their products (Tables 10.2 and 10.3). Banana male flowers contain epigallocatechin and its derivatives, while entisic acid, catechin,

## Table 10.2: Biochemical and Nutritional Composition of Banana (*Musa acuminata* Colla)

| Bioactive Constituents | Function |
|---|---|
| Phenols and phenolic compounds— catechin, epicatechin, gallic acid, anthocyanins, tannins gallocatechin, ferulic, epigallocatechin, myricetin, kaempferol, quercetin, salicylic, gallic, sinapic, vanillic, p-hydroxybenzoic, gentisic, syringic, and p-coumaric acids | Free radical scavenging activity accountable for aging and other issues |
| Carotenoids like β-carotene, lutein, α-carotene, auroxanthin, violaxanthin, isolutein, neoxanthin, α & β-cryptoxanthin | Antioxidants (scavenging singlet oxygen), lowers risk of some cancers, eye diseases, heart problems, improving immunity |
| *Biogenic amines:* Dopamine, serotonin, and norepinephrine | Decreases the plasma oxidative stress, enhances resistance to oxidative variations in low-density lipoproteins, and acts as neurotransmitter for human brain and body, thus influencing mood, concentration, emotional stability, general well-being, and happiness |
| *Phytosterols:* Cycloeucalenol, cycloeucalenone, stigmasterol, cycloartenol, β-sitosterol, and campesterol | Lowers blood cholesterol levels, reducing absorption of cholesterol in intestine Immune system modulator Anticancer properties |

*Source:* From Netshiheni et al. (2019).

caffeic, protocatechuic, cinnamic, and ferulic acids have been isolated from banana pseudostem (Saravanan and Aradhya 2011; Tin et al. 2010). It is a well-known fact that polyphenolic compounds like gallocatechin, cinnamic and caffeic acids, and catechin possess antioxidative, antimicrobial actions, neuroprotective, anticancer, chemo preventive, and antiproliferative properties (Artali et al. 2009; Chanwitheesuk et al. 2007; Chye and Sim 2009; Faried et al. 2007; Jagan et al. 2008; Lu et al. 2006; Mandel et al. 2008; Raina et al. 2008; Shan et al. 2008; Shankar and Mulimani 2007; Wong and Chye 2009). Phytosterols which are naturally available

## Table 10.3: Potential Use as Nutraceuticals of Bioactive Constituents Present in Banana/Plantain By-Products

| Plant Part | Bioactive Constituent | Activity |
|---|---|---|
| Pulp | Putrescine, serotonin, spermidine, dopamine, spermine, tyramine | Stimulants (Adão and Glória 2005) |
| Pseudostem | Entisic acid, catechin, protocatechuic, caffeic, cinnamic, ferulic acids | Antioxidants (Saravanan and Aradhya 2011) |
| Peel | Ascorbic acid, anthocyanins, tocopherols, catecholamines, phytosterols | Antioxidants (González-Montelongo et al. 2010) |
| Peels and pulp | Sterols, esters, tocopherols, steryl glucosides, phenolic compounds | Anti-inflammatory, anti-cholesterol, antioxidants (Oliveira et al. 2008) |
| Peels | β-sitosterol, palmatic acid, succinic acid, 12-hydroxystrearic acid, malic acid, glycoside | Anti-inflammatory, antibacterial, antioxidants, anti-cholesterol (Mokbel and Hashinaga 2005) |
| Petioles, leaves, floral stalk | Campesteryl, sitosteryl 3-β-d-glucopyranoside, 3-β-d-glucopyranoside, and stigmasteryl | Anti-inflammatory, anti-cholesterol (Oliveira et al. 2005; Padam et al. 2012) |

possess a wide range of positive health-related effects which include lowering of blood cholesterol and dropping risk of heart diseases (Miller et al. 2008; Moruisi et al. 2006; Racette et al. 2010; Weingärtner et al. 2008).

A number of bioactive steryl glucosides, i.e., sitosteryl 3-β-d-glucopyranoside, campesteryl, 3-β-d-glucopyranoside, and stigmasteryl 3-β-d-glucopyranoside, are isolated from dichloromethane extraction of *M. acuminata*. Sterols, steryl esters and steryl glucosides are found lavishly in banana indicating its potential to be used as functional food products. The juice of banana pseudostem (*M. paradisiaca*), if administered orally, is considered to increase blood glucose levels both in normal and hyperdiabetic rats signifying a possible cure for hypoglycemic persons suffering from low levels of insulin or consuming hypoglycemic drugs (Oliveira et al. 2005, 2008; Singh et al. 2007).

Anthocyanins found abundantly in fruits and vegetables are looked upon as an imperative component of human nutrition owing to their antioxidative potential (Mertens-Talcott et al. 2008; Zheng et al. 2011). Beside this, anthocyanins also possess anti-inflammatory, anti-carcinogenic, antiviral, cancer chemoprevention properties, and antiproliferative effect (Bowen-Forbes et al. 2010; Karlsen et al. 2007; Kulma and Szopa 2007; Mokbel and Hashinaga 2005; Wang et al. 2006). Banana inflorescence from both cultivated as well as wildly growing varieties are found rich in anthocyanins, hence can serve as a potentially available source of functional food that has a positive effect on health (Kitdamrongsont et al. 2008; Roobha et al. 2011). Dopamine, a catecholamine, is found in large concentrations in the pulp of red bananas (*M. sapientum* var. Baracoa), yellow banana (*M. acuminata*), and peels of Cavendish banana (Adão and Glória 2005; Kulma and Szopa 2007; Mokbel and Hashinaga 2005). These compounds act as free radical scavengers and hence possess strong antimicrobial activities against many microbes like *Staphylococcus aureus, Escherichia coli, Salmonella enteritidis, Bacillus subtilis,* and *Bacillus cereus*. Dopamine, when given to brain dead rats, displayed anti-inflammatory activity consequential in a noteworthy improvement in the rat's blood system and regulation of kidney function (Hoeger et al. 2007).

Use of bioactive constituents present in banana by-products is not only restricted to nutraceutical form for direct consumption by humans but is also used as a natural preservative source for foods. The current scenario of the growing food industry shows increased awareness regarding harmful effects of synthetic preservatives and choosing safe and minimally processed food or using traditional methods of preservation (Tiwari et al. 2009). Many plants including herbs and spices possess natural antimicrobial properties that help in retarding or preventing the growth of food-spoiling microbes and foodborne pathogens strengthening the idea of using naturally occurring substances as food preservatives (Kumar and Tanwar 2011; Kumudavally et al. 2011; Padam et al. 2012; Pillai and Ramaswamy 2012). Antibacterial compounds like 12-hydroxystrearic acid, β-sitosterol, and malic acid extracted out of banana peel act as a suppressant for foodborne pathogens including *B. cereus, S. aureus, E. coli,* and *S. enteritidis* and can possibly be used in food industry systems in the near future (Kitdamrongsont et al. 2008). The preservative capacity of banana peels in slowing down the process of lipid oxidation in raw meat is quite similar to the action of synthetic antioxidant, i.e., butylated hydroxy toluene (BHT), because of presence of antioxidant in peel (Devatkal et al. 2014).

## 10.5 BANANA BY-PRODUCTS AND THEIR NUTRACEUTICALS
### 10.5.1 Banana Peel

Ancient Indian literature documents various medicinal properties of banana and is found to be effective in the treatment of various ailments (Loizzo et al. 2011). Being a staple fruit, availability of banana is there throughout the year and acts as a source

## Table 10.4: Chemical Composition of Banana (*Musa sapientum*) Peel

| Parameter | Content |
| --- | --- |
| Moisture | 6.70% |
| Protein | 0.90% |
| Crude lipid | 1.70% |
| Ash | 8.50% |
| Crude fiber | 31.70% |
| Carbohydrate | 59.00% |
| Potassium | 78.10 mg/g |
| Calcium | 19.20 mg/g |
| Sodium | 24.30 mg/g |
| Iron | 0.61 mg/g |
| Oxalate | 0.51 mg/g |
| Saponins (mg/g) | 24.00 mg/g |
| Oxalate (mg/g) | 0.51 mg/g |
| Phytate (mg/g) | 0.28 mg/g |
| Phenolic compound | 0.90–3 g/100 g |

*Sources:* From Anhwange et al. (2009); Nguyen et al. (2003).

of livelihood security to a large population (Chadha 2002). The peel is the major by-product of the banana industry engaged in its processing which accounts for 30% of the fruit as a potential environmental hazard (Someya et al. 2002) (Table 10.4).

The banana peel contains a high content of dietary fiber and phenolic constituents making them suitable for various uses in nutraceuticals and medicinal industries. According to the National Cancer Standard Institute, extraction from banana peel is considered as nontoxic to human cells making this safe to be used as a naturally occurring source of available antioxidants for the purpose of value addition (Ilori et al. 2007). Even polyphenolic and other bioactive constituents are present in higher amounts in the peel than in the pulp of fruit. There are a number of uses of banana peel, for example, ethanol production by fermentation and hydrolysis, production of biogas, biomass production, antioxidant and antibacterial activities, etc. (Anhwange et al. 2009; Nguyen et al. 2003; Raghavan and Devasagayam 1985). Along with nutraceutical properties, the banana peel contains some enzymes such as superoxide dismutase and oxalate oxidase for their pharmaceutical and medicinal applications. More intense work needs to be carried out to explore commercial uses of banana peel in the food processing industry, pharmaceutical and medicinal areas.

### 10.5.2 Antioxidant Activity in Banana Peels

Oxalate oxidase is one such enzyme present in the peel of banana that degrades renal stones from kidneys and plasma and is used as a phytomedicinal constituent. Availability of oxalate oxidase enzyme in banana peel was first reported by Richardson (Raghavan and Devasagayam 1985). Oxalate is a metabolic end product, and no enzyme is there in the body of the mammalian system that can act upon oxalate. Excess deposition of oxalate in the body causes renal caliculi. Although this condition can be controlled by various approaches, a better and economically effective method is to control the activity of the enzyme oxalate oxidase available in many fruits and vegetables.

Oxalate also hinders the availability of essential minerals like calcium in the body. Furthermore, superoxide dismutase seemingly protects the cell against toxicity of oxygen and inhibits ethylene production from methional. Flavonoids present in banana stimulate the actions of superoxide dismutase (SOD) and catalase which is accountable for reduction in peroxidation level products like hydroperoxides, malondialdehyde, and conjugated dienes. Oxalate oxidase and superoxide dismutase activity of the proteins related to the cupin family possess disease resistance properties (Baker 1976; Fridovich 1972).

Phenolic content in banana peel (*Musa accuminata*, Colla AAA) varies from 0.90–3 g/100 gm of dry weight. Similarly, the concentration of gallocatechin in banana peel is in the range of 160 mg/100 g of dry weight (Nguyen et al. 2003; Someya et al. 2002). Polyphenolic content changes during different stages of ripening and growth. Unripe banana peels possess high antioxidant activity. Polyphenol/flavanones and flavonoids play an important role in these activities (Mokbel and Hashinaga 2005). Also, the content of bioactive compounds and antioxidant activity is also dependent upon the cultivar or variety of banana. For example, Karpooravalli and Red banana are considered rich in bioactive compounds like carotenoids (beta-carotene), carbohydrates, and antioxidative enzymes (Arora et al. 2008). As banana is a tropical plant, it can produce a good amount of antioxidants and can provide a shield from oxidative stress caused by high temperatures and sunshine (González-Montelongo et al. 2010).

### 10.5.3 Antimicrobial Activity

Today's consumer is well aware of concepts related to food safety and does not appreciate and accept the use of synthetic antibacterial agents used in the process of preservation. Natural antimicrobial compounds not only play an important role in the prevention of food borne illnesses, they also render them safe for mass consumption (Conner 1993; Shan et al. 2007). This led to the increased interest to develop antibacterial agents from naturally occurring sources with increased efficiency that are non-toxic in nature. Many phenolic constituents are present in fruit peels which are quite effective against different pathogenic microorganisms (Anagnostopoulou et al. 2006). Tannins and flavonoids both possess antimicrobial activity and are effective in inhibiting the growth of bacteria, fungi, and viruses (Colak et al. 2010) (Table 10.5).

## 10.6 POTENTIAL FOOD APPLICATIONS OF BANANA BY-PRODUCTS

### 10.6.1 Source of Starch, Pectin, and Cellulose

The food industry is using pectin, starch, and cellulose in the form of gelling, stabilizers, and thickening agents. Starch is a set of carbohydrates and exists commercially in the market and is mainly procured from plants like potato, corn, cassava, wheat, and rice. Banana by-products like green culled bananas and the pith of the pseudostem are usually discarded during selection and processing of this fruit but can be utilized for processing into edible starches (Abdul Aziz et al. 2011; Da Mota et al. 2000; Zhang et al. 2005). Amylase contents in banana starches are considered to be relatively low. These starches have low swelling properties, lower retrogradation, and less solubility in water. Banana by-product starches are highly resistant to amylase attack and heating and proved to be a bit superior to modified and unmodified cornstarch, thus giving an edge for potentially higher value in the market (Madhav and Pushpalatha 2006).

Pectin available commercially is a structural heteropolysaccharide categorized under soluble dietary fiber. It is prepared mainly from fruit extract like oranges, apples, citrus peels, and carrots. The methoxyl composition of pectin and gelling quality obtained from banana is somewhat lower than pectin isolated from

## Table 10.5: Antimicrobial Compounds Present in Banana Plant Parts

| Banana Plant Part | Compound | Action |
| --- | --- | --- |
| Banana fruit | Tetradecanoic acid | Antibacterial (Pereira and Maraschin 2015) |
| | Hexadecanoic acid | |
| | Epicatechin | |
| | DL—Limonene | |
| | Gallatocatechin | |
| | Gallocatechin | |
| | Dopamine | |
| Banana peel | Ferulic acid | Antibacterial (Pereira and Maraschin 2015) |
| | Dopamine | |
| | Chlorogenic acid | |
| | Gallic acid | |
| | Hydroxybenzoic acid | |
| | Malic acid | Antimicrobial (Mokbel and Hashinaga 2005) |
| | Gentisic acid | Antifungal |
| Banana pseudostem | Caffeic acid | Antimicrobial (Kandasamy and Aradhya 2014) |
| | Catechin | |
| | Cinnamic acid | |
| | Protocatechuic acid | Antibacterial (Kandasamy and Aradhya 2014) |
| Banana flower | Lupeol | Antimicrobial |

*Source:* From Mostafa (2021).

citrus peels of lime and pomelo (Madhav and Pushpalatha 2006). Pectin can be prepared from discarded or rejected banana peels by using acid extraction and precipitation using ammonium salts or alcohols. Banana peels contain higher pectin content than plantain peels. These fruit peels exhibit a similar or somewhat higher quantity of extractable dietary fibers in comparison to other peels making them suitable as a potentially cheap alternative source of pectin for countries where bananas are produced, reducing their dependence on imported pectin. The high pectin content in the banana peel, which is about 99%–22%, makes it suitable for preparation of non-conventional products by using banana without incorporating any gel additive. Standardizing and developing jellies by incorporating banana peel can be nutritive, beneficial for health and would be more acceptable than any tablets. Jelly is considered to be a favorite sweet course among all, owing to good texture, appearance, and digestibility (Lee et al. 2010). Hence, banana by-products like peels, pseudostem, and green-culled banana can be used as an economical source and raw material for production of high-grade pectin, cellulose, and starch for the food processing industry (Elanthikkal et al. 2010; Emaga et al. 2008b).

### 10.6.2 Natural Bio-Colorant

Anthocyanins, a type of flavonoids, are significant pigments accountable for the violet, red, and purple colors of inflorescence in bananas (Kitdamrongsont et al. 2008). Anthocyanins act as a good bio-colorant because of their attractive colors. These are water-soluble, quite stable in food systems and proven to be good for health (Bagchi et al. 2004; Ferreira Ozela et al. 2007; Konzack and Zhang

2004; Torskangerpoll and Andersen 2005). Anthocyanins can be extracted from purple black chokeberry, sweet potato, bilberry fruits, strawberry, tropical fruits, etc. (Einbond et al. 2004; Fan et al. 2008; Pliszka et al. 2008). The amount of anthocyanins mainly present in banana inflorescence bracts is comprised of cyanidin-3-rutinoside compound which is about 14–32 mg anthocyanin per 100 g of bracts. It can potentially be exploited to be used as an economical ingredient of natural food colorants. The anthocyanin content found in these banana bracts is slightly higher than the anthocyanin content of red cabbage which is available in the market for commercial use. As there is an abundance in the quantity of bracts produced in terms of mass per hectare of land, it offers a sustainable, satisfactory, and better market position for natural bio-colorant from banana by-products (Pazmiño-Durán et al. 2001; Roobha et al. 2011). Anthocyanins are high in demand not only because they are a naturally occurring bio-colorant but also because they possess health-promoting factors and because of an increased demand for natural foods (Rymbai et al. 2011).

### 10.6.3 Biogeneration of Flavor

In the food industry, flavor plays an imperative role. Flavors are the results of several chemical reactions occurring in food during processing and are mainly due to reduction of nitrogen, carbon or sulfur containing mixtures with the formation of organic volatile compounds like aldehydes (Rappert and Müller 2005). Biogeneration of alcohols and aldehydes used in the industry for flavor purposes is occurring naturally through enzymatic pathways in the presence of various enzymes like alcohol dehydrogenase, lipase, hydroperoxide lyase, and lipoxygenase (Gigot et al. 2010). Banana leaves are comprised of a membrane-bound enzyme of 9 lipoxygenase, capable of producing melon-like, oolong tea-like, and cucumber-like fruity flavors upon pickling or when treated with linoleic acid, soybean oil, and linolenic acid, respectively. This is quite comparable to the kinetic properties of lipoxygenase obtained from English peas and canola seeds (Kuo et al. 2006). Hence, there is a huge potential for banana leaves to be used for making natural flavors that can be applied in the food processing industry. Production of nutraceuticals of high value and processing of functional foods are significantly affected by the quality and availability of raw material. There is a substantial variation in the quality of fiber and bioactive constituents attained from banana by-products of diverse varieties and cultivars (Uma et al. 2005). Bananas from numerous varieties and cultivars are being assessed and by-products like rhizome, fruit stalks, pseudostem, leaves, and peel from the commonly grown varieties have a scope for usage as potentially available raw materials in ranges of both food and non-food industrial segments, playing a different role in each application.

## 10.7 CONCLUSION

Banana and by-products judged and considered to partake potential for application as nutraceuticals, food supplements, food additives, feeds fibers, fuel, fertilizers, bioactive constituents source, and organic chemicals need to be further taken up for measuring safety criteria to meet the increasing demands of the market. A standardized procedure for collecting, processing, and storage of banana by-products is desired for addressing in the near future for creation of a suitable setting for available unprocessed raw materials to be used in industrial scale processing. An exponential surge in the world's population and the increasing trend of utilizing eco-friendly and feasible agricultural by-products generates a stable stage for continuous innovation for development of products from the banana by-products and wastage, thus making a supportable income-generating product and providing the users with foods beneficial for health.

## REFERENCES

Abdul Aziz, N.A., L.H. Ho, B. Azahari, R. Bhat, L.H. Cheng, and M.N.M. Ibrahim. 2011. "Chemical and functional properties of the native banana (*Musa acuminata* x *balbisiana* Colla cv. Awak) pseudostem and pseudostem tender core flours". *Food Chemistry* 128:748–753.

Adão, R.C. and M.B.A. Glória. 2005. "Bioactive amines and carbohydrate changes during ripening of 'Prata' banana (*Musa acuminata* × *M. balbisiana*)". *Food Chemistry* 90(4):705–711.

Anagnostopoulou, M.A., P. Kefalas, V.P. Papageorgiou, A.N. Assimopoulou, and D. Boskou. 2006. "Radical scavenging activity of various extracts and fractions of sweet orange peel (*Citrus sinensis*)". *Food Chemistry* 94(1):19–25.

Anhwange, B.A., T.J. Ugye, and T.D. Nyiaatagher. 2009. "Chemical composition of *Musa sapientum* (banana) peels". *Electronic Journal of Environmental, Agricultural and Food Chemistry* 8(6):437–442.

Arora, A., D. Choudhary, G. Agarwal, and V.P. Singh. 2008. "Compositional variation in β-carotene content, carbohydrate and antioxidant enzymes in selected banana cultivars". *International Journal of Food Science & Technology* 43(11):1913–1921.

Artali, R., G. Beretta, P. Morazzoni, E. Bombardelli, and F. Meneghetti. 2009. "Green tea catechins in chemoprevention of cancer: A molecular docking investigation into their interaction with glutathione S-transferase (GST P1-1)". *Journal of Enzyme Inhibition and Medicinal Chemistry* 24(1):287–295.

Arvanitoyannis, I.S. and A. Mavromatis. 2009. "Banana cultivars, cultivation practices, and physicochemical properties". *Critical Reviews in Food Science and Nutrition* 49(2):113–135.

Aurore, G., B. Parfait, and L. Fahrasmane. 2009. "Bananas, raw materials for making processed food products". *Trends in Food Science & Technology* 20(2):78–91.

Bagchi, D., C.K. Sen, M. Bagchi, and M. Atalay. 2004. "Anti-angiogenic, antioxidant, and anti-carcinogenic properties of a novel anthocyanin-rich berry extract formula". *Biochemistry, Moscow* 69(1):75–80.

Baker, J.E. 1976. "Superoxide dismutase in ripening fruits". *Plant Physiology* 58(5):644–647.

Bowen-Forbes, C.S., Y. Zhang, and M.G. Nair. 2010. "Anthocyanin content, antioxidant, anti-inflammatory and anticancer properties of blackberry and raspberry fruits". *Journal of Food Composition and Analysis* 23(6):554–560.

Campos, N.A., R. Swennen, and S.C. Carpentier. 2018. "The plantain proteome, a focus on allele specific proteins obtained from plantain fruits". *Proteomics* 18(3–4):1700227.

Chadha, K.L. 2002. *Banana Handbook of Horticulture.* New Delhi: Directorate of Information & Publications of Agriculture, ICAR;:143–153.

Chanwitheesuk, A., A. Teerawutgulrag, J.D. Kilburn, and N. Rakariyatham. 2007. "Antimicrobial gallic acid from *Caesalpinia mimosoides* Lamk". *Food Chemistry* 100(3):1044–1048.

Chye, F.Y., and K.Y. Sim. 2009. "Antioxidative and antibacterial activities of *Pangium edule* seed extracts". *International Journal of Pharmacology* 5(5):285–297.

Colak, S.M., B.M. Yapici, and A.N. Yapici. 2010. "Determination of antimicrobial activity of tannic acid in pickling process". *Romanian Biotechnological Letters* 15(3):5325–5330.

Conner, D.E. 1993. "Naturally occurring compounds". *Antimicrobials in Foods* 441–468.

Da Mota, R.V., F.M. Lajolo, B.R. Cordenunsi, and C. Ciacco. 2000. "Composition and functional properties of banana flour from different varieties". *Starch-Stärke* 52(2–3):63–68.

De Langhe, E., L.Vrydaghs, P. De Maret, X. Perrier, and T. Denham. 2009. "Why bananas matter: An introduction to the history of banana domestication". *Ethnobotany Research and Applications* 7:165–177.

Devatkal, S.K., R. Kumboj, and D. Paul. 2014. "Comparative antioxidant effect of BHT and water extracts of banana and sapodilla peels in raw poultry meat". *Journal of Food Science and Technology* 51(2):387–391.

dos Santos Alves, L.A.A., J.M. Lorenzo, C.A.A. Gonçalves, B.A. Dos Santos, R.T. Heck, A.J. Cichoski, and P.C.B. Campagnol. 2016. "Production of healthier bologna type sausages using pork skin and green banana flour as a fat replacers". *Meat Science* 121:73–78.

Dotto, J., A.O. Matemu, and P.A. Ndakidemi. 2019. "Nutrient composition and selected physicochemical properties of fifteen Mchare cooking bananas: A study conducted in northern Tanzania". *Scientific African* 6:00150.

Einbond, L.S., K.A. Reynertson, X.D. Luo, M.J. Basile, and E.J. Kennelly. 2004. "Anthocyanin antioxidants from edible fruits". *Food Chemistry* 84(1):23–28.

Elanthikkal, S., U. Gopala Krishna panicker, S. Varghese, and J.T. Guthrie. 2010. "Cellulose microfibres produced from banana plant wastes: Isolation and characterization". *Carbohydrate Polymers*, 80(3):852–859.

Emaga, T.H., C. Robert, S.N. Ronkart, B. Wathelet. and M. Paquot. 2008a. "Dietary fibre components and pectin chemical features of peels during ripening in banana and plantain varieties". *Bioresource Technology* 99(10):4346–4354.

Emaga, T.H., S.N. Ronkart, C. Robert, B. Wathelet, and M. Paquot. 2008b. "Characterisation of pectins extracted from banana peels (*Musa* AAA) under different conditions using an experimental design". *Food Chemistry* 108(2):463–471.

Essien, J.P., E.J. Akpan, and E.P. Essien. 2005. "Studies on mould growth and biomass production using waste banana peel". *Bioresource Technology* 96(13):1451–1456.

Fan, G., Y. Han, Z. Gu, and D. Chen. 2008. "Optimizing conditions for anthocyanins extraction from purple sweet potato using response surface methodology (RSM)". *LWT – Food Science and Technology* 41(1):155–160.

FAO. 2010a. FAOSTAT: Banana Production by Countries 2010, http://faostat.fao.org/site/339/default.aspx [Assessed 27 May 2012].

FAO. 2010b. FAOSTAT: Total World Banana Production 2010, http://faostat.fao.org/site/567/DesktopDefault.aspx?PageID0567#ancor [Assessed 27 May 2012]

Farees, N., D.D. Abateneh, M. Geneto, and N. Naidu. 2017. "Evaluation of banana peel waste as growth medium for probiotic Lactobacillus species". *International Journal of Applied Biology and Pharmaceutical Technology* 8(4):19–23.

Faried, A., D. Kurnia, L.S. Faried, N. Usman, T. Miyazaki, H. Kato, and H. Kuwano. 2007. "Anticancer effects of gallic acid isolated from Indonesian herbal medicine, *Phaleria macrocarpa* (Scheff.) Boerl, on human cancer cell lines". *International Journal of Oncology*, 30(3):605–613.

Ferreira Ozela, E., P.C. Stringheta, and M. Cano Chauca. 2007. "Stability of anthocyanin in spinach vine (*Basella rubra*) fruits". *Ciencia e investigaciónagraria* 34(2):115–120.

Fridovich I. 1972. "Superoxide radical and superoxide dismutase". *Accounts of Chemical Research* 5:321.

Gigot, C., M. Ongena, M.L. Fauconnier, J.P. Wathelet, P. Du Jardin, and P. Thonart. 2010. "The lipoxygenase metabolic pathway in plants: Potential for industrial production of natural green leaf volatiles". *Biotechnology, Agronomy and Society and Environment* 14(3):451–460.

González-Montelongo, R., M.G. Lobo, and M. González. 2010. "Antioxidant activity in banana peel extracts: Testing extraction conditions and related bioactive compounds". *Food Chemistry* 119(3):1030–1039.

Hoeger, S., U. Gottmann, Z. Liu, P. Schnuelle, R. Birck, C. Braun, F.J. Van Der Woude, and B.A. Yard. 2007. "Dopamine treatment in brain-dead rats mediates anti-inflammatory effects: The role of hemodynamic stabilization and D-receptor stimulation". *Transplant International* 20(9):790–799.

Ilori, M.O., S.A. Adebusoye, A.K. Iawal, and O.A. Awotiwon. 2007. "Production of biogas from banana and plantain peels". *Advances in Environmental Biology* 33–39.

Jagan, S., G. Ramakrishnan, P. Anandakumar, S. Kamaraj, and T. Devaki. 2008. "Antiproliferative potential of gallic acid against diethyl nitrosamine-induced rat hepatocellular carcinoma". *Molecular and Cellular Biochemistry* 319(1):51–59.

Jahan, M., M.K. Warsi, and F. Khatoon. 2010. "Concentration influence on antimicrobial activity of banana blossom extract-incorporated chitosan-polyethylene glycol (CS-PEG) blended film". *Journal of Chemical and Pharmaceutical Research* 2(5):373–378.

Jiang, H., Y. Zhang, Y. Hong, Y. Bi, Z. Gu, L. Cheng, Z. Li, and C. Li. 2015. "Digestibility and changes to structural characteristics of green banana starch during in vitro digestion". *Food Hydrocolloids* 49:192–199.

Joshi, R.V. 2007. "Low calorie biscuits from banana peel pulp". *Journal of Solid Waste Technology & Management* 33(3).

Kandasamy, S. and S.M. Aradhya. 2014. "Polyphenolic profile and antioxidant properties of rhizome of commercial banana cultivars grown in India". *Food Bioscience* 8:22–32.

Karlsen, A., L. Retterstøl, P. Laake, I. Paur, S. Kjølsrud-Bøhn, L. Sandvik, and R. Blomhoff. 2007. "Anthocyanins inhibit nuclear factor-κ B activation in monocytes and reduce plasma concentrations of pro-inflammatory mediators in healthy adults". *Journal of Nutrition* 137(8):1951–1954.

Kennedy, J. 2009. "Bananas and people in the homeland of genus Musa: Not just pretty fruit". *Ethnobotany Research and Applications* 7:179–197.

Khawas, P., A.J. Das, K.K. Dash, and S.C. Deka. 2014. "Thin-layer drying characteristics of Kachkal banana peel (*Musa* ABB) of Assam, India". *International Food Research Journal* 21(3).

Khoozani, A.A., J. Birch, and A.E.D.A. Bekhit. 2019. "Production, application and health effects of banana pulp and peel flour in the food industry". *Journal of Food Science and Technology"* 56(2):548–559.

Kitdamrongsont, K., P. Pothavorn, S. Swangpol, S. Wongniam, K. Atawongsa, J. Svasti, and J. Somana. 2008. "Anthocyanin composition of wild bananas in Thailand". *Journal of Agricultural and Food Chemistry* 56(22):10853–10857.

Konzack, I. and W. Zhang. 2004. "Anthocyanins—more than nature's colors". *Journal of Biomedicine and Biotechnology* 5:239–240.

Kookal, S.K. and A. Thimmaiah. 2018. "Nutritional composition of staple food bananas of three cultivars in India". *American Journal of Plant Sciences* 9(12):2480–2493.

Kulma, A. and J. Szopa. 2007. "Catecholamines are active compounds in plants". *Plant Science* 172(3):433–440.

Kumar, R. 1992. "Anti-nutritional factors, the potential risks of toxicity and methods to alleviate them. Legume trees and other fodder trees as protein source for livestock". *FAO Animal Production and Health Paper* 102:145–160.

Kumar, D. and V.K. Tanwar. 2011. "Effects of incorporation of ground mustard on quality attributes of chicken nuggets". *Journal of Food Science and Technology* 48(6):759–762.

Kumudavally, K.V., A. Tabassum, K. Radhakrishna, and A.S. Bawa. 2011. "Effect of ethanolic extract of clove on the keeping quality of fresh mutton during storage at ambient temperature (25±2 C)". *Journal of Food Science and Technology* 48(4):.466–471.

Kuo, J.M., A. Hwang, D.B. Yeh, M.H. Pan, M.L. Tsai, and B.S. Pan. 2006. "Lipoxygenase from banana leaf: Purification and characterization of an enzyme that catalyzes linoleic acid oxygenation at the 9-position". *Journal of Agricultural and Food Chemistry* 54(8):3151–3156.

Lee, E.H., H.J. Yeom, M.S. Ha, and D.H. Bae. 2010. "Development of banana peel jelly and its antioxidant and textural properties". *Food Science and Biotechnology* 19(2):449–455.

Leslie, C.S. 1976. *An Introduction to the Botany of Tropical Crops* (2nd Edition). London: Longman Group Limited; pp. 153–154.

Loizzo, M.R., L.G. Di, E. Boselli, F. Menichini, and N.G. Frega. 2011. "Inhibitory activity of phenolic compounds from extract virgin olive oils on the enzyme involved in diabetes, obesity and hypertension". *Journal of Food Biochemistry* 35:381–399.

Lu, Z., G. Nie, P.S. Belton, H. Tang, and B. Zhao. 2006. "Structure–activity relationship analysis of antioxidant ability and neuroprotective effect of gallic acid derivatives". *Neurochemistry International* 48(4):263–274.

Madhav, A. and P.B. Pushpalatha. 2006. "Characterization of pectin extracted from different fruit wastes". *Journal of Tropical Agriculture* 40:53–55.

Mandel, S.A., T. Amit, L. Kalfon, L. Reznichenko, and M.B. Youdim. 2008. "Targeting multiple neurodegenerative diseases etiologies with multimodal-acting green tea catechins". *Journal of Nutrition*, 138(8)1578S–1583S.

Mertens-Talcott, S.U., J. Rios, P. Jilma Stohlawetz, L.A. Pacheco-Palencia, B. Meibohm, S.T. Talcott, and H. Derendorf. 2008. "Pharmacokinetics of anthocyanins and antioxidant effects after the consumption of anthocyanin-rich acai juice and pulp (*Euterpe oleracea* Mart.) in human healthy volunteers". *Journal of Agricultural and Food Chemistry* 56(17):7796–7802.

Miller, M.R., P.D. Nichols, and C.G. Carter. 2008. "The digestibility and accumulation of dietary phytosterols in Atlantic salmon (*Salmo salar* L.) smolt fed diets with replacement plant oils". *Lipids* 43(6):549–557.

Mokbel, M.S. and F. Hashinaga. 2005. "Antibacterial and antioxidant activities of banana (*Musa*, AAA cv. Cavendish) fruits peel". *American Journal of Biochemistry and Biotechnology* 1(3):125–131.

Moruisi, K.G., W. Oosthuizen, and A.M. Opperman. 2006. "Phytosterols/stanols lower cholesterol concentrations in familial hypercholesterolemic subjects: A systematic review with meta-analysis". *Journal of the American College of Nutrition* 25(1):41–48.

Mostafa, H.S. 2021. "Banana plant as a source of valuable antimicrobial compounds and its current applications in the food sector". *Journal of Food Science* 86(9):3778–3797.

Netshiheni, R.K., A.O. Omolola, T.A. Anyasi, and A.I. Jideani. 2019. "Banana bioactives: Absorption, utilisation and health benefits". In *Banana Nutrition-Function and Processing Kinetics*. Intech Open.

Nguyen, T.B.T., S. Ketsa, and W.G. van Doorn. 2003. "Relationship between browning and the activities of polyphenoloxidase and phenylalanine ammonia lyase in banana peel during low temperature storage". *Postharvest Biology and Technology* 30(2):187–193.

Oliveira, L., C.S. Freire, A.J. Silvestre, and N. Cordeiro. 2008. "Lipophilic extracts from banana fruit residues: A source of valuable phytosterols". *Journal of Agricultural and Food Chemistry* 56(20):9520–9524.

Oliveira, L., C.S.R. Freire, A.J.D. Silvestre, N. Cordeiro, I.C. Torres, and D. Evtuguin. 2005. "Steryl glucosides from banana plant *Musa acuminata* Colla var. Cavendish". *Industrial Crops and Products* 22(3):187–192.

Oyeyinka, B.O. and A.J. Afolayan. 2020. "Potentials of Musa species fruits against oxidative stress-induced and diet-linked chronic diseases: In vitro and in vivo implications of micronutritional factors and dietary secondary metabolite compounds". *Molecules* 25(21):5036.

Padam, B.S., H.S. Tin, F.Y. Chye, and M.I. Abdullah. 2012. "Antibacterial and antioxidative activities of the various solvent extracts of banana (*Musa paradisiaca* cv. Mysore) inflorescences". *Journal of Biological Sciences* 12(2):62–73.

Pazmiño-Durán, E.A., M.M. Giusti, R.E. Wrolstad, and M.B.A. Glória. 2001. "Anthocyanins from banana bracts (*Musa* X paradisiaca) as potential food colorants". *Food Chemistry* 73(3):327–332.

Pereira, A. and M. Maraschin. 2015. "Banana (*Musa* spp.) from peel to pulp: Ethnopharmacology, source of bioactive compounds and its relevance for human health". *Journal of Ethnopharmacology* 160:149–163.

Pillai, P. and K. Ramaswamy. 2012. "Effect of naturally occurring antimicrobials and chemical preservatives on the growth of *Aspergillus parasiticus*". *Journal of Food Science and Technology* 49(2):228–233.

Pliszka, B., G. Huszcza-Ciołkowska, and E. Wierzbicka. 2008. "Effects of extraction conditions on the content of anthocyanins and bioelements in berry fruit extracts". *Communications in Soil Science and Plant Analysis* 39(5–6):753–762.

Ploetz, R.C., A.K. Kepler, J. Daniells, and S.C. Nelson. 2007. "Banana and plantain—An overview with emphasis on Pacific Island cultivars". *Species Profiles for Pacific Island Agroforestry* 1:21–32.

Powthong, P., B. Jantrapanukorn, P. Suntornthiticharoen, and K. Laohaphatanalert. 2020. "Study of prebiotic properties of selected banana species in Thailand". *Journal of Food Science and Technology* 57(7):2490–2500.

Probojati, R.T., D. Listyorini, S. Sulisetijono, and D. Wahyudi. 2021. "Phylogeny and estimated genetic divergence times of banana cultivars (*Musa* spp.) from Java Island by maturase K (mat K) genes". *Bulletin of the National Research Centre* 45(1):1–13.

Qamar, S. and A. Shaikh. 2018. "Therapeutic potentials and compositional changes of valuable compounds from banana—A review". *Trends in Food Science & Technology* 79:1–9.

Racette, S.B., X. Lin, M. Lefevre, C.A. Spearie, M.M. Most, L. Ma, and R.E. Ostlund. 2010. "Dose effects of dietary phytosterols on cholesterol metabolism: A controlled feeding study". *American Journal of Clinical Nutrition* 91(1):32–38.

Raghavan, K.G. and T.P. Devasagayam. 1985. "Oxalate oxidase from banana peel for determination of urinary oxalate". *Clinical Chemistry* 31(4):649.

Raina, K., S. Rajamanickam, G. Deep, M. Singh, R. Agarwal, and C. Agarwal. 2008. "Chemopreventive effects of oral gallic acid feeding on tumor growth and progression in TRAMP mice". *Molecular Cancer Therapeutics* 7(5):1258–1267.

Rappert, S. and R. Mülle. 2005. "Odor compounds in waste gas emissions from agricultural operations and food industries". *Waste Management* 25(9):887–907.

Roobha, J.J., M. Saravanakumar, K.M. Aravindhan, and P.S. Devi. 2011. "The effect of light, temperature, pH on stability of anthocyanin pigments in *Musa acuminata* bract". *Research in Plant Biology* 1(5):5–12.

Rosentrater, K.A., D. Todey, and R. Persyn. 2009. *"Quantifying Total and Sustainable Agricultural Biomass Resources in South Dakota"* A Preliminary Assessment.

Rymbai, H., R.R. Sharma, and M. Srivastav. 2011. "Bio-colorants and its implications in health and food industry—A review". *International Journal of Pharmacological Research* 3(4):2228–2244.

Saravanan, K. and S.M. Aradhya. 2011. "Polyphenols of pseudostem of different banana cultivars and their antioxidant activities". *Journal of Agricultural and Food Chemistry* 59(8):3613–3623.

Shah, M.P., G.V. Reddy, R. Banerjee, P.R. Babu, and I.L. Kothari. 2005. "Microbial degradation of banana waste under solid state bioprocessing using two lignocellulolytic fungi (*Phylosticta* spp. MPS-001 and *Aspergillus* spp. MPS-002)". *Process Biochemistry* 40(1):445–451.

Shan, B., Y.Z. Cai, J.D. Brooks, and H. Corke. 2007. "The in vitro antibacterial activity of dietary spice and medicinal herb extracts". *International Journal of Food Microbiology* 117(1):112–119.

Shan, B., Y.Z. Cai, J.D. Brooks, and H. Corke. 2008. "Antibacterial properties of *Polygonum cuspidatum* roots and their major bioactive constituents". *Food Chemistry* 109(3):530–537.

Shankar, S.K. and V.H. Mulimani. 2007. "α-Galactosidase production by *Aspergillus oryzae* in solid-state fermentation". *Bioresource Technology* 98(4):958–961.

Sidhu, J.S. and T.A. Zafar. 2018. "Bioactive compounds in banana fruits and their health benefits". *Food Quality and Safety* 2(4):183–188.

Singh, S.K., A.N. Kesari, P.K. Rai, and G. Watal. 2007. "Assessment of glycemic potential of *Musa paradisiaca* stem juice". *Indian Journal of Clinical Biochemistry* 22(2):48–52.

Someya, S., Y. Yoshiki, and K. Okubo. 2002. "Antioxidant compounds from bananas (*Musa* Cavendish)". *Food Chemistry* 79(3):351–354.

Subbaraya, U., N. Lutaladio, and W.O. Baudoin. 2006. "Farmer's knowledge of wild Musa in India". *Rome: Plant Production and Protection Division FAO* 1–46.

Sudha, M.L., R. Vetrimani, and K. Leelavathi. 2007. "Influence of fibre from different cereals on the rheological characteristics of wheat flour dough and on biscuit quality". *Food Chemistry* 100(4):1365–1370.

Tin, H.S., B.S. Padam, F.Y. Chye, and M.I. Abdullah. 2010. "Study on the potential of antimicrobial compounds from banana/plantain by-products against foodborne pathogens". In: *National Biotechnology Seminar*, 24th–26th May, Kuala Lumpur, Malaysia.

Tiwari, B.K., V.P. Valdramidis, C.P. O'Donnell, K. Muthukumarappan, P. Bourke, and P.J. Cullen. 2009. "Application of natural antimicrobials for food preservation". *Journal of Agricultural and Food Chemistry* 57(14):5987–6000.

Torskangerpoll, K. and Ø.M. Andersen. 2005. "Colour stability of anthocyanins in aqueous solutions at various pH values". *Food Chemistry*, 89(3):427–440.

Uma, S., S. Kalpana, S. Sathiamoorthy, and V. Kumar. 2005. "Evaluation of commercial cultivars of banana (*Musa* spp.) for their suitability for the fibre industry". *Plant Genetic Resources Newsletter* 142:29.

Vu, H.T., C.J. Scarlett, and Q.V. Vuong. 2018. "Phenolic compounds within banana peel and their potential uses: A review". *Journal of Functional Foods* 40:238–248.

Wang, X., W. Jia, A. Zhao, and X. Wang. 2006. "Anti-influenza agents from plants and traditional Chinese medicine". *Phytotherapy Research: An International Journal Devoted to Pharmacological and Toxicological Evaluation of Natural Product Derivatives* 20(5):335–341.

Weingärtner, O., D. Lütjohann, S. Ji, N. Weisshoff, F. List, T. Sudhop, K. von Bergmann, K. Gertz, J. König, H.J. Schäfers, and M. Endres. 2008. "Vascular effects of diet supplementation with plant sterols". *Journal of the American College of Cardiology* 51(16):1553–1561.

Wong, J.Y. and F.Y. Chye. 2009. "Antioxidant properties of selected tropical wild edible mushrooms". *Journal of Food Composition and Analysis* 22(4):269–277.

Yabaya, A. and S.A. Ado. 2008. "Mycelial protein production by *Aspergillus niger* using banana peels". *Science World Journal* 3(4).

Zhang, P., R.L. Whistler, J.N. BeMiller, and B.R. Hamaker. 2005. "Banana starch: Production, physicochemical properties, and digestibility—A review". *Carbohydrate Polymers* 59(4):443–458.

Zheng, J., C. Ding, L. Wang, G. Li, J. Shi, H. Li, H. Wang, and Y. Suo. 2011. "Anthocyanins composition and antioxidant activity of wild *Lyciumruthenicum* Murr. from Qinghai-Tibet Plateau". *Food Chemistry* 126(3):859–865.

# 11 Orange

*Arun Kumar Gupta, Subhamoy Dhua, Rahul Thakur, Khyali Ncama,
Nkanyiso J. Sithole, Lembe Samukelo Magwaza, Bindu Naik,
and Poonam Mishra*

## CONTENTS

## 11.1 INTRODUCTION

All over the world, citrus fruit is one of the chief crops among fruit varieties (Das et al. 2020). Over the decades, citrus fruits have been processed into several products, from which about 30% are served as juice (Gupta et al. 2021a, 2022). Moreover, the citrus processing industry is placed second all over the world, but it is trailing only the grape industry, which is more concentrated in the processing of wine.

Pomelo, sour orange, kumquat, lime, citron, sweet orange, grapefruit, lemon, and hybrids are some of the most important fruit crops (Gupta et al. 2021b, c; Lu et al. 2021; Zhang et al. 2021 Gupta et al. 2020). *Citrus* belongs to the Rutaceae subfamily, and the genus of Aurantioideae (Wu et al. 2018). This type of fruit variety has been found in Southeast Asia, namely in Southwest China's Yunnan region, Myanmar, and North-Eastern India in the Himalayan slopes (Wu et al. 2018; Gupta et al. 2021d). In most of the tropical and subtropical regions of China, Brazil, and some regions of Europe, the citrus trees are widely farmed, with total annual output of almost 102 million tonnes (USDA 2021). The remaining half of citrus production/exports include tangerines/mandarins (one-third of total citrus output), lemons/limes, and grapefruit (USDA 2021). The *Citrus* genus is well-known for its delicious flavour and richness of bioactive nutrients.

DOI: 10.1201/9781003259213-11

Bioactive compounds, including teraponids such as carotenoids, limonoids, and so on, are abundant in citrus fruits (Lado et al. 2018; Cebadera-Miranda et al. 2019; Lu et al. 2021). Pectin is one of the most vital components present mainly in the citrus fruit walls. In addition to these, vitamins such as C and E, as well as minerals (zinc, manganese, selenium, iron, copper), are all abundant in citrus fruits (Zou et al. 2016; Lado et al. 2018; Cebadera-Miranda et al. 2019; Lu et al. 2021).

Farmers generally gain profits nutritionally and financially from oranges, making them one of the most significant crops in the horticulture industry. The crop is grown, and the productions are higher in tropical and subtropical climates in the United States, South Africa, Spain, Egypt, Brazil, and India. From all types of varieties, Washington navel, Blood, and Valencia are mostly grown as popular oranges. For proper growth, the temperature needs to be from 13°C to 38°C, and the annual rainfall is about 1500 mm. Moreover, the appropriate soil should be in the pH range of 6 to 7, and it should be deep and well-drained.

Several studies have been reported on oranges focusing on the bioactive content and health benefits along with the perspective of its chemical compositions, extraction of bioactive compounds as well as products prepared from the orange. The goal of this chapter is to go through the numerous functional bioactive found in orange fruits, as well as the health benefits they provide. Furthermore, the extraction techniques for bioactive substances are put to the test. Finally, the impact of different processing methods on bioactive compounds is briefly examined in light of future potential.

## 11.2 TYPES AND COMPOSITION OF ORANGE

Even though fresh citrus fruits are widely consumed in all producing nations, processed citrus fruits must be regarded as practically luxury items. Only industrialised countries have breakfast with orange juice. As a result, citrus companies produce high-value goods that are valued for their quality, nutritional content, and purity. Due to the strong relationship between these three features and composition, the citrus constituent analysis is a common subject of scientific activity, encouraged by governments and companies.

Citrus contains a large number of species, and experts are fascinated by the distinctions between them. However, the similarities outnumber the differences when comparing species of the same genus. The economic value of each species varies, and compositional analyses of the most important species are more common. As a consequence, Citrus sinensis (sweet orange) data is more extensive compared to that of Citrus reticulata (tangerine), Citrus limon (lemon), or Citrus paradisi (grapefruit), and data on these species is more in-depth compared to that on other Citrus species. Moreover, several varieties are very popular in each species mentioned above. Of all these varieties, the most commonly used for juice preparation is the Valencia orange, which is another widely known, and most researched, sweet orange. As a result, the majority of the information offered here will be about the juice rather than the whole fruit because the juice, which makes up over half of an orange's total weight, is the most important portion of the fruit and is what people consume the most (Izquierdo and Sendra 2003).

The weight of the peel is about another half of the whole fruit weight, but it is not as important as juice from an orange. Although various by-products (cattle feed, molasses) may be made from the peel, the goal is to eliminate residues and reduce pollution, not to make money. The only peel products utilised in human food, scent, and cosmetics are peel oil which is derived from the extraction process. Pectin is also obtained solely from certain species and varieties (Izquierdo and Sendra 2003).

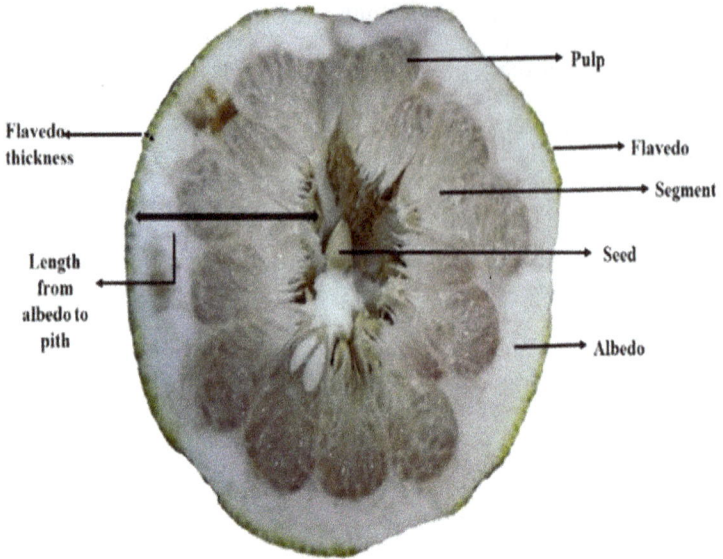

**Figure 11.1** Different parts of citrus fruit. (Image courtesy: Tezpur University, India.)

The juice is almost half of the whole weight of the orange, which is generally stored in juice vesicles in the endocarp. Basically, the fruit peel is composed of epicarp, outer mesocarp, which is combinedly known as flavedo, and inner mesocarp, which is known as albedo, respectively (Figure 11.1). Flavedo and albedo make up around 10% and 25% of the total fruit, individually. The oil is mainly present in the oil sacs of flavedo, while the albedo contains most of the pectin. The remaining weight of the fruit is made up of fibre, pulp, and seeds after juice extraction. Water makes up to 90% of the fruit. Sugars and acids make up the rest and, amino groups, pectin, flavonoids, minerals, and so on, are some minor components present in it. Other citrus fruits have different percentages, but orange fruits have different percentages as well, depending on variety, maturity, location, and cultivation procedures (Izquierdo and Sendra 2003).

## 11.3 DIFFERENT TYPES OF PRODUCTS PREPARED FROM ORANGE

Canned oranges, orange juice, squashes, jam, marmalade, and candies are some common products prepared from oranges and are available in the market. Detailed information about these products is written below.

### 11.3.1 Canned Orange

Canned orange is not as common as other orange-based products. Canned orange is available up to a limited extent. Mostly for canning, "Unshu," "Mandarin," and "Satsuma" varieties of Japan are used and considered as important as these are seedless practically. Among Indian varieties, loose-jacket Mandarin oranges of Nagpur, Assam, etc., which allow easy removal of seeds with avoidable breakages, are recommended for canning. Eventually, it produces a good amount of yield of canned oranges. To get good canned products, proper care, handling, unit operations (peeling, exhausting, processing), and cooling of cans are needed. Loose jacket orange peel is removed easily by hand; however, tight-skinned orange peels are removed prior to dipping the fruit into the boiling water. The adhering fibres are removed after separating the segments. These are dipped in boiling lye solution of 1%–2% strength for 20–30 s, rinsed in warm water to remove the alkali traces, then these are dipped in dilute HCl solution having 0.5%–1.0% strength and eventually rinsed well using cold water. Seed and membranes, if any, also removed by hand. Finally, these processed segments are filled into cans containing some water to protect them from breakage during filling. After filling, the water is drained out of the cans. A little amount of orange flavour can also be added to these before sealing containers in a vacuum double seamer. Alternatively, in a rocking-type pasteuriser in an open tank of water, the filled cans are exhausted and processed simultaneously at 82°C to 87°C for 15 to 20 min. Then in a rocking type of cooler, the processed cans are cooled. Proper precautions need to be taken to avoid the breaking of segments and loss of flavour. Moreover, broken segments are used to make jam, jelly, squash, etc.

### 11.3.2 Orange Juice

Orange juice is quite popular due to its pleasant taste and good nutritional profile (vitamins, minerals, etc.). Until now, orange juice in its raw form is less marketed although these have good nutritive value due to some difficulties like improper storage, taste changes over time, etc. Although synthetic products like orangeade, sherbet, flavoured beverages, etc., are comparatively less nutritive than fresh juice, millions of bottles are still produced over the year.

To produce juice from fresh fruits, some unit operations need to be followed. To begin, fruits are cleaned in a spinning rod cylinder with a helical screw inside that pushes the fruit along with water jets (driven by a centrifugal pump). The fruits are then separated into a woven metal belt that runs the length of the conveyor. Finally, a Taglith style of press is used to remove the juice from the little sacs of loose-jacketed mandarin oranges (developed by Central Food Technological Research Institute, Mysore). However, for the extraction of juices from malta oranges, using a halving and burring machine is necessary. Then the juice is strained and pasteurised, eventually using a flash pasteuriser.

### 11.3.3 Orange Squash

Both loose (Coorg, Nagpur, etc.) and tight-skinned (Sathgudi, Malta, etc.) oranges are preferred for making squash. These two kinds of oranges are processed in differently while squeezing the juice out of the oranges. Basically, tight-skinned oranges are cut into halves either by a halving machine (which contains a circular knife) or by hand with a knife. A rosing machine, fitted with a rose or hand against a revolving bar, is used to press the halves. Then the reamed juice is collected in a vessel. The juice is then filtered using a cloth or by passing through a sieving machine (pulper) as it contains abundant seeds, coarse tissues, etc. Whereas the loose-jacketed oranges are peeled off, and the fibrous rag attached in the segments is removed. Hot lye solution is mostly used to remove the parchment-like material enclosed in the sacs within 0.5 to 1 mm. Then the juice is extracted from the washed segments. Finally, after the juice extraction, squash is prepared using sugar, citric acid, colour, flavouring materials and preservatives. Sugar, water and citric acid are mixed and heated to prepare clean syrup by filtering it using a cloth only after cooling. The clean syrup is blended with juice. Orange flavour is added to it, and the colour is also improved. Then an optimum amount of chemical preservative is added to it. Eventually, the final product is filled into sterilised bottles.

### 11.3.4 Orange Wine

Orange wine-making process is similar to the grape wine-making process. Oranges are first sorted, and the juice is then extracted. Cane sugar is used to sweeten the orange juice. *Saccharomyces ellipsoideus* is added as a starter to ferment the juice, popularly known as "must" in the fermentation industry. To check the activity of bacteria and wild yeasts in the formation of undesirable alcohol formation, sulphur dioxide is added to the "must". The temperature is also maintained. Sugar is passed through various stages in the "must" before being converted into alcohol and finally filled into barrels. The clear wine is syphoned and filled in sealed air-tight containers to exclude all the air after the completion of fermentation. The maturing stage takes 6 to 12 months to acquire the smooth flavour and aroma. During the maturation process, the wine is naturally clarified using egg whites, filter aids, etc. Before packing into bottles, wines are pasteurised to destroy the spoilage organisms, and the bottles are closed using good quality bark corks.

### 11.3.5 Orange Jam

Oranges have high jam-making potential as these are a good source of pectin and acid. Traditionally, jam is prepared by mixing fresh orange slices with pectin, gelling agent, commercial sugar and citric acid. Then the mixture is concentrated to 56% soluble solid content through a boiling process. Briefly, the first step in jam preparation is the selection of fruits and preparation of fruits. Good quality ripe fruits are selected, washed, peeled off and finally cut into small pieces. Then sugar and acid are added to an optimum amount. Generally, 55 parts of sugar are required for 45 parts of fruit. Then the mixture is cooked thoroughly with continuous stirring. The temperature of boiling is kept to 105°C. To check the endpoint of the preparation process, a small portion of the jam is taken out and allowed to fall; if it falls in the form of a sheet rather than falling in a continuous stream, it defines the endpoint of the process, otherwise boiling is continued until the desirable condition reached. Basically, the pH of 3.4 is maintained in an orange jam. Finally, sterilised dry jars are used to pour the hot jam, allowed to cool, closed with the sterilised lid and stored in a cool place.

### 11.3.6 Orange Marmalade

In most cases, marmalade is made by cooking good fruits with their peels, pulps, and juices, with or without water and nutritional sweeteners. While concentrating, the consistency should be maintained until gelatinisation occurs upon cooling the product. The minimum content of total soluble solid fruit content except for peel and peel in suspension should be 65%, 45%, and 5%, respectively. The final product is left overnight to set properly and then filled in sterilised and hermetically sealed containers. However, it is important that the product fill at least 90% of the net weight of the container. Orange marmalades can be of two types: (i) Jelly marmalade and (ii) Jam marmalade. There is no difference in the procedure in making both the marmalades; however, in jelly marmalade, one special attempt has been made to clarify the pectin extract in the fruit.

Nevertheless, candied fruits and crystallised fruits are some other examples of orange products that are commercially available in the market.

### 11.3.7 By-Products of Orange Processing

Approximately 40% of the fruit is utilised by processing industries to develop products from it, and the remaining portion (50%) of the fruit is wasted (seeds, pulp and peels). Moreover, waste parts of oranges contribute to environmental hazards (implying high BOD [biological oxygen demand] and COD [chemical oxygen demand] due to fermentation) without any post-treatment. However, these waste parts are rich sources of fibre, polysaccharides, antioxidants, essential oils, organic acids, pectin, etc. Therefore, waste parts need to be processed so those parts can be utilised properly. Orange pomace from orange juice processing industries is a very common by-product of oranges, which is nowadays utilised to develop flavour, fragrance and non-synthetic food preservative (Dassoff et al. 2021). Other by-products are juice residues, molasses, etc.

## 11.4 NUTRACEUTICALS IN ORANGE

Orange is a rich source of nutraceuticals. Antioxidants (flavonoids), vitamin C, total phenols, fibre, essential oils, carotenes, etc., are present in orange in different proportions in its different parts. Therefore, oranges and its products possess good nutritional value, which promotes human health. Bioactives can be referred to as nutraceuticals. Bioactives are those essential or non-essential compounds that are naturally available and have a significant effect on human health. Generally, bioactives promotes health by preventing life risk causable disease (cancer, cardiovascular disease, etc.) (Biesalski et al. 2009). Orange in the form of juice is an abundant source of bioactive compounds like carotenoids, vitamin C, flavanones, etc. The reason behind the orange pulp and peel's characteristic colour is the presence of carotenoids in enormous amounts. These carotenoids (α-carotene, β-carotene, α-cryptoxanthin, β-cryptoxanthin, zeaxanthin, and lutein) possess good antioxidant activity and serve as a precursor of vitamin A. Flavanones like narirutin, hesperidin, etc., are present in orange juice (Velázquez-Estrada et al. 2013). Most of the products developed from orange juice itself; therefore, the products contain these bioactive compounds in more or less amounts depending upon the processing method. Moreover, the by-products obtained during orange processing also contain the unavoidable amount of bioactive compounds (pectin, essential oils, limonin, etc.). Nowadays, different extraction techniques (ultrasound-assisted extraction, microwave-assisted extraction, pulse electric field extraction, etc.) are adopted by the food processing industries to extract those bioactive compounds rather than wasting them simply as a part of garbage or by using them as cattle food.

Oranges have been shown to reduce heart diseases and arrhythmias. The orange is known to contain an abundant amount of vitamin C as well as beneficial nutrients such as folate, carotenoids, flavonoids, thiamine, minerals, fibre, and limonoids. The fruit is high in macronutrients, micronutrients, minerals, and vitamins that have been proved to be beneficial to one's health. Consumption of oranges aid in the production of collagen, a protein that aids in wound healing and improving skin texture (Chavoshnejad et al. 2021). The consumption of orange juice enhances the ability of the body to absorb iron, which is beneficial in the treatment of anaemia. Oranges are widely used in functional foods either as the main ingredient or an additional ingredient. For instance, orange juice that is fortified with calcium for bone health is commonly found in the market. The value of an orange as a functional food also persists on the orange solely consumed without fortification. The orange contains vitamin C, which is associated with boosting the immune system and reducing the chances of disease infections. Consumption of oranges was demonstrated to moderate the blood pressure of hypertensive patients (Yulia 2020). Oranges also increase blood flow. The increase in blood pressure is aligned with increasing bodily physiological reactions, including improving blood circulation, which results in the stimulation of sexual appetite. Oranges also increase consumers' appetite for food. This can be associated with the increased rates of physiological processes of the body that need continuous fuelling from the food.

## 11.5 DIFFERENT METHODS OF EXTRACTING BIOACTIVE COMPOUNDS

Most bioactive compounds are extracted together with a variety of compounds included in the total soluble solutes. The number and quality of bioactive substances determine their efficacy. Choosing an adequate extraction procedure is critical for quantitative and qualitative analysis of plant-originated bioactive compounds (Azmir et al. 2013). In every bioactive chemical study, extraction is the primary step and has a big influence on the end outcome. The extraction of bioactive substances is influenced by various parameters, including extraction conditions, extraction technique, extraction solvent, and raw materials (Table 11.1).

The soaking method is mainly manipulated by using different solution temperatures and pH levels through various solvents and their concentrations. With the pH level, bases are compared with acidic solvents at different concentrations to observe the conditions that will yield more concentration of the targeted compound. Some researchers use a more pressurised method of extraction, such as compression under different conditions. This method is not widely used, which is attributed to the need for fuel or electricity to run the compressors, that may be expensive for most research institutes compared with the material used for the popular soaking method. Non-conventional and conventional extraction techniques can be distinguished (Figure 11.2). Conventional processes need the use of agitation, organic solvents, and a specific temperature. This method includes things like Soxhlet, maceration, and

## Table 11.1: Extraction Methods for Common Bioactive Compounds Present in the Orange

| Bioactive Compound | Extraction Method | Fruit Section | Reference |
|---|---|---|---|
| Carotenoids | • Juice extractor (shear force extractor and a reamer extractor) | Juice | Li et al. (2021) |
| | • Ultrasound-assisted extraction | Peel | Savic et al. (2021) |
| | • Solvent extraction | Whole fruit | Singh et al. (2021) |
| Flavonoids | • Juice extractor (shear force extractor and a reamer extractor) | Juice | Li et al. (2021) |
| | • Solvent extraction | Peels | Pereira et al. (2017) |
| Phenolic compounds | • Solvent extraction (*methanol:* Water) | Pulp | Iglesias-Carres et al. (2019) |
| | • Solvent extraction (*ethanol:* Water) | Whole fruit | Sir Elkhatim et al. (2018) |
| | • Supercritical fluid extraction and hydro-alcoholic solvent | Pulp | Espinosa-Pardo et al. (2017) |
| Terpenes | • Supercritical $CO_2$ (SC-$CO_2$) | Peel | Jokić et al. (2020) |
| Vitamin C (ascorbic acid) | • Solvent extraction (aqueous, ethyl-alcohol, acetone) | Whole fruit | Dumbravă et al. (2011) |
| | • Ultrasound-assisted hydro-alcohol extraction | Peel | Montero-Calderon et al. (2019) |
| | • Solvent extraction (acetone extraction) | Peel | Senit et al. (2019) |

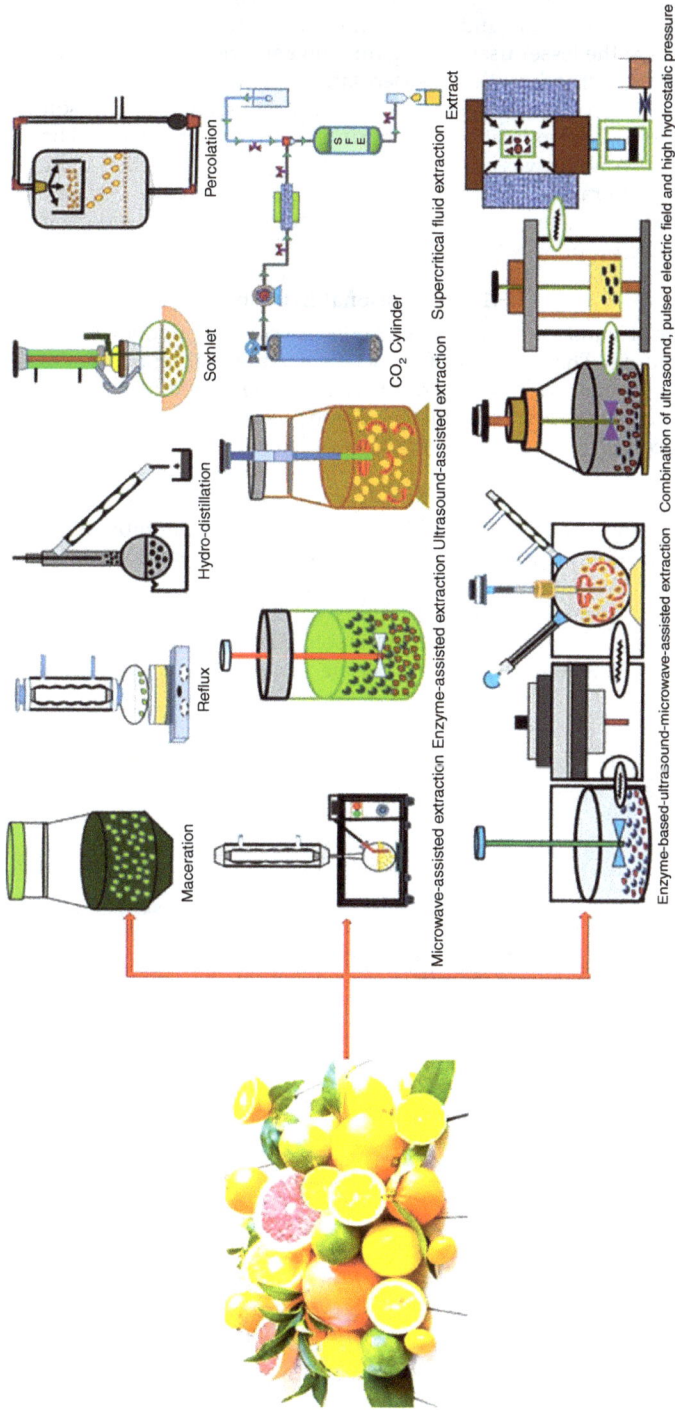

**Figure 11.2** Different extraction techniques of bioactive compounds from citrus fruits.

hydrodistillation. Non-conventional or modern techniques such as supercritical fluid extraction, microwave-assisted extraction, enzyme-assisted extraction, subcritical water extraction, and ultrasound-aided extraction are green or clean processes due to the lesser usage of organic solvents and energy (Soquetta et al. 2018). Advanced methods with increased safety and accuracy have also been introduced. Montero-Calderon et al. (2019) illustrated the use of ultrasound-assisted hydro-alcohol extraction of vitamin C from the orange peel. The extraction of flavonoids was also extracted using solvent extraction with hexane or methanol (Pereira et al. 2017). Some authors utilised pressure extractions, such as the juice extractor used by Li et al. (2021), to extract the flavonoid component from the orange pulp.

### 11.5.1 Conventional Extraction

Using a range of standard extraction methods, bioactive compounds were extracted from plant sources. The efficiency of extraction of various solvents, also the application of heat and/or mixing, are all used in these procedures like Maceration, Soxhlet extraction, and Hydrodistillation. These procedures are the recognised common processes for the extraction of bioactive compounds from plants.

#### *11.5.1.1 Soxhlet Extraction*

Essential bioactive compounds have been extracted from a number of natural sources via Soxhlet extraction. It serves as a comparison point for new extraction processes. Many solvents are used as extractants in this method. The extracted solutes are transported into the bulk liquid by these solvents. The solvent is returned to the plant's solid bed, while the solute is stored in the distillation flask (Figure 11.3). A few studies demonstrated the extraction of bioactive

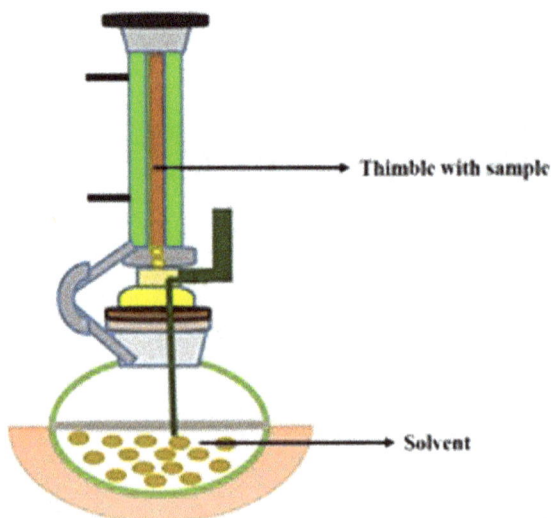

**Figure 11.3** Schematic of Soxhlet assembly: (1) Solid matrix is placed in Soxhlet thimble. The solvent is heated under reflux. (2) Condensation and extraction with "fresh" solvent. Solutes are transferred from the extraction chamber into the reservoir. (3) Continuous repetition of the extraction. (4) Exhaustive extraction is complete.

compounds, especially anthocyanin, by using Soxhlet extraction techniques (Lapornik et al. 2005). The solvent (ethanol, methanol, water), temperature, time, and acidity all affect the degree and rate of extraction of bioactive compounds from plant materials. Although this approach is extensively used for extraction, it requires a large amount of solvent and a long extraction time, which raises the risk of bioactive molecule oxidation (Taofiq et al. 2016). The most frequent method for extracting vitamin C is solvent extraction. Various concentrations of neutral solvents, such as water and acetone, acidic solvents, such as hydrochloric and sulphuric acid, and mixed solvents, such as ethyl alcohol, have been used to extract vitamin C from the whole orange (Dumbravă et al. 2011).

### 11.5.1.2 Maceration

Maceration has long been utilised in the production of tonics at home. It soon gained popularity as a convenient and affordable way to get bioactive compounds and essential oils. For small-scale extraction, maceration is often done in many phases. In the first step of maceration, fine powder of plant materials is made by crushing it to increase the surface area. Getting the solvent to work properly Second, a suitable solvent termed menstruum is used during the maceration operation in a tightly closed container. After squeezing off the liquid, the marc (solid) remains. The trash generated during extraction is pressed to recover massive sums of occluded solutions. The liquid is mixed, and impurities are removed using the number of occluded solutions and the pressed filtration and ensuing strain. Shaking the menstruum occasionally during maceration helps the extraction in two ways: First, it improves the rate of diffusion and removes concentrated solution from the surface of the sample, and second, increasing extraction yield by enabling more solvent to enter the menstruum.

### 11.5.1.3 Hydrodistillation

Hydrodistillation is a method of extracting the volatile fraction from foods using distilled water. Organic solvents are not used in hydrodistillation, which takes 6–8 hours. Hydrodiffusion, hydrolysis, and heat breakdown are the three basic physicochemical processes involved in this approach. In most cases, this method is not employed to extract the heat-sensitive component. Using hydrodistillation, Santana-Méridas et al. (2014) isolated different polyphenols and antioxidants from the solid residue of *Rosmarinus officinalis* L. They discovered phenolic chemicals in the extract that had antioxidant and bioplaguicide properties, such as carnosol, carnosic acid, and cirsimaritin. Hydrodistillation uses a lot of energy and takes a long time. Furthermore, it requires a heating procedure, which limits its use for extracting heat-sensitive bioactive chemicals from plant material (Okoh et al. 2010).

### 11.5.2 Non-Conventional Extraction

Traditional extraction has several limitations, including longer extraction periods, limited extraction selectivity, the requirement for costly and high-quality solvent, evaporation of a significant volume of solvent, and heat breakdown of thermolabile compounds (Wang and Weller 2006). Non-conventional techniques for extraction are applied to overcome these limitations. Ultrasound-assisted extraction, subcritical water extraction, enzyme-assisted extraction, supercritical fluid extraction, pressurised liquid extraction are some of the most promising non-conventional techniques for extraction. A chemical synthesis that is less dangerous, safer chemicals, energy-efficient, safe solvent auxiliaries, fewer derivatives, catalysis, design to minimise degradation, and less

259

time are only a few of these advantages (da Silva et al. 2016). In these techniques, non-conventional processes of extraction are used to extract bioactive compounds.

### 11.5.2.1 Enzyme-Assisted Extraction (EAE)

Enzyme-assisted extraction (EAE) procedures are gaining popularity due to the need for an ecologically friendly extraction process. Plant material has been treated with enzymes before extraction using standard methods. Pectinases, hemicellulases, and cellulases are common enzymes employed to break down the plant cell wall structural integrity, allowing more bioactive to be extracted. These enzymes break down cell wall components, increasing cell permeability and hence increasing bioactive chemical extraction yields (Puri et al. 2012). Xu et al. (2016) and Landbo and Meyer (2001) employed the EAE approach to isolate anthocyanins from leftover black currants and blueberries. On the other hand, this method has several advantages, including increased oxidative stability and antioxidant components such as tocopherols and total phenolic content. However, it has several limitations, such as enzyme separation and cost-efficiency.

In the extraction of essential oil from oranges and grapefruits, when compared to typical extraction methods, EAE increased essential oil yield by 2 to 6 times for grapefruit peel and orange. The hydrolysis of the cell wall is the major action of hemicellulase and cellulase, which results in higher yields and improved cell wall permeability. Enzyme treatment also reduced viscosity, making it simpler to break up emulsions and extract oil from the watery phase (Sowbhagya and Chitra 2010; Chávez-González et al. 2016). The extraction of essential oils from the flavedo of mandarin peels was investigated using a pre-treatment with the Xylanases enzyme (concentrations ranging from 0.1 to 0.3%), accompanied by cold pressing extraction and hydrodistillation. In the comparative study among the samples, it was found that there was a 15% increase in the production of essential oil as compared to the control sample (Mishra et al. 2005; Putnik et al. 2017). Enzymatic activity rupturing the oil sacs/glands results in an extra release of oil from the oil sacs, resulting in increased extraction efficiency.

### 11.5.2.2 Microwave-Assisted Extraction (MAE)

This method has shown to be a reliable and rapid method for extracting bioactive components from citrus wastes and their by-products while using lesser solvents. Figure 11.4 depicts a schematic setup plan for microwave-assisted extraction (MAE) of bioactive substances. For example, in a study to analyse and optimise MAE in the yield of polyphenols from mandarin peels, response surface methodology (RSM) was used. Traditional rotary extraction (RE) and ultrasound-aided extraction were compared to the MAE optimal circumstances. According to the researchers, the greatest yield was attained with an extraction time of 49 s, microwave power of 152 W, a methanol concentration of 66%, and a liquid-to-solid ratio of 16. MAE outperformed the other procedures in terms of the efficiency of extraction and antioxidant activity of the extracts. Some studies in aqueous and aqueous acetone mediums revealed somewhat different results for optimum MAE settings. When MAE was used to extract polyphenols from lemon peels, it produced 15.78 mg Gallic Acid Equivalent (GAE)/g of total phenolic content (TPC), which was similar to the TPC (15.22 mg GAE/g) produced by the ideal conditions of UAE (15.22 mg GAE/g) (Hayat et al. 2009; Ahmad and Langrish 2012; Dahmoune et al. 2013; Nayak et al. 2015; Putnik et al. 2017).

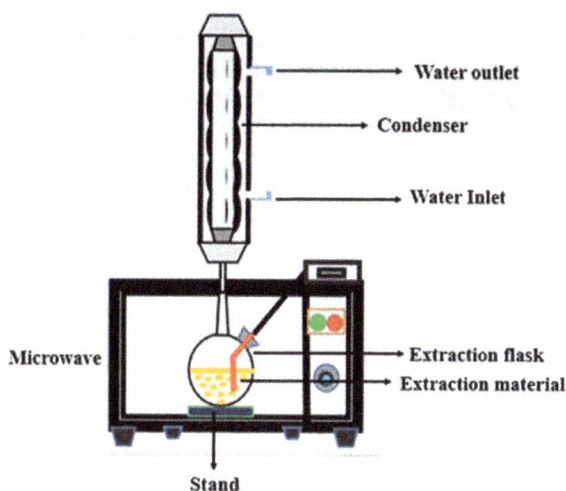

**Figure 11.4** Microwave-assisted extraction assembly for bioactive compound extraction.

Another experiment looked at how MAE affected the recovery of total polyphenols and particular flavonoids from orange peels. The authors compared novel and traditional extractions in 80% ethanol with mechanical agitation at a 5:50 w/v solid-to-liquid ratio. According to the researchers, the best conditions for MAE are 200 W for 180 s and 5:50 w/v solid-to-liquid ratio. On the other hand, antioxidant activity did not perform well in these conditions. At 100 MPa and 300 W, the highest antioxidant value for MAE was obtained (M'hiri et al. 2015). The influence of MAE on the extraction of individual flavonoids, total flavonoids, total phenols, and antioxidant activity from orange peels was investigated by the same research team, and the comparison of obtained results was made using standard extraction methods (Table 11.2). The major flavonoids in orange peel were neohesperidin and hesperidin, which made up around 84% of the total, and their yield was influenced by the extraction procedure. Although MAE produced the highest-yielding extraction, conventional extraction produced the extracts with the maximum antioxidant activity (Putnik et al. 2017).

### 11.5.2.3 Supercritical Fluid Extraction (SFE)

Supercritical fluid extraction (SFE), which is an environmentally friendly process, is mainly used to extract bioactive compounds from natural sources, such as plants, algae, microalgae and food by-products. Due to its affordable, non-toxic, and non-explosive nature, supercritical carbon dioxide ($SC\text{-}CO_2$) is a potential substitute for organic solvents. It has the ability to dissolve lipophilic compounds and may be readily removed from finished products (Wang and Weller 2006; Kumar et al. 2017). Supercritical fluids have a number of advantages over traditional extraction methods, including simpler separation, improved dissolving power, and a greater diffusion coefficient. Supercritical fluids have better transport qualities than liquids due to their high diffusivity and low viscosity and may quickly diffuse through solid materials, resulting in quicker extraction rates. Other benefits include the ability to link directly with analytical

**Table 11.2: In Comparison to Traditional Extraction, the Effect of Ultrasound-Assisted Extraction and Microwave-Assisted Extraction on Antioxidant Bioactive Chemical Extraction from Plant Materials**

Methods of Extraction

| Plant Material | Ultrasound-Assisted Extraction | | | | | |
|---|---|---|---|---|---|---|
| Orange peel | Treatment Conditions | | | | Ethanol/$H_2O$ Ratio (υ/υ) | Extraction Yield |
| | kHz | W | °C | min | | |
| | 25 | 150 | 30 | 15 | 50:50 | • Polyphenols (Caffeic (207%)<br>• p-Coumaric (180%)<br>• Ferulic (192%)<br>• Sinapic acid (66%)<br>• p-Hydroxybenzoic (94%) |
| | 25 | 50–150 | 10–40 | 60 | 20–80:80–20 | • Polyphenols (Naringin (38%)<br>• Hesperidin (42%)<br>• Total phenolic compound (31%) |
| | – | 125 | 35 | 30 | 80:20 | |

| | Microwave-Assisted Extraction | | | | |
|---|---|---|---|---|---|
| | Treatment Conditions | | | Liquid to Solid Ratio | Extraction Yield |
| | W | °C | s | | |
| Orange peel | 500 | <135 | 122 | 25 mL g$^{-1}$ | Polyphenol content (12.20 mg/GAEg$^{-1}$ DW) |
| | 200 | – | 180 | | |
| Lemon peel | 400 | 123 | – | 28:1 mL | Polyphenol content (15.74/GAE g$^{-1}$ DW) |
| Mandarin peel | 400 | <135 | 180 | 1:2 | – |
| | 152 | – | 49 | 16 | |

*Source:* From Putnik et al. (2017).

chromatographic methods like supercritical fluid chromatography (SFC) or gas chromatography (GC), as well as the use of solvents that are generally recognised as safe (GRAS) (Da Silva et al. 2016).

The raw material is put in an extraction container with pressure and temperature controls to maintain the proper environment during the extraction process. A pump then pumps the liquid into the extraction vessel. The products are collected by a tap positioned in the bottom portion of the separators after the fluid and dissolved chemicals have been given to the separators (Figure 11.5). Either the fluid is recycled or discharged into the environment. The selection of supercritical fluids is vital to the performance of the process, and this method can employ a variety of chemicals as solvents (Sihvonen et al. 1999; Kumar et al. 2017).

At 9.5 MPa and 58.6°C, Giannuzzo et al. (2003) discovered that SC-$CO_2$ treated with ethanol extracted more naringin (flavonoid) from citrus waste than pure SC-$CO_2$. When Atti-Santos et al. (2005) used SC-$CO_2$ on milled peels, they discovered the optimal conditions for recovery (30 min, $CO_2$ flow rate of 1 mL/min, 60°C, 90 bar). After supercritical extraction (7.93% w/w) and hydrodistillation (5.45% w/w) on milled peels, they discovered the greatest

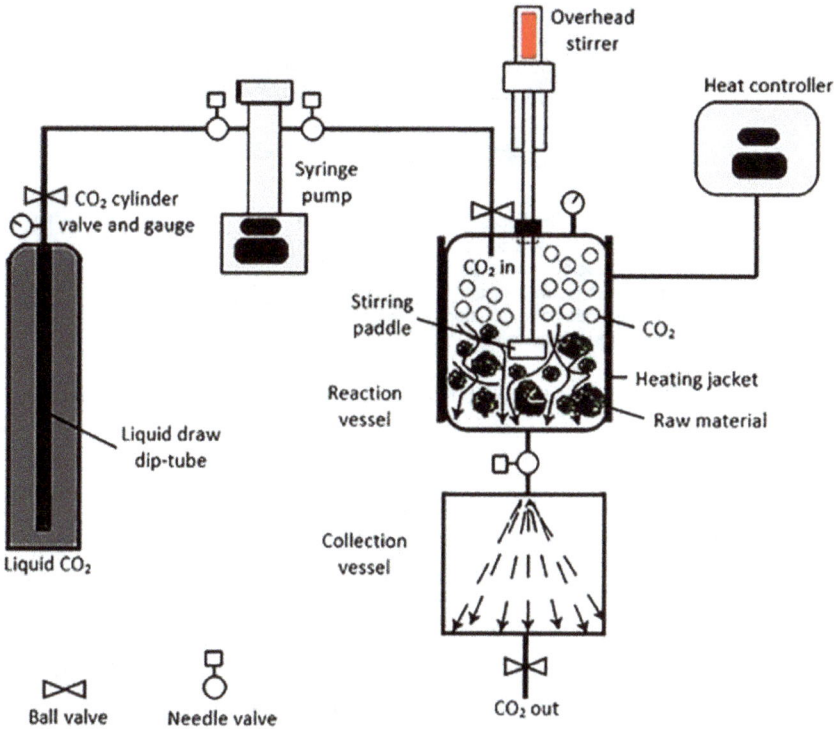

**Figure 11.5** A typical supercritical fluid extraction system. (Adapted from Khaw et al. 2017.)

lime oil yields. Chen and Huang (2016) utilised SC-$CO_2$ technology (6 mL/ min $CO_2$ flow rate, 50°C, 20 MPa,) to extract oleoresin from the peels of three citrus species, speeding up the extraction process by adding alcohol as a solvent helper. According to the researchers, the non-volatile oleoresin isolated from the samples included phytosterols (between 686.1 and 1316.4 g/g), limonoids (between 111.7 and 406.2 mg/g), and polymethoxyflavones (between 86.2 and 259.5 mg/g).

He et al. (2012) studied the antioxidant activity of flavonoid compounds extracted from pomelo peel using SC-$CO_2$ (80°C, 39 MPa). They found that it yielded more flavonoid extract in less time and greater hydroxyl, DPPH*, and ABTS* scavenging capabilities than standard extraction by solvent (Putnik et al. 2017).

The phenolic components extraction from juice collected from the pulp using supercritical fluid extraction of hydro-alcoholic solvents was also demonstrated (Espinosa-Pardo et al. 2017). To enhance the solvent extraction process, Savic Gajic et al. (2021) employed UAE of carotenoids from the orange peel. Over the years, cutting-edge technology has evolved. The solvent extraction approach is now being compared to other technologies to determine the best environmentally friendly and cost-effective way to extract bio-compounds from orange peels. To extract terpenes from powdered orange peel, researchers utilised supercritical $CO_2$, hydrodistillation, and steam explosion (Golmohammadi et al. 2018; Jokić et al. 2020).

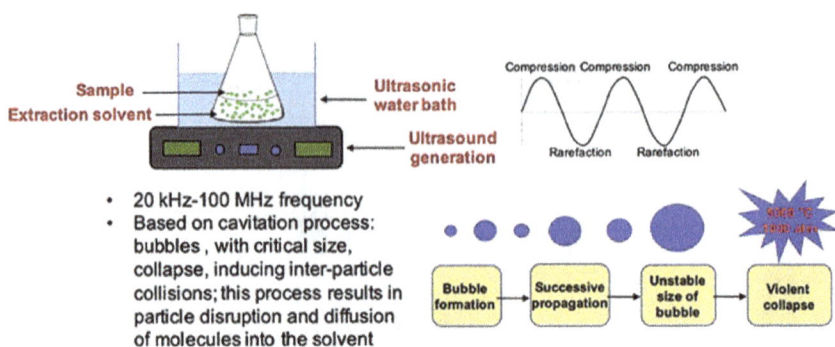

**Figure 11.6** Schematic representations of UAE equipment and characteristics.

### 11.5.2.4 Ultrasound-Assisted Extraction

Heat-sensitive bioactive chemicals may now be extracted using ultrasound-aided extraction, which has been shown to be a cost-effective method (Chemat et al. 2017). Ultrasonic extraction has several benefits over traditional extraction procedures, according to Pingret et al. (2013), including enhanced diffusion, mass transfer, plant cell damage, capillary effects (Sono capillary Effect), and solvent penetration (Figure 11.6). Fragmentation, erosion, capillarity, detexturation, and sonoporation are all independent or linked processes used in ultrasound extraction. The performance of ultrasound-assisted extraction is influenced by a variety of factors, including amplitude, wavelength, sonochemical effects, frequency, ultrasonic reactor size, and medium properties such as solvent type and temperature (Chemat et al. 2017). UAE offers the benefit of saving time, energy, solvent use, and temperature during extraction. The application of the UAE to boost vital oil production has been researched. Researchers used UAE with hydrodistillation to extract essential oils from orange peels (Table 11.2). In comparison to the control samples (without UAE), scientists observed that there is a significant decrease in extraction time while using the UAE. Compared to typical extraction methods, the UAE of oils from Japanese citrus rose by 44% (Mason et al. 2011; Pingret et al. 2014). The cavitation bubbles collapse during ultrasonication will damage essential oil glands, allowing for quicker mass transfer and, eventually, the release of plant essential oil (Li et al. 2014; Putnik et al. 2017). Operating conditions such as treatment time, temperature, pressure amplitude, frequency, and so on all have a big impact on cavitational activity. Essential oils, on the other hand, may be subject to oxidation following extended usage of the sonotrode because of metallic contamination (Putnik et al. 2017).

### 11.5.2.5 Subcritical Water Extraction (SWE)

In the case of subcritical water extraction (SWE), there are four stages of the extraction process. In the first stage, the solute is released from several active sites of the sample matrix at elevated pressure and temperature. The second stage is primarily concerned with the extracts' diffusion into the matrix. Whereas the solutes may diffuse into the extraction solvent after partitioning from the sample matrix in the third stage. Then, finally, the separation and

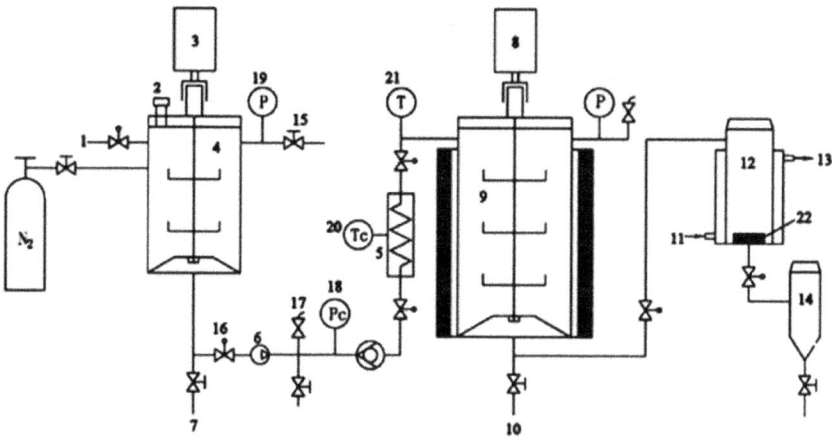

**Figure 11.7** Schematic diagram of subcritical water extraction system. (1) Water inlet; (2) feed inlet; (3) stirring system; (4) solid sample extraction cell; (5) heat exchanger; (6) pressure pump; (7) impounding reservoir; (8) stirring system; (9) solid sample extraction cell; (10) impounding reservoir; (11) cooling water inlet; (12) cooling pan; (13) cooling water outlet; (14) collector; (15) globe valve; (16) spherical valve; (17) safety valve; (18) pressure regulator controller; (19) pressure indicator; (20) temperature regulator controller; (21) temperature indicator; (22) filter plate. (Adapted from Zhang et al. 2020.)

collection of samples from the extraction fluid using chromatography during the fourth stage (Figure 11.7) (Hawthorne et al. 1994; Ong et al. 2006). Moreover, the SWE process has been studied thermodynamically in several previous studies. Basically, the SWE follows two simple steps during the extraction process: One is the release of the desired solutes from their original binding positions inside the sample matrix; another is the removal of these solutes from the sample solution using a front elution chromatography method.

The rise in surface balance damage, greater solubility, and higher mass transfer are basic reasons for the better extraction efficiency of SWE. As the temperature of subcritical fluids rises, so does the capacity of the water to dissolve solutes. This effect is accompanied due to decrease in viscosity as well as a rise in infusibility. Thus, the solute particles are more efficiently released from the sample matrix. During the extraction process in the dynamic mode of SWE, the freshwater is continuously pumped into the system by which both mass transfer efficiency and yield are increased. However, the surface of the treated material may be affected by higher pressure and temperature. Moreover, an increase in temperature may be harmful to chemical bonds such as the hydrogen bonds and van der Waals forces. Also, the active areas in the matrix and dipole interaction between solute and matrix, may be affected (Ong et al. 2006; Cvjetko Bubalo et al. 2015). During SWE, pressure is applied to keep the water in its liquid state as it vaporises above its boiling temperature. Furthermore, by applying pressure, the solutes are prone to dissolve, realising out from the sample matrix.

Over the decades, the recovery of phenolic compounds from various types of food products using SWE has become a trend. Generally, water is known as at the subcritical point when the range of temperature is from 100°C to 374°C, whereas the pressure is set up below 22 MPa to keep the water vapour at its liquid state. SWE is more advantageous than other extraction methods because of its lower extraction time as well as the cost of solvents. Moreover, the better quality of extract and no harm to the environment are some merits of SWE over other extraction methods. Thus, SWE is one of the most promising engineering techniques for extracting various compounds from plants and algae (Herrero et al. 2006; Zakaria and Kamal 2016; Kumar et al. 2017).

In the case of mandarin peel, the researchers utilised ethanol, boiling, and subcritical water to extract bioactive compounds. In this experiment, SWE recovered higher polyphenolic concentrations, although acidic hydrolysis boosted flavonoid and polyphenolic concentrations. The antioxidant activity of carotene and ferric thiocyanate was increased when the environment was acidified (Min et al. 2014; Putnik et al. 2017). Another study investigated citrus pomace to recover total polyphenolic content and antioxidant activity of citrus pomace assisting SWE; this study also analysed the effect of subcritical water on extraction yield. From the result, it colluded the highest recovery of phenolic compounds and antioxidant concentrations during optimal conditions of SWE. Moreover, this extraction method proved to be the best in extracting antioxidants and nutraceuticals, such as poly-methoxylated flavones from citrus pomace (Kim et al. 2009; Putnik et al. 2017).

## 11.6 EFFECT OF PROCESSING ON THE BIOACTIVE COMPOUNDS PRESENT IN ORANGE

### 11.6.1 Thermal Processing

All over the world, orange juice is widely known as a popular consumable beverage, and it is majorly processed since freshly extracted juices are unstable, necessitating heat processing to reduce microbial and enzyme activity (Perez-Cacho and Rouseff 2008). Heat treatment of fruit juice is a common practice by industrial juice processors for their preservation. Although the low pH of orange juice protects it from spoilage caused by microorganisms like bacteria, yeast, and mould, it still needs to be pasteurised to improve its storage stability. Heating orange juice to 85–94°C is enough to reduce the microbial count and prepare it for filling. Several methods of pasteurisation is commercially used for orange juice. One common method is using the tube, which directly provides the juice to a plate heat exchanger so that the juice is not directly in contact with the heating surface. While in some cases, the unpasteurised juice gets into contact with hot, pasteurised juice, and this process is commonly known as preheating, and then preheated juice is further pasteurised by heating with steam or hot water. Treatment of orange juice by flash pasteurisation gives a premium quality beverage by minimising flavour changes due to heat treatment. However, the inactivation of clarifying enzymes like pectinases by pasteurisation results in an aesthetically undesirable beverage (Ibrahim 2007; Aneja et al. 2014).

Fruit juices are heated in a variety of ways, from gently not from concentrate (NFC) to twice heated and reconstituted from concentrate (RCF). Freshly squeezed orange juice has a distinct aroma owing to a diverse blend of volatile chemicals. The flavour of freshly extracted juice is largely influenced by means of the time temperature in thermal processing and storage conditions. The breakdown of aroma molecules geranial and Neral occurs when orange juice is heated, resulting in off-flavours or their precursors from Strecker, Maillard, or acid-catalysed hydration reactions. The components such as p-cymene, 4-vinylguaiacol, and carvone are produced in juice due to these interactions that cause off-flavour (Perez-Cacho and Rouseff 2008).

The pH, total soluble solids, acidity, ascorbic acid content, the activity of pectin methyl esterase (PME), colour, and flavour are some common characteristics of the juices that are affected by different thermal and non-thermal processing methods. These characteristics are usually meant for the estimation of the effects during various processing methods on the characteristics of the treated and non-treated juices. Pasteurisation of orange juice at high temperatures for a short time (HTST) affects the pH, total soluble solids, and colour of the orange juice. It also significantly affects the carotenoid content (Esteve et al. 2009), ascorbic acid content, and the non-enzymatic browning index of the juice. The ascorbic acid content of orange juice is reduced by 80.5% by HTST pasteurisation (Walkling-Ribeiro et al. 2009).

### 11.6.2 Non-Thermal Processing

To overcome the limitations of thermal pasteurisation, non-thermal pasteurisation methods such as high hydrostatic pressure (HPP), pulsed electric field (PEF), ultra-sonication, UV treatment, thermos-sonication, and pulse electric field in combination (TS/PEF), irradiations, supercritical, and dense phase carbon dioxide have been used in fruit juices. Non-thermal processes are appealing because they are expected to result in reduced food quality degradation and improved flavour, colour, taste, and nutrient retention. Minimally processed foods include fresh-squeezed, high-pressure processed (HPP), and pasteurised orange juice. (Wang and Xu 2022). Minimal processing of food products for preservation is an emerging technology. The high quality and safety of minimally processed and preserved products entice the widest possible consumer acceptance.

Thermo-sonication and pulsed electric field in combination (TS/PEF) did not affect the pH or total soluble solid content of the orange juice but had a milder effect on its colour. It also does not show any significant effect on the non-enzymatic browning index of the orange juice, which was significantly affected by HTST treatment. It retains about 96.0% of its ascorbic acid content. Orange juice treated with TS and PEF in combination has a higher residual activity of PME as compared to conventional thermal treatment. However, treatment time and electric field strength increase the residual activity of PME (Walkling-Ribeiro et al. 2009). The content of carotenoids in cold orange juice is less influenced by PEF and HHP than by typical heat treatments (Esteve et al. 2009).

UV therapy is a low-energy method. It has no discernible influence on the orange juice's colour or pH level. Treatment of orange juice with UV (10 J/m$^2$) exposure and thermal sterilisation resulted in the same loss of ascorbic acid (17%). UV processing, unlike heat treatment, does not inactivate the PME. With a short UV exposure (73.8 mJ/cm$^2$), ultraviolet (UV-254 nm) can inactivate most types of bacteria and extend the shelf life of orange juice to 5 days (Tran and Farid 2004).

UV-C, coupled with low-dose nisin treatment, eradicates spores without destroying vitamins and is a possible beverage industry option. However, the length of therapy has an impact on vitamin loss in orange juice (Ferreira et al. 2020).

The pH, °Brix, titratable acidity, and ascorbic acid concentration of the supercritical carbon dioxide treated and unprocessed juices did not differ significantly. SC-CO$_2$ and heat processing inactivated pectin methylesterase in 46.5% and 86.4% of cases, respectively. When compared to fresh and thermally treated juices, the cloud stability of the SC-CO$_2$-processed juice was significantly improved. Yuk et al. (2014) suggest that SC-CO$_2$ processing can increase the microbiological quality of orange juice without causing it to deteriorate, implying that commercialisation is possible.

The taste, colour, and flavour of orange juice are imparted by cloud particles, and cloud stability is determined by colloidal stability as well as suspended particle size and charge. The cloud stability and flavour of orange juice are influenced by the particle size distribution, rheological qualities, and volatile components in the juice. When compared to freshly squeezed and thermally treated orange juice, the dense phase carbon dioxide process (DPCD)-treated juice displays the least amount of physicochemical and flavour component loss. It provides good cloud stability to the juice due to its homogenisation effect. After DPCD treatment, the relative concentrations of ethyl butyrate and trans-2-hexenol declined linearly, but the relative contents of nonanal and citronellol increased, surpassing those of fresh juice and thermally treated juice (Niu et al. 2010). Some of these methods have already been put to use in the marketplace. However, several are still being researched or tested on a small scale for commercial use in the treatment of fruit juices.

## 11.7 ORANGES' BIOACTIVE COMPOUNDS AS TREATMENT FOR CHRONIC DISEASES

Oranges possess a variety of bioactive compounds that prevent, retard, or assist during healing from many chronic disorders (Table 11.3). The high content of vitamin C from oranges assist in protecting the body from

## Table 11.3: Roles of Different Bioactive Components in Ameliorating Chronic Disorders

| Bioactive Compound | Disorder Prevention | Health Promotion | Reference |
|---|---|---|---|
| β-carotene, lycopene, lutein | Alzheimer | Delays dementia through combating stress-induced neuronal damage. | Klatte et al. (2003) |
| Carotenoids, vitamin E, flavonoids, ascorbic acid, lutein, zeaxanthin | Blindness | • Reduces age-related macular degeneration.<br>• Effective for retinitis pigmentation.<br>• Reduces chances of cataract formation. | Khans et al. (2014) |
| Flavonoids | Cardiovascular disease | • Prevents the oxidation of LDL cholesterol.<br>• Improves blood flow.<br>• Reduces arterial blood clots. | Ye (2017) |
| Folate | Dwarfism | Promotes cell division and DNA synthesis. | Ye (2017) |
| Lycopene, carotenoids | Cancer | • Controls cellular DNA damaging factors.<br>• Prevents transcription in tumours. | Radhika et al. (2019) |
| Mg, Cr, Ca, Vitamin D | Diabetes | • Promotes insulin sensitivity.<br>• Promotes glycaemic control. | |
| Polyphenols | Parkinson's disease | • Memory function and hormone secretion. | Chao et al. (2012) |
| Polyphenols, flavonoids and proanthocyanidins | Oral disorders | • Prevention of dental caries, gingivitis, periodontitis, halitosis, malodour.<br>• Alleviates pain of patient with oral lichen planus disease and heals mucosal wound. | Rajat et al. (2012) |
| Vitamin D | Osteoporosis and arthritis | • Improves calcium absorption, muscle strength, and bone mineralisation. | Laird et al. (2010) |
| Vitamin C | Obesity | • Secretion of leptin and other cytokines that reduce LDL and cholesterol. | Conroy et al. (2011) |

damaging free radicals. Vitamin C is also a constituent of collagen, a wound-healing compound that assists in the connections of blood vessels, tendons, ligaments, and bones. A patient with bone illnesses such as osteoporosis or arthritis can benefit from vitamin C content due to these characteristics. Folate is known to play a role in cell division and DNA synthesis (Ye 2017). Cell division is responsible for the growth and development of the entire human body. A person can suffer from dwarfism if this process is inadequate. Consumption of a moderate amount of folate is necessary for growth. The orange fruit also contains thiamine, a vitamin B constituent. Vitamin B is responsible for metabolism, which is necessary for all human physiological processes. The high concentration of various antioxidant compounds in oranges can be associated with the well-documented positive effects of antioxidant compounds. Antioxidants and anti-mutagenic properties directly affect bone health, cardiovascular system, and immune system (Ye 2017).

Benefits from antioxidants such as flavonoids are associated with a properly functioning cardiovascular system, which minimises the chances of developing heart diseases (Muldoon and Kritchevsky 1996). Flavonoids prevent the oxidation of LDL cholesterol and improve blood flow, reducing the possibility of blood clots in the arteries. Flavonoids have gained importance as anticancer agents because of their cytotoxic anticancer agents that promote apoptosis in cancer cells (Abotaleb et al. 2018). Oranges also play vital roles in the immune system. They are widely consumed to heal or reduce the effects of colds. This is attributed to the variety of antioxidant compounds that they possess, which improves the immune system and prevents the multiplication of pathogenic viruses and bacteria in the human body. Terpenes and phenolic compounds possess anti-inflammatory and anti-carcinogenic activity (Codoñer-Franch and Valls-Bellés 2010). These properties can be associated with the retardation of tumour growth and the general reduction of cancer symptoms. Oranges are also known as a rich source of vitamin A. The orange colour of the oranges is derived from the carotenoids that develop as the fruit ripens. The fruit contains high concentrations of β-carotene, which are converted by the body to vitamin A, which is necessary for vision. This enables the consumption of oranges to improve eyesight and prevent the development of blindness. Research has shown that a gradual worsening vitamin A status results in the eye undergoing a series of visual impairments, beginning with night blindness. This reflects the essential role that retinol plays in the formation of rhodopsin. Rhodopsin is the visual pigment essential to the retinal receptors responsible for dark adaptation (Sommer 2008).

## 11.8 FUTURE PERSPECTIVES OF THE ORANGE FRUIT AS A NUTRACEUTICAL AND FUNCTIONAL FOOD

Citrus fruits are widely accepted as highly nutritious snacks that can be consumed as salads or taken as drinks. Over the previous decades, their nutritional status is gradually improved to meet human expectations in terms of the concentrations of bioactive compounds as well as the digestibility of those compounds by the consumer. There is comprehensive research focusing on improving orange nutritional compounds through breeding (Cimen et al. 2021). However, the current technical procedures applied in commercial farms are hindered by using vegetative propagation and the grafting of trees. Breeding experiments are normally efficient on seed-propagated plants. Therefore, the quality of the fresh orange as a nutraceutical and functional food is projected not to change soon. The current status of oranges will remain as is because most farmers will continue using grafting, which interferes with the genes that may be bred to improve bioactive compounds from the fruit.

Alternative ways of improving the accessibility of nutraceutical function from the orange fruit include extracting the necessary compounds. Many products of concentrated active compounds have been developed, including pills, drinks, as well as powders. These products are administered orally strictly to target specific ailments that a consumer wants to release immediately. For chronic diseases, a constant supply of bioactive compounds in low concentrations is necessary as chronic diseases take a longer time to get rid of (Clark 2003). That necessitates longer administration, which may result in other ailments if given in high concentrations. The future of using products concentrated with bioactive compounds of oranges depends on developing new products with concentrations within a healthy threshold that will not result in ailments if consumed for extended periods.

## 11.9 CONCLUSION

For a very long time, citrus fruits have been recognised as a pleasant and healthful supplement to any diet. Orange flavours are among the most well-liked in the world, and it is becoming more and more obvious that orange fruit is healthy and delicious. Orange and orange products are widely known for being rich in vitamins, minerals, and dietary fibre (nonstarch polysaccharides), all of which are necessary for optimal growth and development as well as overall nutritional well-being. An overview of current studies on the health effects of various citrus fruit parts and their primary bioactive components was published. It was intriguing to see that the edible section of the plant and its by-products had a significant biological value. However, it is increasingly becoming clear that these and other physiologically active, non-nutrient molecules present in different citrus can assist in lessening the risk of various chronic illnesses. Orange fruits have a substantial content of polyphenols, which are responsible for a wide variety of positive benefits in humans, and a great number of *in vitro* and *in vivo* studies have suggested an inverse link between increased consumption and decreased risk of chronic illnesses. The extraction of this bioactive component, its incorporation into food, and the production of nutraceuticals are all gaining popularity. Dietary guidelines and recommendations that promote the intake of citrus fruits and their products, when used appropriately, can result in extensive nutritional advantages for the general public.

## REFERENCES

Abotaleb, M., Samuel, S. M., Varghese, E., Varghese, S., Kubatka, P., Liskova, A., & Büsselberg, D. 2018. Flavonoids in cancer and apoptosis. *Cancers, 11*(1):28.

Ahmad, J., & Langrish, T. A. G. 2012. Optimisation of total phenolic acids extraction from mandarin peels using microwave energy: The importance of the Maillard reaction. *Journal of Food Engineering, 109*(1):162–174.

Aneja, K. R., Dhiman, R., Aggarwal, N. K., & Aneja, A. 2014. Emerging preservation techniques for controlling spoilage and pathogenic microorganisms in fruit juices. *International Journal of Microbiology, 2014*:758942.

Atti-Santos, A. C., Rossato, M., Serafini, L. A., Cassel, E., & Moyna, P. 2005. Extraction of essential oils from lime (*Citrus latifolia* Tanaka) by hydrodistillation and supercritical carbon dioxide. *Brazilian Archives of Biology and Technology,* 48:155–160.

Azmir, J., Zaidul, I. S. M., Rahman, M. M., Sharif, K. M., Mohamed, A., Sahena, F., ... & Omar, A. K. M. (2013). Techniques for extraction of bioactive compounds from plant materials: A review. *Journal of food engineering, 117*(4), 426–436.

Biesalski, H. K., Dragsted, L. O., Elmadfa, I., Grossklaus, R., Müller, M., Schrenk, D., ... & Weber, P. 2009. Bioactive compounds: Definition and assessment of activity. *Nutrition, 25*(11–12):1202–1205.

Cebadera-Miranda, L., Domínguez, L., Dias, M. I., Barros, L., Ferreira, I. C., Igual, M., ... & Cámara, M. 2019. Sanguinello and Tarocco (*Citrus sinensis* [L.] Osbeck): Bioactive compounds and colour appearance of blood oranges. *Food Chemistry, 270,* 395–402.

Chao, J., Leung, Y., Wang, M., & Chang, R. C. C. 2012. Nutraceuticals and their preventive or potential therapeutic value in Parkinson's disease. *Nutrition Reviews, 70*(7), 373–386.

Chávez-González, M. L., López-López, L. I., Rodríguez-Herrera, R., Contreras-Esquivel, J. C., & Aguilar, C. N. 2016. Enzyme-assisted extraction of citrus essential oil. *Chemical Papers, 70*(4):412–417.

Chavoshnejad, P., Foroughi, A. H., Dhandapani, N., German, G. K., & Razavi, M. J. 2021. Effect of collagen degradation on the mechanical behavior and wrinkling of skin. *Physical Review E, 104*(3):034406.

Chemat, F., Rombaut, N., Sicaire, A. G., Meullemiestre, A., Fabiano-Tixier, A. S., & Abert-Vian, M. 2017. Ultrasound assisted extraction of food and natural products. Mechanisms, techniques, combinations, protocols and applications. A review. *Ultrasonics Sonochemistry, 34*:540–560.

Chen, M. H., & Huang, T. C. 2016. Volatile and nonvolatile constituents and antioxidant capacity of oleoresins in three Taiwan citrus varieties as determined by supercritical fluid extraction. *Molecules, 21*(12):1735.

Cimen, B., Yesiloglu, T., Incesu, M., & Yilmaz, B. 2021. Studies on mutation breeding in citrus: Improving seedless types of "Kozan" common orange by gamma irradiation. *Scientia Horticulturae, 278*:109857.

Clark, N. M. 2003. Management of chronic disease by patients. *Annual Review of Public Health, 24*:289.

Codoñer-Franch, P., & Valls-Bellés, V. 2010. Citrus as functional foods. *Current Topics in Nutraceutical Research, 8*(4).

Conroy, K. P., Davidson, I. M., & Warnock M. 2011. Pathogenic obesity and nutraceuticals. *The Proceedings of the Nutrition Society. 70*(4):426–438.

Cvjetko Bubalo, M., Vidović, S., Radojčić Redovniković, I., & Jokić, S. 2015. Green solvents for green technologies. *Journal of Chemical Technology & Biotechnology*, *90*(9):1631–1639.

da Silva, B. V., Barreira, J. C., & Oliveira, M. B. P. 2016. Natural phytochemicals and probiotics as bioactive ingredients for functional foods: Extraction, biochemistry and protected-delivery technologies. *Trends in Food Science & Technology*, *50*:144–158.

Da Silva, R. P., Rocha-Santos, T. A., & Duarte, A. C. 2016. Supercritical fluid extraction of bioactive compounds. *Trends in Analytical Chemistry*, *76*:40–51.

Dahmoune, F., Boulekbache, L., Moussi, K., Aoun, O., Spigno, G., & Madani, K. 2013. Valorization of *Citrus limon* residues for the recovery of antioxidants: Evaluation and optimization of microwave and ultrasound application to solvent extraction. *Industrial Crops and Products*, *50*:77–87.

Das, D., Das, D., Gupta, A. K., & Mishra, P. 2020. Drying of *Citrus grandis* (pomelo) fruit juice using block freeze concentration and spray drying. *Acta Alimentaria*, *49*(3):295–306.

Dassoff, E. S., Guo, J. X., Liu, Y., Wang, S. C., & Li, Y. O. 2021. Potential development of non-synthetic food additives from orange processing by-products-A review. *Food Quality and Safety*, *5*.

Dumbravă, D. G., Hădărugă, N. G., Moldovan, C., Raba, D. N., Popa, M. V., & Rădoi, B. 2011. Antioxidant activity of some fresh vegetables and fruits juices. *Journal of Agroalimentary Processes and Technologies*, *17*(2): 163–168.

Espinosa-Pardo, F. A., Nakajima, V. M., Macedo, G. A., Macedo, J. A., & Martínez, J. 2017. Extraction of phenolic compounds from dry and fermented orange pomace using supercritical $CO_2$ and cosolvents. *Food and Bioproducts Processing*, *101*:1–10.

Esteve, M. J., Barba, F. J., Palop, S., & Frígola, A. 2009. The effects of non-thermal processing on carotenoids in orange juice. *Czech Journal of Food Sciences*, *27*(Special Issue 1).

Ferreira, T. V., Mizuta, A. G., de Menezes, J. L., Dutra, T. V., Bonin, E., Castro, J. C., ... & de Abreu Filho, B. A. 2020. Effect of ultraviolet treatment (UV–C) combined with nisin on industrialized orange juice in Alicyclobacillus acidoterrestris spores. *LWT – Food Science and Technology*, *133*, 109911.

Giannuzzo, A. N., Boggetti, H. J., Nazareno, M. A., & Mishima, H. T. 2003. Supercritical fluid extraction of naringin from the peel of *Citrus paradisi*. *Phytochemical Analysis*, *14*(4):221–223.

Golmohammadi, M., Borghei, A., Zenouzi, A., Ashrafi, N., & Taherzadeh, M. J. 2018. Optimization of essential oil extraction from orange peels using steam explosion. *Heliyon*, *4*(11):e00893.

Gupta, A. K., Das, S., Sahu, P. P., & Mishra, P. 2022. Design and development of IDE sensor for naringin quantification in pomelo juice: An indicator of citrus maturity. *Food Chemistry, 377*:131947.

Gupta, A. K., Koch, P., & Mishra, P. 2020. Optimization of debittering and deacidification parameters for pomelo juice and assessment of juice quality. *Journal of Food Science and Technology, 57*(12):4726–4732.

Gupta, A. K., Mishra, P., Senapati, M., & Sahu, P. P. 2021a. A novel electrochemical device for naringin quantification and removal from bitter variety of citrus fruits. *Journal of Food Engineering, 306*:110637.

Gupta, A. K., Pathak, U., Tongbram, T., Medhi, M., Terdwongworakul, A., Magwaza, L. S., ... & Mishra, P. 2021b. Emerging approaches to determine maturity of citrus fruit. *Critical Reviews in Food Science and Nutrition*, 1–22.

Gupta, A. K., Sahu, P. P., & Mishra, P. 2021c. Ultrasound aided debittering of bitter variety of citrus fruit juice: Effect on chemical, volatile profile and antioxidative potential. *Ultrasonics Sonochemistry, 81*:105839.

Gupta, A. K., Yumnam, M., Medhi, M., Koch, P., Chakraborty, S., & Mishra, P. 2021d. Isolation and characterization of naringinase enzyme and its application in debittering of pomelo juice (*Citrus grandis*): A comparative study with macroporous resin. *Journal of Food Processing and Preservation, 45*(5):e15380.

Hawthorne, S. B., Yang, Y., & Miller, D. J. 1994. Extraction of organic pollutants from environmental solids with sub- and supercritical water. *Analytical Chemistry, 66*(18):2912–2920.

Hayat, K., Hussain, S., Abbas, S., Farooq, U., Ding, B., Xia, S., ... & Xia, W. 2009. Optimized microwave-assisted extraction of phenolic acids from citrus mandarin peels and evaluation of antioxidant activity *in vitro*. *Separation and Purification Technology, 70*(1):63–70.

He, J. Z., Shao, P., Liu, J. H., & Ru, Q. M. 2012. Supercritical carbon dioxide extraction of flavonoids from pomelo (*Citrus grandis* [L.] Osbeck) peel and their antioxidant activity. *International Journal of Molecular Sciences, 13*(10):13065–13078.

Herrero, M., Cifuentes, A., & Ibañez, E. 2006. Sub-and supercritical fluid extraction of functional ingredients from different natural sources: Plants, food-by-products, algae and microalgae: A review. *Food Chemistry, 98*(1):136–148.

Ibrahim, R. E. 2007. Storage Induced Changes in the Physico-Chemical and Sensorial Properties of Natural Orange Juice and Drink (Doctoral dissertation, UOFK).

Iglesias-Carres, L., Mas-Capdevila, A., Bravo, F. I., Aragonès, G., Muguerza, B., & Arola-Arnal, A. 2019. Optimization of a polyphenol extraction method for sweet orange pulp (*Citrus sinensis* L.) to identify phenolic compounds consumed from sweet oranges. *PLoS One, 14*(1):e0211267.

Izquierdo, L., & Sendra, J. M. 2003. Citrus fruits composition and characterization. *Encyclopedia of Food Sciences and Nutrition*, 1335–1341.

Jokić, S., Molnar, M., Cikoš, A. M., Jakovljević, M., Šafranko, S., & Jerković, I. 2020. Separation of selected bioactive compounds from orange peel using the sequence of supercritical $CO_2$ extraction and ultrasound solvent extraction: Optimization of limonene and hesperidin content. *Separation Science and Technology*, 55(15):2799–2811.

Khans, R. A., Elhassan, G. O., & Qureshi, K. A. 2014. Nutraceuticals: In the treatment and prevention of diseases—An overview. *Pharma Innovation Journal*, 3(10):47–50.

Khaw, K. Y., Parat, M. O., Shaw, P. N., & Falconer, J. R. 2017. Solvent supercritical fluid technologies to extract bioactive compounds from natural sources: A review. *Molecules*, 22(7):1186.

Kim, J. W., Nagaoka, T., Ishida, Y., Hasegawa, T., Kitagawa, K., & Lee, S. C. 2009. Subcritical water extraction of nutraceutical compounds from citrus pomaces. *Separation Science and Technology*, 44(11):2598–2608.

Klatte, E. T., Scharre, D. W., Nagaraja, H. N., Davis, R. A., & Beversdorf, D. Q. 2003. Combination therapy of donepezil and vitamin E in Alzheimer disease. *Alzheimer Disease & Associated Disorders*, 17(2):113–116.

Kumar, K., Yadav, A. N., Kumar, V., Vyas, P., & Dhaliwal, H. S. 2017. Food waste: A potential bioresource for extraction of nutraceuticals and bioactive compounds. *Bioresources and Bioprocessing*, 4(1):1–14.

Lado, J., Gambetta, G., & Zacarias, L. 2018. Key determinants of citrus fruit quality: Metabolites and main changes during maturation. *Scientia Horticulturae*, 233:238–248.

Laird, E., Ward, M., McSorley, E., Strain, J. J., & Wallace, J. 2010. Vitamin D and bone health; Potential mechanisms. *Nutrients*, 2(7):693–724.

Landbo, A. K., & Meyer, A. S. 2001. Enzyme-assisted extraction of antioxidative phenols from black currant juice press residues (*Ribes nigrum*). *Journal of Agricultural and Food Chemistry*, 49(7):3169–3177.

Lapornik, B., Prošek, M., & Wondra, A. G. 2005. Comparison of extracts prepared from plant by-products using different solvents and extraction time. *Journal of Food Engineering*, 71(2):214–222.

Li, Q., Li, T., Baldwin, E. A., Manthey, J. A., Plotto, A., Zhang, Q., ... & Shan, Y. 2021. Extraction method affects contents of flavonoids and carotenoids in Huanglongbing-affected "Valencia" orange juice. *Foods*, 10(4):783.

Li, Y., Fabiano-Tixier, A. S., & Chemat, F. 2014. *Essential Oils as Reagents in Green Chemistry* (Vol. 1, pp. 71–78). Cham, Switzerland: Springer International Publishing.

Lu, X., Zhao, C., Shi, H., Liao, Y., Xu, F., Du, H., … & Zheng, J. 2021. Nutrients and bioactives in citrus fruits: Different citrus varieties, fruit parts, and growth stages. *Critical Reviews in Food Science and Nutrition*, 1–24.

M'hiri, N., Ioannou, I., Boudhrioua, N. M., & Ghoul, M. 2015. Effect of different operating conditions on the extraction of phenolic compounds in orange peel. *Food and Bioproducts Processing*, 96:161–170.

Mason, T. J., Chemat, F., & Vinatoru, M. 2011. The extraction of natural products using ultrasound or microwaves. *Current Organic Chemistry*, 15(2):237–247.

Min, K. Y., Lee, K. A., Kim, H. J., Kim, K. T., Chung, M. S., Chang, P. S., … & Paik, H. D. 2014. Antioxidative and anti-inflammatory activities of *Citrus unshiu* peel extracts using a combined process of subcritical water extraction and acid hydrolysis. *Food Science and Biotechnology*, 23(5):1441–1446.

Mishra, D., Shukla, A. K., Dixit, A. K., & Singh, K. 2005. Aqueous enzymatic extraction of oil from mandarin peels. *Journal of Oleo Science*, 54(6):355–359.

Montero-Calderon, A., Cortes, C., Zulueta, A., Frigola, A., & Esteve, M. J. 2019. Green solvents and ultrasound-assisted extraction of bioactive orange (*Citrus sinensis*) peel compounds. *Scientific Reports*, 9(1):1–8.

Muldoon, M. F., & Kritchevsky, S. B. 1996. Flavonoids and heart disease. *British Medical Journal*, 24;312(7029):458–459.

Nayak, B., Dahmoune, F., Moussi, K., Remini, H., Dairi, S., Aoun, O., & Khodir, M. 2015. Comparison of microwave, ultrasound and accelerated-assisted solvent extraction for recovery of polyphenols from *Citrus sinensis* peels. *Food Chemistry*, 187:507–516.

Niu, L., Hu, X., Wu, J., Liao, X., Chen, F., Zhao, G., & Wang, Z. 2010. Effect of dense phase carbon dioxide process on physicochemical properties and flavor compounds of orange juice. *Journal of Food Processing and Preservation*, 34:530–548.

Okoh, O. O., Sadimenko, A. P., & Afolayan, A. J. 2010. Comparative evaluation of the antibacterial activities of the essential oils of *Rosmarinus officinalis* L. obtained by hydrodistillation and solvent free microwave extraction methods. *Food Chemistry*, 120(1):308–312.

Ong, E. S., Cheong, J. S. H., & Goh, D. 2006. Pressurized hot water extraction of bioactive or marker compounds in botanicals and medicinal plant materials. *Journal of Chromatography A*, 1112(1–2):92–102.

Pereira, R. M., López, B. G. C., Diniz, S. N., Antunes, A. A., Garcia, D. M., Oliveira, C. R., & Marcucci, M. C. 2017. Quantification of flavonoids in Brazilian orange peels and industrial orange juice processing wastes. *Agricultural Sciences*, 8(07):631.

Perez-Cacho, P. R., & Rouseff, R. 2008. Processing and storage effects on orange juice aroma: A review. *Journal of Agricultural and Food Chemistry*, 56(21):9785–9796.

Pingret, D., Fabiano-Tixier, A. S., & Chemat, F. 2013. Degradation during application of ultrasound in food processing: A review. *Food Control*, 31(2):593–606.

Pingret, D., Fabiano-Tixier, A. S., & Chemat, F. 2014. An improved ultrasound Clevenger for extraction of essential oils. *Food Analytical Methods*, 7(1):9–12.

Puri, M., Sharma, D., & Barrow, C. J. 2012. Enzyme-assisted extraction of bioactives from plants. *Trends in Biotechnology*, 30(1):37–44.

Putnik, P., Bursać Kovačević, D., Režek Jambrak, A., Barba, F. J., Cravotto, G., Binello, A., … & Shpigelman, A. 2017. Innovative "green" and novel strategies for the extraction of bioactive added value compounds from citrus wastes—A review. *Molecules*, 22(5):680.

Rajat, S., Manisha, S., Robin, S., & Sunil, K. 2012. Nutraceuticals: A review. *International Research Journal of Pharmacy*, 3(4):95–99.

Santana-Méridas, O., Polissiou, M., Izquierdo-Melero, M. E., Astraka, K., Tarantilis, P. A., Herraiz-Peñalver, D., & Sánchez-Vioque, R. 2014. Polyphenol composition, antioxidant and bioplaguicide activities of the solid residue from hydrodistillation of *Rosmarinus officinalis* L. *Industrial Crops and Products*, 59:125–134.

Savic Gajic, I. M., Savic, I. M., Gajic, D. G., & Dosic, A. 2021. Ultrasound-assisted extraction of carotenoids from orange peel using olive oil and its encapsulation in Ca-alginate beads. *Biomolecules*, 11(2):225.

Senit, J. J., Velasco, D., Manrique, A. G., Sanchez-Barba, M., Toledo, J. M., Santos, V. E., … & Ladero, M. 2019. Orange peel waste upstream integrated processing to terpenes, phenolics, pectin and monosaccharides: Optimization approaches. *Industrial Crops and Products*, 134:370–381.

Sihvonen, M., Järvenpää, E., Hietaniemi, V., & Huopalahti, R. 1999. Advances in supercritical carbon dioxide technologies. *Trends in Food Science & Technology*, 10(6–7):217–222.

Singh, J., Jayaprakasha, G. K., & Patil, B. S. 2021. Improved sample preparation and optimized solvent extraction for quantitation of carotenoids. *Plant Foods for Human Nutrition*, 76(1):60–67.

Sir Elkhatim, K. A., Elagib, R. A., & Hassan, A. B. 2018. Content of phenolic compounds and vitamin C and antioxidant activity in wasted parts of Sudanese citrus fruits. *Food Science & Nutrition*, 6(5):1214–1219.

Sommer, A. 2008. Vitamin A deficiency and clinical disease: An historical overview. *Journal of Nutrition*, 1;138(10):1835–1839.

Soquetta, M. B., Terra, L. D. M., & Bastos, C. P. 2018. Green technologies for the extraction of bioactive compounds in fruits and vegetables. *CYTA – Journal of Food*, 16(1):400–412.

Sowbhagya, H. B., & Chitra, V. N. 2010. Enzyme-assisted extraction of flavorings and colorants from plant materials. *Critical Reviews in Food Science and Nutrition,* 50(2):146–161.

Taofiq, O., Heleno, S. A., Calhelha, R. C., Alves, M. J., Barros, L., Barreiro, M. F., ... & Ferreira, I. C. 2016. Development of mushroom-based cosmeceutical formulations with anti-inflammatory, anti-tyrosinase, antioxidant, and antibacterial properties. *Molecules,* 21(10):1372.

Tran, M. T. T., & Farid, M. 2004. Ultraviolet treatment of orange juice. *Innovative Food Science & Emerging Technologies,* 5(4): 495–502.

Trejo-Solís C, Pedraza-Chaverrí J, Torres-Ramos M, Jiménez-Farfán D, Cruz Salgado A, Serrano-García N, Osorio-Rico L, Sotelo J. Multiple molecular and cellular mechanisms of action of lycopene in cancer inhibition. Evid Based Complement Alternat Med. 2013;2013:705121. doi: 10.1155/2013/705121. Epub 2013 Jul 21. PMID: 23970935; PMCID: PMC3736525.

United States Department of Agriculture (USDA) Foreign Agricultural Service. Citrus: World Markets and Trade. 2021. Available online: https://www.fas.usda.gov/data/citrus-world-markets-and-trade (accessed on 23 December 2021).

Velázquez-Estrada, R. M., Hernández-Herrero, M. M., Rüfer, C. E., Guamis-López, B., & Roig-Sagués, A. X. 2013. Influence of ultra high pressure homogenization processing on bioactive compounds and antioxidant activity of orange juice. *Innovative Food Science & Emerging Technologies,* 18:89–94.

Walkling-Ribeiro, M., Noci, F., Riener, J., Cronin, D. A., Lyng, J. G., & Morgan, D. J. 2009. The impact of thermosonication and pulsed electric fields on *Staphylococcus aureus* inactivation and selected quality parameters in orange juice. *Food and Bioprocess Technology,* 2(4): 422–430.

Wang, L., & Weller, C. L. 2006. Recent advances in extraction of nutraceuticals from plants. *Trends in Food Science & Technology,* 17(6):300–312.

Wang, K., & Xu, Z. 2022. Comparison of freshly squeezed, Non-thermally and thermally processed orange juice based on traditional quality characters, untargeted metabolomics, and volatile overview. *Food Chemistry,* 373:131430.

Wu, G. A., Terol, J., Ibanez, V., López-García, A., Pérez-Román, E., Borredá, C., ... & Talon, M. 2018. Genomics of the origin and evolution of *Citrus. Nature,* 554(7692):311–316.

Xu, Q., Zhou, Y., Wu, Y., Jia, Q., Gao, G., & Nie, F. 2016. Enzyme-assisted solvent extraction for extraction of blueberry anthocyanins and separation using resin adsorption combined with extraction technologies. *International Journal of Food Science & Technology,* 51(12):2567–2573.

Ye, X. (Ed.). 2017. *Phytochemicals in Citrus: Applications in Functional Foods.* CRC Press.

Yuk, H. G., Sampedro, F., Fan, X., & Geveke, D. J. 2014. Nonthermal processing of orange juice using a pilot-plant scale supercritical carbon dioxide system with a gas–liquid metal contactor. *Journal of Food Processing and Preservation, 38*(1):630–638.

Yulia, R. 2020. Nursing care for hypertension administrative through giving oranges to reduce blood pressure. *Jurnal Keperawatan, 12*(4):1059–1072.

Zakaria, S. M., & Kamal, S. M. M. 2016. Subcritical water extraction of bioactive compounds from plants and algae: Applications in pharmaceutical and food ingredients. *Food Engineering Reviews, 8*(1):23–34.

Zhang, J., Wen, C., Zhang, H., Duan, Y., & Ma, H. 2020. Recent advances in the extraction of bioactive compounds with subcritical water: A review. *Trends in Food Science & Technology, 95*:183–195.

Zhang, M., Zhu, S., Yang, W., Huang, Q., & Ho, C. T. 2021. The biological fate and bioefficacy of citrus flavonoids: Bioavailability, biotransformation, and delivery systems. *Food & Function, 12*(8):3307–3323.

Zou, Z., Xi, W., Hu, Y., Nie, C., & Zhou, Z. 2016. Antioxidant activity of citrus fruits. *Food Chemistry, 196*, 885–896.

# 12 Quince Fruit

*Rifat Bhat, A. Tabish Jehan Been, Sharbat Hussian, Mohammad Amin Mir,
and Mehvish Bashir*

## CONTENTS

## 12.1 INTRODUCTION

Quince (*Cydonia oblonga*) is supposed to be preliminary material for phytochemical
extraction to be exploited in food and nutraceuticals. Recently, it has been
revealed that considerable health risks and benefits are linked mainly to dietary
food preferences (Fulton et al. 2016; Li et al. 2017). To promote healthy life, daily
consumption of fruits and vegetables is advised (Fattouch et al. 2007).

Quince (*Cydonia oblonga* Mill.) is presented in the subfamily Maloideae and
family Rosaceae, in which apples and pears are included, each one being an
economically important fruit. It is hardy, acidic and astringent, hence it is not fit
to be eaten unless processed, but quite often is used for making jam, jelly and
marmalade, and can even be used for making canned products and for making
products after distillation (Costa et al. 2009; Mir et al. 2015).

It has been reported that quince fruit is a great source of organic acids and
polyphenols along with amino acids with well-documented health benefits
(Torkelson 1995; Duke 2002; Postman 2009). Flavonols (kaempferol and quercetin
derivatives), hydroxycinnamic acids and, in a lesser amount, flavanols (catechin
and epicatechin) are the main polyphenols in quince. Quince is recognised for
the compounds potent in antimicrobial, antioxidant and anti-ulcerative action
(Silva et al. 2005a; Khoubnasabjafari and Jouyban 2011; Ashraf et al. 2016; Leonel
et al. 2016). The polyphenolic content obtained from quince fruit peel and seeds
has been documented in a number of studies. Moreover, quite a lot of work has
been done on the phenolic properties and antioxidative capacity of quince, but
the work has mostly been done on the laboratory scale and not on a commercial
or industrial level (Biro and Linder 1999; Souci et al. 2008; Rasheed et al. 2018).

In some countries, the entire fruit is compressed and subjected to high
temperature, followed by the exclusion of the solids that are filtered through
the different sieves. After obtaining the pulp, sugars and additives are added

DOI: 10.1201/9781003259213-12

to it so as to make jam out of quince. The leftover residue is then mostly composed of peel and remains of seeds and sometimes mesocarp as well. It is reported that in the fruit, the skin and seeds contain the highest polyphenolic concentration; hence, they are important from an antioxidant point of view (Torkelson 1995; Li et al. 2017).

Currently, it is said that the antioxidant capacity (AC) cannot be directly predicted from the amount of a particular group of compounds (Sood and Bhardwaj 2015; Gani et al. 2018). This capacity is the result of synergistic and antagonistic effects of the reactions taking place between different polyphenols and with the rest of the parts of what that particular organism eats (Silva et al. 2003). Recently, a new BRT model (Boosted Regression Trees model), a new multivariate statistical method has been devised which is a regression model used to describe and foretell the response of the variable with the help of certain predictors (Lutz-Röder et al. 2002; Silva et al. 2004, 2006; Szychowski et al. 2014).

The effect of food processing on polyphenols does not make an easy relationship which can be cause-effect in its nature (Hopur et al. 2011). Contradictory results have been seen on how the temperature can affect polyphenols. Whereas in grapes and orange juice, green tea, plum, black carrot jam and marmalade and red beetroot jam (Lindberg et al. 1990; Silva et al. 2005; Daneshvand et al. 2012; Karar et al. 2014), it has been seen that with the increase in temperatures, the phenolics and antioxidants increased mostly accounted to the disruption of the integrity of cell wall and membrane and because of the degradation of complexes formed with proteins. On the other hand, beverages made from milk, including fruit beverages, pickled red beetroot and plum and cabbage (Magalhães et al. 2009; Wojdyło et al. 2013) show a negative effect. This is accounted for mostly because of the temperature increase that could have degraded the compounds. The current study is aimed:

- To study the nutraceutical attributes of different parts of quince fruit.

- To study the physiochemical and antioxidant properties of quince fruit as a whole.

## 12.2 ORIGIN AND GEOGRAPHICAL DISTRIBUTION

Quince belongs to Western Asia, and it is believed to have originated from the Trans-Caucasus region and the areas include mostly Asian countries, including Azerbaijan, Iran, Armenia, south-western Russia and Turkmenistan. Quince is believed to have been spread from its native place to the countries near the Himalayan Mountains to the east and all through Europe to the west (Postman 2009). Now it has been disseminated throughout the world. The largest producer of Quince is Turkey, which contributes nearly 25% globally. In India, it is grown in Punjab, Himachal Pradesh and Kashmir, where it is commonly known as *bamchount*. It is also called Baheedana in Urdu, Bihi in Hindi and Safarjalin in Arabic (Khoubnasabjafari and Jouyban 2011).

Quince is shaped like a pear or apple that has a golden yellow-coloured fruit. It has a leathery skin that is non-consumable because of its bitter taste, strong acidity and also because its flesh is a little hard containing grit cells. When the fruit is about to ripen, the hairs on the peel disappear, and this is the stage for taking this fruit into processing in order to make different products like candy, jam, jelly, marmalade and cakes (Silva et al. 2005). It is not a rich source of fat but has a good percentage of some important organic acid, sugar, fibres and minerals such as potassium, phosphorus and calcium (Leonel et al. 2016). *Cydonia oblonga* can be easily grown on grounds or gardens especially when the temperatures are hot and can be easily grown up to a height of 8 m and a width of 4 m. The branches of quince are greyish in colour, and a little pale, with elliptical-shaped leaves, and the flower colour is either pink or white, and its fruits are yellowish in colour and mostly comparable with pears. Furthermore, quince fruits have a particular smell, their flavour is astringent and their seeds are plano-convex that are normally present in two vertical rows. The leaves have a length of 6–11 cm, are elliptical in shape, and have white hairs that are present on the exterior (Ashraf et al. 2016).

## 12.3 QUINCE PROFILE

Quince is not so widely utilised fruit. It has considerable nutritional qualities with a richness of fibre, carbohydrates, proteins, different organic acids, vitamins and minerals (Rasheed et al. 2018). The vitamin C content (10 mg/100 g) is reported to be double the amount as in seen in apples (5 mg/100 g) (Souci et al. 2008). However, according to some reports, the vitamin C content for both of the fruits is at par. Quince has higher mineral content in comparison to apples with Na (9.2 mg), K (189 mg), Ca (66 mg) and Mg (10 mg), while in apples, the content of Na is 2 mg, K is 112 mg, Ca is 5.5 mg and Mg is 6 mg (Biro and Linder 1999).

## 12.4 PHOTOCHEMISTRY OF DIFFERENT PARTS OF QUINCE

### 12.4.1 Fruit (Pulp and Peel)

#### 12.4.1.1 Polyphenols

Quince fruit is as such in which approximately 34 polyphenols are present. These are mostly coumaroylquinic acid derivatives and caffeoylquinic acid derivatives (Karar 2014). Mono- and dicaffeoylquinic acids (3-O-caffeoylquinic, 3,5-O-dicaffeoylquinic acids 4-O-caffeoylquinic and 5-O-caffeoylquinic), kaempferol-3-O-glucoside, kaempferol-3-O-rutinoside, quercetin-3-O-galactoside and quercetin-3-O-rutinoside are those which are present in the quince pulp; while the peels have some more components added to it, which are quercetin and kaempferol derivatives acylated with p-coumaric acid, chlorogenic acid (5-O-caffeoylquinic acid) (37%) and rutin (quercetin 3-O-rutinoside) (36%) are the two most abundantly present phenolic compounds present in the pulp and the peel. On the other hand, the main acid, which is almost 57% in peel and 29% in pulp, is formed by 5-O-caffeoylquinic acid (Magalhães et al. 2009). The fruit is also a rich source of polyphenol oxidase (PPO) enzyme, and it also contains some important phenols like flavan-3-ols, including procyanidin B2, procyanidin trimmers, tetramers, epicatechin, kaempferol, quinic acid and quercetin derivatives (Wojdyło et al. 2014).

#### 12.4.1.2 Organic Acids

Quince is a rich source of various acids. Some of them include ascorbic, oxalic, malic, citric, quinic, shikimic and fumaric acid (Silva et al. 2002; Wojdyło et al. 2014).

#### 12.4.1.3 Volatile Compounds

Apart from being rich in quince C13 non-isoprenoids, there are a lot of volatile compounds present in quince, which include ethyl decanoate, the acetates, like 5-hexenyl acetate, ethyl acetate, (Z)-3-hexenyl acetate, cis and trans marmelo oxide (Tsuneya et al. 1983; Umano et al. 1986; Tateo and Bononi 2010), volatile esters (ethyl-2-octenoate and sesquiterpenes (α-bergamotene and α-farnesene) (Winterhalter and Schreier 1988).

## 12.4.2 Seeds
### 12.4.2.1 Polyphenols

Quince seed is a good source of various polyphenols and these include C-glycosyl flavones, vicenin-2, isoschaftoside, lucenin-2, stellarin-2, schaftoside, 6-C-pentosyl-8-C-glucosyl chrysoeriol and 6-C-glucosyl-8-C-pentosyl chrysoeriol, kaempferol-3-O-rutinoside (Silva et al. 2004) however, rich in 6,8-di-C-glucosyl chrysoeriol (Stellarin-2) (18%).

Some fat-soluble bioactive compounds have also been reported to be present in quince seeds, and these include phytosterols, tocopherols and phenolic acids. Tocopherols consist of α-tocopherol, β-tocopherol and γ-tocopherol which show the highest activity of vitamin C. Amongst the phytosterols, β-sitosterol is responsible for decreasing the levels of LDL cholesterol with specificity towards it (Hegedűs et al. 2013).

### 12.4.2.2 Organic Acids

Quince peel is a rich source of six acids which include citric, ascorbic, malic, quinic, shikimic and fumaric acids and they contribute to about 0.8 g/kg of the sample (Silva et al. 2002). Quince seeds are also rich in other organic acids, including ursolic acid, tormentic acid, β-daucosterol and 34 carbon chromone (Ghopur et al. 2012).

## 12.4.3 Quince Seed Mucilage

A mixture of cellulose and water-soluble polysaccharide is reported to be present in quince seed mucilage. L-arabinose, D-xylose and aldobiouronic acids are also reported in quince seed mucilage which is revealed from acidic hydrolysis (Smith and Montgomery 1959).That part of the mucilage soluble in water is partially O-acetylated (4-O-methyl-D-glucurono) D-xylan and has greater portions of glycuronic acid. Another acid which has also been reported to be present in quince is uronic acid, with a percentage of 35%.

4-O-methyl glucose, D-xylose and D-glucose are the sugars found in the quince mucilage. Wound healing activity is also found in the Quince seed mucilage (Hemmati et al. 2012).

## 12.5 TRADITIONAL MEDICINAL USES OF QUINCE
### 12.5.1 Fruit

Quince can be used to treat nausea, and has anti-inflammatory and ulcer-healing effects. It is believed to be a tonic for gastric, brain and cardiac conditions, and also a tonic for the liver and stomach. They are astringent and are usually appropriate to treat haemorrhoid bleeding (Monka et al. 2014). Hypertension, respiratory system diseases and diseases related to metabolism like diabetes mellitus, hyperlipidaemia, hypercholesterolemia, inflammation of the kidneys, urinary bladder and urinary tract, constipation and bloating can be cured with quince fruit consumption (Vaez et al. 2014). The fruit is also used to treat abdominal pain, leucorrhoea, diarrhoea, uterine haemorrhages, haemoptysis and wounds and finds its use as a sedative, lowering fever, antiseptic, scar healing and hepatoprotective agent (Aslam and Hussain 2013; Al-Snafi 2016).

### 12.5.2 Seeds

A seed of quince is responsible for having an astringent flavour and produces a calming effect. They also find their use in the cure of gastrointestinal (GI) disorders. They are also found to treat sore throat, cough and bronchitis (Aslam and Sial 2014). In order to treat skin wounds, the mucilage of the seeds is very effective (Ghafourian et al. 2015).

## 12.6 PHARMACOLOGICAL USES OF QUINCE
### 12.6.1 Fruit
#### 12.6.1.1 Antiallergy and Anti-Inflammatory Effects
Lemon and quince fruit were researched for their antiallergic properties. Due to the presence of eriocitrin and neochlorogenic acid, the effect of the two extracts resulted in significant basophil degranulation, generation of tumour necrosis factor (TNF) and interleukin-8 (IL-8), and from human mast cells, as demonstrated by LC-MS analysis. (Huber et al. 2012).

It has been reported that Gencydo, which is a mixture of lemon juice and quince fruit extract, is used to reduce histamine, IL-8 and TNF-α release from mast cells induced by Immunoglobulin-E (IgE) and phorbol myristate acetate in allergic disorders. Furthermore, Gencydo is also reported to cause the blockage of eotaxin discharge from human respiratory epithelial cells (Gründemann et al. 2011).

The *in vivo* and *in vitro* testing of hot-water extract of quince fruit was done for the antiallergic properties. The cell culture studies stated a considerable decrease in the release of β-hexosaminidase on the addition of (50, 100 and 200) μg/mL of hot-water extract to cell culture. The control group showed atopic dermatitis, i.e., marks appeared on the face, ear, nose, neck and dorsal skin of mice; however, the quince-treated mice showed significantly lower severity (Sabir et al. 2015).

#### 12.6.1.2 Antidiabetic Activity
The watery fruit extract of quince was potent in overcoming difficulties linked to diabetes. Daily oral intake of extract for about 28 days of about 80 mg/kg, 160 mg/kg and 240 mg/kg of the body weight to male Sprague-Dawley rats was done to induce diabetes by streptozotocin (60 mg/kg). The antidiabetic effect was assessed by estimating their fasting blood glucose level (FBG). The results revealed that the FBG was suppressed according to the dose. Also, a gas chromatography-mass spectrometry assay was carried out to detect the active portion for antidiabetic effect. It was observed that 5-hydroxymethylfurfural or 5-HMF is a part of the active fraction (methanolic fraction) that is somewhat responsible for the antidiabetic effects of quince (Mohebbi et al. 2019).

The effect of an aqueous fruit extract of *Cydoniaoblonga* Miller fruit on the lipid profile and some metabolic parameters of streptozotocin-induced diabetic rats was investigated. Quince fruit extract successfully lowered total cholesterol, serum triglycerides, ALT, AST, ALP and LDL and enhanced HDL in diabetic rats, according to the findings. The extract also prevented diabetes-induced increase in serum urea and creatinine levels, which are indications of renal impairment. In streptozotocin-induced diabetic mice, the aqueous fruit extract of *Cydoniaoblonga* Miller fruit was found to have hypolipidemic, hepatoprotective and renoprotective properties (Mirmohammadlu et al. 2015).

#### 12.6.1.3 Antioxidant Activity
To analyse the radical scavenging potential, the quince extracts were analysed and evaluated against the synthetic antioxidants. It was reported that the strong properties were almost like those obtained from the peel, with a (70%–80%) retarding influence on DPPH radicals (Silva et al. 2006).

The antioxidant functions of quince phenolic extracts evaluated by the linoleic acid peroxidation system and the DPPH radical scavenging system were found to be superior to that of chlorogenic acid and ascorbic acid (Fattouch et al. 2007).

The ability of methanoic pulp, peel and seed extracts to saturate the free radical 2,2'-diphenyl-1-picrylhydrazyl (DPPH) and to prevent 2,2'-azobis (2-amidinopropane) dihydrochloride (AAPH)-induced oxidative hemolysis of human RBCs was determined. The pulp and peel extract's DPPH free radical scavenging capabilities were found to be nearly identical (EC 50 of 0.6 and 0.8 mg/mL, respectively), while the seed extract's antioxidant activity was limited (EC 50 of 12.2 mg/mL). The oxidative activity of AAPH demonstrated that the pulp and peel extracts provided significant protection of the erythrocyte membrane from hemolysis in a time-dependent and concentration-dependent manner (Pacifico et al. 2012).

HPLC/UV was used to examine the phenolic fraction and organic acid fraction of methanolic extracts. When compared to the entire methanolic extract, the phenolic fraction had the strongest antioxidant activity, while the organic acid extract had the poorest. The highest antioxidant capacity was found in the methanolic peel extract, while the strongest antioxidant activity was found in the phenolic seed extract (Magalhães et al. 2009).

### 12.6.2 Seeds
#### 12.6.2.1 Anti-Spasmodic Activity
The anti-spasmodic activity of quince seed extract was investigated using guinea pigs and rabbits. In isolated ileum and jejunum of guinea pig and rabbit, it was discovered that the crude seed extract of quince caused atropine-sensitive spasmodic reactions. When the results were compared to those of a standard $Ca^{2+}$ antagonist, Verapamil, it was discovered that the spasmodic properties of seed extract are due to the presence of a substance in it that causes muscarinic receptor excitation, whereas the $Ca^{2+}$ antagonist phenomenon may lead to antispasmodic actions of the gut and tracheal cells (Janbaz et al. 2013).

#### 12.6.2.2 Anticancer Activity
The quince seed extract has little effect on colon cancer cell development; however, it has a powerful antiproliferative effect against renal cancer cells at higher concentrations (500 g/mL) (Carvalho et al. 2010).

#### 12.6.2.3 Antidiabetic Activity
An L6 skeletal muscle model with insulin resistance was used to test the antidiabetic potential of the quince fruit seed extract. In different L6 myotubes, the extract had a positive effect on insulin-promoted glucose utilisation, lactic acid generation and glycogen production. In L6 myotubes, the extract boosted glycogen production and glucose consumption at a concentration of 12.5 g/mL. The extract showed a beneficial effect on glucose metabolism and a hypoglycemic effect, making it effective in preventing and treating diabetes (Tang et al. 2016).

#### 12.6.2.4 Wound-Healing Activity
The efficacy of quince seeds mucilage cream (QMC) in treating wounds on white Iranian rabbits with cutaneous injuries was examined using concentrations of 5%, 10% and 20% QMC in the eucerin base. It was discovered that using QMC at a 20% concentration for 13 days resulted in complete wound healing (Tamri et al. 2014).

Quince seed extract can be used to treat skin infections. The wound healing rate in mice infected with *Staphylococcus aureus* was compared and assessed using quince seed extract and silver nanoparticles. In comparison to mupirocin and silver nanoparticles, the group treated with quince seed extract (Ethanolic and Acetonic) had a significant impact on wound healing, supporting quince seed extract as an effective choice in wound healing (Alizadeh et al. 2013).

The result of quince seed extract in curing second-degree burn injuries was examined. It was observed that 1% balm of *Cydonia oblonga* seed extract caused 99.5% wound healing in comparison to the sulfadiazine standard (92.97%) (Tajoddini et al. 2013).

Skin infections can be treated using quince seed extract. Using quince seed extract and silver nano particles, the wound healing rate in mice infected with *Staphylococcus aureus* was compared and measured. In compared to mupirocin and silver nanoparticles, the group treated with quince seed extract (ethanolic and acetonic) had a substantial impact on wound healing, indicating that quince seed extract is a viable wound healing option (Sabir et al. 2015).

## 12.7 PROCESSED PRODUCTS MADE FROM QUINCE

Quince cannot be eaten as it is because of its astringent flavour. It cannot be eaten until it is processed because it is a tough fruit. Therefore, it is processed into a large number of products so that it might not remain inedible. These products include jams, jellies, marmalades and candies.

With the use of 50% quince and 50% cactus pear pulp, the production of dehydrated quince fruit sheets has been reported. The mixture was dried up with the application of forced air by a tunnel dehydrator at a temperature of 57°C–60°C for a period of about 6–8 hours. The formulation exhibited a pH value of 4.2, lower acidity of 1.32% and lower vitamin C content as compared to the other formulations. However, the characteristics related to organoleptic properties did not show any major differences in the storage (Sepúlveda et al. 2000).

The Japanese quince (*Chaenomeles japonica*) is quite known because of its processing, and the processed products that have been studied. Various products can be developed from quince, including fruit juice, puree and extracts with aroma. The juices from the fruits were extracted after having proper treatment with pectolytic enzymes. The fruit juice with and without prior treatment with pectolytic enzymes was obtained by crushing and centrifugation or by pressing. Some consumer products, such as ice cream, lemonade, jam, curd and yoghurt, were also developed from the quince fruit. The pectin extracted from the quince was used to improve bread quality. A minimum amount of 0.5% addition of pectin resulted in a 7% increase in bread volume. The pectin was found to have a positive effect on crumb hardness and elasticity (Hellin et al. 2003).

The evaluation of the constituents of peeled quince jams and that of the unpeeled ones and the consequent effect of the processing on the amino acids, phenolics and organic acid profile of the product has been documented. Due to hydrolysis, the thermal processing leads to an alteration in the free amino acid profile. However, there was no major change in the phenolics and the organic acids (Silva et al. 2004).

So a study on the phenols, organic acids and the free amino acids present in the jam of quince, PCA of around 51 varieties was done. The results showed that there was a significant difference between the jams that were made from peeled fruits and those in which there was no peel on the fruit. It was observed that in 3-O- and 5-O-caffeoylquinic acids and all flavonoids, there was a big difference of 37.5% and similarly a difference of 17.0% in the composition of 4-O- and 5-O-caffeoylquinic acids against 3-O-caffeoylquinic and 3,5-dicaffeoylquinic acids. It was concluded that those quince jams that become a part of the market are mostly made from fruits that are not peeled (Silva et al. 2006).

With the application of ohmic heat, the rheological characters of quince nectar were investigated. By use of the concentric viscometer, application of a range of temperature, i.e., 65°C–75°C, was done over different holding times, viz, 0, 10, 15, 20 and 30 minutes. A number of models were fixed to the Shear stress-shear rate data. The results revealed that the best model to fit the experimental rheogram was the Herschel-Bulkley model with regression coefficients (R2) of as much as 0.9997 and low standard errors (SE) of 0.054. The nectar was non-Newtonian and pseudoplastic in the heat range of 20°C–75°C. Therefore, the ohmic heating that did not show any electric outcome could be considered a possible option for heating fruit nectar (Bozkurt and Icier 2009).

Quince, which is considered an underutilised fruit, is used for making jams and jellies, and it has been seen that the jelly made from quince has more pectin and vitamin C than jam. Also, it was seen that both the products were found to be rich sources of phytochemicals like malic acid and ascorbic acid (Sharma et al. 2011).

The fibre products developed from quince pomace have positive physiological and functional properties. The processed products exhibited comparatively more hydrating properties than that of citrus and apple pulps. After evaluating the isolated, dried fractions for chemical composition, functional and physical characters, the dried fractions displayed greater levels of water absorption during the kinetics assay. The absorption of oil was dependent on the micro-structural properties of the fibre powders, while water absorption was based on the material's hydrophilic nature (de Escalada Pla et al. 2010).

Similarly, a viscometer was used in order to study the rheological behaviour of quince puree. It was concluded from the results that quince puree is a non-Newtonian, pseudoplastic fluid. The results showed that the puree's nature was thixotropic, and its viscosity changed with time. This also made it quite obvious that the puree made from quince does not have gel properties that were shown by the change in viscosity with time (Bikić et al. 2012).

A study was conducted to optimise the osmotic–ultrasonic pretreatments and to study the hot-air drying of quince using response surface methodology. Sucrose solutions were used at different doses, i.e., viz, 40°Brix and 60°Brix, the slices of quince fruit were osmo-dehydrated with a processing time set for 1, 1.5 and 2 h, keeping ultrasonication time of 0, 15 and 30 min. Dehydration, solid gain and weight loss parameters were assessed. Ultrasonic time was kept at 27.25 min, osmosis time was 120 min and the concentration of sucrose was kept was 50.52%. It led to a water loss of approximately 34.68 g/100 g fresh sample, a solid gain of about 18.66 g/100 g fresh sample and a reduction in weight of about 16.21 g/100 g fresh sample (Noshad et al. 2012).

A snack made from quince has been reported to be a rich source of prebiotic inulin and a sweetener Stevia. The addition of Stevia into it was responsible for improving its taste apart from the functional properties of the snack that were already improved. It was also seen that the porosity of the fruit was 0.35 cm³/cm³, which meant that the fruit tissue could also be used for vacuum infusion. Also, it was seen that the treatment with ultrasound (US) and vacuum-infusion (VI) treatment was responsible for giving the highest gain in weight and was also responsible for maintaining the higher springiness. However, the changes observed in the colour and the browning index were reduced than that of the non-treated dried quince (Jovanovic-Malinovska et al. 2012).

The effect of some berry and fruit addition in the processing of the quince jam constituents and amount of significant polyphenolic compounds, antioxidant action and properties of quince related to colour and mixed quince jams was evaluated, and it was seen that the content of polyphenols in quince jam was 484.5 mg/100 g. It was seen that the phenolic content and maximum antioxidant activity were seen in the samples that had the addition of chokeberry > blackcurrant > flowering quince. In general, it was seen that the quince jams were not only a good source of antioxidant compounds but were also found very attractive and appealing to consumers (Wojdyło et al. 2013).

The evaluation of the quality of value-added products made from fruit, like Ready-To-Serve beverages (RTS), jam and fruit bars while in storage, was also seen. It was concluded from the results that there was an increase in the soluble solids, titratable acidity and reducing sugars and also a decrease in the ascorbic acid content along with the total sugars. The products that were made could be used up to a storage period of 9 months at normal conditions of temperature and pressure except for RTS beverages. It was also seen that the products were free from microbes also during these 9 months of storage except for RTS beverages (Kumari et al. 2013).

A study on freeze drying quince has been reported in which the drying kinetics of mashed quince was considered. The influence of several actors like heat load power, initial moisture content and the instant of heat application on the dehydration rate and dryer performance were studied. The data of the experiment were subjected to arithmetical models. The results revealed that the dehydration time is considerably lowered by the application of a high-temperature load power at the start of the course (Adhami et al. 2013).

In a study, the antioxidant property and the storage capacity of the phenols present in the juice of quince were studied. The quince juices made from various cultivars grown in Poland were compared among themselves for their polyphenolic compounds and their antioxidant activity. The results concluded that the quince juice that was made from different cultivars showed a great difference in its chemical characteristics. In fact, the phenolic compounds that in the quince fruit were found to be more in comparison to the commonly consumed apple juices (Wojdyło et al. 2014).

The quantification of the biochemical and antioxidant activity of quince fruit and its products was done. It was seen that the hybrid clone C.47 showed more amount of ascorbic acid content of about 55 mg $100 \text{ g}^{-1}$ and in Lichtar (106 mg $100 \text{ g}^{-1}$). Not only that, the cultivar Litchar showed a higher phenolic content (422.6 mg $100 \text{ g}^{-1}$) and greater antiradical activity (12.35 µmol TE/g). In candied quince slices, the range of ascorbic acid content was 116–124 mg $100 \text{ g}^{-1}$ of the product, but a comparatively greater amount was recorded in candied slices of "Lichtar". From the hybrid clone C.47, it was seen that the sugar syrup had a greater amount of vitamin C (56.4 mg 100 g of syrup), and likewise, the slices of the fruit that were candied and were produced from the same had a higher content of phenolic compounds (917 mg $100 \text{ g}^{-1}$) and a higher activity of the antiradical -30.89 µmol TE/g (Rubinskienė et al. 2014).

In a study conducted on how quince tea is developed, the two methods of drying for the antioxidant activity were reported. From the study, it was concluded that the quince that was oven-dried proved to be a better source of phenolics in comparison with the sun-dried quince peel that also had a greater amount of phenols than the quince flesh., Therefore it was concluded that the radical scavenging activity of the sundries and flesh samples was found to be lower than those which were oven-dried and those from the quince peel (Gheisari and Abhari 2014).

Sensory and quality attributes of quince and apple leather were studied. In order to enhance the antioxidant capacity of the leather, it was enriched with maqui extract and was assessed for a number of parameters. It was revealed that leathers had a water content of 17 kg/100 kg, and the total soluble solids were around 70°Brix. The antioxidant-rich extract enhanced the leather's colour and browning index. In quince formulations, total phenols (TP) and antioxidant activity (AOA) were found to be higher (p ≤ 0.05). Almost 45% and 40% increments in AOA and total phenol was observed in apple puree. Antioxidants decreased up to 59% in leathers as compared to fruit puree. During storage, total phenol showed a slight decrease, however, the AOA did not show any change at all (Torres et al. 2015).

The formation of dried slices of quince and the effect of osmotic pre-treatment on the physical characteristics of quince were researched. The results were suggestive of the fact that an osmotic solution of saccharose which was present at a temperature of 60°C, affected the quality of dried quince positively. Also, the results showed that there was a positive effect on the physical characteristics of quince, which resulted in the prevention of fruit tissue darkening during convective drying (Bikić and Mitrevski 2015).

The effect of three distinct packaging materials for packing, i.e., polyethylene pouch, laminate and plastic jar, on antioxidant and physicochemical properties of quince candies that were developed was studied. The consumer acceptability was good with quince candies packed in laminate with a storage period of more than 4 months and possessed better physical and chemical characteristics and antioxidant properties as well when compared to the plastic jar and polyethylene (Mir et al. 2015).

An investigation of the sensory properties and physicochemical changes of the smoothies made during the storage by the amalgamation of apple, quince, pear and flowering quince juices with Sour Cherry Puree was carried out. Seventeen distinct products, viz, 12 smoothies and 5 intermediate products before and after storage were examined for antioxidant activity, phenolic compounds and physical parameters (colour and viscosity) for about 6 months at temperatures of 30°C and 4°C, respectively. The polyphenol content was found to be 517.75 mg of sour cherry/flowering quince smoothie and 333.36 mg/100 g of sour cherry/pear smoothie. A high content of polyphenolic compounds was found in the smoothies added with Flowering Quince Juice and Quince Juice even after 6 months of storage. Also, the smoothies formed were appealing to consumers, particularly those with apple and quince juice addition (Nowicka et al. 2016).

The quince processing to dehydrated slices, jam and candy was reported in which a comparative study of their composition and antioxidant attributes was carried out that exhibited a considerable variation. The processed quince products exhibited greater total phenolic content and antioxidant attributes in comparison to fresh pulp. About 69.12–78.67 mg GAE/100 g of the total phenols were found in the processed quince products. Reducing power, peroxide value ($H_2O_2$), 2,2-Diphenyl-1-picrylhydrazyl (DPPH) and Ferric Reducing Antioxidant Power (FRAP) were found in the range of (70.9–89.5)%, (36.02–51.20)%, (79.91–82.61)% and (1.40 1.68) µM, respectively (Mir et al. 2016).

In order to make a quince jam low in calories, stevioside was used as an artificial sweetener and pectin was used as a stabilising agent. It was found that the jam which was formed had 0.4% pectin, 0.27% stevioside and 50% sugar. The activity of water along with the pH of the jam was increased, but on the other hand, there was a considerable reduction in the amount of monomeric anthocyanin, total phenolic compounds, vitamin C, Brix, viscosity, acidity and a* value. It was concluded from the study that the production of this jam that has low calories can be advised to those people who are very conscious about eating foods that have low calories.

Using a hot air dryer and electro-hydrodynamic method, the quince slices were dried whose effect based on the energy consumption, drying kinetics, phenolic compounds and potent antioxidant activity was investigated on the quince slices. It was revealed that phenolic compounds were 1.3 times greater in hot dried slices compared to electro-hydrodynamic dried slices. Similarly, those slices of quince which were dried had an antioxidant capacity of dried of 1.15 times more than those which had undergone an electro-hydrodynamic process. Thus, revealing that the hot air drying process has a positive effect on the antioxidant activity and the total phenolic compounds of the dried quince (Yousefi et al. 2018).

When maltodextrin was added to the quince powder, which was freeze-dried, the results indicated that with the moisture and the activity of the water reducing, there was an increase in the drying time. It was also seen that there was a change in the colour of the sample when sugar and maltodextrin were added. The two above-mentioned products also affected the values of density, flow and reconstitution properties (Ünlüeroğlugil et al. 2018).

A study was conducted in order to see the effect on the phenolic characters and quality parameters after processed samples were used. The value of total soluble solids (TSS) of puree was 14.4°Brix, which elevated to 75°Brix in the case of bars. The acidity increased to 1.5 g malic acid kg⁻¹ of the fresh weight. P-coumaric acid, quercetin and trans-cinnamic acid were present in fresh puree increased after the thermal processing while, on the other hand, gallic acid content reduced. To achieve the maximum concentration of most of the phenolics, a cooking time should be kept to a minimum of 5 min; nevertheless, a time period of 20 min was observed to be ideal for the p-coumaric acid concentration (Torres et al. 2019).

Dried quince slices developed from four distinct drying procedures (solar drying, drying under the sun, drying using microwave and using a hot air oven) and four distinct pre-treatment techniques (not blanched, blanched, blanched+ascorbic acid and not blanched +ascorbic acid) was done. Each dried slice was filled in low-density poly ethylene (LDPE) packets, retained for 6 months, and kept in observation for microbiological, physico-chemical and sensory attributes. Hot air-dried quince slices exhibited minimum shrinkage, maximum rehydration ratio and highest L* and b* values with the lowest a* value. The maximum reducing sugars content, total sugars content, protein content, mineral content, crude fibre content, the activity of the antioxidants and total concentration of the phenols were also dried slices of quince that were air dried (Munaza 2018).

The manufacture of a nutraceutical formulation, chewing candy (CC), consisting of quince and sea buckthorn juice and juice by-products with the use of agar and gelatine, was reported. It was revealed that the juice and by-products of the juice exhibited antimicrobial activity against every pathogen that was tested. But, the chief zones of inhibition were seen in the case of the quince and sea buckthorn juices against the pathogen *Proteus mirabilis* and *Bacillus*, respectively. The chewing candy made with agar and sea buckthorn by-products (131.7) and with gelatin and quince juice (132.0) resulted in great acceptance. Moreover, adding the juice and juice by-products enhanced the antioxidant activity of CC five-fold (Lele et al. 2018).

The effect of temperature and high-pressure carbon dioxide (HPCD) treatment on the inactivation, aggregation and topological changes of poly phenol oxidase (PPO) were studied on the quince fruit juice. It was observed that HPCD led to the inactivation of PPO at (55°C–65°C) while at the same temperature, thermal processing on its own was not able to slow down PPO activity. In HPCD-treated juice, the rate of browning was seen to be less than in juice that was treated with heat. HPCD induced a reduction in fluorescence intensities and circular dichroism spectra, resulting in the destruction and reorganisation of the configuration of the PPO molecule. On HPCD treatment, a transformation in PPO molecule structure was found that resulted in dissociation initially and following PPO molecule aggregation. Thus, for the activation of the PPO molecule, the HPCD method was revealed to be a highly efficacious thermal treatment. HPCD-treated juices had slightly decreased pH in comparison to the control because of the dissolved $CO_2$ in the quince juice during the HPCD treatment. furthermore, the values of the TSS did not considerably change, but a rise in brightness (L* value) of quince juice was seen (Iqbal et al. 2018).

An investigation on the categorisation and processing of marmalade capacity of quince varieties ("Smyrna," "Fuller," "Portugal," "Mendonza Inta-37," "Provence," "Alaranjado," "CTS 207," "Lajeado," "D'Angers" and "Bereczy") was conducted. The effect on the physical and chemical features, rheological characters and the buyer acceptance of the prepared marmalade was considered. It was observed that different quince cultivars exhibited a huge inconsistency among themselves when physical and physicochemical qualities were taken into consideration. All the cultivars that were investigated for marmalade preparation were alike, with better sensory quality. However, less acceptable marmalade was reported in the cultivar Mendonza Inta-37 (Curi et al. 2018).

A study was conducted in which the quince juice was optimised using the thermosonication technique. The procedure of thermosonication was performed at different temperatures that included (30°C, 35°C, 40°C, 45°C and 50°C), different amplitudes (40%, 45%, 50%, 55% and 60%) and at different time intervals (2, 4, 6, 8 and 10) min so that the bioactive compounds could be optimised that included the total phenols, the total concentration Of ascorbic acid and a total capacity of antioxidants) and values of colour were also determined (L*, a* and b*). It was inferred from the results that quince juice could be optimised at a temperature of 8.7°C, 5.6 minutes and 50.9 amplitude. Total phenolic (591.15 mg GAE/L) and total antioxidant levels (DPPH 0.214 mg TEAC/mL and CUPRAC 0.149 mg TEAC/mL) were greater in that juice of quince, which was thermosonified in comparison to the quince juice that was fresh. However, the process of thermosonication resulted in a decrease in the amount of vitamin C (ascorbic acid 3.78 mg/100 mL). In total, the procedure of thermosonication is believed to be a great technique to improve bioactive components compared to thermal pasteurisation (Yıkmış et al. 2019).

A study was conducted to study the inactivation and changes in the structure of PPO molecule through analysis of the structure in quince juice that was subjected to the treatment of ultrasonification was studied. The results showed that the PPO activity was reduced by about 35% in the juice, which was treated with the help of high ultrasonic intensity (400 W for 20 min) in comparison to the juice that was not treated. The ultrasonic treatment resulted in the inactivation of the PPO molecule due to aggregation of the protein, breakage of tertiary structure, and breakage of the secondary structure of the amino acids. Therefore, it can be conceived that ultrasound processing at high intensity and duration is responsible for the inactivation of the PPO enzyme because of aggregation induction and changes in the topology of the molecule (Iqbal et al. 2020).

## 12.8 FORTIFIED PRODUCTS OF QUINCE *CYDONIA oBLONGA*

Quince is considered a rich source of antioxidants and some nutrients which make it a proper candidate for fortification in foods.

The scalding water of quince, which is believed to be a rich source of antioxidants, including phenols and flavonoids, has been used for the fortification of yoghurt. It was seen that the yoghurt which was formed had greater pH and lower concentration of lactic acid content in comparison to the controlled yoghurts because of its high polyphenolic content. Apart from this, the scalding water of quince also had a considerable effect on the textural and the rheological properties of the fruit (Trigueros et al. 2011).

In yet another study, the effect that the quince powder has on the rheological properties of batter, along with the physical, chemical and sensory properties of sponge cake, were observed. The quince slices were allowed to dry in an infrared-hot air dryer, and the powdered quince was given at five concentrations (control, 5%, 10%, 15% and 20%). Because of the higher level of substitution of quince powder, the cake volume was found to reduce. On increasing the quince powder levels from 0% to 15%, there was an increase in the values of density, consistency and hardness. However, there was an overall decrease in the volume, cohesiveness, resilience, chewiness and crumb L values of the samples. Therefore, 10% quince powder was found to be better for the acceptance of the cake (Salehi and Kashaninejad 2017).

The analysis of the textural profile and stress relaxation parameters of sponge cake modified with (0%, 5%, 10%, 15% and 20%) dried quince powder was studied. The drying of the quince powder was done in an infrared hot air dryer (375 W, 60°C and 1 m/s flow rate). The results were suggestive that Peleg-Normand and four-element Maxwell models were both found to fit the mechanical stress relaxation data of cakes. As far as the values of hardness and consistency of sponge cakes were considered, it was found that there was an increase in the quince powder substitution. Nevertheless, the elasticity, cohesiveness, resilience and chewiness showed a reduction in the values (Salehi and Kashaninejad 2018).

In a study, the effect that is observed by the addition of quince pomace powder (0%–15%) and water content (25%–35%) on the rheological properties of the batter and the physical and chemical characteristics and sensory properties of sponge cake was studied. It was seen in the results that there is a higher concentration of viscosity, batter consistency, dietary fibre, firmness and overall acceptability of cake in comparison with quince pomace. On the other hand, there was a reduction in the moisture content, apart from the density of the cake. It was seen from the RSM results that 12.56% of quince pomace powder and 29.62% of water content showed the desirable physical and chemical quality. The product that was optimised had a total phenol content of 8.32 (mg/g), iron 0.361 (mg/kg dry weight) and calcium 1160 (mg/kg dry weight). It was found that the values were higher than the control. Also, it was seen from the results of SEM that there was uniformity in the cake number of cavities in the cake structure (Anvar et al. 2019).

The result of an amalgamation of freeze-dried Japanese quince fruit (FJQF) (0%–9%) and the cookies so as to enhance their antioxidant qualities, volatile and sensory attributes in storage was observed, which showed that the cookies comprising FJQF had 2–3.5 times more radical scavenging action and had more concentration of volatile compounds like heptanal, hexanal, octanal, 2-heptenal, (E) as compared to control cookies. Also, a higher amount of secondary lipid oxidation products was found in control cookies than in FJQF cookies. Acetic acid was the dominant volatile compound found in the volatile profile of the enriched cookies and ranged from 7.05% to 23.37%. The overall acceptance of the cookies was better, with 1.0% and 1.5% FJQF compared to 6.0% and 9.0% FJQF (Antoniewska et al. 2019).

## REFERENCES

Adhami, S., Rahimi, A. and Hatamipour, M.S. 2013. "Freeze drying of quince (*Cydonia oblonga*): Modelling of drying kinetics and characteristics." *Korean Journal of Chemical Engineering* 30(6):1201–1206.

Alizadeh, H., Rahnema, M., Nasiri, S.S., Ajalli, M. and Rostamkhani, R. 2013. "Effect of *Cydonia oblonga* seed's extract and silver nanoparticles on wound healing in mice infected with *Staphylococcus aureus*."

Al-Snafi, A.E. 2016. "The medical importance of *Cydonia oblonga*-A review." *IOSR Journal of Pharmacy* 6(6):87–99.

Antoniewska, A., Rutkowska, J. and Pineda, M.M. 2019. "Antioxidative, sensory and volatile profiles of cookies enriched with freeze-dried Japanese quince (*Chaenomeles japonica*) fruits." *Food Chemistry* 286:376–387.

Anvar, A., Nasehi, B., Noshad, M. and Barzegar, H. 2019. "Improvement of physicochemical and nutritional quality of sponge cake fortified with microwave-air dried quince pomace." *Iranian Food Science and Technology Research Journal* 15(3):69–79.

Ashraf, M.U., Muhammad, G., Hussain, M.A. and Bukhari, S.N. 2016. "*Cydonia oblonga* M., a medicinal plant rich in phytonutrients for pharmaceuticals." *Frontiers in Pharmacology* 7:163.

Aslam, M. and Hussain, S.Z. 2013. "The effect of hydro-alcoholic extract of *Cydonia oblonga* Miller (Quince) on blood cells and liver enzymes in New Zealand white rabbits." *Inventi Rapid: Ethnopharmacology* 3:1–4.

Aslam, M. and Sial, A.A. 2014. "Effect of hydroalcoholic extract of *Cydonia oblonga* miller (Quince) on sexual behaviour of Wistar rats." *Advances in Pharmacological Sciences* 2014:282698.

Bikić, S., Bukurov, M., Babić, M., Pavkov, I. and Radojčin, M. 2012. "Rheological behavior of quince (*Cydonia oblonga*) puree." *Journal on Processing and Energy in Agriculture* 16(4):155–161.

Bikić, I.P.M.B.S. and Mitrevski, V. 2015. "Effects of osmotic pretreatment on quality and physical properties of dried quinces (*Cydonia oblonga*)." *Journal of Food and Nutrition Research* 54(2): 142–154.

Biro, G. and Lindner, K. 1999. "Nutrient table. Nutrition and nutrient composition." *Medicina Konyvkiado* Rt, Budapest 1999:208–225.

Bozkurt, H. and Icier, F. 2009. "Rheological characteristics of quince nectar during ohmic heating." *International Journal of Food Properties* 12(4):844–859.

Carvalho, M., Silva, B.M., Silva, R., Valentao, P., Andrade, P.B. and Bastos, M.L. 2010. "First report on *Cydonia oblonga* Miller anticancer potential: Differential antiproliferative effect against human kidney and colon cancer cells." *Journal of Agricultural and Food Chemistry* 58(6):3366–3370.

Costa, R.M., Magalhães, A.S., Pereira, J.A., Andrade, P.B., Valentão, P., Carvalho, M. and Silva, B.M. 2009. "Evaluation of free radical-scavenging and antihemolytic activities of quince (*Cydonia oblonga*) leaf: A comparative study with green tea (*Camellia sinensis*)." *Food and Chemical Toxicology* 47(4):860–865.

Curi, P.N., Coutinho, G., Matos, M., Pio, R., Albergaria, F.C. and Souza, V.R.D. 2018. "Characterization and Marmelade processing potential of quince cultivars cultivated in tropical regions." *Revista Brasileira de Fruticultura* 40.

Daneshvand, B., Ara, K.M. and Raofie, F. 2012. "Comparison of supercritical fluid extraction and ultrasound-assisted extraction of fatty acids from quince (*Cydonia oblonga* Miller) seed using response surface methodology and central composite design." *Journal of Chromatography A* 1252:1–7.

De Escalada Pla, M.F., Uribe, M., Fissore, E.N., Gerschenson, L.N. and Rojas, A.M. 2010. "Influence of the isolation procedure on the characteristics of fiber-rich products obtained from quince wastes." *Journal of Food Engineering* 96(2):239–248.

Duke, J.A. 2002. *Handbook of Medicinal Herbs*. CRC Press.

Fattouch, S., Caboni, P., Coroneo, V., Tuberoso, C.I., Angioni, A., Dessi, S., Marzouki, N. and Cabras, P. 2007. "Antimicrobial activity of Tunisian quince (*Cydonia oblonga* Miller) pulp and peel polyphenolic extracts." *Journal of Agricultural and Food Chemistry* 55(3):963–969.

Fulton, S.L., McKinley, M.C., Young, I.S., Cardwell, C.R. and Woodside, J.V. 2016. "The effect of increasing fruit and vegetable consumption on overall diet: A systematic review and meta-analysis." *Critical Reviews in Food Science and Nutrition* 56(5):802–816.

Gani, M., Jabeen, A., Majeed, D., Mir, S.A. and Dar, B.N. 2018. "Proximate composition, mineral analysis and antioxidant capacity of indigenous fruits and vegetables from temperate region of Indian Himalayas." *Journal of Food Measurement and Characterization* 12(2):1011–1019.

Ghafourian, M., Tamri, P. and Hemmati, A. 2015. "Enhancement of human skin fibroblasts proliferation as a result of treating with quince seed mucilage." *Jundishapur Journal of Natural Pharmaceutical Products* 10(1).

Gheisari, H.R. and Abhari, K.H. 2014. "Drying method effects on the antioxidant activity of quince (*Cydonia oblonga* Miller) tea." *Acta Scientiarum Polonorum Technologia Alimentaria* 13(2):129–134.

Ghopur, H., Usmanova, S.K., Ayupbek, A. and Aisa, H.A. 2012. "A new chromone from seeds of *Cydonia oblonga*." *Chemistry of Natural Compounds* 48(4):562–564.

Gründemann, C., Papagiannopoulos, M., Lamy, E., Mersch-Sundermann, V. and Huber, R. 2011. "Immunomodulatory properties of a lemon-quince preparation (Gencydo®) as an indicator of anti-allergic potency." *Phytomedicine* 18(8–9):760–768.

Hegedűs, A., Papp, N. and Stefanovits-Bányai, É. 2013. "Review of nutritional value and putative health-effects of quince (*Cydonia oblonga* Mill.) fruit." *International Journal of Horticultural Science* 19(3–4):29–32.

Hellin, P., Jordan, M.J., Vila, R., Gustafsson, M., Göransson, E., Åkesson, B., Gröön, I., Laencina, J. and Ros, J.M. 2003 "Processing and products of Japanese quince (Chaenomeles japonica) fruits." *Japanese quince—Potential fruit crop for northern Europe. Final report of FAIR-CT97-3894. Swedish University of Agricultural Sciences, Alnarp* (2003): 169–175.

Hemmati, A.A., Kalantari, H., Jalali, A., Rezai, S. and Zadeh, H.H. 2012. "Healing effect of quince seed mucilage on T-2 toxin-induced dermal toxicity in rabbit." *Experimental and Toxicologic Pathology* 64(3):181–186.

Hopur, H., Asrorov, A.M., Qingling, M., Yili, A., Ayupbek, A., Nannan, P. and Aisa, H.A. 2011. "HPLC analysis of polysaccharides in quince (*Cydonia oblonga* Mill. var. maliformis) fruit and PTP1B inhibitory activity." *The Natural Products Journal* 1(2):146–150.

Huber, R., Stintzing, F.C., Briemle, D., Beckmann, C., Meyer, U. and Gründemann, C. 2012. "In vitro antiallergic effects of aqueous fermented preparations from *Citrus* and *Cydonia* fruits." *Planta Medica* 78(04):334–340.

Iqbal, A., Murtaza, A., Marszałek, K., Iqbal, M.A., Chughtai, M.F., Hu, W., Barba, F.J., Bi, J., Liu, X. and Xu, X. 2020. "Inactivation and structural changes of polyphenol oxidase in quince (*Cydonia oblonga* Miller) juice subjected to ultrasonic treatment." *Journal of the Science of Food and Agriculture* 100(5):2065–2073.

Iqbal, A., Murtaza, A., Muhammad, Z., Elkhedir, A.E., Tao, M. and Xu, X. 2018. "Inactivation, aggregation and conformational changes of polyphenol oxidase from quince (*Cydonia oblonga* Miller) juice subjected to thermal and high-pressure carbon dioxide treatment." *Molecules* 23(7):1743.

Janbaz, K.H., Shabbir, A., Mehmood, M.H. and Gilani, A.H. 2013. "Insight into mechanism underlying the medicinal use of *Cydonia oblonga* in gut and airways disorders." *Journal of Animal and Plant Sciences* 23:330–336.

Jovanovic-Malinovska, R., Velickova, E., Kuzmanova, S. and Winkelhausen, E. 2012. "Development of a quince snack enriched with inulin and stevia."

Karar, M.G.E., Pletzer, D., Jaiswal, R., Weingart, H. and Kuhnert, N. 2014. "Identification, characterization, isolation and activity against *Escherichia coli* of quince (*Cydonia oblonga*) fruit polyphenols." *Food Research International* 65:121–129.

Khoubnasabjafari, M. and Jouyban, A. 2011. "A review of phytochemistry and bioactivity of quince (*Cydonia oblonga* Mill.)." *Journal of Medicinal Plants Research* 5:3577–3594.

Kumari, A., Dhaliwal, Y.S., Sandal, A. and Badyal, J. 2013. "Quality evaluation of *Cydonia oblonga* (Quince) fruit and its value added products." *Indian Journal of Agricultural Biochemistry* 26(1):61–65.

Lele, V., Monstaviciute, E., Varinauskaite, I., Peckaityte, G., Paskeviciute, L., Plytnikaite, M., Tamosiunaite, V., Pikunaite, M., Ruzauskas, M., Stankevicius, R. and Bartkiene, E. 2018. "Sea buckthorn (*Hippophae rhamnoides* L.) and quince (*Cydonia oblonga* L.) juices and their by-products as ingredients showing antimicrobial and antioxidant properties for chewing candy: Nutraceutical formulations." *Journal of Food Quality* 2018(1):1–8.

Leonel, M., Leonel, S., Tecchio, M.A., Mischan, M.M., Moura, M.F. and Xavier, D. 2016. "Characteristics of quince fruits cultivars' (*Cydonia oblonga* Mill.) grown in Brazil." *Australian Journal of Crop Science* 10(5):711–716.

Li, L., Pegg, R.B., Eitenmiller, R.R., Chun, J.Y. and Kerrihard, A.L. 2017. "Selected nutrient analyses of fresh, fresh-stored, and frozen fruits and vegetables." *Journal of Food Composition and Analysis* 59:8–17.

Lindberg, B., Mosihuzzaman, M., Nahar, N., Abeysekera, R.M., Brown, R.G. and Willison, J.M. 1990. "An unusual (4-O-methyl-D-glucurono)-D-xylan isolated from the mucilage of seeds of the quince tree (*Cydonia oblonga*)." *Carbohydrate Research* 207(2):307–310.

Lutz-Röder, A., Schneider, M. and Winterhalter, P. 2002. "Isolation of two new ionone glucosides from quince (*Cydonia oblonga* Mill.) leaves." *Natural Product Letters* 16(2):119–122.

Magalhães, A.S., Silva, B.M., Pereira, J.A., Andrade, P.B., Valentão, P. and Carvalho, M. 2009. "Protective effect of quince (*Cydonia oblonga* Miller) fruit against oxidative hemolysis of human erythrocytes." *Food and Chemical Toxicology* 47(6):1372–1377.

Mir, S.A., Wani, S.M., Ahmad, M., Wani, T.A., Gani, A., Mir, S.A. and Masoodi, F.A. 2015. "Effect of packaging and storage on the physicochemical and antioxidant properties of quince candy." *Journal of Food Science and Technology* 52(11):7313–7320.

Mir, S.A., Wani, S.M., Wani, T.A., Ahmad, M., Gani, A., Masoodi, F.A. and Nazir, A. 2016. "Comparative evaluation of the proximate composition and antioxidant properties of processed products of quince (*Cydonia oblonga* Miller)." *International Food Research Journal* 23(2).

Mirmohammadlu, M., Hosseini, S.H., Kamalinejad, M., Gavgani, M.E., Noubarani, M. and Eskandari, M.R. 2015. "Hypolipidemic, hepatoprotective and renoprotective effects of *Cydonia oblonga* Mill. fruit in streptozotocin-induced diabetic rats." *Iranian Journal of Pharmaceutical Research: IJPR* 14(4):1207.

Mohebbi, S., Naserkheil, M., Kamalinejad, M., Hosseini, S.H., Noubarani, M., Mirmohammadlu, M. and Eskandari, M.R. 2019. "Antihyperglycemic activity of quince (*Cydonia oblonga* Mill.) fruit extract and its fractions in the rat model of diabetes." *International Pharmacy Acta* 2(1): e7.

Monka, A., Grygorieva, O., Chlebo, P. and Brindza, J. 2014. "Morphological and antioxidant characteristics of quince (*Cydonia oblonga* Mill.) and Chinese quince fruit (*Pseudocydonia sinensis* Schneid.)." *Slovak Journal of Food Science* 8:333–340.

Munaza, B. 2018. "*Optimization of drying conditions for development of value added products from quince (Cydonia oblonga Miller)*" (Doctoral dissertation, Ph. D thesis, Sher-e-Kashmir University of Agricultural Sciences and Technology of Jammu, Jammu & Kashmir, India).

Noshad, M., Mohebbi, M., Shahidi, F. and Ali Mortazavi, S. 2012. "Multi-objective optimization of osmotic–ultrasonic pretreatments and hot-air drying of quince using response surface methodology." *Food and Bioprocess Technology* 5(6):2098–2110.

Nowicka, P., Wojdyło, A., Teleszko, M. and Samoticha, J. 2016. "Sensory attributes and changes of physicochemical properties during storage of smoothies prepared from selected fruit." *LWT – Food Science and Technology* 71:102–109.

Pacifico, S., Gallicchio, M., Fiorentino, A., Fischer, A., Meyer, U. and Stintzing, F.C. 2012. "Antioxidant properties and cytotoxic effects on human cancer cell lines of aqueous fermented and lipophilic quince (*Cydonia oblonga* Mill.) preparations." *Food and Chemical Toxicology* 50(11):4130–4135.

Postman, J. 2009. "*Cydonia oblonga*: The unappreciated quince." *Arnoldia* 67(1):2–9.

Rasheed, M., Hussain, I., Rafiq, S., Hayat, I., Qayyum, A., Ishaq, S. and Awan, M.S. 2018. "Chemical composition and antioxidant activity of quince fruit pulp collected from different locations." *International Journal of Food Properties* 21(1):2320–2327.

Rubinskienė, M., Viškelis, P., Viškelis, J., Bobinaitė, R., Shalkevich, M., Pigul, M. and Urbonavičienė, D. 2014. "Biochemical composition and antioxidant activity of Japanese quince (*Chaenomeles japonica*) fruit, their syrup and candied fruit slices." *Sodininkystė ir daržininkystė* 33(1–2):45–52.

Sabir, S., Qureshi, R., Arshad, M., Amjad, M.S., Fatima, S., Masood, M. and Chaudhari, S.K. 2015. "Pharmacognostic and clinical aspects of *Cydonia oblonga*: A review." *Asian Pacific Journal of Tropical Disease* 5(11):850–855.

Salehi, F. and Kashaninejad, M. 2017. "The effect of quince powder on rheological properties of batter and physico-chemical and sensory properties of sponge cake." *Journal of Food Biosciences and Technology* 7(1):1–8.

Salehi, F. and Kashaninejad, M. 2018. "Texture profile analysis and stress relaxation characteristics of quince sponge cake." *Journal of Food Measurement and Characterization* 12(2):1203–1210.

Sepúlveda, E., Sáenz, C. and Álvarez, M. 2000. "Physical, chemical and sensory characteristics of dried fruit sheets of cactus pear (*Opuntia ficus indica* (L) Mill) and quince (*Cydonia oblonga* Mill)." *Italian Journal of Food Science* 12(1):47–54.

Sharma, R., Joshi, V.K. and Rana, J.C. 2011. "Nutritional composition and processed products of quince (*Cydonia oblonga* Mill.)."

Silva, B.M., Andrade, P.B., Ferreres, F., Domingues, A.L., Seabra, R.M. and Ferreira, M.A. 2002. "Phenolic profile of quince fruit (*Cydonia oblonga* Miller) (pulp and peel)." *Journal of Agricultural and Food Chemistry* 50(16):4615–4618.

Silva, B.M., Andrade, P.B., Ferreres, F., Seabra, R.M., Beatriz, M., Oliveira, P.P. and Ferreira, M.A. 2005a. "Composition of quince (*Cydonia oblonga* Miller) seeds: Phenolics, organic acids and free amino acids." *Natural Product Research* 19(3):275–281.

Silva, B.M., Andrade, P.B., Gonçalves, A.C., Seabra, R.M., Oliveira, M.B. and Ferreira, M.A. 2004. "Influence of jam processing upon the contents of phenolics, organic acids and free amino acids in quince fruit (*Cydonia oblonga* Miller)." *European Food Research and Technology* 218(4):385–389.

Silva, B.M., Andrade, P.B., Martins, R.C., Seabra, R.M. and Ferreira, M.A. 2006. "Principal component analysis as tool of characterization of quince (*Cydonia oblonga* Miller) jam." *Food Chemistry* 94(4):504–512.

Silva, B.M., Andrade, P.B., Martins, R.C., Valentão, P., Ferreres, F., Seabra, R.M. and Ferreira, M.A. 2005b. "Quince (*Cydonia oblonga* Miller) fruit characterization using principal component analysis." *Journal of Agricultural and Food Chemistry* 53(1):111–122.

Silva, B.M., Casal, S., Andrade, P.B., Seabra, R.M., Oliveira, M.B. and Ferreira, M.A. 2003. "Development and evaluation of a GC/FID method for the analysis of free amino acids in quince fruit and jam." *Analytical Sciences* 19(9):1285–1290.

Smith, F. and Montgomery, R. 1959. "Chemistry of plant gums and mucilages and some related polysaccharides."

Sood, S. and Bhardwaj, M. 2015. "Nutritional evaluation of quince fruit and its products." *Journal of Krishi Vigyan* 3(2s):67–69.

Szychowski, P.J., Munera-Picazo, S., Szumny, A., Carbonell-Barrachina, Á.A. and Hernández, F. 2014. "Quality parameters, bio-compounds, antioxidant activity and sensory attributes of Spanish quinces (*Cydonia oblonga* Miller)." *Scientia Horticulturae* 165:163–170.

Tajoddini, A., Rafieian-Kopaei, M., Namjoo, A.R., Sedeh, M., Ansari, R. and Shahinfard, N. 2013. "Effect of ethanolic extract of *Cydonia oblonga* seed on the healing of second-degree burn wounds." *Armaghane Danesh* 17(6):494–501.

Tamri, P., Hemmati, A. and Boroujerdnia, M.G. 2014. "Wound healing properties of quince seed mucilage: *In vivo* evaluation in rabbit full-thickness wound model." *International Journal of Surgery* 12(8):843–847.

Tang, D., Xie, L., Xin, X. and Aisa, H. 2016. "Antidiabetic action of *Cydonia oblonga* seed extract: Improvement of glucose metabolism via activation of PI3K/AKT signaling pathway." *Journal of Pharmacognosy and Phytochemistry* 4(2):7–13.

Tateo, F. and Bononi, M. 2010. "Headspace-SPME analysis of volatiles from quince whole fruits." *Journal of Essential Oil Research* 22(5):416–418.

Torkelson, A.R. 1995. *Cross Name Index of Medicinal Plants* (Vol. 2). CRC Press.

Torres, C.A., Romero, L.A. and Diaz, R.I. 2015. "Quality and sensory attributes of apple and quince leathers made without preservatives and with enhanced antioxidant activity." *LWT – Food Science and Technology* 62(2):996–1003.

Torres, C.A., Sepúlveda, G. and Concha-Meyer, A.A. 2019. "Effect of processing on quality attributes and phenolic profile of quince dried bar snack." *Journal of the Science of Food and Agriculture* 99(5):2556–2564.

Trigueros, L., Pérez-Alvarez, J.A., Viuda-Martos, M. and Sendra, E. 2011. "Production of low-fat yogurt with quince (*Cydonia oblonga* Mill.) scalding water." *LWT – Food Science and Technology* 44(6):1388–1395.

Tsuneya, T., Ishihara, M., Shiota, H. and Shiga, M. 1983. "Volatile components of quince fruit (*Cydonia oblonga* Mill.)." *Agricultural and Biological Chemistry* 47(11):2495–2502.

Umano, K., Shoji, A., Hagi, Y. and Shibamoto, T. 1986. "Volatile constituents of peel of quince fruit, *Cydonia oblonga* Miller." *Journal of Agricultural and Food Chemistry* 34(4):593–596.

Ünlüeroğlugil, Ö., Yüksel, H., Çalışkan Koç, G. and Dirim, S. 2018. "Freeze dried quince (*Cydonia oblonga*) puree with the addition of different amounts of maltodextrin: Physical and powder properties." In *IDS 2018. 21st International Drying Symposium Proceedings* (pp. 1293–1300). Editorial Universitat Politècnica de València.

Vaez, H., Hamidi, S. and Arami, S. 2014. "Potential of *Cydonia oblonga* leaves in cardiovascular disease." *Hypothesis* 12(1):1–10.

Winterhalter, P. and Schreier, P. 1988. "Free and bound C13 norisoprenoids in quince (*Cydonia oblonga*, Mill.) fruit." *Journal of Agricultural and Food Chemistry* 36(6):1251–1256.

Wojdyło, A., Oszmiański, J., and Bielicki, P. 2013a. "Polyphenolic composition, antioxidant activity, and polyphenol oxidase (PPO) activity of quince (*Cydonia oblonga* Miller) varieties." *Journal of Agricultural and Food Chemistry* 61(11):2762–2772. https://doi.org/10.1021/jf304969b

Wojdyło, A., Teleszko, M. and Oszmiański, J. 2014. "Antioxidant property and storage stability of quince juice phenolic compounds." *Food Chemistry* 152:261–270.

Yıkmış, S., Aksu, H., Çöl, B.G. and Alpaslan, M. 2019. "Thermosonication processing of quince (*Cydonia oblonga*) juice: Effects on total phenolics, ascorbic acid, antioxidant capacity, color and sensory properties." *Ciência e Agrotecnologia* 43.

Yousefi, M., Hossein Goli, S.A. and Kadivar, M. 2018. "Physicochemical and nutritional stability of optimized low-calorie quince (*Cydonia oblonga*) jam containing stevioside during storage." *Current Nutrition & Food Science* 14(1):79–87.

# 13 The Role of Grapes in Nutraceuticals and Functional Foods

*Santwana Palai*

## CONTENTS

## 13.1 INTRODUCTION

The global demand for health-promoting foods is rising as more people become aware of the relationship between diet and healthiness. Grapes (*Vitis vinifera* L.) have been used in health care and disease treatment for over 6,000 years due to their numerous uses in food and nutrition, health and medicinal value along with high economic implications (Martin et al. 2020). The grape originated in the Mediterranean region and spread to entire temperate regions. Approximately 85% of grapes are utilised to make wine, with the majority produced in Argentina, South Africa, Spain, California, Chile, and France. Grapes can be taken as raw or juice or fermented into wine. Grapes are used in various ways, like direct consumption of table grapes, wine production through wine grapes, and stored as dried grapes (raisins). Grape processing during wine production generates a large amount of waste, such as grape seeds, grape pomace, wine lees, etc. These wastes contain grape phytochemical compounds possessing nutritional benefits for better well-being (Sadh et al. 2018).

Grape phytochemicals found in grape seed extracts help to maintain a healthy state by modulating inflammation and reducing the expression of inflammation-related factors. Phytochemicals improve dysbiosis (gut microbiota complicated through metabolic syndrome) and regulate inflammatory diseases caused by TNF-α creation. After absorption, flavonoids travel in glucuronide form through

DOI: 10.1201/9781003259213-13

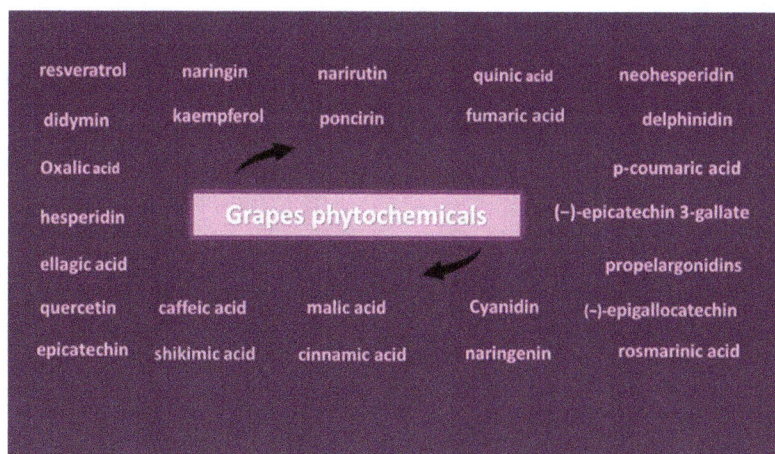

| | | | | |
|---|---|---|---|---|
| resveratrol | naringin | narirutin | quinic acid | neohesperidin |
| didymin | kaempferol | poncirin | fumaric acid | delphinidin |
| Oxalic acid | | | | p-coumaric acid |
| hesperidin | **Grapes phytochemicals** | | | (–)-epicatechin 3-gallate |
| ellagic acid | | | | propelargonidins |
| quercetin | caffeic acid | malic acid | Cyanidin | (–)-epigallocatechin |
| epicatechin | shikimic acid | cinnamic acid | naringenin | rosmarinic acid |

**Figure 13.1**   Various types of phytochemicals present in grapes.

the bloodstream to inflammatory sites, like the liver and lungs, where they are activated (Santa et al. 2019).

These phytochemicals found in grapes like phenolic acids, stilbenes, flavanols, flavanones, flavones, flavan-3-ols, isoflavonoids, anthocyanins, and proanthocyanidins increase antioxidant activity. Grapes and their products consist mainly of p-coumaric acid, ellagic acid, caffeic acid, quercetin like phenolic compounds, resveratrol like stilbenes, quercetin, kaempferol, myricetin, naringin, naringenin, hesperidin like flavonoids, cyanidin, peonidin, delphinidin, petunidin like anthocyanidins and propelargonidins, prodelphinidins, and procyanidins like proanthocyanidins or grape tannins (Figure 13.1 and Table 13.1).

## 13.2  VARIOUS TYPES OF NUTRACEUTICALS IN GRAPES

Grape pomace has significant amounts of anthocyanins. The skin and seeds of various grape cultivars contain phytochemicals like carotenoids, terpenoids, and flavonoids (Ðilas et al. 2009). Grape phytochemicals are primarily composed of flavonoids, which include flavon-3-ols (quercetin kaempferol, and myricetin), flavonoid glycosides (narirutin, naringin, naringenin, hesperidin, neohesperidin), flavan-3-ols (catechins) and flavones (luteolin and apigenin), anthocyanins (cyanidin), tannins and proanthocyanidins (procyanidins), and stilbenes (resveratrol) (De Ancos et al. 2015), which extend various health benefits (Table 13.2). Grape phenolics like catechins, anthocyanins, tannins, and flavonols have high antioxidant activity and aid in preventing oxidative damage. (Peña-Neira 2017). Grape phenolic compounds have anti-inflammatory properties due to the presence of flavonols, flavanols, stilbenes (resveratrol), and procyanidins (oligomeric flavonoids). Grape flavonoids are also antiallergic and anti-inflammatory. Red wine and red grapes possess flavonoids having antioxidant effects, which can lower heart cancer and neurodegenerative disease risk (Prakash et al. 2012). Wine contains quercetin and other polyphenols that protect low-density lipoproteins from oxidation. Resveratrol is an antioxidant, antimutagen, and inducer of phase II drug-metabolising enzymes. It also facilitated anti-inflammatory properties and reserved hydroperoxidase and cyclooxygenase roles. Grape antioxidants reduce the hazard of various

## Table 13.1: Structure and Effects of Phytochemicals Present in Grapes

| Sl. No. | Grape Phytochemicals | Common Name | Structure | Effect | Reference |
|---|---|---|---|---|---|
| 1 | p-Coumaric acid | 4-Hydroxycinnamic acid | | Anticancer, antiulcer, antiplatelet, anti-inflammatory, antioxidant, antidiabetic activities | Ilavenil et al. (2016) |
| 2 | Caffeic acid | 3,4-Dihydroxy cinnamic acid | | Anti-inflammatory, antioxidant, anti-carcinogenic activity | Espíndola et al. (2019) |
| 3 | Ferulic acid | 4-Hydroxy-3-methoxycinnamic acid | | Anti-inflammatory, anticancer, antimicrobial, antioxidant properties | Zduńska et al. (2018) |
| 4 | Ellagic acid | – | | Anti-carcinogenic, antioxidant, neuroprotective, antiproliferative activity | Mirsane (2017) |

(Continued)

**Table 13.1: Structure and Effects of Phytochemicals Present in Grapes (Continued)**

| Sl. No. | Grape Phytochemicals | Common Name | Structure | Effect | Reference |
|---|---|---|---|---|---|
| 5 | Sinapic acid | 3,5-Dimethoxy-4-hydroxycinnamic acid | | Antiglycaemic, antimutagenic, antioxidant, anticancer, neuroprotective, antibacterial activities | Chen (2016) |
| 6 | Cinnamic acid | — | | Antioxidant, anticancer, anti-inflammatory activities | Adisakwattana (2017) |
| 7 | Gallic acid | 3,4,5-Trihydroxybenzoic acid | | Antiulcer, anticancer, antibacterial, antifungal, antiviral, anticholesterol activities | Badhani et al. (2015) |
| 8 | Vannilic acid | 4-Hydroxy-3-methoxybenzoic acid | | Antibacterial, anti-inflammatory, antimicrobial, analgesic, chemopreventive effects | Calixto-Campos et al. (2015) |
| 9 | Syringic acid | — | | Antioxidant, anti-inflammatory, endothelium-dependent vasodilation, antiendotoxic, antimicrobial activities | Huang et al. (2021) |

(Continued)

**Table 13.1: Structure and Effects of Phytochemicals Present in Grapes (Continued)**

| Sl. No. | Grape Phytochemicals | Common Name | Structure | Effect | Reference |
|---------|---------------------|-------------|-----------|--------|-----------|
| 10 | Protocatechic acid | – | | Anticancer, analgesic, antidiabetic, antiaging, antioxidant, antiviral, antibacterial, antiulcer, antiatherosclerotic, antifibrotic, anti-inflammatory, hepatoprotective, cardioprotective, neuroprotective, and nephroprotective | Kakkar and Bais (2014) |
| 11 | Resveratrol | 3,4′,5-Trans-trihydroxystilbene, 3,5,4′-cis-trihydroxystilbene, 3,5,4′-trihydroxy-trans-stilbene | | Phytoestrogenic cardioprotective, anti-inflammatory, anti-carcinogenic, vasorelaxant, neuroprotective effects | Salehi et al. (2018) |
| 12 | Piceid | Resveratrol 3-β-mono-D-glucoside | | Antioxidant, antiatherosclerotic, anti-inflammatory, cardioprotective effects | Romero-Pérez et al. (1999) |
| 13 | Quercetin | 3,3′,4′,5,7-Pentahydroxyflavone | | Antihypercholesterolemic anti-inflammatory, anti-obesity, vasodilator, antihypertensive, antiatherosclerotic activities | David et al. (2016) |

*(Continued)*

**Table 13.1: Structure and Effects of Phytochemicals Present in Grapes (Continued)**

| Sl. No. | Grape Phytochemicals | Common Name | Structure | Effect | Reference |
|---|---|---|---|---|---|
| 14 | Kaempferol | 3,4′,5,7-Tetrahydroxyflavone | | Cardioprotective, anti-inflammatory, antibacterial, antiviral, anticoagulant antiplatelet, antitumour, antifungal, anti-neuroinflammatory activity | Silva dos Santos et al. (2021) |
| 15 | Myricetin | 3,5,7,3′,4′,5′-Hexahydroxyflavone | | Antioxidant, antiviral, antidiabetic, anticancer, antibacterial, antiamyloidogenic, anti-inflammatory effects | Park et al. (2016) |
| 16 | Didymin | Isosakuranetin 7-O-rutinoside | | Antitumour, antioxidative stress, anti-inflammatory, antinociceptive, hepatic cytoprotective, neuroprotective, anxiolytic-like effects | Yao et al. (2018) |

*(Continued)*

**Table 13.1: Structure and Effects of Phytochemicals Present in Grapes (Continued)**

| Sl. No. | Grape Phytochemicals | Common Name | Structure | Effect | Reference |
|---|---|---|---|---|---|
| 17 | Narirutin | – | | Anti-inflammatory, angiogenic functions in vascular disease, antioxidant, anti-inflammatory; improve antitubercular potency | Singh et al. (2020) |
| 18 | Naringin | – | | Antihepatitis C virus production, anticancer, antioxidant, cardiovascular protective effects | Mandial et al. (2018) |
| 19 | Naringinen | – | | Antiatherogenic, antioxidant, anti-inflammatory effects, carbohydrate metabolism promoter, immunomodulator | Salehi, et al. (2019) |

(Continued)

**Table 13.1: Structure and Effects of Phytochemicals Present in Grapes (Continued)**

| Sl. No. | Grape Phytochemicals | Common Name | Structure | Effect | Reference |
|---|---|---|---|---|---|
| 20 | Hesperidin | – | | Cardioprotective, antihypertensive, antidiabetic, antihyperlipidemic activities | Ahmadi and Shadboorestan (2016) |
| 21 | Neohesperidin | – | | Antioxidative, anti-inflammatory, antiapoptosis effects | Shi et al. (2015) |
| 22 | Poncirin | Isosakuranetin-7-neohesperidoside | | Antiosteoporotic, antitumour, anti-inflammatory, anticolitic effect | Afridi et al. (2019) |

(Continued)

**Table 13.1: Structure and Effects of Phytochemicals Present in Grapes (Continued)**

| Sl. No. | Grape Phytochemicals | Common Name | Structure | Effect | Reference |
|---|---|---|---|---|---|
| 23 | Apigenin | 4′,5,7-Trihydroxyflavone | | Antioxidant, anti-inflammatory, blood pressure modulator, antibacterial, antiviral properties | Yan et al. (2017) |
| 24 | Chrysin | 5,7-Chrysin, 5,7-Dihydroxyflavone | | Neuroprotective, hepatoprotective, renoprotective, cardioprotective, antiviral, anticancer, antidiabetic, gastrointestinal, respiratory, reproductive, ocular, and skin protective effects | Talebi et al. (2021) |
| 25 | Luteolin | 3′,4′,5,7-Tetrahydroxyflavone | | Anti-inflammation, antiallergy, anticancer, antioxidant or pro-oxidant-like effects | Lin et al. (2008) |

*(Continued)*

**Table 13.1: Structure and Effects of Phytochemicals Present in Grapes (Continued)**

| Sl. No. | Grape Phytochemicals | Common Name | Structure | Effect | Reference |
|---------|----------------------|-------------|-----------|--------|-----------|
| 26 | Catechin | 3,3′,4′,5,7-Pentahydroxyflavan | | Anticancer, anti-infectious, anti-obesity, antidiabetic, hepatoprotective, neuroprotective, cardioprotective effect | Isemura (2019) |
| 27 | Gallocatechin | – | | Antioxidant, antibacterial, antiallergic, anti-inflammatory activities | Afzal et al. (2015) |
| 28 | Epigallocatechin | Flavan-3,3′,4′,5,5′,7-hexol | | Anti-obesity, antidiabetic, antibacterial, antiatherosclerotic, anticancer, antiviral effects | Wu et al. (2009) |

*(Continued)*

**Table 13.1: Structure and Effects of Phytochemicals Present in Grapes (Continued)**

| Sl. No. | Grape Phytochemicals | Common Name | Structure | Effect | Reference |
|---|---|---|---|---|---|
| 29 | Epicatechin 3-o-gallate | – | | Radical scavenging, anti-carcinogenic, antiapoptotic, antioxidant, metal chelating, good radical scavenging, metal chelation, neurorescue neuroprotective action | Singh et al. (2015) |
| 30 | Epicatechin | – | | Antioxidant, antiangiogenic, cytotoxicity properties | Abdulkhaleq et al. (2017) |
| 31 | Genistein | – | | Anti-inflammatory activities, antioxidant, neuroprotective, cytotoxic, anticancer, antidiabetic, lipid metabolism, depression, and bone and cardiovascular diseases | Sharifi-Rad et al. (2021) |
| 32 | Diadazein | – | | Antidiabetic, anticancerous, neuroprotective, cardioprotective, skin and bone-protective effects | Sun et al. (2016) |

*(Continued)*

## Table 13.1: Structure and Effects of Phytochemicals Present in Grapes (*Continued*)

| Sl. No. | Grape Phytochemicals | Common Name | Structure | Effect | Reference |
|---------|----------------------|-------------|-----------|--------|-----------|
| 33 | Cyanidin | – | | Antidiabetic, antitoxicity, anti-inflammatory, anticancer, neuroprotective, cardioprotective capacities | Liang et al. (2021) |
| 34 | Peonidin | – | | Anti-obesity, anticancer, anti-inflammatory, neuroprotective, antidiabetic, cardioprotective disease | Li et al. (2017) |
| 35 | Delphinidin | – | | Antioxidant, anti-inflammatory, antimutagenesis, antiangiogenic | Shrestha et al. (2012) |

(*Continued*)

**Table 13.1: Structure and Effects of Phytochemicals Present in Grapes (*Continued*)**

| Sl. No. | Grape Phytochemicals | Common Name | Structure | Effect | Reference |
|---|---|---|---|---|---|
| 36 | Petunidin | – | | Anti-osteoclastogenic, antioxidative, anti-inflammatory | Nagaoka et al. (2019) |
| 37 | Malvidin | – | | Antioxidant capacity, free radical scavenging, antihypertensive activity | Huang et al. (2016) |
| 38 | Procyanidins | – | | Antioxidant, anticancer, anti-inflammatory, immunosuppressive antivirus activity | Dasiman et al. (2022) |

(*Continued*)

## Table 13.1: Structure and Effects of Phytochemicals Present in Grapes (Continued)

| Sl. No. | Grape Phytochemicals | Common Name | Structure | Effect | Reference |
|---|---|---|---|---|---|
| 39 | Propelargonidins | 3,5,7,4′-tetrahydroxylation | | Antigenotoxic, antioxidative, anticancer, anti-inflammatory, antiproliferative agents | Falleh et al. (2011) |
| 40 | Prodelphinidins | – | | Antiviral, antitumour, anti-inflammatory effects | Zuckerkandl and Pauling (1965) |

**Table 13.2: Role of Phytochemicals of Grapes as Nutraceuticals and Functional Foods**

| Sl. No. | Phytochemicals | Source | Group | Disease | Mechanism of Action/Important Roles | Reference |
|---|---|---|---|---|---|---|
| 1 | p-Coumaric acid, caffeic acid, ellagic acid, sinapic acid, cinnamic acid, ferulic acid | Grape skins, pulp, flesh of fruit | Hydroxy-cinnamic acid (phenolic acid) | Cardiovascular diseases, cancer, inflammation, ageing, microbial infections | • Lipid peroxidation<br>• Hydroperoxides inhibition<br>• Antimicrobial activity<br>• More efficiently causes haemolysis of the erythrocyte's membrane | Nile et al. (2013) |
| 2 | Gallic acid, vanillic acid, syringic acid, protocatechuic acid | Grape skins, pulp, flesh of fruit | Hydroxy-benzoic acid (phenolic acid) | | | Gómez-Mejía et al. (2021) |
| 3 | Resveratrol and piceid | Pulp of grapes, grape skin | Stilbenes | Cardiovascular diseases, oxidative stress, viral diseases, inflammation, liver diseases, neurodegenerative diseases | • Reduce atherosclerosis, ischemic heart disease risk<br>• Lengthen life by inducing longevity genes, lowering morbidity, and mortality risk after cardiovascular complications | Bertelli and Das (2009) |
| 4 | Quercetin, kaempferol, myricetin, didymin | Skins, seeds | Flavonols (flavanoids) | Cancer, cardiovascular, type 2 diabetes mellitus, and neurodegenerative diseases | Modulation of iNOS, COX-2, and CRP leads to anti-inflammatory effects through mechanisms involving NF-kappaB activation and the subsequent up-regulation of pro-inflammatory genes | García-Mediavilla et al. (2007) |
| 5 | Narirutin, naringin, naringenin, hesperidin, neohesperidin, poncirin | Grape skins, seeds, and stems of the fruit | Flavanones (flavanoids) | Type 2 diabetes mellitus, allergy, ulcer, cancer, cardiovascular, metabolic syndrome, obesity, neurodegenerative diseases | CPT-1, AMPK- and PPARα- mediated fat utilisation and mitochondria preservation, inhibition of the TNF-α-facilitated inflammatory course and tissue injury in the liver and blood vessels | Fantini et al. (2015) |

*(Continued)*

**Table 13.2: Role of Phytochemicals of Grapes as Nutraceuticals and Functional Foods (Continued)**

| Sl. No. | Phytochemicals | Source | Group | Disease | Mechanism of Action/Important Roles | Reference |
|---|---|---|---|---|---|---|
| 6 | Apigenin, chrysin, luteolin | Grape skin, seed oil | Flavones (flavanoids) | Oxidative stress-related conditions, cancer, neurodegenerative diseases, age-related inflammation | Inhibit oxidative stress by up-regulating GCLM, HO-1, and GCLC, gene transcription via ERK2/Nrf2/ARE signalling pathways, directly inhibiting the release of inflammatory molecules in the brain | Huang et al. (2013) |
| 7 | Catechin, epicatechin 3-O-gallate, epicatechin, gallocatechin, epigallocatechin | Grape seeds | Flavan-3-ols | Hepatic fibrosis, UV-injury, osteoporosis, photoaging of the skin, cancer, cardiovascular disorders | Inhibiting NF-B to reverse the peritoneal fibrosis process, increasing nitric oxide production, and decreasing endothelin-1, an oxidative stress marker | Chu et al. (2017) |
| 8 | Genistein, diadazein | Grape seed | Isoflavonoids | Sex hormone-dependent cancer, cardiovascular diseases | Reduces biological activity and oestrogen levels by stimulating the production of plasma sex hormone-binding globulin, weak estrogenic properties, and lower plasma total and LDL cholesterol | Poschner et al. (2017); Pan et al. (2001) |
| 9 | Cyanidin, peonidin, delphinidin, petunidin, and malvidin | Grape skin, wine | Anthocyanidins | Aging, memory loss, cancer, diabetes, obesity, cardiovascular disorders, neurodegenerative diseases | Inhibit the mitogen-activated protein kinase signalling cascade by suppressing the activation of nuclear factor kappa B | Salehi et al. (2020); Zhang et al. (2019) |
| 10 | Procyanidins, propelargonidins, prodelphinidins procyanidins, propelargonidins | Grape seeds | Proanthocyanidins (grape tannins) | Neurodegenerative diseases, cancer, eye affections, cardiovascular diseases, osteoarthritis | Reduce the production of pro-inflammatory mediators like TNF-α and reactive oxygen species like iNOS activity antagonising the NF-κB signalling pathway, potent inhibitors of kinases including MLCK | Unusan (2020) |

315

age-related chronic diseases like heart disease, cataracts, dementia, cancer, etc. Traditionally, red grape leaves treated diarrhoea, uterine haemorrhage, and heavy menstrual bleeding. Resveratrol and ellagic acid lower the risk of coronary heart disorders. Proanthocyanidins present in the grape seed can help prevent and treat vascular complications in diabetics (Zhang et al. 2015).

Grape phytochemical contents (flavonoid, phenolic, saponin, proanthocyanidin) are completely related to antioxidant activities, which are measured using various methods (CUPRAC, FRAP, DPPH, and ABTS radical scavenging). Red grape seeds had the highest polyphenol content as well as activity, with the highest levels of epicatechin, myricetin, catechin, caffeic acid, gallic acid, ferulic acid, etc. Being high in phytochemicals, grape extracts can be established as a nutraceutical and functional foods (Wongnarat and Srihanam 2017).

Grape phenolics are antibacterial and antiviral in nature. Grape phytochemicals like salicylic acid, gallic acid, hydroxybenzoic acid, and protocatechuic acid are antibacterial in nature. Some viruses have been shown to be resistant to chlorogenic acid and epicatechin. Phenolic compounds with anticancer effects aid in the prevention of cancers of the colon, lung, liver, oesophagus, skin, and mammary gland. Resveratrol can prevent cancer by preventing DNA damage, improving DNA repair, slowing tumour growth, slowing cell conversion to cancerous, etc. (Chen et al. 2006).

Because of their phytochemical compositions and antioxidant activities, grapes can be considered a valuable source of nutraceutical and functional foods. Grapes and their derivatives can be used as raw materials or additives in various foods to impart beneficial properties. Grape skins and seeds can make novel health food products known as functional foods because grape phytochemicals help to prevent inflammatory diseases such as intestine-related inflammatory diseases. Grapes and grape derivatives can improve the functional qualities of numerous foods in developing novel nutraceutical and functional foods (Fernández-Marín et al. 2017). Grape phytochemicals have bioaccessibility and bioavailability with potentially beneficial health effects (Table 13.2). Grape constituents' biological activities account for the global importance of grape production as well as the potential of grape products as nutraceuticals in complementary and alternative medicine. This article presents recent research on isolated functional ingredients of grapes and its derivatives that can be used for the progress of novel as a nutraceutical and functional foods.

## 13.3 MOST RECENT RESEARCH RELATED TO THE BIOACTIVE COMPOUNDS PRESENT IN THE GRAPES
### 13.3.1 Antioxidant Effects

Polyphenols chelate metal ions and scavenge radicals like quercetin chelates iron ions. Both quercetin and rutin have the ability to complex metals between aglycones and glycosides are the chelators of transition metals. Flavonoids with 4-oxo, 5-OH, and 3,4-catechol configurations substantially prevent Fenton-induced oxidation. Between, or chelating complexes containing divalent cations can form between the 3- and 4-OH groups or 5-OH and 4-oxo groups. Polyhydroxylated flavonoids may be useful as Fenton reaction inhibitors in vivo because of their metal-chelating characteristics and radical scavenging capability. Owing to their metabolism, these polyphenols are generally more efficient regulators of metal-induced oxidation than non-metal-induced oxidation. (Heim et al. 2002).

Red grape polyphenols, resveratrol inhibit COX, peroxisome proliferator-activated receptor-, and endothelial NOS, which is evident through in vivo and in vitro investigations with mouse and rat macrophages (Mohar and Malik 2012). Resveratrol analogues trigger antioxidant systems by inhibiting the respiratory chain in mitochondria, adenosine triphosphatase, and xanthine oxidase (Huang et al. 2008).

Two other flavonoids found in red grapes, like EGCG and quercetin, inhibit the release of growth factors, chemokines, adhesion molecules, and proinflammatory cytokines by inactivating nuclear factor kappa-light-chain-enhancer of activated B cells in epithelial cells and monocytes. The use of quercetin partly sorted out the molecular pathways involved in the deactivation of NF-B nuclear translocation. This flavonoid blocked the nuclear translocation of NF-B subunits p50 and p65 and the phosphorylation of IB kinase (IB) proteins in macrophages (Magrone et al. 2019).

### 13.3.2 Antiatherosclerotic Effects

The antiatherosclerotic effects of grape products are due to their antioxidant and antiplatelet qualities. Grape seed and skin contain many phenolic complexes. The effects of grape seed and skin fractions on low-density lipoprotein oxidation in vitro, platelet aggregation, and comparative binding of phenolics to low-density lipoprotein were investigated to sort the proportional contributions of phenolic classes of grape products. Platelet aggregation was dramatically increased in the presence of oligosaccharides, low molecular weight PGPFs anthocyanins, hydroxycinnamic acids, and flavonols. The binding of low-density lipoprotein, platelet aggregation, and low-density lipoprotein oxidation were efficiently inhibited, demonstrating the major role of polymeric PGPFs in grape products. Phenolics may sometimes lower the grape products' net biological efficacy and can have negative impacts on cardiovascular disease risk factors (Shanmuganayagam et al. 2012).

### 13.3.3 Anti-Inflammatory Effects

Chronic inflammation causes chronic diseases like arthritis, diabetes, autoimmune diseases, cancer, neurological disorders, cardiovascular diseases, autoimmune diseases, neurological disorders, Alzheimer's, and pulmonary diseases. Grape polyphenols can reduce chronic inflammation via modulating inflammatory pathways or lowering reactive oxygen species (ROS) levels. Grape flavonoids and proanthocyanidins are natural molecules that can mark many pathways to alleviate chronic inflammation, making them more effective than available synthetic anti-inflammatory drugs with a single target (Zhang et al. 2015).

In comparison with the commercial non-steroidal anti-inflammatory medicine (like indomethacin), hydroxycinnamic acid derivatives, anthocyanins, proanthocyanidins, and flavonoids demonstrated stronger anti-inflammatory efficacy. Proanthocyanidins in grape seeds have also been shown to have potent anti-inflammatory properties since they avert lipid peroxidation, hunt free radicals, and limit pro-inflammatory cytokines generation (Farzaei et al. 2015).

Procyanindin extract is a combination of polyphenols derived from grape seed, primarily procyanidins, with anti-inflammatory properties. Procyanidin extract inhibits NO and PGE2 generation, suppresses iNOS expression, and inhibits NFkB translocation in activated macrophages, all influencing the inflammatory response. Thus, grape seed procyanidins have an immunomodulatory activity, and hence a potential health benefit in inflammatory diseases characterised by an excess of NO and $PGE_2$ (Terra et al. 2007).

Grape seed extract can generate novel anti-inflammatory medications. An extract of grape seed suppressed LPS-induced RAW264.7 macrophages Grape seed extract improves the anti-inflammatory properties of LPS-activated mice macrophage RAW264.7 cells. The grape seed extract contains flavan-3-ols (epicatechin, epigallocatechin gallate, catechin, procyanidin b1, b2, b4), flavonols (myricitrin, kaempferol, and quercetin), and phenolic acid (gallic acid).

In RAW264.7 cells, grape seed extract reduced cytokine expression. In the inflammatory response, grape seed extract reduced the MAPK pathway, and NF-B stimulation. In LPS-stimulated RAW 264.7 cells, grape seed extract dramatically reduced gene expression and protein production of interleukin-6, tumour necrosis factor-$\alpha$, the inducible isoform of nitric oxide synthase and nitric oxide. The downregulation of inflammatory cascade proteins like mitogen-activated protein kinase and nuclear factor kappa B resulted in decreased inflammation. Thus, grape seed extract is potent in generating novel anti-inflammatory medications. Still, more research is needed to extract its precise components to fight inflammation (Harbeoui et al. 2019).

The flavonols like myricetin, quercetin, and kaempferol can inhibit pro-inflammatory enzymes like cyclooxygenase-2, inducible NO synthase, lipoxygenase, NF-B, and activating protein-1. Activation of phase II antioxidant detoxifying enzymes like mitogen-activated protein kinase, nuclear factor-erythroid 2- related factor, and protein kinase C are the proposed molecular mechanisms for flavonoids. Quercetin and kaempferol inhibit cyclooxygenase-2 in macrophages of rat peritoneum. Catechin moderately prevents cyclooxygenase-2. Flavonols like quercetin, morin, myricetin, and kaemferol are more effective at inhibiting lipoxygenase than flavones (Serafini et al. 2010).

### 13.3.4 Immunomodulatory Effects
The immunological function of red wine polyphenols of Negroamaro, an Italian red wine, was demonstrated through in vitro potential for promoting the pro-inflammatory and anti-inflammatory cytokines and nitric oxide release for maintaining the host's immune homeostasis. These Negromaro polyphenols can activate extracellular regulated kinase and p38 kinase while inhibiting lipoxygenase more than flavones. The NF-kappa B pathway is activated over time by increasing the production of the I-kappa B-alpha phosphorylated form. These processes could be crucial molecular events in the pro-inflammatory cascade and atherogenesis inhibition. Thus, moderate red wine consumption is defending the host in preventing many age-related disorders from occurring due to its immunomodulating capabilities (Magrone and Jirillo 2010).

### 13.3.5 Antiplatelet Effects
Although purple grape juice and red wine include polymeric flavonoids having antioxidant characteristics that can protect against cardiovascular events, their medical usage has been limited due to their alcohol and sugar concentrations. Increased inflammation and thrombosis are also linked to acute cardiac events. When seeds and skins were combined, platelet aggregation was inhibited significantly, NO production was increased, and superoxide production was reduced. The inflammatory mediator soluble CD40 ligand release was immediately reduced after incubating with seed or skin extracts. Pharmacologically relevant concentrations of purple grape skins and seed extracts can decrease platelet activity and platelet-dependent inflammatory reactions. These findings imply that purple grape-derived flavonoids have antithrombotic and anti-inflammatory actions that are dependent on platelets (Vitseva et al. 2005).

Grape products, which are high in polyphenolics, help prevent platelet aggregation, increasing the risk of coronary artery disease. Mixing grape seed and grape skin extracts, which are both important sources of grape polyphenolics that are proven to reduce platelet aggregation independently, would increase their antiplatelet effects. Thus, grape seed and skin components have a stronger antiplatelet effect when combined prior to consumption, as in red wine, grape juice, or a commercial product containing both grape seed and skin extracts (Shanmuganayagam et al. 2002).

The synthesis of nitric oxide by platelets and endothelial cells is boosted by red wine and purple grape juice. Purple grape juice and red wine possess flavonoids which suppress atherosclerosis. The benefits of drinking purple grape juice or red wine when consumed daily need years to show their full effect on heart health. Owing to the beneficial antiplatelet and antioxidant effects of purple grape juice and red wine that improve endothelial function, the American Heart Association recommends moderate consumption of purple grape juice or red wine daily with vegetables and fruit servings for diminishing cardiovascular disease risk (Folts 2002).

### 13.3.6 Antimicrobial Effects

The principal polyphenols and the total polyphenolic content of grape (*Vitis vinifera*) berries extracts, and their vinification by-products were assessed and quantified. The grape seed extracts have substantial levels of flavan-3-ols and their derivatives, whereas grape pomace and grape stem extracts have large amounts of phenolic acids, stilbenes, and flavonoids. The grape seed and stem extracts of the red cultivar Mandilaria were found to have the most potent in vitro antilisterial activity. The plate count methodology and an automated technique with conductance measurements and a conventional dilution method were successfully used to assess the antimicrobial effects with the MIC estimation. The minimum inhibitory concentrations (MICs) utilising Malthus equipment for seeds and stems indicated these extracts as a cheap source of potent natural antilisterial combinations. These extracts can be incorporated or combined into food systems to the prevention of *Listeria monocytogenes* growth (Anastasiadi et al. 2009).

### 13.3.7 Antiallergic Effects

Quercetin is a grape polyphenol with immunomodulatory and bronchodilatory effects. It has the potential to develop as an antiasthmatic medication (Moon et al. 2008). After allergen exposure, quercetin reduces allergen-induced development of airway hyperresponsiveness, goblet cell metaplasia, lung eosinophilia, TH2 responses in the lung, etc. The treatment with quercetin reduced the production of inflammatory cytokines, tracheal ring relaxation, bronchoalveolar lavage fluid cells, and eosinophil peroxidase in the lungs. It can also reduce the synthesis of periostin and periostin-induced eosinophil chemoattractants, improving the clinical condition of allergic rhinitis. Thus, it can be an excellent supplement for the therapy and prophylaxis of allergic illnesses like allergic asthma, atopic dermatitis, and allergic rhinitis (Jafarinia et al. 2020).

Kaempferol, isorhamnetin, and quercetin found in *Elaeagnus pungens* leaf can effectively treat chronic bronchitis and asthma. They act on the leukocyte, eosinophil and neutrophil recruitment, and cytokine concentrations in bronchoalveolar lavage fluid, showing anti-inflammatory and antitussive activities. It decreases the gravest diseases of asthma and chronic bronchitis through bronchial epithelial cell activation, collagen, and mucus synthesis, and airway hyperactivity (Zhu et al. 2018; Mlcek et al. 2016).

### 13.3.8 Antiulcer Effects

Procyanidins present found in grape seeds have antioxidative properties showing beneficial biological effects (Busserolles et al. 2006). Rats were used to test the antiulcer properties of grape seed extracts and procyanidins. The stomach protective effect of various procyanidins augmented with a rise in catechin unit's polymerisation. Longer oligomers than tetramers possess significant protective effects against injury in stomach mucosa (Wang et al. 2007).

Grape seed extracts resulted in the highest reductions in gastric malondialdehyde. The antiulcer activity mechanism shields the stomach surface from radical harm by radical scavenging. The defence action of procyanidins is through covering the stomach surface owing to their strong ability to bind protein (Saito et al. 1998).

The capacity of grape seed extracts to reduce lipid peroxidation in the stomach mucosa may then be linked to its gastroprotective properties on ethanol- and aspirin-induced stomach ulcers in rats (Cuevas et al. 2011).

### 13.3.9 Antimutagenesis Effects

Both organic and conventional grapevine leaf extracts possess antigenotoxic, antimutagenic, and antioxidant effects, as well as significant in vitro biological effects. The antigenotoxic activity was determined using the alkaline comet assay and the enzymes endonuclease III and formamidopyrimidine DNA glycosylase. The antimutagenic property was evaluated using micronucleus formation. The antioxidant activities were determined using the 2',7'-dichlorodihydrofluorescein diacetate assay, as well as the radical scavenging, superoxide dismutase, and catalase assays. The ascorbic acid levels and phenolic content of both extracts were also determined. Organic leaf extract clearly decreased intracellular reactive oxygen species levels in V79 cells and demonstrated better ability for DPPH scavenging as well as greater SOD and CAT activities than conventional leaf extract. This could be because organic leaf extract has higher phenolic and ascorbic acid concentrations, resulting in significant in vitro biological effects (Trindade et al. 2016).

Phytochemicals like ellagic acid have grown in popularity due to its powerful anti-carcinogenic, antimutagenic, and hepatoprotective properties. It works either as an antioxidant to counteract the negative effects of oxidative stress directly or indirectly by triggering antioxidant enzyme systems of cells (Vattem and Shetty 2005).

## 13.4 HEALTH ELEMENTS OF GRAPES' BIOACTIVE COMPOUNDS AS A TREATMENT FOR VARIOUS CHRONIC DISORDERS

Dietary polyphenols have favourable impacts on human health, like prevention and/or reduction of cardiovascular, inflammatory, neurodegenerative, and neoplastic illnesses. Flavonols, including kaemferol, quercetin, morin, and myricetin, are proven to be more effective grape phytochemicals (Figure 13.2).

### 13.4.1 Grape Phytochemicals as Anticancer Agents

Cancer is a diverse sickness with uninhibited cell multiplication resulting in a disrupted cell cycle forming aberrant cells that metastasise to different body parts. The key characteristics of cancer cells are altered metabolism, angiogenesis promotion, disrupted cell cycles, chronic inflammation, resistance to immune response, metastasis formation, and frequent mutations (Aktipis et al. 2015).

Flavonoids are polyphenolic chemicals like anthocyanidins, flavanones, flavones, flavonols, flavanols, and isoflavonoids. Flavonoids show anticancer properties through their ability to control reactive oxygen species, scavenging enzyme effects, contributing to cell cycle arrest, induction of cell death, and reducing cancer cell propagation and intrusiveness. While dealing with ROS homeostasis, flavonoids operate as antioxidants and potential pro-oxidants

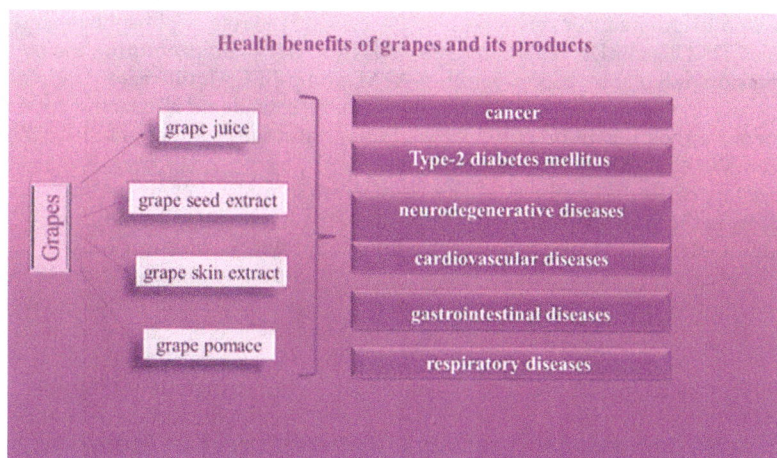

**Figure 13.2**   Health benefits of grapes and its products.

in cancerous cells, activating apoptotic paths (Dias et al. 2021). Owing to the existence of phenolic hydroxyl groups and their tendency to stabilise free radicals, flavonoids straightly scavenge ROS and chelate metal ions. Indirectly flavonoid activates antioxidant enzymes, suppresses pro-oxidant enzymes, and stimulates the production of antioxidant enzymes and phase II detoxifying enzymes. Flavonoid anticancer effects include both antioxidant and pro-oxidant activities (Kopustinskiene et al. 2020).

Grape-related antitumoural action spans a diverse set of biological pathways and cellular targets, ultimately resulting in cell growth stoppage and amplified apoptosis in various cancer cell lines, including colon, bladder, breast, lung, leukaemia, and prostate malignancies. These effects are most likely controlled at the molecular level by selectively altering the redox balance and exhibiting both antioxidant and pro-oxidant properties (Dinicola et al. 2014).

Grape seed extract-related anticancer effect is primarily based on the induction of reactive oxygen species and coordinated down- and up-regulation of numerous critical biochemical pathways like metalloproteinases, cytoskeleton proteins, NF-kB, PI3K/Akt, MAPK kinases, etc. In vitro and animal studies imply that grape seed extract is highly relevant as a source of possible novel anticancerous pharmacological compounds to be further researched clinically (Karami et al. 2018).

By stabilising or inducing p53, quercetin, an antioxidant flavonoid, can induce cell cycle arrest and death in hepatocellular carcinoma cells. Quercetin dramatically reduced HepG2 cell proliferation and decreased intracellular ROS levels, but not Huh7 cells. The action of quercetin on HepG2 cells reveals that quercetin's antiproliferative effect on hepatocellular carcinoma cells can be achieved via lowering intracellular ROS, which is independent of p53 expression (Jeon et al. 2019).

**Bladder cancer** is the most prevalent malignant bladder carcinoma among numerous plant-based diets with high kaempferol content. Kaempferol repressed the propagation of malignant bladder cells by triggering programmed cell death and S phase arrest and displayed substantial antioxidant activity on erythrocytes. Kaempferol has a substantial repressing effect on bladder cancer cells while being extremely safe on normal cells of the bladder. Kaempferol inhibited bladder cancer cell spread by preventing the role of phosphorylated Mcl-1, CDK4, CyclinD1, Bcl-xL, Bid, and AKT (p-AKT), and promoting the expression of Bax, Bid, p53, p38, p21, p-ATM, and p-BRCA1, ultimately causing apoptosis and S phase arrest. Kaempferol may be considered a bioactive food element for the prevention of oxidative damage and the treatment of bladder cancer (Wu et al. 2018).

**Prostate cancer** is an important cause of death in males. When medications that target the androgen receptor are utilised, recurrence of the condition is common. Natural chemicals have the ability to inhibit the progression and spread of certain cancer cells. Naringenin, a citrus-derived natural antioxidant flavonoid, reduced spread and passage while triggering programmed cell death and ROS generation in prostate cancer cells. Also, naringenin caused a loss of mitochondrial membrane potential as well as an increase in Bax and a drop in Bcl-2 proteins in PC3 cells but not in LNCaP cells. Naringenin inhibited the phosphorylation of P70S6K, P38ERK1/2, and S6 proteins in PC3 cells and ERK1/2, P53, P38, and JNK proteins in LNCaP cells. Thus, naringenin induced AKT phosphorylation in both PC3 and LNCaP cells. Thus, naringenin improved the efficacy of paclitaxel in suppressing the evolution of prostate cancer cell lines, recommending it as a viable chemotherapeutical agent for treating prostate cancer (Lim et al. 2017).

**Gall bladder cancer** remains unexplored due to the lack of an effective experimental model. Gall bladder cancer cell proliferation was significantly inhibited after one day of hesperidin exposure. Hesperidin administration resulted in enhanced ROS production and nuclear condensation. Hesperidin's promising efficacy is demonstrated through cellular apoptosis and mitochondrial membrane potential loss in primary cells derived from surgically excised malignant gall bladder tissues. Caspase-3 activation and G2/M cell cycle arrest were also enhanced in a dose-dependent manner. Thus, hesperidin may act as an anticancer agent in gall bladder cancer treatment (Pandey et al. 2019).

### 13.4.2 Grape Phytochemicals against Type 2 Diabetes Mellitus

Type 2 diabetes is distinguished through impaired glucose disposal in bordering tissues due to insulin resistance, overrun of glucose in the liver, abnormalities in pancreatic beta-cell function, and diminished beta-cell mass. Overweightness, lack of physical activity, and high glycaemic index of meal consumption are all key risk features for type 2 diabetes. Diabetes individuals are suggested to follow a low-glycaemic index diet since it improves diabetes symptoms. Grapes have a low glycaemic load and glycaemic index. Grapes include many polyphenols, stilbenes like resveratrol and flavanol like quercetin, catechins, and anthocyanins that can improve beta-cell activity, reduce hyperglycaemia, and protect against beta-cell loss. Thus, grapes and its products can be beneficial to type 2 diabetics owing to their low mean glycaemic index and glycaemic load (Zunino 2009).

Early intervention with grape seed proanthocyanidins can alleviate diabetic peripheral neuropathy in rats with type 2 diabetes mellitus. They also maintain normal morphology of nervous tissues while alleviating hyperglycaemia and reversing $Ca^{2+}$ overload in sciatic nerves by increasing $Ca^{2+}$-ATPase activity. Proanthocyanidins reduced low-density lipoprotein levels and increased nerve conduction velocity in Sprague-Dawley type 2 diabetic rats given low-dose streptozotocin and a high-carbohydrate/high-fat diet (Testa et al. 2016).

Epigallocatechin-gallate is an antioxidant flavanol. By lowering lipid peroxidation, it can protect cellular DNA from reactive oxygen species. Diabetes causes oxidative stress in the neurons of the nociceptive spinal cord. Antioxidant therapy with EGCG can prevent long-term effects such as oxidative stress damage and neuronal hyperactivity in the spinal cord, as well as improve behavioural symptoms of diabetic peripheral neuropathy (Raposo et al. 2015).

### 13.4.3 Grape Phytochemicals against Neurodegenerative Diseases

Alzheimer's disease is a lingering neurological illness with no effective therapy. The current medications offer symptomatic relief while postponing or stopping the development of age-related neurocognitive damage. Grape extracts show various biological properties that mitigate the neurological damage caused by Alzheimer's disease (Ozkur et al. 2020). Grape extracts are natural reservoirs of polyphenols with anti-inflammatory, antioxidative, neuromodulating, antiamyloidogenic, and antiacetylcholinesterase properties. Grape polyphenol like resveratrol and other components, particularly from grape leaves and seed extract, involves modulation of many Alzheimer's disease-related mechanisms, including neuroinflammation, oxidative stress, and Aβ-plaque formation. So, grape-extract-derived polyphenols are considered great candidates for combating Alzheimer's disease's multifactorial character (Fouad and Zaki Rizk 2019).

Grape polyphenols have an effect on the life span of C57BL/6 mice as well as behavioural and neuroinflammatory changes observed in a transgenic mouse model of Parkinson's disease having A53T-mutant human α-synuclein overexpression. Grape polyphenol concentrate had a considerable on the survived impact on mice and greatly increased the average life span in mice. the grape polyphenol diet improved memory reconsolidation and decreased memory extinction in a transgenic Parkinson's disease animal seen in a passive avoidance test. A decrease followed the behavioural effects of grape polyphenols therapy in α-synuclein buildup in the frontal cortex and a decrease in neuroinflammatory marker expression in the frontal cortex and hippocampus. Thus, a grape polyphenol-rich diet can be advised as gifted purposeful nutrition for aging and individuals having neurodegenerative illnesses (Tikhonova et al. 2020).

Resveratrol is a stilbene that is mostly found in the grapevine's skins. Stilbenes are low molecular weight phytoalexins created by plants as a defence strategy after an infective bout. Water-soluble resveratrol has the capability to cross the blood-brain barrier and have neuromodulatory actions in the brain, hence improving neurocognitive decline. As a result, resveratrol is a multi-target polyphenol exerting neuroprotective actions by increasing brain redox imbalance, interacting through signalling pathways associated with the neuronal role and its existence, inhibiting Aβ-oligomerization, suppressing cholinesterase action, and lastly, preventing neurodegeneration (Ahmed et al. 2017).

Grape seed extract with polyphenols can slow neurodegeneration in transgenic Alzheimer's disease mice by growing the bioavailability of the flavan-3-ol molecules in the brain, which stimulates antioxidant mechanisms. These extracts improved memory in both mid-age and older rats (Devi and Chamoli 2020). An improved understanding of polyphenols' neuroprotective effects and the various mechanisms of action acting in the nervous system can aid in the development of more effective drugs for the treatment of neurodegenerative diseases (Moosavi et al. 2016).

Grape polyphenols protect against Alzheimer's disease by obstructing Aβ-oligomerisation, inhibiting the creation of neurotoxic oligomers, and preventing Aβ membrane interactions. Because of their ability to interrelate with brain proteins, grape polyphenols are neuroprotective (Fouad and Zaki Rizk 2019; Figueira et al. 2017).

### 13.4.4 Grape Phytochemicals against Cardiovascular Diseases

Grapes and their derivatives can be high in natural bioactive compounds like hydroxycinnamic acids, anthocyanins, proanthocyanidins, and stilbenes. Grape consumption lowers the risk of cardiovascular disease and associated risk factors like hypertension. Grapes and its products can be functional foods in the reduction of hypertension. Grapes' antihypertensive effects may be mediated by a decrease in angiotensin II and endothelin 1 like vasoconstricting molecules and an increase in the vasodilating molecule nitric oxide, and a reduction in inflammation and oxidative stress (Sabra et al. 2021).

The by-products of winemaking, like grape pomace, are a rich source of dietary fibre, having beneficial effects like the regulation of glucose absorption and prevention of obesity, blood cholesterol, and cardiovascular risk. Therefore, grape by-products constitute potential, owing to their nutritional and biological properties to act as an anti-inflammatory agent for the stoppage of cardiovascular illness (Coelho et al. 2020).

### 13.4.5 Grape Phytochemicals against Gastrointestinal Diseases

Grape pomace is high in dietary fibre (primarily cellulose, with minor amounts of pectins and hemicelluloses), and nutritional benefits (vitamins and minerals, bio-actives like flavonoids and lycopene). Grape pomace, which contains fibre, can regulate bowel functions and water retention through functional properties like amplified water holding and binding, gelling, and thickening (O'Shea et al. 2012).

Grape seeds have been shown to be anticolitis. It provided additional protection by suppressing inflammation and apoptosis. The hydroalcoholic black grape seed extract and oil provide protection by lowering the ulcer index, colon weight, and total colitis index. Grape root extract protects against oxidative DNA damage caused by hydrogen peroxide on human colonic adenocarcinoma cells (HT-29 cells) by preventing $H_2O_2$-induced-DNA damage, as demonstrated by the comet assay (Insanu et al. 2021).

The inclusion of grape pomace in various plant food products, meat products, fish, and dairy products increased the total polyphenolic content in the final fortified products. These fortifications caused colour fluctuations into darker, bluish and reddish. The upsurge in total polyphenols increases the oxidative stability of fortified products of meat and fish products and prolongs their shelf life (Antonić et al. 2020).

### 13.4.6 Grape Phytochemicals against Respiratory Diseases (COVID)

Respiratory inflammation can be caused by an air-mediated disease through smoke, polluted air, viruses, and bacteria leading to many air-mediated sicknesses, including asthma, pulmonary diseases, chronic bronchitis, etc. The COVID-19 pandemic is a viral respiratory disease-causing serious bronchiole, pharynx lungs and damages resulting in oxygen shortage. Resveratrol from grapes is a well-known anti-inflammatory agent for the lungs (Timalsina et al. 2021). The stilbene resveratrol suppresses asthmatic parameters like eosinophilia, airway hyperresponsiveness, mucus hypersecretion, and cytokine release, thus aiding in the respiratory illness treatment (Lee et al. 2009).

Resveratrol is a triphenolic stilbene having antioxidant and anti-inflammatory effects abundantly found in red grapes. It works in tandem with zinc to boost our immune-inflammatory viral response. In vitro, resveratrol effectively inhibited SARS-CoV-2. Resveratrol-zinc nanoparticles have a significant pharmacokinetic advantage for COVID-19 and can be used as nutraceuticals for COVID-19 and related immune inflammation (Kelleni 2021).

## 13.5 FUTURE PERSPECTIVES

Combating chronic diseases such as cancer, type 2 diabetes mellitus, and COVID-19 related to inflammation, immunity, and oncogenesis can be attempted using grape phytochemicals in combination with readily available therapeutics. More research is needed to improve the bioavailability of phytochemicals for the cure of diseases like Alzheimer's disease. The mechanisms causing grape polyphenol-induced improvements need to be researched.

## 13.6 CONCLUSION

In recent years, grapes have been used to produce various food additives and nutritional supplements on a global scale. The majority of these commercialised goods are derived from pomace left from grape wine or juice production. Grapes and its products, like grape extracts, grape skin, dry seed, pomace powder, and anthocyanin colourants, should be promoted as being a source of vitamins as a nutritious food to include in our daily diet. The unique combination of polyphenols comprising anthocyanins, stilbenes, proanthocyanins, and flavonoids makes grapes a viable source for novel nutraceutical product development to be used as food supplements. The inclusion of grapes and its products as food supplements in our regular diets can aid health substantially.

## REFERENCES

Abdulkhaleq, L. A., M. A. Assi, M. H. M. Noor, R. Abdullah, M. Z. Saad, and Y. H. Taufiq-Yap. 2017. "Therapeutic uses of epicatechin in diabetes and cancer." *Veterinary World* 10(8): 869.

Adisakwattana, S. 2017. "Cinnamic acid and its derivatives: Mechanisms for prevention and management of diabetes and its complications." *Nutrients* 9(2): 163.

Afridi, R., A. U. Khan, S. Khalid, B. Shal, H. Rasheed, M. Z. Ullah, O. Shehzad, Y. S. Kim, and S. Khan. 2019. "Anti-hyperalgesic properties of a flavanone derivative poncirin in acute and chronic inflammatory pain models in mice." *BMC Pharmacology and Toxicology* 20(1): 1–16.

Afzal, M., Safer, A. M., and Menon, M. 2015. "Green tea polyphenols and their potential role in health and disease." *Inflammopharmacology*, 23, 151–161. https://doi.org/.org/10.1007/s10787-015-0236-1

Ahmadi, A., and A. Shadboorestan. 2016. "Oxidative stress and cancer; the role of hesperidin, a citrus natural bioflavonoid, as a cancer chemoprotective agent." *Nutrition and Cancer* 68 (1): 29–39.

Ahmed, T., S. Javed, S. Javed, A. Tariq, D. Šamec, S. Tejada, S. F. Nabavi, N. Braidy, and S. M. Nabavi. 2017. "Resveratrol and Alzheimer's disease: Mechanistic insights." *Molecular Neurobiology* 54(4): 2622–2635.

Aktipis, C. A., A. M. Boddy, G. Jansen, U. Hibner, M. E. Hochberg, C. C. Maley, and G. S. Wilkinson. 2015. "Cancer across the tree of life: Cooperation and cheating in multicellularity." *Philosophical Transactions of the Royal Society B: Biological Sciences* 370(1673): 20140219.

Anastasiadi, M., N. G. Chorianopoulos, G. J. E. Nychas, and S. A. Haroutounian. 2009. "Antilisterial activities of polyphenol-rich extracts of grapes and vinification by products." *Journal of Agricultural and Food Chemistry* 57(2): 457–463.

Antonić, B., S. Jančíková, D. Dordević, and B. Tremlová. 2020. "Grape pomace valorization: A systematic review and meta-analysis." *Foods* 9(11): 1627

Badhani, B., N. Sharma, and R. Kakkar. 2015. "Gallic acid: A versatile antioxidant with promising therapeutic and industrial applications." *RSC Advances* 5(35): 27540–27557.

Bertelli, A. A. A., and D. K. Das. 2009. "Grapes, wines, resveratrol, and heart health." *Journal of Cardiovascular Pharmacology* 54(6): 468–476.

Busserolles, J., E. Gueux, B. Balasinska, Y. Piriou, E. Rock, Y. Rayssiguier, and A. Mazur. 2006. "In vivo antioxidant activity of procyanidin-rich extracts from grape seed and pine (*Pinus maritima*) bark in rats." *International Journal for Vitamin and Nutrition Research*. 76(1):22–27.

Calixto-Campos, C., T. T. Carvalho, M. S. N Hohmann, F. A. Pinho-Ribeiro, V. Fattori, M. F. Manchope, A. C. Zarpelon, M. M., Baracat, S. R. Georgetti, R. Casagrande, and W. A. Verri Jr. 2015. "Vanillic acid inhibits inflammatory pain by inhibiting neutrophil recruitment, oxidative stress, cytokine production, and NFκB activation in mice." *Journal of Natural Products* 78(8): 1799–1808.

Chen, C. 2016. "Sinapic acid and its derivatives as medicine in oxidative stress-induced diseases and aging." *Oxidative Medicine and Cellular Longevity* 2016:3571614. https://doi.org/10.1155/2016/3571614

Chen, J. Y., P. F. Wen, W. F. Kong, Q. H. Pan, J. C. Zhan, J. M. Li, S. B. Wan, and W. D. Huang. 2006. "Effect of salicylic acid on phenylpropanoids and phenylalanine ammonia-lyase in harvested grape berries." *Postharvest Biology and Technology* 1;40(1):64–72.

Chu, C., J. Deng, Y. Man, and Y. Qu. 2017. "Green tea extracts epigallocatechin-3-gallate for different treatments." *BioMed Research International* (2017). https://doi.org/10.1155/2017/5615647

Coelho, M. C., R. N. Pereira, A. S. Rodrigues, J. A. Teixeira, and M. E. Pintado. 2020. "The use of emergent technologies to extract added value compounds from grape by-products." *Trends in Food Science & Technology* 106(2020): 182–197.

Cuevas, V. M., Y. R. Calzado, Y. P. Guerra, A. O. Yera, S. J. Despaigne, R. M. Ferreiro, and D. C. Quintana. 2011. "Effects of grape seed extract, vitamin C, and vitamin E on ethanol-and aspirin-induced ulcers." *Advances in Pharmacological Sciences*. https://doi.org/10.1155/2011/740687

Dasiman, R., N. M. Nor, Z. Eshak, S. S. M. Mutalip, N. R. Suwandi, and H. Bidin. 2022. "A review of procyanidin: Updates on current bioactivities and potential health benefits." *Biointerface Research in Applied Chemistry* 12(5): 5918–5940.

David, A. V. A., R. Arulmoli, and S. Parasuraman. 2016. "Overviews of biological importance of quercetin: A bioactive flavonoid." *Pharmacognosy Reviews* 10 (20): 84.

De Ancos, B., C. Colina-Coca, D. González-Peña, and C. Sánchez-Moreno. 2015. "Bioactive compounds from vegetable and fruit by-products." *Biotechnology of Bioactive Compounds. Sources and Applications*. I. 22:3–6.

Devi, S. A., and A. Chamoli. 2020. "Polyphenols as an effective therapeutic intervention against cognitive decline during normal and pathological brain aging." *Advances in Experimental Medicine and Biology* 1260: 159–174.

Dias, M. C., D. C. G. A. Pinto, and A. Silva. 2021. "Plant flavonoids: Chemical characteristics and biological activity." *Molecules* 26 (17): 5377.

Đilas, S., J. Čanadanović-Brunet, and G. ćetković. 2009. "By-products of fruits processing as a source of phytochemicals." *Chemical Industry and Chemical Engineering Quarterly/CICEQ* 15(4): 191–202.

Dinicola, S., A. Cucina, D. Antonacci, and M. Bizzarri. 2014. "Anticancer effects of grape seed extract on human cancers: A review." *Journal of Carcinogenesis and Mutagenesis* 8: 005. doi: 10.4172/2157-2518.S8-005

Espíndola, K. M. M., R. G. Ferreira, L. E. M. Narvaez, A. C. R. Silva Rosario, A. H. M. da Silva, A. G. B. Silva, A. P. O. Vieira, and M. C. Monteiro. 2019. "Chemical and pharmacological aspects of caffeic acid and its activity in hepatocarcinoma." *Frontiers in Oncology* 9: 541.

Falleh, H., S. Oueslati, S. Guyot, A. B. Dali, C. Magné, C. Abdelly, and R. Ksouri. 2011. "LC/ESI-MS/MS characterisation of procyanidins and propelargonidins responsible for the strong antioxidant activity of the edible halophyte *Mesembryanthemum edule* L." *Food Chemistry* 127 (4): 1732–1738.

Fantini, M., M. Benvenuto, L. Masuelli, G. V. Frajese, I. Tresoldi, A. Modesti, and R. Bei. 2015. "In vitro and in vivo antitumoral effects of combinations of polyphenols, or polyphenols and anticancer drugs: Perspectives on cancer treatment." *International Journal of Molecular Sciences* 16 (5): 9236–9282.

Farzaei M. H., M. Abdollahi, and R. Rahimi. 2015. "Role of dietary polyphenols in the management of peptic ulcer". *World Journal of Gastroenterology* 7;21(21): 6499–6517.

Fernández-Marín, M.I., R. F. Guerrero, B. Puertas, M. C. García-Parrilla, E. Cantos-Villar. 2013. "Functional grapes." In: K. Ramawat and J. M. Mérillon (eds.), *Natural Products*. Springer, Berlin, Heidelberg. https://doi.org/10.1007/978-3-642-22144-6_69

Figueira, I., R. Menezes, D. Macedo, I. Costa, and C. N. dos Santos. 2017. "Polyphenols beyond barriers: A glimpse into the brain." *Current Neuropharmacology* 15(4): 562–594.

Folts, J. D. 2002. "Potential health benefits from the flavonoids in grape products on vascular disease." *Flavonoids in Cell Function* 95–111.

Fouad, G. I., and M. Zaki Rizk. 2019. "Possible neuromodulating role of different grape (*Vitis vinifera* L.) derived polyphenols against Alzheimer's dementia: Treatment and mechanisms." *Bulletin of the National Research Centre* 43(1): 1–13.

García-Mediavilla, V., I. Crespo, P. S. Collado, A. Esteller, S. Sánchez-Campos, M. J. Tuñón, and J. González-Gallego. 2007. "The anti-inflammatory flavones quercetin and kaempferol cause inhibition of inducible nitric oxide synthase, cyclooxygenase-2 and reactive C-protein, and down-regulation of the nuclear factor kappaB pathway in Chang liver cells." *European Journal of Pharmacology* 557(2007): 221–229.

Gómez-Mejía, E., C. L. Roriz, S. A. Heleno, R. Calhelha, M. I. Dias, J. Pinela, N. Rosales-Conrado, M. E. León-González, I. C. Ferreira, and L. Barros. 2021. "Valorisation of black mulberry and grape seeds: Chemical characterization and bioactive potential." *Food Chemistry*. 337: 127998

Harbeoui, H., A. Hichami, W. Aidi Wannes, J. Lemput, M. Saidani Tounsi, and N. A. Khan. 2019. "Anti-inflammatory effect of grape (*Vitis vinifera* L.) seed extract through the downregulation of NF-κB and MAPK pathways in LPS-induced RAW264. 7 macrophages." *South African Journal of Botany* 125: 1–8.

Heim, K. E., A. R. Tagliaferro, and D. J. Bobilya. 2002. "Flavonoid antioxidants: Chemistry, metabolism and structure-activity relationships." *Journal of Nutritional Biochemistry* 13(10): 572–584.

Huang, X. F., H. Q. Li, L. Shi, J. Y. Xue, B. F. Ruan, and H. L. Zhu. 2008. "Synthesis of resveratrol analogues, and evaluation of their cytotoxic and xanthine oxidase inhibitory activities." *Chemistry & Biodiversity* 5(4): 636–642.

Huang, C. S., C. K. Lii, A. H. Lin, Y. W. Yeh, H. T. Yao, C. C. Li, T. S. Wang, and H. W. Chen. 2013. "Protection by chrysin, apigenin, and luteolin against oxidative stress is mediated by the Nrf2-dependent up-regulation of heme oxygenase 1 and glutamate cysteine ligase in rat primary hepatocytes." *Archives of Toxicology* 87(1): 167–178.

Huang, Y., M. Xu, J. Li, K. Chen, L. Xia, W. Wang, P. Ren, and X. Huang. 2021. "Ex vivo to in vivo extrapolation of syringic acid and ferulic acid as grape juice proxies for endothelium-dependent vasodilation: Redefining vasoprotective resveratrol of the French paradox." *Food Chemistry* (2021): 130323. https://doi.org/10.1016/j.foodchem.2021.130323.

Huang, W., Z. Yunming, L. Chunyang, S. Zhongquan, and M. Weihong. 2016. "Effect of blueberry anthocyanins malvidin and glycosides on the antioxidant properties in endothelial cells." *Oxidative Medicine and Cellular Longevity* 2016. https://doi.org/10.1155/2016/1591803.

Ilavenil, S., D. H. Kim, S. Srigopalram, M. V. Arasu, K. D. Lee, J. C. Lee, J. S. Lee, S. Renganathan, and K. C. Choi. 2016. "Potential application of p-coumaric acid on differentiation of C2C12 skeletal muscle and 3T3-L1 preadipocytes—An in vitro and in silico approach." *Molecules* 21(8): 997.

Insanu, M., H. Karimah, H. Pramastya, and I. Fidrianny. 2021. *"Phytochemical Compounds and Pharmacological Activities of Vitis vinifera L.: An Updated Review."* 11(5): 13829–13849. https://doi.org/10.33263/BRIAC115.1382913849

Isemura, Mamoru. 2019. "Catechin in human health and disease." *Molecules* 24(3): 528.

Jafarinia, M., M. S. Hosseini, N. Kasiri, N. Fazel, F. Fathi, M. G. Hakemi, and N. Eskandari. 2020. "Quercetin with the potential effect on allergic diseases." *Allergy, Asthma & Clinical Immunology* 16: 1–11.

Jeon, J. S., S. Kwon, K. Ban, Y. K. Hong, C. Ahn, J. S. Sung, and I. Choi. 2019. "Regulation of the intracellular ROS level is critical for the antiproliferative effect of quercetin in the hepatocellular carcinoma cell line HepG2." *Nutrition and Cancer* 71(5): 861–869.

Kakkar, S., and S. Bais. 2014. "A review on protocatechuic acid and its pharmacological potential." *International Scholarly Research Notices* (2014). http://dx.doi.org/10.1155/2014/952943

Karami, S., M. Rahimi, and A. Babaei. 2018. "An overview on the antioxidant, anti-inflammatory, antimicrobial and anticancer activity of grape extract." *Biomedical Research and Clinical Practice* 3(2): 1–4.

Kelleni, M. T. 2021. "Resveratrol-zinc nanoparticles or pterostilbene-zinc: Potential COVID-19 mono and adjuvant therapy." *Biomedicine & Pharmacotherapy* 139: 111626. https://doi.org/10.1016/j.biopha.2021.111626

Kopustinskiene, D. M., V. Jakstas, A. Savickas, and J. Bernatoniene. 2020. "Flavonoids as anticancer agents." *Nutrients* 12(2): 457.

Lee, M., S. Kim, O. K. Kwon, S. R. Oh, H. K. Lee, and K. Ahn. 2009. "Anti-inflammatory and anti-asthmatic effects of resveratrol, a polyphenolic stilbene, in a mouse model of allergic asthma." *International Immunopharmacology* 9(4): 418–424.

Li, D., P. Wang, Y. Luo, M. Zhao, and F. Chen. 2017. "Health benefits of anthocyanins and molecular mechanisms: Update from recent decade." *Critical Reviews in Food Science and Nutrition* 57(8): 1729–1741.

Liang, Z., H. Liang, Y. Guo, and D. Yang. 2021. "Cyanidin 3-O-galactoside: A natural compound with multiple health benefits." *International Journal of Molecular Sciences* 22(5): 2261.

Lim, W., S. Park, F. W. Bazer, and G. Song. 2017. "Naringenin-induced apoptotic cell death in prostate cancer cells is mediated via the PI3K/AKT and MAPK signaling pathways." *Journal of Cellular Biochemistry* 118(5): 1118–1131.

Lin, Yong, Ranxin Shi, Xia Wang, and Han-Ming Shen. 2008. "Luteolin, a flavonoid with potential for cancer prevention and therapy." *Current Cancer Drug Targets* 8(7): 634–646.

Magrone, T., and E. Jirillo. 2010. "Polyphenols from red wine are potent modulators of innate and adaptive immune responsiveness." *Proceedings of the Nutrition Society* 69(3): 279–285.

Magrone, T., M. Magrone, M. A. Russo, and Jirillo, E. 2019. "Recent advances on the anti-inflammatory and antioxidant properties of red grape polyphenols: In vitro and in vivo studies." *Antioxidants (Basel, Switzerland)* 9(1): 35. https://doi.org/10.3390/antiox9010035

Mandial, D., P. Khullar, H. Kumar, G. K. Ahluwalia, and M. S. Bakshi. 2018. "Naringin–chalcone bioflavonoid-protected nanocolloids: Mode of flavonoid adsorption, a determinant for protein extraction." *ACS Omega* 3(11): 15606–15614.

Martin, M. E., E. Grao-Cruces, M. C. Millan-Linares, and S. Montserrat-De la Paz. 2020. "Grape (*Vitis vinifera* L.) seed oil: A functional food from the winemaking industry." *Foods* 9(10): 1360.

Mirsane, S. 2017. "Benefits of ellagic acid from grapes and pomegranates against colorectal cancer." *Caspian Journal of Internal Medicine* 8(3): 226–227.

Mlcek, J., T. Jurikova, S. Skrovankova, and J. Sochor. 2016. "Quercetin and its anti-allergic immune response." *Molecules* 21(5): 623.

Mohar, D. S., and S. Malik. 2012. "The sirtuin system: The holy grail of resveratrol?" *Journal of Clinical & Experimental Cardiology* 3(11): 216. https://doi.org/10.4172/2155-9880.1000216

Moon, H., H. H. Choi, J. Y. Lee, H. J. Moon, S. S. Sim, and C. J. Kim. 2008. "Quercetin inhalation inhibits the asthmatic responses by exposure to aerosolized-ovalbumin in conscious guinea-pigs." *Archives of Pharmacal Research* 31(6): 771–778.

Moosavi, F., R. Hosseini, L. Saso, and O. Firuzi. 2016. "Modulation of neurotrophic signaling pathways by polyphenols." *Drug Design, Development and Therapy* 10: 23–42. https://doi.org/10.2147/DDDT.S96936

Nagaoka, M., T. Maeda, S. Moriwaki, A. Nomura, Y. Kato, S. Niida, M. C. Kruger, and K. Suzuki. 2019. "Petunidin, a b-ring 5'-O-methylated derivative of delphinidin, stimulates osteoblastogenesis and reduces srankl-induced bone loss." *International Journal of Molecular Sciences* 20(11): 2795.

Nile, S. H., S. H. Kim, E. Y. Ko, and S. W. Park. 2013. "Polyphenolic contents and antioxidant properties of different grape (*V. vinifera, V. labrusca*, and *V. hybrid*) cultivars." *BioMed Research International* (2013). https://doi.org/10.1155/2013/718065

O'Shea, N., E. K. Arendt, and E. Gallagher. 2012. "Dietary fibre and phytochemical characteristics of fruit and vegetable by-products and their recent applications as novel ingredients in food products." *Innovative Food Science & Emerging Technologies* 16(2012): 1–10.

Ozkur, M., N. Benlier, I. Saygili, and E. Ogut. 2020. "Technological advances in improving bioavailability of phytochemicals for the treatment of Alzheimer's disease." In *Nutrients and Nutraceuticals for Active & Healthy Ageing*, 265–277. Springer, Singapore.

Pan, W., K. Ikeda, M. Takebe, and Y. Yamori. 2001. "Genistein, daidzein and glycitein inhibit growth and DNA synthesis of aortic smooth muscle cells from stroke-prone spontaneously hypertensive rats." *Journal of Nutrition* 131(4): 1154–1158.

Pandey, P., U. Sayyed, R. K. Tiwari, M. H. Siddiqui, N. Pathak, and P. Bajpai. 2019. "Hesperidin induces ROS-mediated apoptosis along with cell cycle arrest at G2/M phase in human gall bladder carcinoma." *Nutrition and Cancer* 71(4): 676–687.

Park, K. S., Y. Chong, and M. K. Kim. 2016. "Myricetin: Biological activity related to human health." *Applied Biological Chemistry* 59(2): 259–269.

Peña-Neira, A. 2017. "Grapes." In *Fruit and Vegetable Phytochemicals: Chemistry and Human Health*, 2nd Edition, 1041–1054.

Poschner, S., A. Maier-Salamon, M. Zehl, J. Wackerlig, D. Dobusch, B. Pachmann, K. L. Sterlini, and W. Jäger. 2017. "The impacts of genistein and daidzein on estrogen conjugations in human breast cancer cells: A targeted metabolomics approach." *Frontiers in Pharmacology* 8: 699.

Prakash, D., C. Gupta, and G. Sharma. 2012. "Importance of phytochemicals in nutraceuticals." *Journal of Chinese Medicine Research and Development* 1(3): 70–78.

Raposo, D., C. Morgado, P. Pereira-Terra, and I. Tavares. 2015. "Nociceptive spinal cord neurons of laminae I-III exhibit oxidative stress damage during diabetic neuropathy which is prevented by early antioxidant treatment with epigallocatechin-gallate (EGCG)." *Brain Research Bulletin* 110, 68–75

Romero-Pérez, A. I., M. Ibern-Gómez, R. M. Lamuela-Raventós, and M. C. de la Torre-Boronat. 1999. "Piceid, the major resveratrol derivative in grape juices." *Journal of Agricultural and Food Chemistry* 47(4): 1533–1536.

Sabra, A., T. Netticadan, and C. Wijekoon. 2021. "Grape bioactive molecules, and the potential health benefits in reducing the risk of heart diseases." *Food Chemistry* 12: 100149. https://doi.org/10.1016/j.fochx.2021.100149

Sadh, P. K., S. Kumar, P. Chawla, and J. S. Duhan. 2018. "Fermentation: A boon for production of bioactive compounds by processing of food industries wastes (by-products)." *Molecules* 23: 2560. http://dx.doi.org/10.3390/molecules23102560

Saito, M., H. Hosoyama, T. Ariga, S. Kataoka, and N. Yamaji. 1998. "Antiulcer activity of grape seed extract and procyanidins." *Journal of Agricultural and Food Chemistry* 46(4): 1460–1464.

Salehi, B., P. V. T. Fokou, M. Sharifi-Rad, P. Zucca, R. Pezzani, N. Martins, and J. Sharifi-Rad. 2019. "The therapeutic potential of naringenin: A review of clinical trials." *Pharmaceuticals* 12(1): 11.

Salehi, B., A. P. Mishra, M. Nigam, B. Sener, M. Kilic, M. Sharifi-Rad, P. Fokou, N. Martins, and J. Sharifi-Rad. 2018. "Resveratrol: A double-edged sword in health benefits." *Biomedicines* 6(3): 91. https://doi.org/10.3390/biomedicines6030091

Salehi, B., J. Sharifi-Rad, F. Cappellini, Ž. Reiner, D. Zorzan, M. Imran, B. Sener, M. Kilic, M. El-Shazly, N. M. Fahmy, and E. Al-Sayed. 2020 "The therapeutic potential of anthocyanins: Current approaches based on their molecular mechanism of action." *Frontiers in Pharmacology* 11: 1300. https://doi.org/10.3389/fphar.2020.01300

Santa, K., Y. Kumazawa, and I. Nagaoka. 2019. "The potential use of grape phytochemicals for preventing the development of intestine-related and subsequent inflammatory diseases." *Endocrine, Metabolic & Immune Disorders-Drug Targets (Formerly Current Drug Targets-Immune, Endocrine & Metabolic Disorders)* 19(6): 794–802.

Serafini, M., I. Peluso, and A. Raguzzini. 2010. "Flavonoids as anti-inflammatory agents." *Proceedings of the Nutrition Society* 69(3): 273–278.

Shanmuganayagam, D., M. R. Beahm, M. A. Kuhns, C. G. Krueger, J. D. Reed, and J. D. Folts. 2012. "Differential effects of grape (*Vitis vinifera*) skin polyphenolics on human platelet aggregation and low-density lipoprotein oxidation." *Journal of Agricultural and Food Chemistry* 60 (23): 5787–5794.

Shanmuganayagam, D., M. R. Beahm, H. E. Osman, C. G. Krueger, J. D. Reed, and J. D. Folts. 2002. "Grape seed and grape skin extracts elicit a greater antiplatelet effect when used in combination than when used individually in dogs and humans." *Journal of Nutrition* 132(12): 3592–3598.

Sharifi-Rad, J., C. Quispe, M. Imran, A. Rauf, M. Nadeem, T. A. Gondal, B. Ahmad, M. S. Mubarak, O. Sytar, and O. M. Zhilina, et al. 2021. "Genistein: An integrative overview of its mode of action, pharmacological properties, and health benefits." *Oxidative Medicine and Cellular Longevity* (2021). https://doi.org/10.1155/2021/3268136

Shi, Q., X. Song, J. Fu, C. Su, X. Xia, E. Song, and Y. Song. 2015. "Artificial sweetener neohesperidin dihydrochalcone showed antioxidative, anti-inflammatory and anti-apoptosis effects against paraquat-induced liver injury in mice." *International Immunopharmacology* 29(2): 722–729.

Shrestha, B., M. L. S. Theerathavaj, S. Thaweboon, and B. Thaweboon. 2012. "In vitro antimicrobial effects of grape seed extract on peri-implantitis microflora in craniofacial implants." *Asian Pacific journal of Tropical Biomedicine* 2(10): 822–825.

Silva dos Santos, J., J. P. Goncalves Cirino, P. de Oliveira Carvalho, and M. M. Ortega. 2021. "The pharmacological action of kaempferol in central nervous system diseases: A review." *Frontiers in Pharmacology* 11: 2143.

Singh, N. A., A. K. A. Mandal, and Z. A. Khan. 2015. "Potential neuroprotective properties of epigallocatechin-3-gallate (EGCG)." *Nutrition Journal* 15(1): 1–17.

Singh, B., J. P. Singh, A. Kaur, and N. Singh. 2020. "Phenolic composition, antioxidant potential and health benefits of citrus peel." *Food Research International* 132: 109114.

Sun, M. Y., Y. Ye, L. Xiao, K. Rahman, W. Xia, and H. Zhang. 2016. "Daidzein: A review of pharmacological effects." *African Journal of Traditional, Complementary and Alternative Medicines* 13(3): 117–132.

Talebi, M., M. Talebi, T. Farkhondeh, J. Simal-Gandara, D. M. Kopustinskiene, J. Bernatoniene, and S. Samarghandian. 2021. "Emerging cellular and molecular mechanisms underlying anticancer indications of chrysin." *Cancer Cell International* 21(1): 1–20.

Terra, X., J. Valls, X. Vitrac, J. M. Mérrillon, L. Arola, A. Ardèvol, C. Bladé, J. Fernández-Larrea, G. Pujadas, J. Salvadó, and M. Blay. 2007. "Grape-seed procyanidins act as antiinflammatory agents in endotoxin-stimulated RAW 264.7 macrophages by inhibiting NFkB signaling pathway." *Journal of Agricultural and Food Chemistry* 55(11): 4357–4365.

Testa, R., A. R. Bonfigli, S. Genovese, V. De Nigris, and A. Ceriello. 2016. "The possible role of flavonoids in the prevention of diabetic complications." *Nutrients* 8(5): 310.

Tikhonova, M. A., N. G. Tikhonova, M. V. Tenditnik, M. V. Ovsyukova, A. A. Akopyan, N. I. Dubrovina, T. G. Amstislavskaya, and E. K. Khlestkina. 2020. "Effects of grape polyphenols on the life span and neuroinflammatory alterations related to neurodegenerative Parkinson disease-like disturbances in mice." *Molecules* 25(22): 5339.

Timalsina, D., K. P. Pokhrel, and D. Bhusal. 2021. "Pharmacologic activities of plant-derived natural products on respiratory diseases and inflammations." *BioMed Research International* 2021: 1636816. https://doi.org/10.1155/2021/1636816

Trindade, C., G. V. Bortolini, B. S. Costa, J. C. Anghinoni, T. N. Guecheva, X. Arias, M. V. Césio, H. Heinzen, D. J. Moura, J. Saffi, and M. Salvador. 2016. "Antimutagenic and antioxidant properties of the aqueous extracts of organic and conventional grapevine Vitis labrusca cv. Isabella leaves in V79 cells." *Journal of Toxicology and Environmental Health, Part A* 79 (18): 825–836.

Unusan, N. 2020. "Proanthocyanidins in grape seeds: An updated review of their health benefits and potential uses in the food industry." *Journal of Functional Foods* 67: 103861.

Vattem, D. A., and K. Shetty. 2005. "Biological functionality of ellagic acid: A review." *Journal of Food Biochemistry* 29(3): 234–266.

Vitseva, O., S. Varghese, S. Chakrabarti, J. D. Folts, and J. E. Freedman. 2005. "Grape seed and skin extracts inhibit platelet function and release of reactive oxygen intermediates." *Journal of Cardiovascular Pharmacology* 46(4): 445–451. doi: 10.1097/01.fjc.0000176727.67066.1c. PMID: 16160595.

Wang, G. Z., G. P. Huang, G. L. Yin, G. Zhou, C. J. Guo, C. G. Xie, B. B. Jia, and J. F. Wang. 2007. "Aspirin can elicit the recurrence of gastric ulcer induced with acetic acid in rats." *Cellular Physiology and Biochemistry* 20: 205–212.

Wongnarat, C., and P. Srihanam. 2017. "Phytochemical and antioxidant activity in seeds and pulp of grape cultivated in Thailand." *Oriental Journal of Chemistry* 33(1): 113–121.

Wu, P. P., S. C. Kuo, W. W. Huang, J. S. Yang, K. C. Lai, H. J. Chen, K. L. Lin, Y. J. Chiu, L. J. Huang, and J. G. Chung. 2009. "(-)-Epigallocatechin gallate induced apoptosis in human adrenal cancer NCI-H295 cells through caspase-dependent and caspase-independent pathway." *Anticancer Research* 29(4): 1435–1442.

Wu, P., X. Meng, H. Zheng, Q. Zeng, T. Chen, W. Wang, X. Zhang, and J. Su. 2018. "Kaempferol attenuates ROS-induced hemolysis and the molecular mechanism of its induction of apoptosis on bladder cancer." *Molecules* 23(10): 2592.

Yan, X., M. Qi, P. Li, Y. Zhan, and H. Shao. 2017. "Apigenin in cancer therapy: Anticancer effects and mechanisms of action." *Cell & Bioscience* 7(1): 1–16.

Yao, Q., M. T. Lin, Y. D. Zhu, H. L. Xu, and Y. Z. Zhao. 2018. "Recent trends in potential therapeutic applications of the dietary flavonoid didymin." *Molecules* 23(10): 2547.

Zduńska, K., A. Dana, A. Kolodziejczak, and H. Rotsztejn. 2018. "Antioxidant properties of ferulic acid and its possible application." *Skin Pharmacology and Physiology* 31(6): 332–336.

Zhang, J., G. B. Celli, and M. S. Brooks. 2019. "Natural sources of anthocyanins." In *Anthocyanins from Natural Sources: Exploiting Targeted Delivery for Improved Health* 1–33. doi: 10.1039/9781788012614-00001

Zhang Y. J., R. Y. Gan, S. Li, Y. Zhou, A. N. Li, D. P. Xu, and H. B. Li. 2015. "Antioxidant phytochemicals for the prevention and treatment of chronic diseases." *Molecules.* 20(12): 21138–21156.

Zhu, J. X., L. Wen, W. J. Zhong, L. Xiong, J. Liang, and H. L. Wang. 2018. "Quercetin, kaempferol and isorhamnetin in *Elaeagnus pungens* Thunb. leaf: Pharmacological activities and quantitative determination studies." *Chemistry & Biodiversity* 15(8): e1800129.

Zuckerkandl, E., and L. Pauling. 1965. "Evolutionary divergence and convergence in proteins." In *Evolving Genes and Proteins,* 97–166. Academic Press.

Zunino, Susan J. 2009. "Type 2 diabetes and glycemic response to grapes or grape products." *Journal of Nutrition* 139(9): 1794S–1800S.

# 14 Regulatory Aspects of Global Nutraceuticals and Functional Foods for the Utilization of Fruits – An Insight

*Monika Choudhary and Amarjeet Kaur*

## CONTENTS

## 14.1 INTRODUCTION

Nutraceuticals are comprised of food or food products that have additional benefits for human health. Precisely, these are less than pharmaceuticals and more than food. The perception of nutraceuticals varies from country to country as there is no single accepted definition across the world that actually describes these products in a similar fashion. Many countries assume nutraceuticals as part of dietary supplements. In developed nations, about 50%–70% of the population consume nutraceuticals, and consumption is rising with age. Going by the safety of nutraceuticals, these are reliable products for consumption regardless of their approval by concerned authorities. Several research studies have been conducted to validate the safety and effectiveness of nutraceuticals. However, nutraceuticals may pose a certain risk if these are to be used without medical control, as interactions with medication can be harmful, especially in vulnerable groups. A nutraceutical may range from specific diets to isolated nutrients and herbal products. It also includes dietary supplements, processed foods (soups, beverages, and cereals), and genetically engineered foods. Likewise, most commonly cultivated fruits and underutilized fruits are considered functional foods or these serve as an important source of nutraceutical components (Tables 14.1 and 14.2).

With the advancement in cellular-level nutraceuticals, embryonic models are being set up by researchers for amalgamation and considering information from clinical trials on unconventional therapies into conscientious medical practice (Health Canada 1998). Further, functional food represents the addition of a novel ingredient to a food product that has an added positive role to play in human health (Health Canada 1998). Few civilizations, such as Asians, Egyptians, and Sumerians, have provided data recommending that food can be efficiently used as medicine in the treatment as well as prevention of diseases. The Institute of Medicine's Food and Nutrition Board has defined

DOI: 10.1201/9781003259213-14

## Table 14.1: Nutraceuticals Derived from Commonly Consumed Fruits

| Fruit | Scientific Name | Nutraceutical | Properties | References |
|---|---|---|---|---|
| Anona | *Annona squamosa* | Annonaceous acetogenins | Antitumor | Han et al. (2015) |
| Apple | *Malus domestica* (Borkh) | Kaempferol, rutin, quercetin, procyanidins epicatechin, caffeic acid, 3-hydroxyphloridzin, coumaric acid, phloridzin, quercetin-3-O-arabinoside | • Bone health<br>• Weight management<br>• Asthma and pulmonary function<br>• Positive effects on aging and cognitive decline<br>• Gastrointestinal health | Hyson (2011) and Walia et al. (2016) |
| Banana | *Musa paradisica* L. (Musaseae) | Serotonin, vitamin B6, norepinephrine | • Antioxidant<br>• Combat depression | Kanazawa and Sakakibara (2000) |
| Citrus | *Citrus sinensis* | Hesperidin, naringin, limonoides | • Antibacterial<br>• Antifungal<br>• Anticancer<br>• Antioxidant | Russo et al. (2016) and Alam et al. (2014) |
| Guava | *Psidium guajava* | Essential oils, lycopene, vitamin C, minerals such as iron, calcium, phosphorus | • Anti-inflammatory<br>• Anticancer<br>• Prevents skin damage and prostate cancer | Joseph and Priya (2011) and Weng (2010) |
| Jamun | *Syzygium cumunii* | β-Sitosterol, lupeol, stigmasterol, 12-oleanen-3-Ol-3β-acetate | Antidiabetic | Alam et al. (2012) |
| Papaya | *Carica papaya* | Benzyl glucosinates, papain, carotenoids, polyphenols, isothiocyanates | • Antioxidant<br>• Gelatinolytic properties | Bertuccelli et al. (2016) and Manosroi et al. (2014) |
| Pineapple | *Ananas comosus* | Bromelein | Relieves diarrhea, osteoarthritis, and cardiovascular disorders | Pavan et al. (2012) |
| Mango | *Mangifera indica* L. | Anthocyanins, β-glucogallin, vitamin C, carotene, gallic acids, quercetin, isoquercetin, mangiferin, ellagic acid | • Antioxidant<br>• Antimicrobial<br>• Antihyperlipidemic | Stoilova et al. (2005) and Muruganandan et al. (2005) |
| Mangosteen | *Garcinia mangostana* | Xanthonoids | • Decrease visceral fat<br>• Treat skin implications | Morton (1987) and Hayamizu et al. (2003) |

functional food as "any food and food ingredients that may provide a health benefit beyond the traditional nutrition that it contains". It may be obtained from plant or animal sources. And the term nutraceutical was also coined by the United States, which describes foods with the potential to cure disease

**Table 14.2: Nutraceuticals Obtained from Underutilized Fruits**

| Fruit | Scientific Name | Nutraceutical | Properties | References |
|---|---|---|---|---|
| Pawpaw fruit | *Asimina triloba* (L.) Dunal | Ellagic acid, caffeic acid, vitamin C, ferulic acid | Antitumor efficacy | Coothankandaswamy et al. (2010) and Kobayashi et al. (2008) |
| Azarole fruit | *Crataegus azarolus* L. | Anthocyanidins, flavonoids, catechins, terpenoids, phenolic acids | • Hypotensive<br>• Antiarrhythmic<br>• Hypolipidemic<br>• Antioxidant | Belkhir et al. (2013) |
| Goji fruit | *Lycium barbarum* L. | Flavonoids, zeaxanthin, phenolic acids, minerals, alkaloids | • Antitumor<br>• Antioxidant<br>• Immunomodulation<br>• Cytoprotection | Amagase and Farnsworth (2011) and Donno et al. (2016) |
| Mulberry | *Morus nigra* L. | Anthocyanins, carotenoids, flavonoids | • Hypertension<br>• Arthritis<br>• Diabetes<br>• Anemia | Calin-Sanchez et al. (2013) and Sánchez-Salcedo et al. (2015) |
| Shadblow service-berry | *Amelanchier canadensis* (L.) Medicus | Anthocyanins, chlorogenic acid, lutein rutin, catechins, tocopherols, sterols | • Antidiabetic<br>• Regulate lipid metabolism | Juríková et al. (2013); Ozga et al. (2007); Bakowska-Barczak and Kolodziejczyk (2008) and Bakowska-Barczak et al. (2007) |

or specific disease conditions (Brendler et al. 2009; Brower 1998; Hardy 2000; Kalra 2003). Collectively, nutraceuticals and functional foods and beverages have been referred to as "NFx."

About two centuries ago, sugar could be accessible only from medical stores (Brillat-Savarin 1862). Today, it is one of the most established nutritional products in the market, which has captivated end users from a very young age. On one side, people are consuming food products of compromised nutritive value due to processing (Tovey and Hobsley 2004). On the other hand, people lack time to consume a balanced meal. Thereby, nutraceuticals are a must in today's dietary regime so as to compensate for these losses (Burdock et al. 2006; Choi et al. 2006; Olmedilla-Alonso et al. 2006; Sieber 2007). So, the primary step is to ascertain the short as well as long-term safety of nutraceuticals in preclinical and clinical settings. Therefore, properly planned human studies must be conducted to support these health ingredients with evidence. For this, double-blind intervention trials and epidemiological studies may play a pivotal role. Also, the duration of the trials must be long, and the subject's size should also be large to authenticate the results. The quantities of food used in studies must be pertinent to actual life and provide measurable effects in the selected indicators. These clinical trials must be carried out by involving different communities belonging to different cultures to reveal food properties in varied environments. The studies should also take into account the individual's physical activity level. So, health claims of nutraceuticals must be authenticated by suitable as well as adequate research results. There are beliefs that this evidence must be as meticulous as in the case of drugs. Thus, the amalgamation of conventional knowledge and research outcomes will bring about an improvement in healthy foods and novel therapeutic strategies.

## 14.2 REGULATORY ASPECTS

Food regulations are often facilitated by consumer behavior, food research, and product and process innovation and development. Many nations have focused on setting up a framework of food regulations prescribing different standards pertaining to food preservatives and additives and labeling. Gradually, the understanding of food regulations is noticeable through increased consumption of dietary supplements, which possess remedial significance in the prevention and treatment of particular diseases. In each country, food laws form the foundation of laws for all types of food, such as nutraceuticals, functional food, dietary supplements, and health foods. For instance, the Food and Drug Administration (FDA) in the United States regulates dietary supplements differently than conventional foods and drug products. As per the Dietary Supplement Health and Education Act of 1994 (DSHEA), the dietary supplement maker is answerable for ensuring the safety of dietary supplements prior to commercialization. In case of any ambiguity, the FDA is authorized to take action against any questionable product even after its marketing. In general, it is not necessary for companies to get registration and approval for the products under FDA prior to manufacturing or marketing dietary supplements. Nevertheless, it is their responsibility to ensure the correct labeling of that product. The responsibilities of the FDA after marketing include monitoring safety. For example, product information includes labeling, any nutrition or health claim, and supplementary literature and adverse event reporting, if any (FDA 2003). The Federal Trade Commission regulates dietary supplement advertising.

Regulatory aspects pertinent to nutraceuticals and functional foods across the globe are discussed below.

### 14.2.1 USA

The Dietary Supplement Health and Education Act (DSHEA) was launched by The United States in 1994 so as to endorse substantial suppleness between medicines and foods found in other regions across the world (Office of Inspector General 2003). According to DSHEA, a dietary supplement may contain "a herb or other botanical" or "a concentrate, metabolite, constituent, extract or combination of any ingredient from the other categories." The American food regulatory system is more centralized than the European one. Generally, the United States Department of Agriculture (USDA) and the Food and Drug Administration (FDA) are the main food regulatory bodies in the United States. These two central authorities cover all phases of the food regulatory system, such as evaluation, investigation, regulation, inspection, and sanction. Still, there are opinions that the USDA and the FDA should be merged into one agency for more efficiency. Moreover, all domestic and foreign companies dealing in the business of dietary supplements must act in accordance with guidelines for quality assurance. Even more, companies dealing with testing, quality assurance, and distribution of food supplements in the United States should also meet the terms. In addition, all the stakeholders involved in this segment of business, manufacturer to distributor, need to report to the FDA regarding any adverse event. The DHSEA has set up a framework for FDA regulation regarding supplements which provides more freedom to the manufacturers of dietary supplements and also gives required information to consumers (Bagchi 2014).

## 14.2.2 Japan

FOSHU, Foods for Special Dietary Uses, was established by the Japanese Ministry of Health and Welfare (MHW) in 1991 to regulate the labeling of specific foods. The word functional was not drawn due to its existence in the definition of "pharmaceuticals". And these may influence the build-up or functions of the body. FOSHU is an authorized structure for labeling derived from medical and nutritional science, which enables manufacturers to claim foods that are appropriate for a specific health condition or may maintain it. Hence, scientific validation comprising clinical trials, nutrition-based studies, and analytical data is required to attain FOSHU permission which prescribes the health efficiency of the food or the components in terms of safety and stability. At the outset, many companies were not interested in FOSHU owing to these obligations, but nowadays, MHW has taken a deregulation process to support manufacturers so as to expand the FOSHU market (FOSHU System 1991).

In Japan, there is a diversity of healthy foods which implicate health ingredients with biological and nutritional effects based on scientific documentation. Among them, micronutrients have been given special consideration and categorized as dietary supplements. Still, it is debatable to quote them as functional foods based on scientific literature. The market value is approximately 750 billion yen of health foods (FOSHU System 1991). The drive in Japan has emerged on the right track facilitating the whole world with a suitable podium for future progress.

## 14.2.3 Canada

Products containing micronutrients and herbs are recognized as natural health products (NHPs) in Canada. These products are regulated as a specific regulation incorporated under the Canadian Food and Drugs Act (the Act). The Natural Health Products Regulations (NHPR) consider the exceptional nature and characteristics of these products. Moreover, Health Canada has approved about 61,000 NHPs for sale in Canada since 2004 and 1250 manufacturing sites for these products (Nestmann et al. 2006). NHP refers to a cluster of health products with regulations comprising micronutrients, conventional medicines, and plant-based products, including herbal products, enzymes, probiotics, homeopathic medicines, and a few self-care products containing natural ingredients. As discussed above, NHPs are regulated according to NHPR, and several unprocessed applications were reported after its implementation. Hence, Health Canada has been enthusiastically making amendments to its organizational processes to certify that submissions are processed with competence. For the sake of transformation of the NHPs regulations in Canada, a set of principles was published in 2012 to enable strengthening innovation and growth of the NHP sector (Health Canada 2012). This was set out by Health Canada to achieve balance in consumer accessibility for safe products.

Similar to the United States, Canadian regulations have also been comprised of innovative models for regulating NHPs and dietary supplements. Basically, NHPs regulations consist of five key components: A three-class system of NHPs based on risk, site licensing modifications, requirements, and pathways for licensing NHPs, compliance transition over time, and quality guidance redevelopment for NHPs (Health Canada 2012). NHPs' three-class system is a risk-based set-up built-up of understanding regarding ingredients, claims, and blends of NHPs that the NHPD has assessed in past years.

Class 1 includes products with the uppermost assurance and contributes 75% of all NHPs, such as micronutrients and various herbal products. Class 2 holds reasonable certainty, with 20%–24% of NHPs having a minimum of one claim and/or ingredients supported by PCI. Further, Class 3 holds the lowest assurance comprising 1%–5% of NHPs with no claim or ingredient supported by PCI, e.g., a new product developed for the prevention of rheumatoid arthritis. So, this claim should be supported by enough clinical evidence with complete premarket consideration. At present, there are more than 55,000 products in the Canadian NHP category. Canadian regulatory programs and policies for NHPs are going through substantial modifications; so far, the major assured objective of the NHPD remains to give end users the well-versed option for those personal products that are safe and sound, effective and manufactured under good manufacturing processes.

### 14.2.4 European Union (EU)

EU legislation does not distinguish nutraceuticals/functional foods as a distinctive class as these are considered in other countries such as Japan. Moreover, there is no authorized characterization for NFx in Europe. This depicts that functional foods or nutraceuticals must meet all the requirements premeditated by food legislation in terms of ingredients, labeling, health or nutrition claims, etc. In 1995, the United Kingdom Ministry of Agriculture, Fisheries, and Food (MAFF, now DEFRA) defined functional food to distinguish it from fortified foods and dietary supplements (Ministry of Agriculture, Fisheries and Food 1995). The definition describes functional food with an ingredient incorporated into it to give a specific medical or physiological benefit other than a merely dietetic effect (Milner 2002). Nutraceutical regulations are basically taking shape in the scaffold of European legislation. Currently, European health authorities have increasingly recognized nutraceuticals in the field of health and nutrition claim claims. In view of this, a plan for the provision of information on food products, such as labeling, and advertising to consumers (European Commission 2008) was adopted by the EC in 2008. This plan was a collective approach by Directive 2000/13/EC and Directive 90/496/EEC while projecting it as a single instrument. The EU Regulation prohibits any foodstuff to be not referred with properties of prevention and curing of disease. This rule is also applicable to the presentation of food products in terms of packaging or packaging material, the appearance of foodstuff, and its display.

### 14.2.5 Russia

The Russian Federation Food Security Doctrine, approved by Order No.120 by the President of the Russian Federation on 30.01.10, is a pedestal document that shelters state guarantees in relation to food. One of the chief objectives put by the Doctrine is to attain and preserve the accessibility of safe foods in the quantity and variety equivalent to sufficient dietary recommendations linked to a dynamic and healthy standard of living.

Russian Federation is constantly improvising its food regulation to refine food quality for the efficient management of different nutritional disorders. Consequently, a committee, named Technical Standardization Committee No. 036 Functional Foods, was fashioned in 2008 for implementation of the Central Law "On Technical Regulation" (No. 184-FZ dt. 27.12.2002) and a formation of a structure of scientific committees for standardization of nutraceuticals and functional foods. This committee is comprised of three subcommittees (SC): SC1 – Functional Foods of Plant Origin, SC2 – Functional Foods of Animal Origin, and SC3 – Evaluation of Functional Foods and Functional Ingredients Efficacy. The main objectives include guaranteeing conformity between the governmental and food regulation of the Russian Federation and their coordination with the global prerequisites and regulations of other nations, categorizing components with functional prospective and their share in foods; developing a method of validation and prevention of bogus events; organizing the system for consumer awareness regarding functional foods, and demonstrating interests of the Russian Federation in worldwide organizations.

The standardization of functional foods was supported by the Interstate Council for Standardization, Metrology, and Certification, which commenced and permitted the formation of Interstate Technical Standardization Committee (ITC) No. 526 Functional Foods in 2011. The board takes into account the functional foods of plant origin (plus probiotics and fortified foods), animal origin (plus probiotics and fortified foods), and functional food components of both plant and animal origin (including probiotics, prebiotics, and synbiotics). Furthermore, the Russian Federal Law No 29-FZ on food safety and quality categorizes dietary supplements as food products. The law defines biologically active food supplements (BAFS) as "natural (identical to natural) biologically active substances designed for consumption with food or introduction into the composition of food products."

The authorized scaffold for spreading the utilization of food supplements in Russia continues to develop and progress. Companies are accountable for product safety and quality and for the reliability and wholeness of information about their products. Moreover, Russia has prepared negative lists of compounds, substances, microorganisms, tissues, and animals in a distinctive manner from other nations so as to prohibit their use in dietary supplements. These comprise medicinal plants with no evidence of human consumption in food history. Also, restrictions have been imposed on the use of supplements such as micronutrients, probiotics, and prebiotics in the diets of children. Russia does have a positive list of components as well, containing 166 approved components, for instance, micronutrients, fatty acids, amino acids, and biologically active components that have suggested and upper limit intake levels. Moreover, an efficient, approved, and well-adopted methodology has been developed for analyzing these elements in food supplements (Tutelyan and Sukhanov 2008).

### 14.2.6 India

Fruit and vegetables are grown in abundance in India, but processing is only 2% compared to 80% in the United States (Keservani and Sharma 2015). Poor infrastructure and rigid food regulations are major obstacles to the growth of the food processing sector. Earlier, there were different laws and regulations for different processing sectors in India. This diversity fetched the attention of public experts and members of the Standing Committee of Parliament, which suggested the convergence of scattered food laws under a single regulatory authority responsible for food safety in the interest of public health. In addition, a specific focus was drawn towards nutraceuticals which was not well-defined sector earlier but had full potential to grow in order to provide health benefits to end users. Ultimately, the Indian Food Safety Standard Bill 2005 was passed with an assurance to provide the foremost implication for the Indian food processing industry. In 2006, the Indian Food Safety and

Standard Act (FSSAI) was implemented. FSSAI is a modern integrated food law to serve as a single reference point in relation to the regulation of food products, including nutraceuticals, dietary supplements, and functional food. Chiefly, it is aimed at the establishment of a single statute with regard to food and the provision of a basic framework for the systematic growth of the food processing industry. Yet, FSSAI needs significant improvisation in terms of infrastructure and suitable stewardship so as to be equivalent to food laws and standards in the United States and Europe. A significant expansion is necessary for the act to pose an evident impact on the Indian functional food and nutraceutical industry the way DSHEA in the United States had on the nutraceutical industry in 1994. The implementation of FSSAI is a noteworthy initial step, but a lot of efforts have to be made to mitigate overlapping in rules with the previous regulatory system.

Functional foods have yet to be characterized individually in India as in Japan, the United States, and Europe. In India, functional foods may include fruits and nutritionally improved foods and their food products, herbal extracts, and spices. Undoubtedly, FSSAI has incorporated the prominent requirements of the Prevention of Food Adulteration Act 1954 and is also based on international legislations, Instrumentalities and the Codex Alimentarius Commission. Basically, the liability of designing and regulating nutraceuticals standards lies with the FSSAI as framed by Food Safety Act 2006. This authority will cover nutraceuticals, functional foods, dietetic food products, and other related food products (FICCI 2007). Further, FSSAI 2006 consists of 12 chapters. Chapter IV, Article 22 of the act deals with nutraceutical, functional food, and dietary supplements in terms of the regulation of these products. It regulates in such a way that any interested individual can produce, vend, or allocate or import products, including novel foods, food for special dietary uses, organic food, genetically modified food, and dietary supplements. And Articles 23 and 24 are basically focused on the packaging and labeling of food and the restriction of advertisements regarding foods. According to FSSAI, the following foods have been categorized into nutraceutical or dietary supplements and specific dietary uses:

1. Food that is particularly manufactured so as to assure specific dietary needs that subsist due to specific physiological conditions. And foods that are processed in such a way so as to distinguish the formulation of these products from common food of equivalent nature. And, if these common foods contain the following ingredients as a major or minor component- Micronutrients and protein as per the recommended dietary allowances or enzymes, plants or herbs as a single ingredient or in combination in any form such as powder or concentrates, or extracts in water or alcohol and ingredients of animal origin. Non-conventional foods in the form of powders, liquids, jelly, granules, tablets, and capsules are intended to be used only through oral route. Foods that are not drugs as defined under Section 3 of the Drugs and Cosmetics Act 1940. Also, it does not include a narcotic drug or psychotropic substance as described under the Narcotic Drugs and Psychotropic Substances Act 1985 and the ingredients listed under the Drugs and Cosmetics Rules 1945.

2. Organic foods or products that are manufactured as per specified standards for organic production.

3. Proprietary and novel food which are safe for consumption and do not contain any prohibited ingredients in their formulations.

The Indian Government, unlike the United States, is continuing efforts to design and develop a law to ensure standardized manufacturing, importing, and marketing of nutraceuticals or functional foods.

### 14.2.7 China

In 2003, China transferred that administrative permission for health foods from the Ministry of Health (MOH) to the State Food and Drug Administration (SFDA). The SFDA established a set of strategies and requirements for regulating health food registration and re-registration. It also includes a novel plan to alter the present scope of health claims and processes for new claims. In the meantime, the Chinese health food industry has swiftly gone upwards to RMB 100 billion Yuan (Li and Li 2011). Moreover, China has also become a supplier of imperative raw materials across the world in the health industry. With the implementation of the Food Hygiene Law, Functional food or health food was launched first in China in the mid-1990s. Article 22 of this law has defined health food as food with a specific health function. The law described that health food, with its instruction, should be submitted to the concerned authority for its estimation and authorization. When SFDA took up the directorial assessment and authorization of functional, the definition of health food or functional food was further illustrated as foods with specific health claims or micronutrient supplements and foods that are suitable for human consumption with particular regulatory functions of the body (Yang 2008) provided it will not be claimed for any treatment and also will not cause any mild or severe risk to the human body (SFDA 2005). Further, Food Safety Law was implemented in 2009 to overtake Food Hygiene Law. And it was ensured that the concerned regulatory departments shall carry out their assigned duties and take up their responsibilities per the guidelines law. Food with health claims will not cause any type of chronic hazard to the human body. The labeling will not give any description about the prevention or treatment of disease. Further, the information must be correct and evidently specify the suitability and functionality; similarly, product formulations must comply with the labeling instructions.

So, China has described health foods as foods that are used for only maintaining or improving health conditions and not for therapeutic purposes. Apart from this, raw materials used in health food production should also comply with national standards. As it was observed that about one-sixth of applications related to health foods received rejection due to non-compliance of raw materials with food safety regulations. Generally, ordinary food ingredients are permitted to be used in the development of health foods. But China has allowed the use of raw materials that have been enlisted in the Chinese database pertaining to food composition, food additives, nutritional fortification substances, and certain pharmaceuticals listed in China Pharmacopoeia.

Currently, there is no authorized synchronized description or coordination of the technological requirements and course of action for functional foods in Asia. Researchers and food industries usually recognize functional foods to incorporate or to be fortified with nutrients or other active components that assist in maintaining good health. These foods in Asia are regulated as per the conformist food classification with two basic claims, such as nutrient content claims stating the amount of certain nutrients on the product label and comparative nutrient claims describing nutritive value proportionate to other analogous foods. Besides, disease risk reduction claims recognized by the Codex Alimentarius are usually not endorsed in Asia. Nevertheless, northern Asian countries use these claims as they have a set-up of functional food regulations. Still, the regulatory environment for health claims is at the embryonic stage, and noteworthy changes are expected in the near future.

### 14.2.8 Africa

In Africa, nutraceuticals describe the use of complete or fragmented plants, plant foods, algae, lichens, and botanical preparations. Basically, these foods in Africa have grown contrary to a range of ecological and cultural segments. Thus, it is significant to describe and execute thorough standardized measures, quality control, and assurance systems. The assessment of these products and guaranteeing their safe and proficient use through documentation and food regulation is not an easy task. The legal position regarding Nfx and phytochemicals differs from nation to nation. Most African countries have not formulated any regulation or registration system to recognize herbal medicines. On the other hand, countries that have given some kind of recognition lack budgeting to assist the proper functioning of the regulatory system. Moreover, another aspect of conventional medicine communities is that they do not operate under the country's legislation structure for assortment and their business in wild species (Sharma et al. 2011). Though herbal preparations are commonly used in the African population, still many countries do not have a set-up to register these formulations. In view of that, WHO has designed several standard courses of action, including general regulations and laws to augment the registration, advertising, and delivery of conventional medicine formulations of guaranteed value in the WHO African region (Sharma et al. 2011).

The modifications in dietary patterns for an improvement in health and any disease condition have resulted in an immense interest from researchers and health organizations during current times. The demand for nutraceuticals and functional foods is burgeoning in developed and developing countries (Verbeke 2005). A similar trend is happening in Africa with respect to health and nutrition claims related to food packaging. As discussed above, functional foods and nutraceuticals are termed traditional foods, dietary supplements, foods for special dietary use, and medical foods or drugs in the regulatory systems of Asia, Canada, Europe, and the United States. But the African regulatory system pertinent to nutraceuticals is still in an embryonic state which seeks authorized essential steps for the development of reliable legislation.

### 14.3 CODEX: AN INTERNATIONAL REGULATORY SYSTEM

In 1962, FAO and WHO unanimously created uniform Rome-based health food standards and named it as Codex Alimentarius (food code) Commission (Codex). Codex aimed at motivating sound international trade while designing an international mechanism for the encouragement of health and monetary gains of end users. Codex is the biggest organization in the world of health food standards, comprising more than 150 member countries and global institutes that unite and share ideas as well as information pertaining to the food industry and safety issues (Winickoff and Bushey 2009). According to the FAO, Codex members correspond to 98% of the world's population and are also members of the FAO and WHO. In simple words, the Codex Alimentarius is an anthology of principles, guidelines, codes of practice, and other proposals or recommendations. Few of these are generalized, and few are specified. Some manage all-inclusive requirements associated with food or food groups, and others handle the function and running of manufacturing procedures or the administrative process of regulatory arrangements for food quality as well as the security of end users.

Worldwide, the food code or codex has to be an indicator for end users, food manufacturers and processors, food regulations, and business. Not only has the codex posed a massive impact on the manufacturer's vision but also the consciousness of the consumers. Its impact has been extended to each and every continent, and its gigantic involvement in public health security and realistic customs in the food industry or trade is evident. This food code provides an exclusive platform for all nations to come together under one umbrella at an international level so as to formulate and harmonize food standards and to ensure their implementation at the global level. It also accommodates them to encompass a responsibility in the improvisation of codes related to hygienic manufacturing or processing procedures and recommendations with reference to conformity with those standards. The implication of the food code for consumer security in terms of their health was emphasized in 1985 by the UN Resolution 39/248, wherein guiding principles had been employed to intensify and strengthen strategies related to the protection of end users.

At present, the codex contains more than 200 standards, covering different areas of concern such as food labeling, food additives, analytical methodologies, and sampling procedures, food certification and inspection during import and export, residues and contaminants in foods. Codex also takes care of foods for special dietary uses, including dietary supplements. In this regard, the Commission for Nutrition and Foods for Special Dietary Uses (CNFSDU) of Codex has formulated the subsequent responsibilities to:

1. Study explicit nutrition-related problems allotted by the Commission and give recommendations to the Commission on common nutrition issues.

2. Frame general necessities, as suitable, relating to the nutritional facets of all foods.

3. Formulate standards, principles, or relevant text for foods for special dietary uses, in coordination with other working groups where it is needed.

4. Think about, improve if required, and support necessities on nutrition-related aspects projected for the inclusion of Codex standards and associated documents.

It does not deal with herbals, amino acids, metabolites, concentrates, and several other non-essential nutrients. In the early 1990s, the Codex Committee on Nutrition and Foods for Special Dietary Uses (CCNFSDU) initiated the debate on strategies for micronutrient supplements. Later on, the Committee concluded work on outlining the principles and guidelines for micronutrient food Supplements and submitted them to the Codex Alimentarius Commission (CAC) for its adoption. The guidelines are relevant to supplements that include micronutrients, where these commodities are recognized as foods. The guidelines deal with the safety, wholesomeness, composition, and bioavailability of the sources of micronutrients. The guidelines also do not denote upper limits in these supplements but offer standards for ascertaining the maximum quantity of micronutrients per portion of supplement consumed daily, as suggested by the company. The criterion indicates that large amounts ought to be adapted, taking into consideration the systematic risk assessment based on, by and large, acknowledged scientific data and also taking into account the varying degrees of the suitability of diverse communities. The guidelines also take care of the packaging and labeling of dietary supplements (Boutrif 2003).

## 14.4 INTERNATIONAL ALLIANCE OF DIETARY FOOD SUPPLEMENT ASSOCIATIONS

The International Alliance of Dietary Food Supplement Associations (IADSA) was conceptualized in 1998. Since its conception, IADSA has expanded over six continents through partnerships with more than 50 dietary supplement alliances. Currently, more than 9500 companies have become members of IADSA. The efficiency of IADSA as an association is rooted in its capability to disseminate information and ideas throughout the world. IADSA covers food regulators, scientific organizations, national organizations, consumer associations, and food companies. During a workshop held in Japan in 2007 (Richardon and Group 2007), drafts on food regulations to be implemented for food products throughout the world and their prospects for application and benefits of functional foods were shared. The major activities of IADSA were announced in the presence of 300 delegates representing different nations. These are:

1. To provide a swift stream of dogmatic and strategy statistics on dietary supplements so as to ensure that there is consciousness and perception of innovative expansions.

2. To coordinate policy and course of action on regulatory concerns worldwide, specifically relative to Codex on micronutrient supplements, food additives, and health claims.

3. To broaden as well as intensify the systems of alliances worldwide by serving the development of new companies or organizations dealing in dietary supplements and endorsing existing alliances.

4. To organize international and provincial events to endorse conversations on the technical and regulatory issues behind the global market of dietary supplement.

Resolutions and strategies framed by international regulatory bodies such as CODEX, FAO, and WHO have become progressively more authoritative for the companies involved in the business of functional foods, nutraceuticals, and dietary supplements. And IADSA works closely with these global bodies to make sure that the observations of the health industry are taken into consideration in policymaking.

## 14.5 CONCLUSION

Nutraceutical regulatory system is evolving a little slowly in comparison to the increasing number of products that are available in the market across the world. The FDA in the United States focuses on the safety aspects and food supplements, recognizes the term nutraceutical, and implements a different set of regulations in contrast with traditional foods and drugs. In Canada, nutraceuticals are acknowledged as more of a drug than a food product. Other countries have definite legislation; for instance, Indian legislation does not attribute any precise legal status to nutraceuticals. The government of India established FSSA in 2006 to initiate a legislation system. FSSA does not distinguish dietary supplements, nutraceuticals, and functional foods, but rather each is described as a food for a special dietary application. Japan is among the first countries to face the regulating matter with regard to food supplements and foodstuffs by issuing the Foods for Specified Health Use (FOSHU). Generally, many countries, such as China, control nutraceuticals merely as a food category, and the national regulations applicable for food apply. Also, countries like Brazil and China have strict requisites, and an inclusive animal or human clinical trial is required before registration. Based on this information, it is predictable that a safety measurement and complete clinical study may be obligatory before any nutraceutical is launched in the market. Moreover, a health claim should be endorsed and credited only after a complete clinical trial is projected to the appropriate authority for authorization to validate its efficacy and safety with regard to the claimed health effect based on perceptive of the mechanism of action and nonexistence of unwanted side effects.

## REFERENCES

Alam, M. R., A. B. Rahman, M. Moniruzzaman, M. F. Kadir, M. A, Haque, M. R. U. H. Alvi, and M. Ratan. 2012. "Evaluation of antidiabetic phytochemicals in *Syzygium cumini* (L.) Skeels (Family: Myrtaceae)". *Journal of Applied Pharmaceutical Science* 2: 94–98.

Alam, M. A., N. Subhan, M. M. Rahman, S. J. Uddin, H. M. Reza, and S. D. Sarker. 2014. "Effect of citrus flavonoids, naringin and naringenin, on metabolic syndrome and their mechanisms of action". *Advances in Nutrition* 5: 404–417.

Amagase, H., and N. R. Farnsworth. 2011. "A review of botanical characteristics, phytochemistry, clinical relevance in efficacy and safety of *Lycium barbarum* fruit (goji)". *Food Research International* 44: 1702–1717.

Bagchi, D. 2014. *Neutraceutical and Functional Food Regulations in the United States and around the World*. Academic Press, USA.

Bakowska-Barczak, A. M, and P. Kolodziejczyk. 2008. "Evaluation of Saskatoon berry (*Amelanchier alnifolia* Nutt.) cultivars for their polyphenol content, antioxidant properties, and storage stability". *Journal of Agricultural and Food Chemistry* 56: 9933–9940.

Bakowska-Barczak, A. M., M. Marianchuk, and P. Kolodziejczyk. 2007. "Survey of bioactive components in Western Canadian berries". *Canadian Journal of Physiology and Pharmacology* 85: 1139–1152.

Belkhir, M., O. Rebai, K. Dhaouadi, F. Congiu, C. I. G Tuberoso, M. Amri, and S. Fattouch. 2013. "Comparative analysis of Tunisian wild *Crataegus azarolus* (yellow azarole) and *Crataegus monogyna* (red azarole) leaf, fruit, and traditionally derived syrup: Phenolic profiles and antioxidant and antimicrobial activities of the aqueous-acetone extracts". *Journal of Agricultural and Food Chemistry* 61: 9594–9601.

Bertuccelli, G., N. Zerbinati, M. Marcellino, N. S. N. Kumar, F. He, V. Tsepakolenko, J. Cervi, A. Lorenzetti, and F. Marotta. 2016. "Effect of a quality-controlled fermented nutraceutical on skin aging markers: An antioxidant-control, double-blind study". *Experimental and Therapeutic Medicine* 11: 909–916.

Boutrif, E. 2003. "The new role of Codex Alimentarius in the context of WTO/ SPS agreement". *Food Control* 14: 81–88.

Brendler, T., L. D. Phillips, and S. Spiess. 2009. *A Practical Guide to Licensing Herbal Medicinal Products*. Pharmaceutical Press.

Brillat-Savarin, J. A. 1862. *"Physiologie du gout"*. *Librairie des Bibliophiles*, u. Trykkeaar.

Brower, V. 1998. "Nutraceuticals: Poised for healthy slice of healthcare market?" *Nature Biotechnology* 16: 728–731.

Burdock, G. A., I. G. Carabin, and J. C. Griffiths. 2006. "The importance of GRAS to the functional food and nutraceutical industries". *Toxicology* 221: 17–27.

Calin-Sanchez, A., J. Martinez-Nicolas, S. Munera-Picazo, A. Carbonell-Barrachina, P. Legua, and F. Hernandez. 2013. "Bioactive compounds and sensory quality of black and white mulberries grown in Spain". *Plant Foods for Human Nutrition* 68: 370–377.

Choi, Y. M., S. H. Bae, D. H. Kang, and H. J. Suh. 2006. "Hypolipidemic effect of lactobacillus ferment as a functional food supplement". *Phytotherapy Research* 20:1056–1060.

Coothankandaswamy, V., Y. Liu, S. C. Mao, J. B. Morgan, F. Mandi, M. B. Jekabsons, D. G. Nagle, and Y. D. Zhou. 2010. "The alternative medicine pawpaw and its acetogenin constituents suppress tumor angiogenesis via the HIF-1/ VEGF pathway". *Journal of Natural Products* 73: 956–961.

Donno, D., M. G. Mellano, E. Raimondo, A. K. Cerutti, Z. Prgomet, and G. L. Beccaro. 2016. "Influence of applied drying methods on phytochemical composition in fresh and dried goji fruits by HPLC fingerprint". *European Food Research and Technology* 242: 1961–1974.

European Commission. 2008. Proposal for a Regulation of the European Parliament and of the Council on the provision of Food Information to Consumers. COM (2008), Brussels of 30.01.08, 2008/028 (CODE).

FDA. 2003. "Consumer Health Information for Better Nutrition Initiative". Task Force Final Report.

FICCI. 2007. Study on Implementation of Food Safety and Standard Act 2006: An Industry Perspective.

FOSHU. 1991. The FOSHU System. Nutrition Improvement Law Enforcement Regulation Ministerial Ordinance No. 41; July 1991. https://www.researchgate. net/publication/296377503

Han, B., T. D. Wang, S. M. Shen, Y. Yu, C. Mao, Z. J. Yao, and L. S. Wang. 2015. "Annonaceous acetogenin mimic AA005 induces cancer cell death via apoptosis inducing factor through a caspase-3-independent mechanism". *BMC Cancer* 15: 1–11.

Hardy, G. 2000. "Nutraceutical and functional food: Introduction and meaning". *Nutrition* 16: 688–689.

Hayamizu, K., Y. Ishii, I. Kaneko, M. Shen, Y. Okuhara, N. Shigematsu, H. Tomi, M. Furuse, G. Yoshino, and H. Shimasaki. 2003. "Effects of *Garcinia cambogia* (hydroxycitric acid) on visceral fat accumulation: A doubleblind, randomized, placebo-controlled trial". *Current Therapeutic Research – Clinical and Experimental* 23: 551–567.

Health Canada 1998. Nutraceuticals/Functional Foods and Health Claims on Foods: Policy Paper. [Health Canada, 1998]. Hc-sc.gc.ca. https://www.canada.ca/en/health-canada/services/food-nutrition/food-labelling/health-claims/nutraceuticals-functional-foods-health-claims-foods-policy-paper.html (Retrieved on 6 March 2011).

Health Canada 2012. A new approach to natural health products.

Hyson, D. A. 2011. "A comprehensive review of apples and apple components and their relationship to human health". *Advances in Nutrition* 2: 408–420.

Joseph, B., and M. Priya. 2011. "Phytochemical and biopharmaceutical aspects of *Psidium guajava* (L.) essential oil: A review". *Research Journal of Medicinal Plants* 5.

Juríková, T., S. Balla, J. Sochor, M. Pohanka, J. Mlcek, and M. Baron. 2013. "Flavonoid profile of saskatoon berries (*Amelanchier alnifolia* Nutt.) and their health promoting effects". *Molecules* 18: 12571–12586.

Kalra, E. K. 2003. "Nutraceutical: Definition & introduction". *AAPS PharmSci* 5: Article 25. doi:10.1208/PS/0500225.

Kanazawa, K., and H. Sakakibara. 2000. "High content of dopamine, a strong antioxidant, in Cavendish banana". *Journal of Agricultural and Food Chemistry* 48: 844–848.

Keservani, R. K., and A. K. Sharma. 2015. Ch19: Nutraceutical and Functional Food Regulations in India.

Kobayashi, H., C. Z. Wang, and K. W. Pomper. 2008. "Phenolic content and antioxidant capacity of pawpaw fruit *(Asimina triloba* L.) at different ripening stages". *Hortscience* 43: 268–270.

Li, J., and D. Li. 2011. "Current status of Chinese legal system and standard system for health food". *Food Science* 32: 318–323.

Manosroi, A., C. Chankhampan, K. Pattamapun, and K. Pattamapun. 2014. "Antioxidant and gelatinolytic activities of papain from papaya latex and bromelain from pineapple fruits". *Chiang Mai Journal of Science* 41: 635–648.

Milner, J. A. 2002. "Functional foods and health: A US perspective". *British Journal of Nutrition* 88 (Supplement 2): S15–S18.

Ministry of Agriculture, Fisheries and Food (MAFF). 1995. Food standards and labelling division discussion paper on functional foods and health claims. MAFF Publication, August 1995. https://food.ec.europa.eu/system/files/2016-10/labelling_nutrition-claims-consumer_group-fl_com9158_en.pdf

Morton, F. J. 1987. *Fruits of Warm Climates*, 301–304. Purdue University.

Muruganandan, S., K. Srinivasan, S. Gupta, P. K. Gupta, and J. Lal. 2005. "Effect of mangiferin on hyperglycemia and atherogenicity in streptozotocin diabetic rats". *Journal of Ethnopharmacology* 97: 497–500.

Nestmann, E. R., M. Harwood, and S. Martyres. 2006. "An innovative model for regulating supplement products: Natural health products in Canada". *Toxicology* 221:50–58.

Office of Inspector General. 2003. "Dietary Supplement Labels: Key Elements" (PDF). U.S. Department of Health and Human Services.

Olmedilla-Alonso, B., F. Granado-Lorencio, C. Herrero-Barbudo, and I. Blanco-Navarro. 2006. "Nutritional approach for designing meat-based functional food products with nuts". *Critical Reviews in Food Science and Nutrition* 46: 537–542.

Ozga, J. A., A. Saeed, W. Wismer, and D. M. Reinecke. 2007. "Characterization of cyanidin-and quercetin-derived flavonoids and other phenolics in mature saskatoon fruits (*Amelanchier alnifolia* Nutt.)". *Journal of Agricultural and Food Chemistry* 55: 10414–10424

Pavan, R., S. Jain, Shraddha, and A. Kumar. 2012. "Properties and therapeutic application of bromelain: A review". *Biotechnology Research International* 2012: 976203

Richardon, D. P., and I. S. Group. 2007. "Nutrition, health ageing and public policy". *Brussels: International Alliance of Dietary Food Supplement Associations (IADSA)*: 1–71

Russo, M., A. Arigò, M. L. Calabrò, S. Farnetti, L. Mondello, and P. Dugo. 2016. "Bergamot (*Citrus bergamia* Risso) as a source of nutraceuticals: Limonoids and flavonoids". *Journal of Functional Foods* 20: 10–19.

Sánchez-Salcedo, E. M., P. Mena, C. García-Viguera, J. J. Martínez, and F. Hernández. 2015. "Phytochemical evaluation of white (*Morus alba* L.) and black (*Morus nigra* L.) mulberry fruits, a starting point for the assessment of their beneficial properties". *Journal of Functional Foods* 12: 399–408.

SFDA 2005. Interim Administrative Measures of Health Food Registration - Decree No.19, 2005.

Sharma, S., M. Patel, M. M. Bhunch, M. Chatterjee, and S. Shrivastava. 2011. "Regulatory status of traditional medicines in Africa region". *International Journal of Research in Ayurveda and Pharmacy* 2:103–110.

Sieber, C. C. 2007. "Functional food in elderly persons". *TherapeutischeUmschau* 64: 141–146.

Stoilova, I., S. Gargova, A. Stoyanova, and L. Ho. 2005. "Antimicrobial and antioxidant activity of the polyphenol mangiferin". *Herba Polonica* 51: 37–44.

Tovey, F. I., and M. Hobsley. 2004. "Milling of wheat, maize and rice: Effects on fibre and lipid content and health". *World Journal of Gastroenterology* 10: 1695–1696.

Tutelyan, V., and B. Sukhanov. 2008. "Biologically active food supplements: Modern approaches to quality and safety assurance". *VoprPitaniya* 77: 4–15.

Verbeke, W. 2005. "Consumer acceptance of functional foods: Socio-demographic, cognitive and attitudinal determinants". *Food Quality and Preference* 16: 45–57.

Walia, M., S. Kumar, and V. K. Agnihotria. 2016. "UPLC-PDA quantification of chemical constituents of two different varieties (golden and royal) of apple leaves and their antioxidant activity". *Journal of the Science of Food and Agriculture* 96: 1440–1450.

Weng, K. K. 2010. "Lycopene content and antioxidant properties of pink guava industry by-products". Master of Science thesis submitted to Universiti Putra Malaysia, Malaysia.

Winickoff, D. E., and D. M. Bushey. 2009. "Science and power in global food regulation: The rise of the Codex Alimentarius". *Science, Technology & Human Value* 35: 356–381.

Yang, Y. 2008. "Scientific substantiation of functional food health claims in China". *Journal of Nutrition* 138: 1199S–1205S.

# 15 Summary of Natural Products in the Nutraceutical Industry

*Bharti Mittu, Renu Sharma, Abida Bhat, Mahaldeep Kaur, and Sandaldeep Kaur*

## CONTENTS

## 15.1 INTRODUCTION

The nutraceutical industry first emerged in the early 1990s. The annual average growth rate of 7.3% of the nutraceutical industry between 1999 and 2002, the growth rate of this industry has been explosive in the past few years, which has doubled to 14.7%. The primary stimulus for the drastic growth of the nutraceutical industry is consumer demand. The global nutraceutical market has an approximate worth of USD 117 billion. Some of the fundamental strategies of the modern nutraceutical industry, therefore, involve enhancing the investment in research and development projects to find innovative ways towards nutraceutical, validating health

DOI: 10.1201/9781003259213-15

claims of the products and market research. Consumers are willing to follow healthy lifestyles and obtain sufficient nutrition to avoid diseases such as diabetes, high blood pressure, cancer, and obesity. Currently, the world's largest nutraceutical markets are the United States, European Union, and India, and China is likely to join the race by 2030. Nutraceutical food supplements are considered beneficial for human health as they provide the necessary elements for fighting diseases. Stephen De Felipe coined this term in 1989 and defined it as food or part of food with health benefits. The Nutraceutical market provides a wide range of products, such as vitamins, antioxidants, herbs, seeds, prebiotics, and many more. Consumption of these foods is increasing in developed cities/countries to fulfill nutrient requirements. Advancements in modern biotechnology techniques have successfully developed genetically modified microorganisms/plants that produce valuable natural substances such as prebiotics, insulin, chondroitin sulfate, etc. Nutraceuticals fall into many categories, which include nutrients, probiotics, herbals, phytochemicals, prebiotics, dietary fiber, and enzymes. Many scientific studies have supported the fact that these nutraceutical components improve the body's immune system for defending against pathogens. These studies have also shown promising outcomes with the use of nutraceuticals in treating chronic diseases such as diabetes, hypertension, neurodegeneration, and cancer with minimum side effects. Fruits have a special space in the nutraceutical industry. Most fruits contain beneficial compounds like polyphenolic components that can promote antioxidant, anti-inflammatory, antibacterial, antifungal, and chemopreventive effects. Xanthones, carotenoids, and saponins also exhibit beneficial health effects. This chapter discusses the various nutraceutical natural products in detail with their functional aspects on human health.

### 15.1.1 Nutraceuticals

A dietary supplement is a product that is intended to supplement the diet that bears or contains one or more ingredients like vitamin, mineral, herb, amino acid or a concentrate, metabolite, constituent, extract, or combinations of these. India's nutraceutical industry is growing at a fast speed, predicted to grow exponentially, and expected to hold at least 3.5% of the global market share by 2023. Fruits are the cheapest and most common source of nutrients, *viz.* carbohydrates, proteins, vitamins, minerals, and essential amino acids (Bumgarner 2012; Murphy et al. 2012). Apart from that, they can also be helpful in treating various diseases (Mahima et al. 2012). Fruits vary in their composition, and a variety of colorful fruits and vegetables gives your body a wide range of nutrients/ phytochemicals that are important for good health. A fruit consumed in our daily diet is associated with reduced risk of cancers, and additive/ synergistic effects of phytochemicals in fruits are responsible for their potent antioxidant and anticancer activities.

Nutrients are broadly categorized into two types, namely, macronutrients and micronutrients. Macronutrients are nutrients required by the body in huge quantities, whereas micronutrients are nutrients that are required by the body in lesser quantities. Examples of macronutrients include lipids, proteins, and carbohydrates that the body requires to carry out various functions, such as metabolic and structural activities. Micronutrients (vitamins and minerals are required for the appropriate functioning of the body (Akram et al. 2020; Derbyshire 2018). For example, micronutrients are required for the proper formation and growth of the fetus, even during intrauterine life. Deficiencies of vitamin D, iron, iodine, and folic acid resulted in congenital disorders or even death. Previous studies reported the daily-required allowance of various vitamins and minerals, but the requirements of micronutrients are not fixed. Physical activity, childhood, adolescence, old age, pregnancy, and specific diets (e.g., vegan) are the factors that influence the need for micronutrients. As a result, assessing micronutrient necessities and the consequences of micronutrient deficits is critical in explaining their role in health and disease (Hans and Jana 2018).

## 15.2 VITAMINS

Vitamins are mainly present in natural foods and are essential for the body's regular growth, development, and maintenance. These are organic compounds, and the term vitamin is derived from the Latin words "vita" and "amine", which mean "life" and "nitrogen", respectively. Vitamins act as a catalyst in the proper utilization of carbohydrates and fats and help in the production of energy. Vitamins are necessary for the survival of humans, but the human body cannot produce a majority of them. Meat, fruits, and leafy vegetables are excellent sources of vitamins (Schaefer 2014).Vitamins contribute a major part to the nutraceutical industry. Among nutraceuticals, Vitamin D, Vitamin C, and Zinc are on the top of the list since they help manage Covid-19 and prevent severe infection. According to the All India Organization of Chemists and Druggists (AIOCD)—AWACS report, Indians bought almost Rs 15,000 crore worth of vitamin supplements.

### 15.2.1 Types of Vitamins

Vitamins are necessary for the proper functioning and development of the human body. There are two types of vitamins: Fat-soluble vitamins (A, C, D, E, and K) and water-soluble vitamins (Vitamin B complex; thiamine (B1), riboflavin (B2), niacin (B3), pantothenic acid (B5), pyridoxine (B6), cyanocobalamin (B12), biotin, and folate/folic acid, and vitamin C as mentioned in Table 15.1 and Figure 15.1 (Akram et al. 2020).

### 15.2.2 Fat-Soluble Vitamins

The fat-soluble vitamins (A, D, E, and K) can dissolve in fats and oils. These vitamins are absorbed along with fats upon consumption of diet and can be stored in the fatty tissues of the body. Plant and animal foods, as well

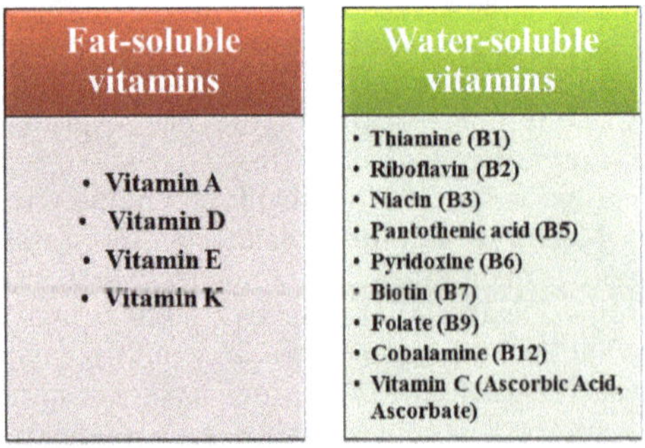

| Fat-soluble vitamins | Water-soluble vitamins |
|---|---|
| • Vitamin A<br>• Vitamin D<br>• Vitamin E<br>• Vitamin K | • Thiamine (B1)<br>• Riboflavin (B2)<br>• Niacin (B3)<br>• Pantothenic acid (B5)<br>• Pyridoxine (B6)<br>• Biotin (B7)<br>• Folate (B9)<br>• Cobalamine (B12)<br>• Vitamin C (Ascorbic Acid, Ascorbate) |

**Figure 15.1** Types of vitamins. (From Akram et al. 2020.)

**Table 15.1: Types, Functions, Sources, and Deficiencies of Vitamins**

| Vitamins | Functions | Food Sources | Deficiency Disease | References |
|---|---|---|---|---|
| Vitamin A (retinol) | • Aids in vision<br>• Growth and development. Proper functioning of immune system and reproduction<br>• Formation of red blood cells and skin | Green leafy vegetables (tomatoes, carrots, broccoli)<br>Fruits (guava, watermelon, mangoes, and oranges), milk and nuts, and fish liver oils | • Impairment of vision<br>• Bitot's spots<br>• Xerophthalmia<br>• Keratomalacia<br>• Anorexia follicular hyperkeratosis<br>• Retardation of growth<br>• Infection of the respiratory and intestinal system<br>• Myelin sheaths started degenerating | Akram et al. (2020) |
| Vitamin D<br>*Active form:*<br>1,25-dihydroxyvitamin D) | • Helps in contraction of nerves<br>• Proper functioning of all the body cells<br>• Helps in the absorption of calcium, thereby maintaining bone and muscle health | Salmon, cheese, cereals, milk, egg yolk, and fortified milk are the source of the preformed vitamin D. 7-Dehydrocholesterol is the precursor of this vitamin, made in the skin after exposure to sunlight | • Rickets and fragile bones<br>• Osteomalacia<br>• Skeletal deformities | Bleizgys (2021) |
| Vitamin E (α-tocopherol) | • Antioxidant<br>• Blood vessels formation<br>• Boost the immune function | Nuts (almonds, peanuts, and hazelnuts) and vegetable oils (sunflower, wheat germ, safflower, corn, and soybean oils)<br>Green, leafy vegetables (spinach and broccoli) | • Cystic fibrosis<br>• Ataxia<br>• Abetalipoproteinemia<br>• Hemolysis of RBCs and resulted in macrocytic anemia in premature infants | Ungurianu et al. (2021) |
| Vitamin K<br>K1 (phylloquinone)<br>K2 (menaquinone) | • Helps in clot formation<br>• Proper functioning of several proteins involved in various physiological processes | Green vegetables (spinach, broccoli)<br>Vegetable oils (soybean, rapeseed, and olive), peanut, corn, sunflower, and safflower<br>Animal liver, fermented foods (cheese, soybean (Japanese natto) | • Generalized bleeding<br>• Hemorrhagic condition of the newborn<br>• Clotting time is prolonged in adults | Akram et al. (2020)<br>Akram et al. (2020) |

*(Continued)*

**Table 15.1: Types, Functions, Sources, and Deficiencies of Vitamins (Continued)**

| Vitamins | Functions | Food Sources | Deficiency Disease | References |
|---|---|---|---|---|
| B1 (thiamine) | • Key role in cerebral metabolism<br>• Cofactor for enzymes involved in energy metabolism | Beef, liver, seeds, dried milk, oats, pork nuts, oranges, eggs, legumes, and yeast | Beriberi (dry, wet and infantile) | Gibson et al. (2016) |
| B2 (riboflavin) | • Conversion of carbohydrates into glucose for the production of energy<br>• Antioxidant (neutralizes free radicals) | Plant foods and animal sources (poultry, meat, fish, and dairy products such as milk, eggs, and cheese)<br>Green vegetables (turnips, collard greens) | • Ariboflavinosis (desquamation around mouth skin mouth)<br>• Glossitis (sparkly red and sore tongue)<br>• Eye disturbances<br>• Soreness of lips<br>• Photophobia (light sensibility)<br>• Scrotal dermatitis | Buehler (2011) |
| B3 (niacin) | • Helps in lowering LDL cholesterol<br>• Reduces the risk of cardiovascular diseases<br>• Eases arthritis | Animal sources (lean red meat, poultry, butter, and liver), whole grain cereals, maize, bread tea, coffee | Pellagra | Shah et al. (2013) |
| B5 (pantothenic acid) | • Component of CoA<br>• Transports acyl groups for enzymatic processes | Peanut butter, liver, kidney, almonds, wheat bran, cheese and lobster | • Dermatological conditions (alopecia, dermatitis) or adrenal insufficiency<br>• Enteritis | Tardy et al. (2020) |
| B6 (pyridoxine) | Co-factor for various biochemical reactions that regulate cellular metabolism | Fish, beef liver and other organ meats, starchy vegetables, fruits potatoes | • Seborrheicdermatitis<br>• Peripheral neuropathy<br>• Glossitis<br>• Cheilosis<br>• Depression, confusion, and seizure in adults | Stach et al. (2021) |

*(Continued)*

**Table 15.1: Types, Functions, Sources, and Deficiencies of Vitamins (Continued)**

| Vitamins | Functions | Food Sources | Deficiency Disease | References |
|---|---|---|---|---|
| B7 (biotin) | • Converts food into glucose for energy production<br>• Production of fatty acids and amino acids (the building blocks of protein)<br>• Aids in the stimulation of protein/amino acid metabolism in the hair roots and fingernail cells | Egg yolk, mushroom, almonds, sweet potatoes, cheese, spinach, cauliflower | Unknown | Lipner (2018) |
| B9 (folate) | • Replication of DNA<br>• Breakdown of vitamins and amino acids<br>• Reduces spinal bifida (neural tube defects) in neonates taken by pregnant mothers | Dark green leafy vegetables (spinach), liver, pear, avocado, orange paw-paw fruits, beans and nuts | • Defects in the neural tube<br>• Pregnant women receive supplements of folate as a preventive method<br>• Causes megaloblastic anemia, a type of macrocytic anemia | Sobczyńsk-Malefora and Harrington (2018) |
| Vitamin B12 (cyanocobalamin) | • Cellular metabolism<br>• Synthesis of DNA<br>• Methylation and metabolism of mitochondria<br>• Functioning of brain and synthesis of RBCs | Meat (especially liver and shellfish), milk products, and eggs | • Myelin damage<br>• Neurological disorders (ataxia, neuropathy)<br>• Megaloblastic anemia<br>• Dementia (neuropsychiatric symptoms) | Oh et al. (2021) |
| C (ascorbic acid) | • Antioxidant property, cardiovascular diseases, common cold, age-related muscular degeneration, helps in enzyme activation, and immune function and cataract | Fresh fruits and vegetables, gooseberry, citrus fruits (limes, oranges, and lemons), tomatoes, green and red peppers, potatoes, papaya, kiwi, strawberries and cantaloupes, green leafy vegetables (broccoli, fortified cereals and its juices). Animal source (liver part) | • Scurvy (produced collagen is not stable)<br>• Joint swelling, muscle pain, and bleeding | Mittu et al. (2022) |

as nutritional supplements, are the primary sources of these vitamins. These vitamins are critical for the proper working of the body. Deficiencies associated with these vitamins have been linked to various disorders or health problems. The RDAs (Recommended Daily Allowance) for the fat-soluble vitamins A, D, E, and K are 8000–1000, 8000–5000, 8–10, and 70–140 g/day, respectively (Rafeeq et al. 2020).

### 15.2.3 Water-Soluble Vitamins

The water-soluble vitamins such as Vitamin B and C dissolve easily in water and are absorbed by the body very quickly. These vitamins are transported to various tissues but are not stored by the body. Meat, eggs, milk, legumes, cereal grains, poultry, fish, and fresh vegetables are excellent sources of vitamin B-complex. The source of vitamin C includes citrus fruits, strawberries, peppers, kiwis, and broccoli. However, the RDA of these vitamins includes thiamin (1 mg/day), riboflavin (1.2 mg/day), pyridoxine (2–2.2 mg/day), niacin (13 milli-equivalents), biotin (100–200 µg/day), ascorbic acid (60 µg/day), and pantothenic acid (4–7 mg/day) (Akram et al. 2020).

### 15.2.4 List of Vitamins and Their Functions

Table 15.1 highlights the significance, sources, and deficiency associated with the vitamins.

### 15.3 MINERALS

Minerals are inorganic elements that the body cannot synthesize and must be obtained through diet. They occur naturally in soil and water. Some are necessary for living organisms, while others are extremely toxic. Plants absorb a large amount of minerals from the environment, which are usually passed through the food chain to the animals. A lack of such nutritionally important minerals is usually fatal. Minerals are essential components of the human body. They are required for the formation and function of vital biomolecules in the human body. Although minerals are not a source of energy in the body, they are required for the normal functioning of biochemical processes. These essential minerals are classified as either macro or micro (trace) minerals based on the requirements of the body (Akram et al. 2020).

### 15.3.1 Types of Minerals

Two kinds of minerals are known, including macrominerals and trace minerals. Table 15.2 enlists the functions, sources, and deficiencies associated with the minerals.

1. Minerals like sodium, calcium, phosphorus, magnesium, and potassium are examples of macro minerals. The average requirement of these macronutrients in adults is more than 100 mg/day (Prashanth et al. 2015).

2. Trace elements are minerals that are required in small amounts for daily metabolic processes in the human body. The average requirement of these minerals in adults is less than 100 mg/day. However, a lack of any trace elements resulted in serious health-related issues. Iron, copper, zinc, iodine, manganese, and other trace minerals are a few such examples (Prashanth et al. 2015).

**Table 15.2: List of Minerals and Their Functions**

| Minerals | Function of Minerals | Sources | Deficiency Disease | References |
|---|---|---|---|---|
| Calcium | Essential for the immune system for healthier bones and teeth | Soybeans, egg, milk, blackberries, wheat Dates, almonds, pomegranate, and sesame seeds | • Bones become brittle<br>• Osteoporosis<br>• Hypocalcemia<br>• Cataracts<br>• Brain alterations | Reid et al. (2015) |
| Sodium | Regulate blood pressure and blood volume for proper functioning of muscles and nerves | Onions, sweet potato, broccoli, fresh fruits, pumpkin seeds, eggs, and milk | • Seizures<br>• Hypernatremia<br>• Fatigue<br>• Apathy<br>• Coma<br>• Cramps in the muscles | Cogswell et al. (2016) |
| Iodine | • Important for healthy skin, nails, hair, and teeth<br>• Maintains growth and body weight regulation | Food growing in iodine-rich places, seafood, milk, and iodized salt | Goiter and enlargement of the thyroid | Akram et al. (2020) |
| Phosphorus | Bones and teeth formation | Pomegranate, passion fruits, beef Dates, oats, and tuna | • Osteomalacia in adults<br>• Rickets in children<br>• Hypophosphatemia | Arai and Sakuma (2015) |
| Magnesium | • Working of muscles<br>• Helps metabolism and growth of bone | Vegetables (spinach, broccoli, legumes) and sunflower seeds, cashews, seeds, whole-wheat bread, halibut, milk | • Rapid heartbeat<br>• Fatigue<br>• Poor memory<br>• Numbness<br>• Muscle twitching<br>• Tingling<br>• Irritability | Allen and Dror (2018) |

*(Continued)*

**Table 15.2: List of Minerals and Their Functions (Continued)**

| Minerals | Function of Minerals | Sources | Deficiency Disease | References |
|---|---|---|---|---|
| Iron (Fe) | • Supports formation of heme<br>• Transports proteins required for oxygen to RBCs, other enzymes, flavoproteins | Meats, egg yolks, red meat, dried fruits,<br>Legumes, leafy greens, cereals, iron-enriched breads, fish, fortified cereals, shellfish, and poultry | • Weakness, insomnia, tiredness and lethargy, headaches, palpitations, breath shortness, cracked lips, and brittle nails | Akram et al. (2020) |
| Copper (Cu) | • Part of metalloenzymes<br>• Formation of red blood cell and connective tissues | Liver, kidney, shellfish, nuts, and wholegrain cereals. Passing of water (soft or acidic) through copper pipes add Cu to the food | • Dry skin<br>• Hair problems<br>• Anemia<br>• Deficiency of vitamin C | Patil et al. (2013) and Akram et al. (2020) |
| Zinc (Zn) | • Cell-mediated immunity<br>• Formation of bone<br>• Growth of tissue<br>• Functioning of brain<br>• Fetus and child growth | Whole grains, fish meat, oysters, poultry, vegetables | • Loss of taste<br>• Retardation of growth<br>• Slow healing of wounds<br>• Delayed sexual development in children | Bagherani and Smoller (2016) |
| Iodine | • Required for healthy hair, skin, nails, and teeth<br>• Regulates growth and weight of the body | Seafood, iodized salt, food in iodine-rich places, and milk | • Goiter<br>• Enlargement of the thyroid gland | Akram et al. (2020) |
| Selenium | • Antioxidant<br>• Efficient working of the immune system<br>• Inhibited the development of HIV to AIDS<br>• Helps the motility of sperm and reduces miscarriage risk | Cereals, seafood, meats, seafood, grains, vegetables, fruits, and beverages | • Necrosis of muscle<br>• Hemolytic anemia<br>• Cardiomyopathy | Akram et al. (2020) |

*(Continued)*

**Table 15.2: List of Minerals and Their Functions (Continued)**

| Minerals | Function of Minerals | Sources | Deficiency Disease | References |
|---|---|---|---|---|
| Chromium (Cr) | • Antioxidant<br>• Decreases resistance of insulin in diabetic patients | Cheese, brewer's yeast, whole grain breads, pork kidney, cereals spices, molasses, and some bran cereals, beef, eggs, oysters, and turkey | Impacts insulin potency in regulating sugar balance | Tulasi and Rao (2014) |
| Manganese (Mn) | Activates various enzymes (hydrolases, transferases, kinases, decarboxylases), that plays a key role in clotting of blood and hemostasis in conjunction with vitamin K | Oysters, nuts, whole grains, soybeans, mussels, rice, leafy vegetables, legumes, coffee, tea, and spices such as black pepper | • Problems in metabolizing carbohydrates<br>• Nervous irritability<br>• Dermatitis<br>• Poor memory<br>• Heavy menstrual periods<br>• Blood sugar problems<br>• Fragile bones and fatigue | Buchman (2014) |
| Fluoride (F) | Bone and teeth formation, stops dental caries and decay | Drinking water, beverages, fish, oral toothpaste | Teeth and bones become weak | O'Mullane et al. (2016) |
| Molybdenum (Mo) | Act as a cofactor for enzymes xanthine oxidase, aldehyde oxidase, sulfite oxidase and mitochondrial amidoxime | Nuts, legumes; breads and grains; green vegetables leafy, liver, and milk | Unknown | Akram et al. (2020) |

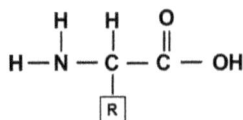

**Figure 15.2**  General structure of amino acid.

## 15.4 AMINO ACIDS

Amino acids are organic acids which humans use as building blocks of protein. Amino acids are organic compounds and the building elements of proteins containing the amino ($NH_2$) and carboxyl (COOH) functional groups and side chain (R or alkyl group) specific to each group of amino acid. Carbon (C), hydrogen (H), oxygen (O), and nitrogen are the four main elements in amino acids. In addition, amino acid side chains are attached to other elements. In general, the molecular formulae of amino acids are $H_2NCHRCOOH$, where 'R' is the side chain (Figure 15.2). The amino acid has a net positive charge at a physiological pH of 7.2–7.4, wherein the amino group is in protonated form. In contrast, the amino acid bears a net negative charge at a physiological pH of 7.2–7.4, wherein the carboxyl group is in deprotonated form. The chemical behavior of an amino acid is characterized by the properties of its side chain (thus classified as acidic, basic, polar, or nonpolar) (Akram et al. 2011; Lopez and Mohiuddin 2020).

Amino acids are of three different types. Nonessential amino acids are made by the body whereas essential amino acids should be taken by a diet with enough essential amino acids. Amino acid supplements contain one or more of the nine essential amino acids which body does not produce on its own. These include Lysine, Leucine, Tryptophan, Histidine, Isoleucine, Methionine, Phenylalanine, Threonine, and Valine. Nutraceutical supplementation with essential amino acids and branched-chain amino acids (BCAAs) regulates metabolism and energy balance. Amino acid supplementation promotes skeletal and cardiac muscle mitochondrial biogenesis, inhibits oxidative damage, increases protein synthesis in muscles and physical endurance, reduces body weight, and enhances immune function. They have a crucial place in the nutraceutical industry (Bifari et al. 2017).

### 15.4.1 General Features of Amino Acids

Amino acids are white, crystalline solids that dissolve in water but are insoluble in solvents such as organic solvents. They have been associated with very high melting and boiling points. They are sweet, tasteless, or have bitter flavor (Lopez and Mohiuddin 2020).

Amino acids are classified as Essential and Non-Essential Amino Acids. Essential amino acids are not formed by the body and are thus obtained by humans and other animals via dietary sources for good health. Examples of essential amino acids include Histidine, Isoleucine, Leucine, Lysine, Methionine, Phenylalanine, Threonine, Tryptophan, and Valine. In contrast, amino acids that are synthesized by the body via various biochemical reactions are called non-essential amino acids. Non-essential amino acids include Alanine, Asparagine, Arginine, Aspartic acid, Cysteine, Glutamic acid, Glutamine, Glycine, Proline, Selenocysteine, Serine, and Tyrosine (Kamble et al. 2021; Lopez and Mohiuddin 2020). Based on R-group chemistry, amino acids are classified into various

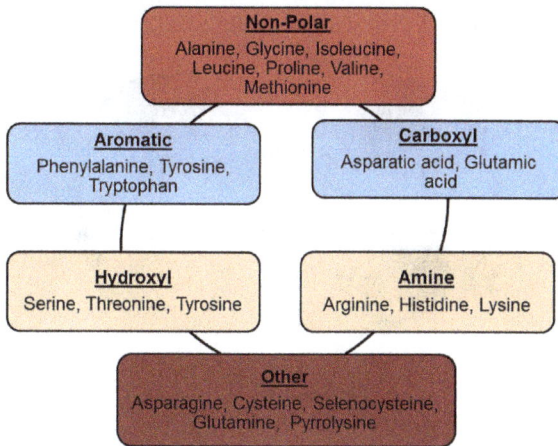

**Figure 15.3** Classification of amino acid on the basis of R-group. (From Kamble et al. 2021.)

groups, namely, Non-Polar, Carboxyl, Amine, Aromatic, Hydroxyl, and others, as mentioned in Figure 15.3.

Various food groups that are a rich source of amino acids are mentioned in Table 15.3. The aforementioned products help in the growth and development of individuals.

### 15.4.2 Functions of Amino Acids

Amino acids play a vital function in the human body. These are associated with various functions such as structural, hormonal, digestive, immune

## Table 15.3: Food Source of Amino Acids

| Food Categories | Food Products |
| --- | --- |
| Meat and its products | Beef, pork, sheep, goat veal, processed red meat products, minced meat, liver, and organ meat |
| Grain products | Bread and rolls, rice, cereal grains, wheat flour, pasta, macaroni, noodles, pizza |
| Milk and dairy products | Whole milk, powdered milk, cheese, yogurt, milkshakes, cottage cheese |
| Seafood | Fresh, chilled, or frozen shellfish, fish and shellfish products |
| Fruits | Apples, bananas, berries, citrus fruits, peaches and nectarines, dry fruits, and nuts |
| Fats and oils | Olive oil, margarine, and plant and animal fats |
| Eggs | Eggs |
| Snacks and sweets | Chocolate, powdered cacao, ice cream, chips, cake, pies, and honey |
| Sugars and salt | Jams, syrup, marmalade, salt |
| Beverages and non-alcoholic | Fruit juices, mixed juices, other non-alcoholic beverages, coffee, tea, beer, wine, cocktails |

*Source:* From Górska-Warsewicz et al. (2018).

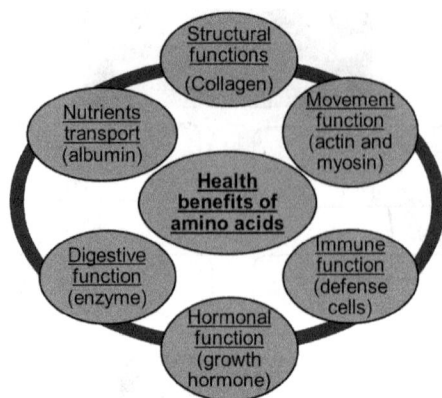

**Figure 15.4** Health benefits of amino acids. (From Lopez and Mohiuddin 2020.)

function, nutrient transport, and movement functions, as mentioned in Figure 15.4 (Kamble et al. 2021; Lopez and Mohiuddin 2020).

### 15.4.3 Deficiencies Related to Amino Acids

As previously stated, amino acids are the building blocks of proteins, and proteins play a critical role in almost all life processes. As a result, it is necessary to include all essential amino acids in our daily diet in order to maintain healthy and proper body functions. Different pathological disorders may occur as a result of amino acid deficiency, some of which are listed in Figure 15.5 (Rose 2019).

A proportional relationship exists between a nutraceutical supplement and a health condition or disease. Arginine supplements (ergogenic) essential amino acid improve human metabolism and physiology in various diseases such as coronary heart disease, hypertension, and myocardial infarction, as mentioned in Table 15.4 (Sharma et al. 2016).

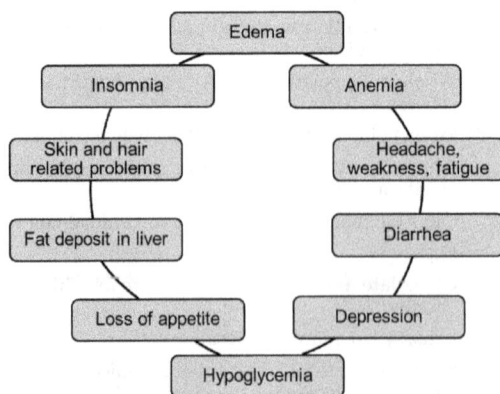

**Figure 15.5** Deficiency diseases due to amino acids. (From Rose 2019.)

## Table 15.4: Various Nutraceutical Amino Acids, Their Sources, and Uses

| # | Nutraceutical Amino Acids | Source | Uses |
|---|---|---|---|
| 1 | Glutamic acid | Protein foods like fish, dairy, eggs, and meat | Anticancer |
| 2 | Tryptophan | Turkey, light meat, wheat bread, sweet chocolate, tryptophan | Mood and depression, smoking cessation |
| 3 | Valine | *Animal origin*: Meat, poultry, fish, dairy, cheese<br>*Plant origin*: Lentils, peanuts, soy, mushrooms, sesame seeds | Muscle metabolism, tissue repair, mental vigor, muscle coordination, calm emotions |
| 4 | Arginine | Seafood | Anti-inflammatory, migraines, phosphorus helps calcium build bones and teeth |
| 5 | Arginine | Wheat flour, whole-grain | Breast cancer. heart disease, promote health |
| 6 | Arginine | Garlic, raw | Antibacterial, antiviral, anticancer |
| 7 | Arginine | Onion, raw | Anti-inflammatory, anticancer |
| 8 | Arginine | Pork loin | Boost immunity, heart health, fat burning, digestion, high blood pressure |
| 9 | Arginine | Chicken | Boost sperm production, heart attack, boosting immunity |
| 10 | Arginine | Lentils | Weight loss |
| 11 | Arginine | Soy | Cardiovascular benefits, anticancer, hot flashes, bone health, obesity, type 2 diabetes |
| 12 | Arginine, Caffeine | Vitamin A, C, E, calcium, cholesterol, arginine | Boost blood flow |
| 13 | Arginine | Spirulina | Type 2 diabetes, strokes, chronic, kidney disease, allergic rhinitis |
| 14 | Oleic, palmitoleic acids, carotenes | Nuts (almonds, peanuts, almonds, cashew nut) | Anti-inflammatory, rheumatoid arthritis, Alzheimer's disease |

*Source:* From Sharma et al. (2016).

## 15.5 FATTY ACIDS

These are an essential element of lipids found in plants, animals, and microorganisms. It generally includes a straight chain with an even number of carbon atoms and hydrogen atoms present alongside the chain length and at the one end of the chain. Whereas a carboxyl group (—COOH) is located at the other end. Mainly, a fatty acid is known to be an acid due to the existence of the carboxyl group in the chain. The acid is known to be saturated when all the carbon-to-carbon bonds are single, whereas the acid is said to be unsaturated when double or triple bonds are present in the chain. Some fatty acids contain branched chains, whereas others have ring structures (e.g., prostaglandins) (Chen and Liu 2020). These are not found in nature in free form; instead, they are commonly found in combination with glycerol (alcohol) in the form of triglycerides (Figure 15.6). Long-chain polyunsaturated fatty acids (PUFAs) such as α-linolenic acid and linoleic acid cannot be synthesized by humans and are deemed essential. The nutraceutical products of these acids, such as DHA, which are important for neurological and visual development are extremely important to human well-being.

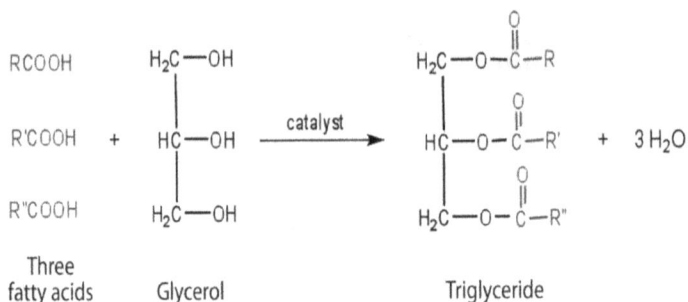

**Figure 15.6** Structure of fatty acid.

### 15.5.1 Types of Fatty Acids

1. Fatty acids are classified as saturated or unsaturated (Figure 15.7), depending upon the existence of carbon-carbon single or double bonds or the nature of the chain. Saturated fatty acids are the most basic type, consisting of unbranched, linear chains of $CH_2$ groups connected by carbon-carbon single bonds with a terminal carboxylic acid. The term 'saturated' refers to the greater number of hydrogen atoms attached to each carbon atom in a fat molecule. The formula of saturated fatty acids is $C_nH_{2n+1}COOH$. Animal-derived fatty acids are generally even-numbered linear chains of saturated fatty acids. This type of fatty acid has been associated with a higher melting point, remains solid at room temperature, and is found in animal fats such as butter, meat, and whole milk. In contrast, Unsaturated fatty acids are more complex types of fatty acids consisting of a bent hydrocarbon chain connected by one or more carbon-carbon double bonds with a terminal carboxylic acids group. The term 'unsaturated' refers to the fact that they do not have the maximum possible hydrogen atoms bound to carbon atoms. It exists in two confirmations, namely, cis and trans form, depending upon the presence of a double bond. When two hydrogen atoms adjacent to the double bond remain on the same side of the chain, then the

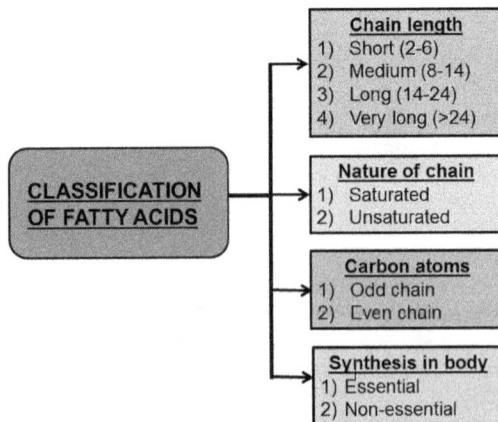

**Figure 15.7** Classification of fatty acid. (From Kaur et al. 2014.)

configuration is called cis-configuration. In the case of the cis isomer, the rigidity of the double bond freezes its conformation and causes the chain to bend, thus restricting the conformational freedom of fatty acid. In contrast, a trans arrangement, on the other hand, implies that the two adjacent hydrogen atoms are on opposite sides of the chain, there is no bending of the chain, and their form is identical to straight saturated fatty acids. Unsaturated fatty acids exist mainly in the cis conformation in the human body. This type of fatty acid has been associated with a lower melting point compared to saturated fatty acids, and thus they are present in the liquid state at room temperatures. Vegetable oils and fish oils are the rich sources of these fatty acids (Lawrence 2021).

2. Furthermore, these are classified as Essential and Non-Essential Fatty Acids based on the synthesis of fatty acids by the body. Essential fatty acids are not synthesized by the body, they are obtained by humans and animals via dietary sources for good health. The most common examples of essential fatty acids are Linoleic acid (an omega-6 fatty acid that helps in the formation of blood clots) and alpha-linolenic acid (an omega-3 fatty acid that reduces blood clot formation). Some leafy vegetables, seeds, nuts, grains, vegetable oils, and meats are good sources of omega-6 fatty acids. However, vegetable oils, nuts and seeds, shellfish, and fish are all good sources of omega-3 fatty acids. In contrast, fatty acids that are synthesized by the body via various biochemical reactions are known as Non-Essential Fatty Acids. Arachidic acid, stearic acid, and palmitic acid are the most common examples of these acids (Kaur et al. 2014).

3. Based on the length of the fatty acid chain, these are categorized as short-chain, medium-chain, long-chain, and very long-chain fatty acids. Short-chain fatty acids (SCFAs) are fatty acids with aliphatic tails of five or fewer carbons (e.g., butyric acid). Whereas medium-chain fatty acids (MCFAs) are fatty acids that have 6 to 12 carbon aliphatic tails and can form medium-chain triglycerides. Long-chain fatty acids (LCFAs) are fatty acids with carbon aliphatic tails ranging from 13 to 21 carbons. In contrast, very long-chain fatty acids (VLCFAs) are aliphatic-tail fatty acids with 22 or more carbons (Heil et al. 2019).

Furthermore, fatty acids have been associated with various health benefits when consumed in dietary composition, as mentioned in Figure 15.8.

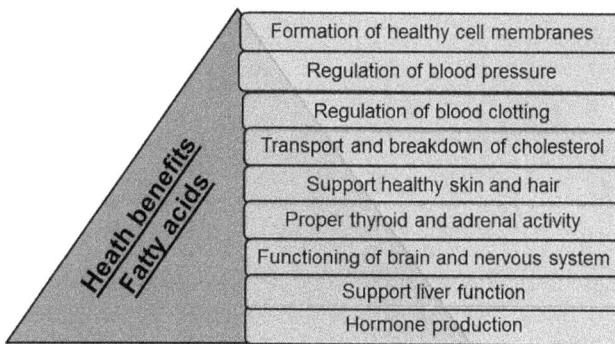

**Figure 15.8**  Health benefits of fatty acids. (From Bajželj et al. 2021.)

## Table 15.5: List of Important Nutraceutical Compounds Found in Oils and Fat Sources with Health Benefits

| Source | Nutraceutical Compound | Applications |
| --- | --- | --- |
| Rice bran oil, olive oil, wheat germ oil, shark liver oil | Squalene | Anticancer properties |
| Soybean oil | Isoflavones | Health benefits against heart ailments, aging, osteoporosis, hormonal imbalance |
| Borage oil, evening primrose, hempseed, black currant seed oil | GLA (gamma-linolenic acid) | Anti-inflammatory properties |
| Salmon, fresh tuna, algal oil, mackerel | EPA (eicosapentaenoic acid), DHA (docosahexaenoic acid) | Anti-inflammatory properties |
| Soybeans | Lecithin | Natural emulsifier, antioxidant properties |
| Flaxseeds, sesame, pumpkin seeds | Lignans such as SDG (secoisolariciresinol diglucoside), MAT (matairesinol), etc. | Antioxidant and anticancer properties |
| Rice bran oil | Oryzanol | Reduce serum cholesterol levels |

*Source:* From Dhara and Chakrabarti (2020).

### 15.5.2 Deficiency of Fatty Acids

Essential fatty acid deficiency in cystic fibrosis is well documented and was previously thought to be caused by mal-absorption, and abnormalities in CF are caused by CFTR dysfunction, as CFTR may play a role in cellular fatty acid metabolism. The clinical signs of deficiency of essential fatty acids are dry scale rash, reduced growth in children and infants, and a decrease in wound healing ability. The symptoms that are associated with the deficiency of an omega-3 fatty acid include visual problems and sensory nerve disorders ('neuropathy'). Animal studies have revealed that a lack of omega-3 fatty acids has a significant impact on learning and memory. DHA (docosahexaenoic acid) is required for proper brain development and visual function. During early infant development, adequate DHA composition allows for optimal function in areas such as visual acuity and attention span, IQ, and visuospatial learning (Pipoyan et al. 2021). A list of such fatty acids containing nutraceutical compounds with their applications is provided in Table 15.5.

### 15.6 OMEGA-3 FATTY ACIDS

Omega-3 fatty acids are one of the essential fats that our bodies require for a variety of tasks but cannot produce on their own. Omega-3 fatty acids are obtained from a variety of foods. Cod liver oil, fish, vegetable oils, walnuts, flaxseed oil, and leafy vegetables are all high in omega-3 fatty acids. Omega-3 fatty acids have many advantages, including a reduced risk of cancer, protection against cardiovascular disease, and a critical function in the creation of hormones that control blood coagulation, inflammation, and other processes. In this chapter, we will discuss the chemical aspects of omega-3 fatty acids as well as their health benefits for human beings (Visioli and Agostoni 2022).

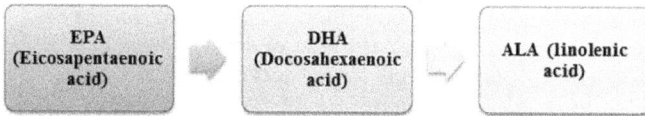

**Figure 15.9** Forms of omega-3 fatty acids. (From Calvo et al. 2017.)

### 15.6.1 What Are Omega-3 Fatty Acids?

Omega-3 fatty acids are polyunsaturated fatty acids with a carbon-carbon double three atoms away from the terminal -$CH_3$ (methyl group) in their carbon atom chain.

Omega-3 fatty acids are essential for human physiology and animal lipid metabolism. Because mammals are unable to synthesize these necessary chemical substances, they must get them through their diet (Visioli and Agostoni 2022).

### 15.6.2 Structure of Omega-3 Fatty Acids

Multiple double bonds exist between carbon atoms in omega-3 fatty acid molecules. It must have a double bond between the 3rd and 4th carbon atoms from the carbon atom chain's end in each molecule. The carbon atom chain of omega-3 fatty acids with 18 or fewer carbon atoms is known as short chain omega-3 fatty acid,' whereas the carbon atom chain of omega-3 fatty acids with 20 or more carbon atoms is known as 'long chain omega-3 fatty acid (Calvo et al. 2017) (Figure 15.9)

Fatty acid chains have two ends: One is carboxylic (-COOH), and the other is methyl (-$CH_3$). The carboxylic end is referred to as the 'alpha' of the chain, whereas the methyl end is referred to as the 'omega' of the chain. Its molecular formula is $C_{60}H_{92}O_6$, and its molecular weight is 909.4 g.mol$^{-1}$ (Calvo et al. 2017; Visioli and Agostoni 2022).

### 15.6.3 Sources of Omega-3 Fatty Acids

One must include foods having a greater amount of omega-3 fatty acids in diet because human body cannot synthesize them and they have essentially vital roles (Figure 15.10). Fatty fish, green vegetables, walnuts, seaweed and some forms of algae, milk, blue eye cod, shark, broccoli, eggs, strawberry, kiwi, red meat, shrimp, tuna, oysters, hemp and flax and so on, are all good sources

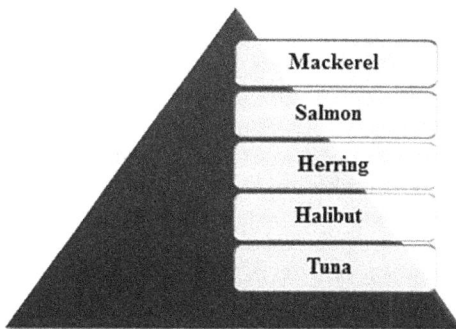

**Figure 15.10** Sources of omega-3 fatty acids. (From Sartorio et al. 2022.)

of omega-3 fatty acids. Flaxseed, often known as linseed, contains 11.4 g of omega-3 per 85 g of serving. Hemp is the second most rich source of omega-3 fatty acids, with 11 g of omega-3 per 85 g of serving (Ponnampalam et al. 2021; Sartorio et al. 2022).

Although fish oils are a good source of these fatty acids, they should be used with caution because they can cause heavy metal poisoning in the body. Metals such as mercury, lead, nickel, and other heavy metals can be found in refined fish oil supplements. These build up in our bodies over time and long-term intake, resulting in heavy metal poisoning. Contaminants in fish oil have been determined to be acceptable by the World Health Organization (Ponnampalam et al. 2021; Sartorio et al. 2022).

### 15.6.4 Benefits of Omega-3 Fatty Acids

These are important not only for the growth and development of the body but also for the prevention of a variety of disorders. Many studies reported the benefits that are associated with omega-3 fatty acids in preventing heart disease (Djuricic and Calder 2021). Consumption of these fatty acids lowers the risk of cancer. It aids in decreasing blood pressure and hypertension, and improving blood circulation. They are efficient in reducing inflammation, help relieve rheumatoid arthritis symptoms, aid in the body's physiological development, are used to treat autism, ADHD, and other conditions, treatment of sadness and anxiety, help with visual difficulties, treatment of bipolar disorder, beneficial in the treatment of Alzheimer's disease because they are somewhat effective against cognitive difficulties. Moreover, children's asthma attacks can be prevented by taking omega-3 supplements, which help in various metabolic syndrome and autoimmune illnesses and can be used to treat insomnia.

### 15.7 DIETARY FIBER

Dietary fiber is a form of carbohydrate (indigestible) with a primary source from plants. Dietary habits, which mainly involve junk foods or food with less fiber content, contribute to weight gain. Obesity is the leading cause of various chronic diseases such as diabetes, hypertension, cardiovascular effects, dyslipidemia, and cancer (Figure 15.11). Classification of dietary fiber is mainly into two categories based on their solvable property in water-insoluble and soluble fibers. Water-soluble fibers are mainly sourced from fruits and vegetables, whereas water-insoluble comes from whole grains and cereals. Daily intake of dietary fiber correlates with efficient metabolic function with appetite regulation, improved gut microflora function, and weight management (Barber et al. 2020). Dietary fiber is beneficial for controlling blood glucose and lipids management. Various clinical research studies and trials support the fact that dietary fiber reduces the risk of diabetes with improved glycemic control (Redondo-Blanco et al. 2020). Dietary fiber provides therapeutic improvement in gastrointestinal (GI) tract ailments such as chronic diarrhea, inflammatory bowel disease (IBD), irritable bowel syndrome (IBS), and functional constipation (Cronin et al. 2021; Gill et al. 2021). Dietary fiber is also linkto in modulating cardio-metabolic outcomes by lowering the risks of cardiovascular diseases (CVD) and coronary heart diseases (CHD) with reduced LDL cholesterol levels in the blood (Bozzetto et al. 2018). Dietary fiber also shows potential anticancer effects, as shown in a research study on ovarian cancer patients (Huang et al. 2018). The composition of dietary fiber based on its two groups include cellulose, lignin, and resistant starch (insoluble fiber group); glucans, inulin, pectin, gums, arabinoxylans, and mucilage (soluble fiber group) (Ciudad-Mulero et al. 2019).

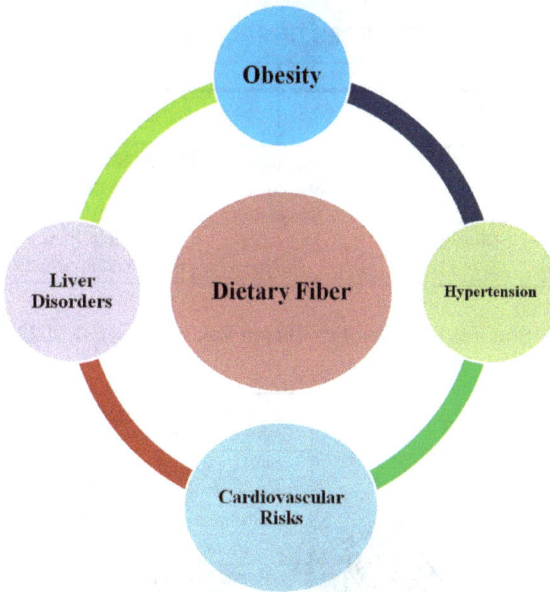

**Figure 15.11** Representation of dietary fiber function in lowering the risks of human health disorders. (From Ciudad-Mulero et al. 2019.)

## 15.8 PROBIOTICS

"**Probiotics**" is derived from the Greek phrase "for life." It was given by Lilly and Stillwell discovered it in 1965, and is defined as "live microorganisms that confer a health benefit to the host when administered in adequate amounts." The health benefits of probiotic cultures are known to vary depending on the strains. It is critical to choose them based on their resistance towards acid and bile salts, as well as their tendency to live transit through the stomach and small intestine to reach the large intestine. *Lactobacilli* and *Bifidobacteria* are mainly found in commercial probiotics (Kaur et al. 2013; Ranjha et al. 2021).

### 15.8.1 Characteristics of Probiotics

A microbial strain must possess numerous particular properties to be considered a probiotic. This is divided into three categories: Safety, performance, and technological aspects. The factors are further dependent on the specific purpose of the strains and the site for the expression of the particular property. Considering the safety, the origin of the probiotic strain should be human, collected from the gastrointestinal tract (GIT) of a fit individual. It should be GRAS (generally recognized as safe), nonpathogenic, and not associated with infectious endocarditis or gastrointestinal disorders. It should not carry genes that confer resistance to antibiotics. It should not elicit an immune response in the host, implying that the host must be immune-tolerant to it. Moreover, it should be non-pathogenic, non-toxic, non-allergic, non-mutagenic, or non-carcinogenic. It must be associated with anti-mutagenic and anti-carcinogenic and should not cause any inflammation in humans. It should have an advantageous antibiogram profile. Probiotic strains must be stable genetically and free of plasmid transfer mechanisms (Palanivelu et al. 2022).

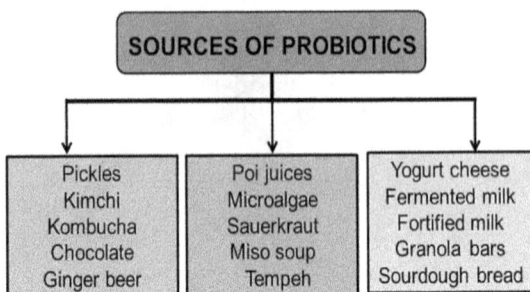

**Figure 15.12** Sources of probiotics. (From Palanivelu et al. 2022.)

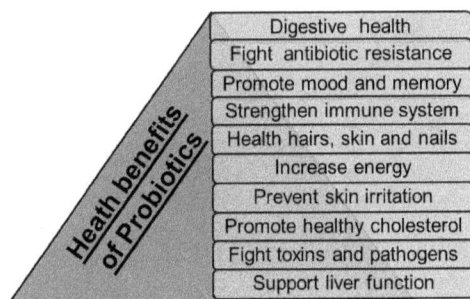

**Figure 15.13** Health benefits of probiotics. (From Ranjha et al. 2021.)

There are various sources of probiotics that directly confer health benefits mentioned in Figures 15.12 and 15.13.

### 15.8.2 Types of Probiotics

Both yeast and bacteria are comprised of probiotics. However, bacteria are the most widely used. A list of the most commonly used probiotics is mentioned in Table 15.6 (Kaur et al. 2013; Mittu and Girdhar 2015).

## Table 15.6: Most Commonly Used Probiotics

| Microbial Strains | | Location/Presence | Function |
|---|---|---|---|
| Lactobacillus | L. acidophilus | Small intestine and vagina | Fights off harmful bacteria |
| | L. reuteri | Mouth and intestine | Helps the digestive system and prevents tooth decay |
| Bifidobacteria | B. animalis | Commonly used in food supplements | Boosts immune system and fights harmful food-borne bacteria |
| | B. breve | Digestive tract and vagina | Absorb nutrients by fermenting sugar and breaking plant fiber |
| | B. lactis | Raw milk | Catalyzes the reaction that produces buttermilk, cottage cheese (paneer) |
| | B. longum | Gastrointestinal tract | Breaks down carbohydrates and also acts as an antioxidant |

*Source:* From Binda et al. (2020).

## 15.9 ANTIOXIDANTS

Antioxidant's protective role against oxidative stress in the human body gained importance in the nutraceutical and pharmaceutical industry. The main principle/function of antioxidants is to inhibit oxidation by scavenging ROS (reactive oxygen species), thus preventing oxidative damage. Natural sources of antioxidants are generally from plant secondary metabolites in which phenolic compounds (tocopherols, flavonoids, and phenolic acids) serve as the major source (Gulcin 2020). These natural antioxidants in the nutraceutical industry provide beneficial protection against life-threatening diseases (Loizzo et al. 2019). Compared to natural, synthetic antioxidants (butylated hydroxytoluene [BHT], gallates, butylated hydroxyanisole [BHA], tertiary butyl hydroquinone) derivatives of phenolic compounds are utilized in the food industry as stabilizing agents, in cosmetics as preservatives and pharmaceutical industry. Synthetic antioxidants are grouped according to their nature of activities, such as chelating agents, oxygen scavengers, and free radical terminators during oxidative stress. Food sources for natural antioxidants include fruits, dark chocolate, nuts, whole grains, berries, herbs, and spices. Extraction methods for isolating these valuable plant antioxidants involve different mechanisms, such as microwave-assisted, ultrasound-assisted, and pressurized liquid-assisted with the aim of higher yield at shorter extraction times (Khan et al. 2019). Class of antioxidants (phenolic acids, flavonoids, astaxanthin, ergosterol, etc.) from the sea source derived from different diversities of microalgae are promising in the nutraceutical and pharmaceuticals industry (Sansone and Brunet 2019). Some species from microalgae diversity, such as *Dunaliella salina, Haematococcuspluvialis, Botryococcusbraunii,* and *Spirulinaplatensis* are valuable nutraceutical biosources (Santhakumaran et al. 2020). Nutraceutical antioxidants' stability and bioavailability are enhanced by their encapsulation with nanoparticles such as nanoliposomes, nanogels, niosomes, hexosome, cyclodextrin, etc, with their controlled antioxidant activity (Maqsoudlou et al. 2020). Nanocarrier technology is effective in maintaining the shelf life and functional structure of antioxidants with increased bioavailability in nutraceutical bio-foods. The nanoliposome antioxidant (vitamins C and E) combination provides an effective combination in reducing oxidative stress at the biological membranes with synergetic antioxidant delivery (Khorasani et al. 2018). Apart from plants and microalgae, microorganisms are also a good source of antioxidants for the nutraceutical industry with controlled growth conditions. Microbial-origin antioxidants in the nutraceutical industry are potential sources of therapeutics for their non-cytotoxic/mutagenic properties (Rani et al. 2021). The microbial diversity of known secondary metabolites is 23,000 known with 42% produced from actinomycetes, fungi, and 16% by eubacteria (Chandra et al. 2020). Nutraceutical antioxidants provide beneficial protection against many diseases, such as Alzheimer's, depression, myocardial disorder, neurological disorder, schizophrenia, and cancer (Table 15.7). Antioxidant property for scavenging ROS with a principal focus on ferroptosis is the main biological function of nutraceutical antioxidants (Mao et al. 2018).

## Table 15.7: List of Nutraceutical Antioxidants with Their Biological Roles

| Antioxidant | Source | Chemical Nature | Bioactivity |
|---|---|---|---|
| Ergothioneine | Microorganisms | 2-Mercapto-histidine trimethylbetaine | Prevents oxidative stress, and lowers the risk of coronary disease |
| Betacyanins | *Opuntiaficus indica* (L.) Mill. | Betanidin-5-O-beta-glucoside | Anti-angiogenic, antioxidant, and cytoprotective |

*(Continued)*

## Table 15.7: List of Nutraceutical Antioxidants with Their Biological Roles (*Continued*)

| Antioxidant | Source | Chemical Nature | Bioactivity |
| --- | --- | --- | --- |
| Resveratrol | Grapes | Natural phenol (3,5,4-trihydroxy-trans-stilbene) | Antioxidant, anti-inflammatory, antiangiogenic, and lowers cholesterol |
| Rosmainic acid | Rosemary | Polyphenol | Anti-inflammatory, antioxidant, antiviral, antibacterial |
| EGCG | Green tea | Flavonoid (epigallocatechin-3-gallate) | Antioxidant and neuroprotective |
| Quercetin | Plants | Flavonoid (3,3,4,5,7-pentahydroxyflavone) | Antioxidant, anti-inflammatory, cytoprotective |
| Curcumin | Plants | Phenolic pigments (diferuloylmethane) | Anti-inflammatory, antioxidant, and repair damaged tissue |
| Allicin | *Allium sativum* L. (garlic) | Diallylthiosulfinate | Antioxidant, lowers cholesterol, cytoprotective, antimicrobial |
| Vitamin E | Plants and animals | Tocopherols and tocotrienols | Antioxidant |
| Vitamin C (ascorbic acid) | Fruits | L-threo-Hex-2-enono-1,4-lactone | Antioxidant and cardioprotective |
| Lipoic acids | Plants and animals | Alpha-lipoic acid or thioctic acid | Antioxidant, reduce diabetic peripheral neuropathy. |

*Sources:* From Borodina et al. (2020); Kelsey et al. (2010); Smeriglio et al. (2019).

### 15.10 POLYPHENOLIC COMPOUNDS

Secondary metabolites', especially polyphenols, role in the nutraceutical industry are considered beneficent for human health. Their presence in the diet helps to counter the effects of dreadful diseases such as neurodegenerative, cardiovascular, diabetes, and cancer. Nutraceutical polyphenolic compounds' principal function is claimed to be antioxidant in nature with a potential chemotherapeutic role. As a major source, plants contain various phenols and polyphenols whose characterization and isolation need to be properly exploited (Figure 15.14). Advanced knowledge of different analytical methods such as MSI (mass spectrometry imaging), AMS (ambient mass spectrometry), and MALDI-MSI (matrix-assisted laser desorption ionization) increased the understanding of the biological role of polyphenols having nutraceutical potential (Piccolella et al. 2019). Natural polyphenols sources include spices, tea, dark chocolate, wine, herbs, and red berries. Plant polyphenol compounds have a vast composition of classification represented in a given figure.

Nutraceutical supplements such as *Camellia sinensis* (green tea), *Rubus idaeus* (raspberry), *Vaccinium macrocarpon* (cranberry), and *Vitis vinifera* (grapes) extracts contain a variety of phenolics with anti-inflammatory, antiaging, and antioxidant properties (Vidal-Casanella O et al. 2021). Various experimental methods have shown the role of polyphenol nutraceuticals in combating oxidative imbalance by modulating the gut microbiota (Vamanu 2019). Among the different antioxidants, polyphenols (such as hydroxytyrosol and maqui) play a regulatory role against lipid/glucose dysmetabolism, thus reducing risk factors

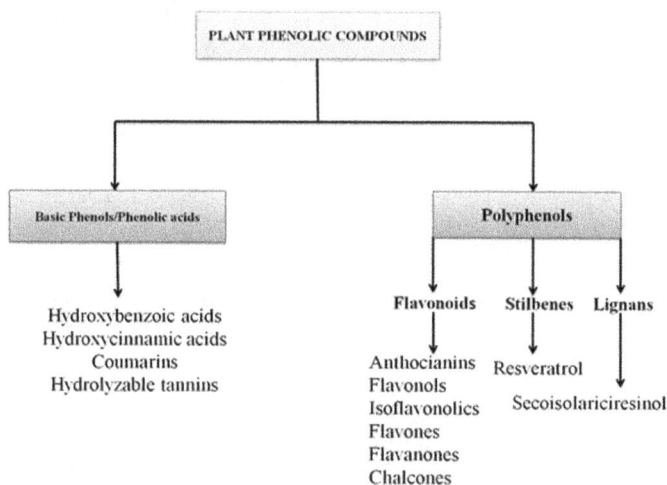

**Figure 15.14** Classification of phenolic compounds. (From Ranjha et al. 2021.)

associated with metabolic disorders. Results generated in a pilot study showed polyphenol MCN (multicomponent nutraceutical) such as Eonlipid improved antioxidant potential with reducing factors associated with atherogenesis (Roberto Corsi et al. 2017). Polyphenols (lycopene, catechism, curcumin, resveratrol) have a beneficial role in nutraceuticals shown by experimental studies (in vivo/in vitro) presented them to have a neuroprotective role against neurodegenerative disorders such as Alzheimer's (Sawikr et al. 2017). RCT (randomized controlled trials) that are being conducted or under process based on polyphenol nutraceuticals present them to be used as an adjunct therapy for cardiovascular diseases whose further clinical evaluation and dosage effectiveness need further to be checked (Tome-Carneiro and Visioli 2016). In nutraceutical foodstuffs, phenolic compounds add color, oxidative stability, and taste perception. Clinical trials (NCT01886989, NCT03049631, NCT01766570, NCT04847999, NCT02650726, NCT01923597, NCT02035592) of polyphenolic compounds showed the efficacy of these compounds in clinical diabetic studies (Fernandes et al. 2022). Dietary polyphenols (thymol, flavan-3-ols, resveratrol, curcumin) play a role in weight management, thus reducing the effects like obesity and diabetes (Silvester et al. 2019). Studies conducted on the biological role of polyphenols support their beneficial effect on human health, but still, there are some limitations to their synergistic interactions, absorption and metabolism (Tresserra-Rimbau et al. 2018).

## 15.11 PHYTOCHEMICALS

Plant phytochemical components show varied biological activities with positive effects on human health. These compounds exert protection against different chronic diseases such as cancer, heart ailment, diabetes, and hypertension. They are considered non-essential in the diet, but because of their defense nature, these are included in nutraceutical foods. Nearly 4,000 plant phytochemicals exist with diversified classifications having different chemical/physical and biological functions (Sharma et al. 2019). Plant seeds (cucumber, mango, pumpkin, and papaya) are enriched with these phytochemicals (phytosterols, flavonoids, triterpenoids, terpenes, lactones, and furanones) for which they are incorporated in nutraceutical fruit and nut spreads (Rohini et al. 2021). Dietary phytochemicals from coffee, grapes, cocoa, and wine show evidence of cognitive decrease in aging (Howes et al. 2020). Nutraceutical phytochemicals, similar to the other plant secondary metabolites, show anti-inflammatory and antioxidant properties (Howes 2018). These secondary metabolites in the nutraceutical/pharmacological industry make the goal of a healthy lifestyle achievable (Rijai 2019). Phytochemicals (terpenoids, essential oils, and other secondary metabolites) are also being used in the food processing industry for their anti-fungal properties to inhibit the spoilage of food items (Redondo-Blanco et al. 2020). Encapsulation of secondary metabolites with nanoparticles increases the efficacy and potential of these compounds. Phytochemicals' bioefficacy is an important parameter for their bioavailability inside the human body to perform biological functions. Phytochemical nanocarriers (SPIONs (superparamagnetic iron-oxide nanoparticle), mesoporous nanoparticle, liposomes, micelles, niosomes, bilosomes, archaeosomes, and gold/silver nanoparticle) have increased stability and bioavailability which make them useful in nanomedicine, cosmetic industry, and nutraceutical food items (Ahmad et al. 2021). Phytochemicals with a range of therapeutic potentials find a place in ancient and modern medicine (Velu et al. 2018).

## 15.12 NON-FLAVONOIDS

Non-flavonoid compounds (stilbenes, hydroxycinnamic acids, and hydroxybenzoic acids), also called phenolic acids, are the most common non-flavonoids. The plant polyphenols group is classified into flavonoid and non-flavonoid sub-categories (Leri et al. 2020). Non-flavonoids also contain hydrolyzable tannins from common sources, such as fruits, tea, wine and nuts (Vidal-Casanella et al. 2021). As compared to other polyphenols, these compounds also display anti-inflammatory, antioxidant, anticancer, and antimicrobial activities. Structurally these compounds contain a single carboxylic moiety. Food sources of these compounds include fruits, seeds, leaves of vegetables, and tea. These compounds act as a precursor for other biomolecules, which they find an important need in the food industry, nutraceutical foods, cosmetics, and therapeutics (Kumar and Goel 2019).

## 15.13 CONCLUSION

The nutraceutical term falls between food supplements and pharmaceuticals. They add value to health and protect against pathological and chronic disorders. These food supplements are added to the normal diet in the form of tablets, capsules, liquids, and powder form. Their beneficial and toxicological effects are studied in models (in vitro/in vivo) before entering them into the dietary supplements. Various bioactive compounds especially plant and animal-derived SMs (secondary metabolites) play an essential role in these nutraceuticals' health benefits. These phytochemicals primarily exhibit antioxidant properties as nutraceuticals which reduce oxidative stress-related effects. The modern generation is more concerned with attaining a healthy lifestyle which increased the popularity of nutraceutical foods. When added to the dietary supplements, they act as antidiabetic, antifungal, antibacterial, anticancer, and immunity boosters. Modern approaches to encapsulating these bioactive compounds with different nanocarriers have improved the bioefficacy of these nutraceuticals. Nutraceutical industries are growing, with new companies joining the market to meet nutritional deficiencies. But this growth need to concern safety and efficacy of these nutraceuticals before entering into the market. Thus regulatory bodies to check up on these nutraceuticals are important to regulate them worldwide.

## REFERENCES

Ahmad, R., Srivastava, S., Ghosh, S., & Khare, S. K. 2021. "Phytochemical delivery through nanocarriers: A review." *Colloids and Surfaces B: Biointerfaces* 197:111389.

Akram, M., Asif, H. M., Uzair, M., Akhtar, N., Madni, A., Shah, S. A., & Hasan, Z. 2011. "Amino acids: A review article." *Journal of Medicinal Plants Research* 5(17).

Akram, M., Munir, N., Daniyal, M., Egbuna, C., Găman, M. A., Onyekere, P. F., & Olatunde, A. 2020. "Vitamins and minerals: Types, sources and their functions." In *Functional Foods and Nutraceuticals* 149–172. Springer, Cham.

Allen, L. H., & Dror, D. K. 2018. "Introduction to current knowledge on micronutrients in human milk: Adequacy, analysis, and need for research." *Advances in Nutrition,* 9:275S–277S.

Arai, H., & Sakuma, M. 2015. "Bone and nutrition. Bone and phosphorus intake." *Clinical Calcium* 25(7):967–972.

Bagherani, N., & Smoller, B. R. 2016. "An overview of zinc and its importance in dermatology – Part I: Importance and function of zinc in human beings." *Global Dermatology* 3(5):330–336.

Bajželj, B., Laguzzi, F., & Röös, E. 2021. "The role of fats in the transition to sustainable diets." *Lancet Planetary Health* 5(9):e644–e653.

Barber, T. M., Kabisch, S., Pfeiffer, A. F. H., & Weickert, M. O. (2020). "The health benefits of dietary fibre." *Nutrients, 12*(10), 3209. https://doi.org/10.3390/nu12103209

Bifari, F., Ruocco, C., Decimo, I., Fumagalli, G., Valerio, A., & Nisoli, E. 2017. "Amino acid supplements and metabolic health: A potential interplay between intestinal microbiota and systems control." *Genes & Nutrition* 12(1):1–2.

Binda, S., Hill, C., Johansen, E., Obis, D., Pot, B., Sanders, M. E., & Ouwehand, A. C. 2020. "Criteria to qualify microorganisms as 'probiotic' in foods and dietary supplements." *Frontiers in Microbiology* 1662.

Bleizgys, A. 2021. "Vitamin D dosing: Basic principles and a brief algorithm (2021 Update)". *Nutrients* 13(12):4415.

Borodina, I., Kenny, L. C., McCarthy, C. M., Paramasivan, K., Pretorius, E., Roberts, T. J., van der Hoek, S. A., & Kell, D. B. 2020. "The biology of ergothioneine, an antioxidant nutraceutical." *Nutrition Research Reviews* 32:190–217.

Bozzetto, L., Costabile, G., Della Pepa, G., Ciciola, P., Vetrani, C., Vitale, M., Rivellese, A. A., & Annuzzi, G. 2018. "Dietary fibre as a unifying remedy for the whole spectrum of obesity-associated cardiovascular risk." *Nutrients, 10*(7), 943.

Buchman, C. A., Dillon, M. T., King, E. R., Adunka, M. C., Adunka, O. F., & Pillsbury, H. C. (2014). "Influence of cochlear implant insertion depth on performance: A prospective randomized trial." *Otology & Neurotology: Official Publication of the American Otological Society, American Neurotology Society [and] European Academy of Otology and Neurotology*, 35(10), 1773–1779.

Buchman, A. R. 2014. "Manganese." In: Catharine, A., Ross, B. C., Robert, J., Tucker K. L., & Ziegler T. R. (eds.), *Modern Nutrition in Health and Disease*, 11th edn, 238–244. Baltimore; Lippincott Williams & Wilkins.

Buehler, B. A. 2011. "Vitamin B2: Riboflavin." *Journal of Evidence-Based Complementary & Alternative Medicine* 16(2):88–90.

Bumgarner, N. R., Scheerens, J. C., & Kleinhenz, M. D. 2012. "Nutritional yield: A proposed index for fresh food improvement illustrated with leafy vegetable data." *Plant Foods for Human Nutrition* 67(3), 215–222.

Calvo, M. J., Martínez, M. S., Torres, W., Chávez-Castillo, M., Luzardo, E., Villasmil, N., ...& Bermúdez, V. 2017. "Omega-3 polyunsaturated fatty acids and cardiovascular health: A molecular view into structure and function." *Vessel Plus* 1:116–128.

Chandra, P., Sharma, R. K., & Arora, D. S. 2020. "Antioxidant compounds from microbial sources: A review." *Food Research International* 129:108849.

Chen, J., & Liu, H. 2020. "Nutritional indices for assessing fatty acids: A mini-review." *International Journal of Molecular Sciences* 21(16):5695.

Cogswell, M. E., Mugavero, K., Bowman, B. A., & Frieden, T. R. 2016. "Dietary sodium and cardiovascular disease risk—Measurement matters." *New England Journal of Medicine* 375(6):580.

Ciudad-Mulero, M., Fernández-Ruiz, V., Matallana-González, M. C., & Morales, P. 2019. "Dietary fiber sources and human benefits: The case study of cereal and pseudocereals." In: *Advances in Food and Nutrition Research* 90: 83–134. https://doi.org/10.1016/bs.afnr.2019.02.002

Derbyshire, E. 2018. "Micronutrient intakes of British adults across mid-life: A secondary analysis of the UK national diet and nutrition survey." *Frontiers in Nutrition* 5:55.

Desai, A. https://health.economictimes.indiatimes.com/news/pharma/nutraceutical-industry-a-consumer-driven-market/84365994.

Dhara, O., & Chakrabarti, P. P. 2020. Lipid based nutraceuticals and nanoformulations: Emerging applications in pharmaceuticals and cosmetics industries.

Djuricic, I., & Calder, P. C. 2021. "Beneficial outcomes of omega-6 and omega-3 polyunsaturated fatty acids on human health: An update for 2021." *Nutrients* 13(7):2421.

Fernandes, I., Oliveira, J., Pinho, A., & Carvalho, E. 2022. "The role of nutraceutical containing polyphenols in diabetes prevention." *Metabolites* 12(2):184.

Gibson, G. E., Hirsch, J. A., Fonzetti, P., Jordan, B. D., Cirio, R. T., & Elder, J. 2016. "Vitamin B1 (thiamine) and dementia." *Annals of the New York Academy of Sciences* 1367(1):21–30.

Górska-Warsewicz, H., Laskowski, W., Kulykovets, O., Kudlińska-Chylak, A., Czeczotko, M., & Rejman, K. 2018. "Food products as sources of protein and amino acids—The case of Poland." *Nutrients* 10(12):1977.

Gulcin İ. 2020. "Antioxidants and antioxidant methods: An updated overview." *Archives of Toxicology* 94(3):651–715.

Hans, K. B., & Jana, T. 2018. "Micronutrients in the life cycle: Requirements and sufficient supply." *NFS Journal* 11:1–11.

Heil, C. S., Wehrheim, S. S., Paithankar, K. S., & Grininger, M. 2019. "Fatty acid biosynthesis: Chain-length regulation and control." *ChemBioChem* 20(18):2298–2321.

Howes, M. J. 2018. "Phytochemicals as anti-inflammatory nutraceuticals and phytopharmaceuticals." In *Immunity and Inflammation in Health and Disease* 363–388. Academic Press.

Howes, M. J., Perry, N. S., Vásquez-Londoño, C., & Perry, E. K. 2020. "Role of phytochemicals as nutraceuticals for cognitive functions affected in ageing." *British Journal of Pharmacology* 177(6):1294–1315.

Huang, X., Wang, X., Shang, J., Lin, Y., Yang, Y., Song, Y., & Yu, S. 2018. "Association between dietary fiber intake and risk of ovarian cancer: A meta-analysis of observational studies." *Journal of International Medical Research*, 46(10), 3995–4005.

Kamble, C., Chavan, R., & Kamble, V. 2021. "A review on amino acids." *Research & Reviews: A Journal of Drug Design & Discovery* 8(3):19–27

Kaur, B., Balgir, P. P., Mittu, B., Kumar, B., & Garg, N. 2013. "Biomedical applications of fermenticin HV6b isolated from Lactobacillus fermentum HV6b MTCC10770." *BioMed Research International*.

Kaur, N., Chugh, V., & Gupta, A. K. 2014. "Essential fatty acids as functional components of foods-a review." *Journal of Food Science and Technology* 51(10):2289–2303.

Kelsey, N. A., Wilkins, H. M., & Linseman, D. A. 2010. "Nutraceutical antioxidants as novel neuroprotective agents." *Molecules* 15(11):7792–7814.

Khan, M. K., Paniwnyk, L., & Hassan, S. 2019. "Polyphenols as natural antioxidants: Sources, extraction and applications in food, cosmetics and drugs." In *Plant Based "Green Chemistry 2.0"* 197–235. Singapore: Springer.

Khorasani, S., Danaei, M., & Mozafari, M. R. 2018. "Nanoliposome technology for the food and nutraceutical industries." *Trends in Food Science & Technology* 79:106–115.

Kumar, N., & Goel, N. 2019. "Phenolic acids: Natural versatile molecules with promising therapeutic applications." *Biotechnology Reports* 24:e00370.

Lawrence, G. D. 2021. "Perspective: The saturated fat–unsaturated oil dilemma: Relations of dietary fatty acids and serum cholesterol, atherosclerosis, inflammation, cancer, and all-cause mortality." *Advances in Nutrition* 12(3):647–656.

Leri, M., Scuto, M., Ontario, M. L., Calabrese, V., Calabrese, E. J., Bucciantini, M., & Stefani, M. 2020. "Healthy effects of plant polyphenols: Molecular mechanisms." *International Journal of Molecular Sciences* 21(4):1250.

Lipner, S. R. 2018. "Rethinking biotin therapy for hair, nail, and skin disorders." *Journal of the American Academy of Dermatology* 78(6):1236–1238.

Loizzo, M. R., & Tundis, R. 2019 "Plant antioxidant for application in food and nutraceutical industries." *Antioxidants* 8(10):453.

Lopez, M. J., & Mohiuddin, S. S. 2020. "Biochemistry, essential amino acids *In: StatPearls* Internet https://www.ncbi.nlm.nih.gov/books/NBK557845/

Mao, X. Y., Jin, M. Z., Chen, J. F., Zhou, H. H., & Jin, W. L. 2018. "Live or let die: Neuroprotective and anticancer effects of nutraceutical antioxidants." *Pharmacology & Therapeutics* 183:137–151.

Mahima, R. A., Deb, R., Latheef, S. K., Abdul Samad, H., Tiwari, R., Verma, A. K., Kumar, A., & Dhama, K. 2012. "Immunomodulatory and therapeutic potentials of herbal, traditional/indigenous and ethnoveterinary medicines." *Pakistan Journal of Biological Sciences*, 15(16), 754–774.

Maqsoudlou, A., Assadpour, E., Mohebodini, H., & Jafari, S. M. 2020. "Improving the efficiency of natural antioxidant compounds via different nanocarriers." *Advances in Colloid and Interface Science* 278:102122.

Mittu, B., Bhat, Z. R., Chauhan, A., Kour, J., Behera, A., & Kaur, M. 2022. "Ascorbic acid." In *Nutraceuticals and Health Care* 289–302. Academic Press.

Mittu, B., & Girdhar, Y. 2015. "Role of lactic acid bacteria isolated from goat milk in cancer prevention." *Autoimmune Diseases* 1(2): 2470-1025.108.

Murphy, M. M., Barraj, L. M., Herman, D., Bi, X., Cheatham, R., & Randolph, R. K. 2012. "Phytonutrient intake by adults in the United States in relation to fruit and vegetable consumption." *Journal of the Academy of Nutrition and Dietetics, 112(2),* 222–229.

O'Mullane, D. M., Baez, R. J., Jones, S., Lennon, M. A., Petersen, P. E., Rugg Gunn, A. J., Whelton, H., & Whitford, G. M. 2016. "Fluoride and oral health." *Community Dental Health* 33:69–99.

Oh, S., Cave, G., & Lu, C. 2021. "Vitamin B12 (cobalamin) and micronutrient fortification in food crops using nanoparticle technology." *Frontiers in Plant Science* 1451.

Palanivelu, J., Thanigaivel, S., Vickram, S., Dey, N., Mihaylova, D., & Desseva, I. 2022. "Probiotics in functional foods: Survival assessment and approaches for improved viability." *Applied Sciences* 12(1):455.

Patil, M., Sheth, K. A., Krishnamurthy, A. C., & Devarbhavi, H. 2013. "A review and current perspective on Wilson disease. *Journal of Clinical and Experimental Hepatology* 3(4):321–336.

Piccolella, S., Crescente, G., Candela, L., & Pacifico, S. 2019. "Nutraceutical polyphenols: New analytical challenges and opportunities." *Journal of Pharmaceutical and Biomedical Analysis* 175:112774.

Pipoyan, D., Stepanyan, S., Stepanyan, S., Beglaryan, M., Costantini, L., Molinari, R., & Merendino, N. 2021. "The effect of trans fatty acids on human health: Regulation and consumption patterns." *Foods* 10(10):2452.

Ponnampalam, E. N., Sinclair, A. J., & Holman, B. W. 2021. "The sources, synthesis and biological actions of omega-3 and omega-6 fatty acids in red meat: An overview." *Foods* 10(6):1358.

Prashanth, L., Kattapagari, K. K., Chitturi, R. T., Baddam, V. R. R., & Prasad, L. K. 2015. "A review on role of essential trace elements in health and disease." *Journal of Dr. NTR University of Health Sciences* 4(2):75.

Rafeeq, H., Ahmad, S., Tareen, M. B. K., Shahzad, K. A., Bashir, A., Jabeen, R., & Shehzadi, I. 2020. "Biochemistry of fat soluble vitamins, sources, biochemical functions and toxicity." *Haya: The Saudi Journal of Life Sciences*.

Rani, A., Saini, K. C., Bast, F., Mehariya, S., Bhatia, S. K., Lavecchia, R., & Zuorro, A. 2021. "A microorganisms: A potential source of bioactive molecules for antioxidant applications." *Molecules* 4:1142.

Ranjha, M. M. A. N., Shafique, B., Batool, M., Kowalczewski, P. Ł., Shehzad, Q., Usman, M., & Aadil, R. M. 2021. "Nutritional and health potential of probiotics: A review." *Applied Sciences* 11(23):11204.

Redondo-Blanco, S., Fernandez, J., Lopez-Ibanez, S., Miguelez, E. M., Villar, C. J., & Lombo, F. 2020. "Plant phytochemicals in food preservation: Antifungal bioactivity: A review." *Journal of Food Protection* 83(1):163–171.

Reid, I. R., Bristow, S. M., & Bolland, M. J. 2015. "Calcium supplements: Benefits and risks." *Journal of Internal Medicine* 278(4):354–368.

Review Nutraceuticals in Periodontal Health: A Systematic Review on the Role of Vitamins in Periodontal Health Maintenance Alfonso Varela-López 1 ID, María D. Navarro-Hortal 2, Francesca Giampieri 1 ID, Pedro Bullón 3 ID, Maurizio Battino 1 ID and José L. Quiles 2, ID, Received: 25 April 2018; Accepted: 17 May 2018; Published: 20 May 2018 *Molecules* 2018, 23(5), 1226; https://doi.org/10.3390/molecules23051226 Received: 25 April 2018/Revised: 16 May 2018/Accepted: 17 May 2018/Published: 20 May 2018

Rijai, L. 2019 "Review of phytochemicals and its biological activities and contemporary nutraceuticals." *Journal of Tropical Pharmacy and Chemistry* 4(6):298–310.

Roberto Corsi, M. D., Giovanni Mosti, M. D., Attilio Cavezzi, M. D., Elena Fioroni, M. S., Roberto Colucci, B. S., & Valentina Quinzi, M. S. 2017. "A polyphenol-based multicomponent nutraceutical in dysmetabolism and oxidative stress: Results from a pilot study." *Journal of Dietary Supplements* 15(1):34–41.

Rohini, C., Geetha, P. S., Vijayalakshmi, R., & Mini, M. L. 2021. "Phytochemicals characterization of nutraceutical enriched fruits and nuts spread." *Journal of Applied and Natural Science* 13(SI):124–129.

Rose, A. J. 2019. "Amino acid nutrition and metabolism in health and disease." *Nutrients* 11(11):2623.

Sansone, C., & Brunet, C. 2019. "Promises and challenges of microalgal antioxidant production." *Antioxidants* 8(7):199.

Santhakumaran, P., Ayyappan, S. M., & Ray, J. G. 2020. "Nutraceutical applications of twenty-five species of rapid-growing green-microalgae as indicated by their antibacterial, antioxidant and mineral content." *Algal Research* 47:101878.

Sartorio, M. U. A., Pendezza, E., Coppola, S., Paparo, L., D'Auria, E., Zuccotti, G. V., & BerniCanani, R. 2022. "Potential role of omega-3 polyunsaturated fatty acids in pediatric food allergy." *Nutrients* 14(1):152.

Sawikr, Y., Yarla, N. S., Peluso, I., Kamal, M. A., Aliev, G., & Bishayee, A. 2017. "Neuroinflammation in Alzheimer's disease: The preventive and therapeutic potential of polyphenolicnutraceuticals." *Advances in protein chemistry and structural biology* 108:33–57.

Schaefer, B. 2014. "Vitamins." In: *Natural Products in the Chemical Industry*. Berlin, Heidelberg: Springer. https://doi.org/10.1007/978-3-642-54461-3_7.

Shah, T. Z., Ali, A. B., Jafri, S. A., & Qazi, M. H. 2013. "Effect of nicotinic acid (Vitamin B3 or Niacin) on the lipid profile of diabetic and non–diabetic rats." *Pakistan Journal of Medical Sciences* 29(5):1259.

Sharma, D. R., Kumar, S., Kumar, V., & Thakur, A. 2019. "Comprehensive review on nutraceutical significance of phytochemicals as functional food ingredients for human health management." *Journal of Pharmacognosy and Phytochemistry* 8(5):385–395.

Sharma, V., Singh, L., Verma, N., & Kalra, G. 2016. "'The nutraceutical amino acids' Nature's fortification for robust health." *British Journal of Pharmaceutical Research* 11(3):1–20.

Silvester, A. J., Aseer, K. R., & Yun, J. W. 2019. "Dietary polyphenols and their roles in fat browning." *Journal of Nutritional Biochemistry* 64:1–2.

Smeriglio, A., Bonasera, S., Germanò, M. P., D'Angelo, V., Barreca, D., Denaro, M., Monforte, M. T., Galati, E. M., & Trombetta, D. 2019. "*Opuntiaficus-indica* (L.) Mill. fruit as source of betalains with antioxidant, cytoprotective, and anti-angiogenic properties." *Phytotherapy Research* 33(5):1526–1537.

Sobczyńska-Malefora, A., & Harrington, D. J. 2018. "Laboratory assessment of folate (vitamin B9) status." *Journal of Clinical Pathology* 71(11):949–956.

Stach, K., Stach, W., & Augoff, K. 2021. "Vitamin B6 in health and disease." *Nutrients* 13(9):3229.

Tardy, A. L., Pouteau, E., Marquez, D., Yilmaz, C., & Scholey, A. 2020. "Vitamins and minerals for energy, fatigue and cognition: A narrative review of the biochemical and clinical evidence." *Nutrients* 12(1):228.

Tome-Carneiro, J., & Visioli, F. 2016. "Polyphenol-based nutraceuticals for the prevention and treatment of cardiovascular disease: Review of human evidence." *Phytomedicine* 23(11):1145–1174.

Tresserra-Rimbau, A., Lamuela-Raventos, R. M., & Moreno, J. J. 2018. "Polyphenols, food and pharma. Current knowledge and directions for future research." *Biochemical Pharmacology* 156:186–195.

Tulasi, G, & Rao, K. J. 2014. "Essentiality of chromium for human health and dietary nutrition." *Journal of Entomology and Zoology* 2(1):107–108.

Ungurianu, A., Zanfirescu, A., Nițulescu, G., & Margină, D. 2021. "Vitamin E beyond its antioxidant label." *Antioxidants* 10(5):634.

Vamanu, E. 2019. "Polyphenolicnutraceuticals to combat oxidative stress through microbiotamodulation." *Frontiers in Pharmacology* 10:492.

Velu, G., Palanichamy, V., & Rajan, A. P. 2018. "Phytochemical and pharmacological importance of plant secondary metabolites in modern medicine." In *Bioorganic Phase in Natural Food: An Overview* 135–156. Springer, Cham.

Vidal-Casanella, O., Núñez, O., Granados, M., Saurina, J., & Sentellas, S. 2021. "Analytical methods for exploring nutraceuticals based on phenolic acids and polyphenols." *Applied Sciences* 11(18):8276.

Visioli, F., & Agostoni, C. 2022. "Omega 3 fatty acids and health: The little we know after all these years." *Nutrients* 14(2):239.

# Index

Note: Locators in *italics* represent figures and **bold** indicate tables in the text.

For Product Safety Concerns and Information please contact our EU
representative GPSR@taylorandfrancis.com
Taylor & Francis Verlag GmbH, Kaufingerstraße 24, 80331 München, Germany

www.ingramcontent.com/pod-product-compliance
Lightning Source LLC
Chambersburg PA
CBHW060750220326
41598CB00022B/2388

* 9 7 8 1 0 3 2 1 9 4 9 1 2 *